Human Sexuality

A NURSING PERSPECTIVE

with a chapter by:
WILLIAM D. BALL, Pharm.D.

Oncology Specialist
Lederle Laboratories
Formerly Clinical Pharmacist in Medicine
Department of Pharmacy Services
University Hospitals, Cleveland, Ohio

and a chapter by:
MYRON G. EISENBERG, Ph.D.

Chief, Psychology Service
Hampton Virginia Veterans Administration Medical Center
Hampton, Virginia

Human Sexuality

A NURSING PERSPECTIVE

Second Edition

Rosemarie Mihelich Hogan, R.N., M.S.N.

Associate Professor, School of Nursing
Kent State University
Kent, Ohio

 APPLETON-CENTURY-CROFTS/Norwalk, Connecticut

0-8385-3957-2

85 86 87 88 89 / 10 9 8 7 6 5 4 3 2 1

Prentice-Hall International, Inc., London
Prentice-Hall of Australia, Pty. Ltd., Sydney
Prentice-Hall of India Private Limited, New Delhi
Prentice-Hall of Japan, Inc., Tokyo
Prentice-Hall of Southeast (Asia) (Pte.) Ltd., Singapore
Whitehall Books Ltd., Wellington, New Zealand

Library of Congress Cataloging in Publication Data

Hogan, Rosemarie Mihelich.
  Human sexuality.

  Includes bibliographies and index.
  1. Sexual disorders—Nursing. 2. Sex. 3. Sex
(Psychology) I. Ball, William D. II. Eisenberg,
Myron G. III. Title. [DNLM: 1. Nursing. 2. Sex
Behavior—nurses' instruction. 3. Sex Disorders—
psychology—nurses' instruction. WY 87 H714h]
RC877.H63 1984   616.6'9   84–12297
ISBN 0–8385–3957–2

Design: Lynn M. Luchetti

PRINTED IN THE UNITED STATES OF AMERICA

*to Frank, Jackie, Bob,
John, Kathy, Val*

Contents

Preface to
the Second Edition

In reviewing the preface in the first edition of *Human Sexuality, A Nursing Perspective,* there seems little to change in relation to my philosophy as it relates to sexuality. It is a quality of being human and does indeed influence nurse–client interaction. Nurses are becoming more knowledgeable about the topic, but myths and misconceptions and a paucity of information still burden the nursing profession in some areas.

The second edition contains updated information about all facets of sexuality for nursing students and nurses in all settings. Additional and more recent research findings are included whenever they are available.

The first edition of the book attempted to present an objective approach to the topic of sexuality focusing on diverse opinions and data so that readers could analyze and develop their own informed opinion. Response from readers indicated success in this goal since there was very little criticism that biased accounts were presented, although the chapters on homosexuality and abortion were questioned by several readers who argued one viewpoint or another believing that the author should do so also. I continue to believe, however, that all facets and views about topics must be presented, not necessarily because I agree with some viewpoints, but because my philosophy of education holds that the true scholar has the broader picture, as well as in-depth knowledge, on which to base decisions. The objective of this text continues to be, therefore, presentation of information from many viewpoints.

The format of the book remains the same, but information has been updated, added and in some cases condensed. Many additional sources have been cited including information available since 1980. Nursing implications have been expanded in some chapters, giving practical information applicable to client care. The annotated bibliography was placed at the end of the book but the reader is urged to consult the reference notes at the end of each chapter for more in-depth information about a particular subject. Careful referencing has been done to expedite literature search by students and others interested in gaining greater knowledge of sexuality.

My thanks is extended to my many new professional colleagues at Kent State University who continue to help me question and think as well as to my "old" friends and colleagues who provide me with support. My family continues to support my efforts, and as before, without the help of my husband, Frank, this book would not be "brought forth."

Sandra Reba Evancho, my typist, again deserves my gratitude for her ability to decipher my handwriting, type a readable text, and meet all deadlines. She is a blessing!

Preface to the First Edition

Sexuality is a quality of being human and it influences patient/client care to a degree that may not always be readily perceivable. Fortunately nurses are recognizing that their sexuality and that of their patients/clients are unavoidably interrelated. However, many nurses suffer from the same paucity of information and the same myths and misconceptions about sexuality that afflict the larger society.

The objective of this text is to supply needed information and to correct misinformation within a bio-psycho-social and nursing process framework that will be helpful to nursing students and to graduate nurses in diverse settings. A nursing process approach is utilized for the presentation of nursing implications of health deviations and sexual problems, since it provides the important systematic approach that helps promote high quality nursing care.

When possible, research findings are presented as one source of information. In addition, effort was made to present an objective approach to the topic of sexuality; rather than arguing for or against any particular sexual behavior or viewpoint, diverse opinions and data are presented so that readers can develop their own informed opinion.

However, there are two basic tenets underlying this text. The first is that nurses, although entitled to their own beliefs and behavior in relation to sexuality, have a serious obligation not to penalize by word or deed those who hold to different beliefs and practices. Sexuality is so sensitive a subject, and so integral to our being, that it is easy for health care practitioners to penalize by inadequate, sporadic, or superficial care those who express their sexuality differently.

The second basic belief is that sexuality encompasses more than physical sexual activity. It involves our identities and our roles as women and men. Consequently, psychologic and sociocultural factors are as important as biologic factors to insure healthy sexuality, which must be viewed in the context of total human relationships and being.

With this in mind, Unit I presents the bio-psycho-social information that is the "underpinning" necessary for nursing care of individuals in relation to their sexuality.

Unit II presents the general assessment parameters and process as well as information about teaching and counseling that are necessary care components of persons of any age or in any setting. The general sexual reponses of individuals to illness and hospitalization are also presented—information that is especially important for Unit V.

Unit III focuses on the problems that may complicate the healthy growth and development of sexuality, while Unit IV focuses on the reproductive consequences of sexual expression.

Finally, Unit V presents the effects of specific health deviations and their therapies on sexuality and information for nurses to help persons attain, maintain, or regain sexual health.

Writing a book has many parallels with pregnancy. Beforehand, one debates whether the physical and emotional stress that may accompany the event and the life changes that the birth of a child may necessitate are desired and if the outcome will be worth the effort. If the decision is made to proceed, many months of excitement and joy, coupled at times with discomfort and something approaching regret, may follow. Moreover, the culmination of the process, whether a child or a book, is not necessarily what was initially envisioned, but still brings its own joy and satisfaction and the knowledge that part of oneself has been shared and communicated. Either process requires the involvement of others.

Without the consistent approval and encouragement of my husband, Frank, this book would not have been "brought forth." His support was unwavering. In their own inimitable ways my former professional colleagues also made this book possible, whether they were aware of the fact or not: Kathryn Baker, Linda Broseman, Deanna Carroll, Dorothy Kuhn, Barbara Long, Lynn Chenoweth, Mary Alice Robinson, Teresa Trump, and Mary Wyper all deserve my heartfelt thanks.

Finally, my thanks to all the typists. Sandra Reba Evancho, who typed the initial manuscript from my notoriously illegible handwriting, deserves special accolades and my eternal gratitude for her patience and forbearance.

Bio-Psycho-Social Aspects of Sexuality

Chapter 1

Human Sexuality—An Overview

Human sexuality has been described in many ways, depending on the beliefs and the biases of the author. Definitions may be limited or multifaceted in scope. The common denominator in all definitions is the recognition that sexuality is an intrinsic part of our being. Sexuality is much more than the sex act. Jeanne Fonseca has called it the quality of being human, all that we are as men and women.[1] The term has also been described as encompassing the "most intimate feelings and deepest longings of the human heart to find meaningful relationships."[2] Sexuality connotes the totality of human being, unlike the word *sex,* which connotes a physiologic act. The broader term includes the biologic as well as the sociocultural, psychologic, and ethical components of sexual behavior.

In society, sexuality may be used or abused. It may bring pleasure or pain, happiness or despair. George Hohmann has succinctly described this multifaceted concept. Sexuality can be considered a biologic act that involves the buildup of both autonomic nervous system and striated muscle activity that culminates in orgasm. It is a biologic force that is necessary for the procreation of the human race, but it is also much more.

Psychosocial goals of individuals may be attained by sexual means. Wavering or faltering self-esteem may be supported or increased. Sexuality may also be used to manipulate and control another who is important to the individual's life. Implicit in these goals of sexual behavior is the reality that "hidden agendas" may be as important or more important than some of the more obvious ends of human sexual interactions.

Finally, sexuality is the expression of two individual personalities and their merging in both symbolic and physical feelings of tenderness, respect, and concern for each other and their pleasure.[3] There is mutuality—focus on the other as well as the self. Sexuality is not confined to the bedroom or to areas of the body. It is what we do, but it is also what we are.

To state that sexuality is more than a biologic sex act is not to diminish the importance of sexual activity, whether penile–vaginal intercourse or other forms of sexual activity that provide sexual tension reduction, satisfaction, and pleasure for an individual. Additional factors must also be considered. If sexual activity exists not only for reproduction but also for pleasure, then masturbation, oral–genital contact, and emotional and physical relationships between members of the same sex are legitimate means of sexual expression.

Sexuality is so multidetermined and so multidimensional that one must study and integrate its biologic, psychologic, sociologic, and ethical aspects. Conceptualization of human sexuality is especially difficult, since these factors, if studied as entities, must also be considered as they interface with each other and contribute to sexual health or sexual disequilibrium.

This chapter presents a general over-

3

view of sexuality and introduces the reader to the topic of gender identity and the biologic, psychologic, and sociocultural concomitants of sexuality. A historical overview of societies' sexual practices, attitudes, and beliefs is presented to enable the reader to see the variability of ideas about sexuality over time. Finally, the place of sex and sexuality in Abraham Maslow's schema of basic needs is presented to complete the picture of sexuality.

BIO-PSYCHO-SOCIAL ASPECTS OF SEXUALITY

Biologic Aspects

The biologic aspects of sexuality include the anatomic and physiologic "givens"—the sex organs, hormones, nerves, and brain centers. Biologic aspects also encompass the concept of instinct, part of the larger reproductive instinct to mate and perpetuate the species.[4]

Psychologic Aspects

Sexuality involves not only gender identity but also sexual self-image or self-concept. Positive sexual self-concept is characterized by acceptance of, comfort with, and value of oneself as male or female. These attitudes toward self are formed through interactions with others and profoundly affect interactions with others. Individuals with positive self-concept are more open with others, presenting less of a facade and more willing to share self, than those with poor self-esteem. Body image, the internalized picture that an individual has of the physical appearance of his body, is closely allied with self-concept.[5] Change or disturbance in body image may negatively affect sexual self-concept.

Sociocultural Aspects

Gender and *sexual identity* are terms used to describe one's internal sense of masculinity or femininity; the awareness of "I am male" or "I am female," in contrast to the term *sex,* which summarizes the biologic attributes that characterize the male or female. At times, sexual identity may be referred to as *core gender identity,* the conviction (usually by the age of two or three) that one belongs to the male or female sex. It is a psychologic state, part of identity, but it is not synonymous with belonging to one's sex (i.e., the biologically assigned sex) but rather the conviction that one does so belong[6]

Core gender identity is the result of (1) biologic factors (embryologic and central nervous system centers); (2) genital anatomy, which signals to the parents that they have a boy or a girl; and (3) sex assignment and rearing, including society's attitudes toward what is masculine and feminine. Robert Stoller believes that "imprinting," such as seen in some birds and mammals, may be a factor and that classic conditioning also influences core gender identity.[7]

If gender identity is the internal feeling of maleness or femaleness, *gender* or *sexual role behavior* may be defined as all we do to disclose ourselves as male or female to others—the external behavior that identifies us. Gender role is not established at birth but is built up cumulatively through experience, planned or unplanned, and through explicit but more frequently implicit instruction.

How do we learn our sexual role? There are three major sources of information. Some information is usually learned in a formal manner through school and parents. A far greater influence is the sexual value system of the family and the community. There may be clusters of negative values that represent public sexual norms and that exert far greater influence than that of planned learning. Children learn to see and evaluate their parents' attitudes toward many facets of life, politics, religion, and—of greater importance—sexuality. There may be a pattern of repression and avoidance of sexual topics by many parents. Children's attitudes are shaped by these factors, and information from the third source of sexual learning, the peer group, is filtered through this parental value system to the child.[8]

Peer learning is probably the most pervasive type of sexual learning. Too often, unfortunately, sexual relationships are learned through an exchange of gestures and cues rather than open discussion and direct experimentation. Traditionally, males obtain information that is only indirectly sexually informative. The male gets an image of a sexual self rather than of sexuality. Stories of sexual prowess may be a central topic, with much emphasis on heterosexual expertise and exploits. Penis size becomes important and frightening, and orgasms are counted and compared. The male learns to be the technical expert, the aggressor, the leader in the sex act.

Traditionally, the female has learned a complementary role. Girls exchange information about affections and love. If the male is the expert, there is a cultural constraint on the girl to limit her role in sexual activity, since she is not knowledgeable (at least theoretically) about the sex act. If the male is the aggressor then the female must be passive; if he is the leader, she must be subservient. Many problems are inherent in these stereotypes; the male may become concerned if he is not "manly" as defined by society's stereotypes of manliness; the woman may be concerned if she does not fit the current conception of "femininity."

Changing roles and relationships in society seem to be freeing many men from the pressure of being "masculine" and many women from the stereotype of being "feminine." Jung stated that we are both anima and animus—in us we have both the spirit of man and the spirit of woman.[9] We are not male or female, we are human.

CHANGING PRACTICES, ATTITUDES, AND BELIEFS—A HISTORICAL PERSPECTIVE

In discussing sexual roles, it must be emphasized that it is not so important what these roles are, as long as they are understood and accepted by individuals. The critical factors is not what we do but whether we are comfortable in our sexuality. Our comfort is asso-

ciated with the cultural milieu in which we are located, and this is in a constant state of flux. Attitudes and beliefs and practices of sexuality have varied throughout history.

Role conflict occurs when there is lack of congruence between individuals' perception of their sexual roles and the role prescription of society. Traditionally, for example, women have been less concerned about orgasm. In some areas of the Middle East, frigidity is not a concern but sterility is. Moreover, patterns of sexual behavior that have been condemned in one era have been considered normal in another.

A review of sexual behavior in society throughout history indicates that sexual practices have not varied considerably, although attitudes, values, beliefs, and what is officially prohibited or encouraged may change over time. Periods of sexual freedom have been followed by periods of sexual repression and restriction.

Sexuality has always had a major role in human affairs and has had a prominent place in customs, religious acts, morality, and law. Much of our standards, attitudes, and laws have been derived from the Old Testament Judaic pattern, which highly regarded sexual activity as a means of reproduction and pleasure but subjected it to strict regulation. A second major influence was early Christian teaching, which added some negative attitudes toward sexuality but emphasized the need for love and affection. Finally, the Judeo–Christian sexual tradition was transmitted in an intensified form by the Puritan tradition and the antisexual pattern that has been its official morality code.

The 1970s were a period of sexual revolution. More sophisticated information about sex and sexuality was available than ever before. The sex act was recognized as a vital physical expression of attachment to others—as a type of communication that could be fun, playful, serious, or passionate. Sexuality has been called one of the propelling forces of humankind, possessing the same kind of force as birth, death, and life itself.[10]

Sexuality has become a far more open

subject, and therapy for sexual problems is an integral part of health care. New treatment methods such as sexual reassignment for gender identity disturbance are being used. Treatment of sexual dysfunctions by the use of techniques developed by Masters and Johnson has been successful in alleviating problems that have been refractory to traditional psychotherapeutic methods.

Oral contraceptives and the intrauterine devices are most effective methods of fertility control, and their discovery has made possible the separation of reproductive effects of sexual activity from its social, libidinal, and recreational aspects. Male–female relationships have changed. With the advent of the Women's Liberation Movement, women have demanded a greater role in all sectors of business and society. Changes have taken place in attitudes toward premarital sexual activity. Yet society can still be sexually confused and repressive. Women especially may still find it difficult to speak frankly about sexuality.

Criticism has been directed toward the sexuality presented by magazines such as *Playboy, Penthouse,* and *Oui.* Although sex is presented as fun, such portrayal is also unrealistic. Cox in *The Secular City* states

> It is precisely because these magazines are antisexual that they deserve the most searching kind of theological criticism. . . . For *Playboy's* man, others—especially women— are *for* him. They are his leisure accessories, his playthings.[11]

Novelist–theologian Frederick Buechner has presented another viewpoint. He has stated, "Contrary to Mrs. Grundy, sex is not sin. Contrary to Hugh Hefner, it is not salvation either."

Some argue that the sin in sex today is that it has been publicized, profaned, and vulgarized. Still, in the 1970s there was an increasing openness and comfort with sexuality.

The 80s have seen a continuation of the sexual life styles of the 70s but with a growing volume of dissent from those who argue that earlier values in regard to sexual behavior must return. The Moral Majority and others preach a traditional role for women as homemakers and mothers, condemn abortion and campaign for its abolition. The Equal Rights Amendment to the Constitution was not ratified, and Ronald Reagan was overwhelmingly elected president on a platform that included emphasis on the return to "traditional" values.

San Fransisco has a large, open, politically powerful homosexual community, but in West Virginia the attorney general's office has ruled that because homosexuality is considered immoral in most West Virginia communities, teachers may be discharged for their *reputation* of homosexuality, even if not observed in overt homosexual acts.[12]

Editors of *Psychology Today* question whether we have not begun a new infatuation with romance. They speculate that the sexual revolution may be over and that social forces are turning us back to traditional romance.[13]

The continued increase in venereal diseases—especially herpes and acquired immune deficiency syndrome (AIDS)—and the publicity that surrounds them has caused some to question or modify their sexual lifestyles. Others assert that these diseases are the result of and punishment for what they consider our society's promiscuity and immoral sexual behavior. (See Chapter 22.)

It is too soon to see whether the proverbial pendulum is swinging back to a more restrictive view of acceptable sexual behavior in the 1980s. One can only watch and speculate.

SEXUALITY AND THE BASIC NEEDS

Sexuality has been described earlier in the chapter as a quality of being human with bio-psycho-social aspects. As such, its relationship to other human needs must be considered.

Abraham Maslow has proposed a theory of human motivation based on the concept of needs that must be satisfied if health is to be attained and maintained. These needs are ranked in a hierarchy of prepotency. Those that are considered basic physiologic needs include the needs for oxygen, food and fluids, elimination, rest and activity, shelter, and sex. These are labeled *survival needs,* since they are necessary for existence. However, the need for sexual activity is an exception to the grouping, since it is not necessary for individual survival, but for species survival. The other higher-order needs identified by Maslow include security–safety, love–belonging, esteem, and finally, self-actualization.[14] Sexuality is a significant part of each.

Sex may be studied as a pure physiologic need, but ordinarily sexual behavior is multidetermined; that is, it is determined not only by the sexual but by other needs, chief of which is the need for love and affection.[15] Love is not considered synonymous with sex, but the need for human contact is essential to combat feelings of alienation and loneliness.

Sexual behavior is complex in its unconscious purposes. One individual may wish to assert masculinity. Another's sexual behavior may be directed toward impressing or seeking affection. Maslow believes the sexual drive is given by heredity, but the choice of sexual object and choice of behavior is acquired or learned in the course of the life history.

Although sex is considered one of the basic physiologic needs, its satisfaction, along with satisfaction of other basic needs, may be given up for high ideals, values, or social standards. In addition, if these needs are satisfied in earlier years, individuals develop exceptional power to withstand present and future thwarting. High frustration tolerance is present.[16]

Sexual deprivation per se does not necessarily have psychopathologic effects. Celibacy becomes pathogenic only when the individual feels that it represents rejection by the opposite sex, lack of respect, or thwarting of other basic needs. Sexual deprivation is easily tolerated by the individual for whom it does not have these implications.[17]

Sexuality is also an important element in the needs for psychologic security, self-esteem, love, and belonging. The individual's feelings of worth as a male or female and feeling of psychologic security, i.e., freedom from anxiety, have profound implications for sexual functioning and the development of sexual relationships.

SELF-ACTUALIZATION AND SEXUALITY

Maslow has described self-actualization as synonymous with health and the self-actualized individual as one in whom sex and love are more perfectly fused than in others. Sexual pleasure and orgasm are not just passing pleasures but a kind of basic strengthening and revivifying experience. Sex is not sought for its own sake. Maslow is not positive, but he has noted that the self-actualized individual may give up sex or reject it if it is offered without love and affection.[18] The absence of sexual activity is more easily tolerated in such an individual. Living at a higher level makes lower needs and their frustration or satisfaction less important, less central, and more easily neglected. Paradoxically, the self-actualized individual enjoys sex more wholeheartedly when the sex need is gratified.[19]

Finally, the self-actualized individual makes no sharp distinction or differentiation between the roles and personalities of the two sexes. The female can be active and aggressive, eschewing the traditional role behavior without feeling threatened. The male does not mind being passive if the situation warrants it.[20]

The self-actualized individual is described as one in whom love and sex are more closely fused. What is the relationship of sexuality to love?

LOVE AND SEXUALITY

Sexuality must be seen in the context of the individual's whole life. To some, sex is a pivot point, to others, it seems virtually unimportant. To some, love must be a necessary condition before sex. To others, the two are considered separate entities that may or may not coexist. Love, like sexuality, is a complex phenomenon. There are different kinds of love, all of which affect sexuality and its development. The maternal love for the child is one example of motherly love for the weak and helpless. Friendly love between equals is considered brotherly love.[21] Love of humanity (*agape*) is the love a person has for all people. It is selfless and nonsexual. Finally, *eros* is the sexual attraction between two people. These types of love may differ more in degree of feeling than in substance.

According to Freud, eros is present in all relationships to some extent. Some element of sexual pleasure can be experienced by the mother while nursing her child. (See Chapter 21.)

Love, defined as the affectional feelings for others, has a developmental aspect. Each type of love relationship prepares the individual for the next phase. Problems in one phase will cause problems in others. Katchadourian and Lunde identify five basic phases: (1) maternal love, (2) paternal love, (3) infant–mother love, (4) peer or age-mate love, and (5) heterosexual love. These are integrated and interdependent affectional systems and have sexual components.[22] Problems related to sexuality may develop when these love relationships are inadequate, poorly-developed, or interrupted. (See Chapters 15 through 18.)

Love is essential for growth, being, and becoming. Love and sex have traditionally been associated. However, the new sexual "freedom" is dichotomizing the two, and women particularly are affected. Traditionally they have been brought up to subordinate sex needs to love needs and to express sexuality only in a loving relationship. The double standard is giving way, so that some women are expressing their sex life as separate from their love life. The danger is that women may express liberal sexual viewpoints, actively participate in the new sexual freedom, and then realize that their unconscious has lagged behind. Guilt, anxiety, and dissatisfaction may follow.

The new freedom results in more open talk and more sexual activity, but often less emotional attachment to sexual activity. Rosenbaum points out that when sex is fused with feelings of love and intimacy we have the most intense human experience—true lovemaking. She feels that some seek out sex not because of love and intimacy, but perhaps as a result of their lack. Sex may be a desperate attempt to feel close to another.[23]

NOTES

1. Fonseca JD: Sexuality—a quality of being human. Nurs Outlook 18:25, November 1970
2. Brower L: Character education: A guideline for discussion of sexual behavior. J School Health 39:715–722, December 1967
3. Hohmann GW: Considerations in management of psychosexual readjustment in the cord injured male. Rehabil Psychol 19:50–58, 1972
4. Katchadourian HA, Lunde DT: Fundamentals of Human Sexuality. New York, Holt, 1975, p 2
5. Kneisl CR: Body image its meaning to self. J NY State Nurses 2:29–35, Spring 1971
6. Stoller RJ: Gender Identity. In Sadock BJ, Kaplan HI, Freedman AM: The Sexual Experience, Baltimore, Williams and Wilkins, 1976, pp 182–195
7. Ibid
8. American Medical Association Committee on Human Sexuality: Human Sexuality. Chicago, American Medical Association, 1972, p 29
9. Jung C: Psychological Types. New York, Harcourt, 1923, pp 594–599
10. Boston Women's Book Collective: Our Bodies, Ourselves, 2nd ed. New York, Simon and Schuster, 1976, p 38

11. Cox H: The Secular City. New York, Macmillan, 1965, p 177
12. Plain Dealer, March 11, 1983 p 5A
13. Rubenstein C: Love and Romance. Psychology Today. 17(2):60–63, February, 1983
14. Maslow A: Motivation and Personality. New York, Harper and Bros, 1954
15. Ibid, p 45
16. Ibid, p 58
17. Ibid, p 107
18. Ibid, p 187
19. Ibid, p 189
20. Ibid, p 189
21. Fromm E: The Art of Loving. New York, Harper and Bros, 1956
22. Katchadourian HA, Lunde DT: Fundamentals of Human Sexuality. New York, Holt, 1975, pp 245–249
23. Rosenbaum MB: Female sexuality, or why can't a woman be more like a woman. In Oaks WW, Melchisde GA, Ficher I (eds): Sex and the Life Cycle. New York, Grune and Stratton, 1976, p 94

Chapter 2

Nursing and Human Sexuality

Sexuality is intrinsic to our being—a basic need and an aspect of humanness that cannot be divorced from life events. It influences our thoughts, actions, and interactions and is involved in aspects of physical and mental health. As a basic need, it is one of the essential focuses of health care. Unfortunately, too often nurses have inadequate knowledge, understanding, and comfort with their own sexuality and that of their patient/client. This is not surprising since nurses are the members of a society that has been restrictive of discussion and investigation of sexuality and sexual problems.

Society's attitude is changing, and patients/clients are asking for help in many areas of sexuality. Not all nurses need to be prepared as sex therapists, but all nurses can integrate sexuality into health care, focusing on preventive, therapeutic, and educational interventions to assist individuals attain or maintain sexual health.

The purpose of this chapter is to present a brief historical review of nursing as it has been affected by society's sexual beliefs and practices, as well as a review of nurses' role in promoting and maintaining the sexual health of patients/clients. Problems that face the nursing profession in the areas of sexuality are identified and discussed, including sexual stereotyping and sexism within the profession. Finally, a vision of nursing care of the future as it relates to sexuality is presented.

HISTORICAL OVERVIEW

The first nurses were monks who integrated care of the sick with service to God. In contrast, early nurses in England were prostitutes who cared for the ill to augment their usual income. Although the work of Florence Nightingale ushered in modern nursing, nursing orders of Catholic sisters preceded her in trying to deliver high-standard sick care. Thus, early nursing was characterized by male and female, the sexual ascetic and the sexually promiscuous, delivering care to the sick.

Nurses' sexuality has been suppressed and repressed. Florence Nightingale's rules prohibited jewelry, ribbons, or ornaments of any kind. Nurses were to live in dormitories under the close supervision of a matron and were permitted out only when accompanied by another nurse. Students were chosen partly on the basis of a homely appearance![1]

Practice has changed, so that an attractive appearance does not disqualify the nursing school candidate. However, enhancing one's appearance by the use of jewelry or ornaments and make-up is discouraged in some nursing services.[2] These rules and regulations may have been related to nurses' traditionally accorded right to touch the body in order to carry out hygiene and other care, while still maintaining personal "purity" and asexuality.

The norm of cleanliness and neatness continued after the time of Florence Nightingale. A review of an early nursing journal reveals articles devoted to the maintenance of cleanliness of the patient and the ward. The only literature remotely connected with sexuality had the enticing title of "The Relation of Syphilis and the Nursing Profession." The author, a physician, related cases of nurses contracting syphilis from kissing syphilitic infants with open lesions and admonished them to halt the practice.[3] A review of nursing textbooks from the early 1930s until 1977 indicated little if any increase in information related to sexuality per se. Bertha Harmer, in 1934, includes the statement that the orderly is usually responsible for the male patients.[4] The connotation of nurses as pure and asexual as well as the prevailing cultural mores served to prohibit the topic of sexuality in a nursing education that was rigid, hierarchical in control, and strictly disciplined.

A holistic approach to care supposedly focused on meeting physical, emotional, and spiritual needs, but the patient as a sexual being was essentially ignored. In the late 60s, nursing literature began to reflect increased awareness of the individual's sexuality as a proper concern for nursing. Articles related to masturbation, homosexuality, and communicating about sexual topics began to appear. In 1970, *Nursing Outlook* devoted an entire issue to human sexuality.

In the late 70s and early 80s, nursing literature and research on sexuality increased as did calls to include content in the nursing curriculum.[5] Descriptions of elective courses and integration of content in existing courses appeared in nursing literature.[6-8] Models of intervention levels[9] were also developed to indicate the level of education required for various levels of care.

The number of nurses participating in scholarly workshops, seminars, and continuing education courses has also grown. Nurses have functioned in leadership roles for nonnursing sexually-oriented organizations such as the American Association of Sex Educators, Counselors, and Therapists (AASECT), the Society for the Scientific Study of Sex (SSSS), and the Society for Sex Therapy and Research (SSTAR).[10]

Progress has been made in moving nurses into the mainstream of sexual health care, but there are discordant notes. In a 1983 study[11] involving 120 nurses caring for oncology patients, results of the Sex Knowledge and Attitude Test (SKAT) indicated that their knowledge scores were significantly lower and that they were more conservative in their attitudes toward heterosexual relationships, masturbation, and abortion than a group of nurses tested in 1972. One isolated study does not indicate a trend, but it does raise questions. Are nurses part of a conservative trend? How committed to promoting sexual health are nurses who practice direct patient care? If nurses are moving into the mainstream of sex education and research, are there still "pockets" of resistance to the topic in schools of nursing and among some nurse educators and administrators?

A Challenge to Nursing

In 1973, the World Health Organization studied the curricula of medical and nursing schools throughout the world to identify whether any content was devoted to human sexuality. Their findings indicated that little information was being offered. In 1974, a short book, *The Teaching of Human Sexuality in Schools for Health Professionals,* was published by WHO to help schools introduce this type of subject matter into the curriculum. The book sets out the knowledge, skills, and attitudes that are needed for counseling and teaching human sexuality.[12]

Nurses knowledgeable about and comfortable with the topic of sexuality and comfortable with their own sexuality have the opportunity to promote sexual health. However, in an area as sensitive and personal as sexuality, conflicts about role exist. Some nurses may have strong and committed religious beliefs about the immorality of certain sexual practices. Conflict inevitably ensues when nurses are confronted with the care of individuals whose practices do not conform to these beliefs. A young public health nurse identified one aspect of this conflict when she described her feelings about caring for homosexual persons in her case load. "I believe the Bible. Homosexuality is wrong—it's a sin. I can give them the physical care they need but my inclination is to try and help them see the error of their life—and try to convert them. . . . I sometimes wonder if I should be giving them care." She mirrored what is the honest dilemma of many nurses. In addition to feeling that some behavior and practices are wrong, nurses may be repulsed, embarrassed, or shocked by some, if not most, sexual behavior that does not fit their norms.

Talking about sexuality is difficult, since many, if given any sexual facts at all by parents, were told, "but nice girls (or boys) don't talk about these things in public." We learned early that sexuality was a taboo topic. Some nurses have firm and honest convictions that sexuality is a personal matter and that, apart from reproduction, is not an area of nursing concern. Others recognize that if nurses do indeed care for the whole person, sexuality, a quality of being human, is indeed an important part of their professional domain.

RESEARCH—NURSES AND SEXUALITY

Early research on sexuality by nurses focused on two areas: knowledge and attitudes of nurses, students, and faculty and the effects of sexuality courses in these areas.[13-15] Findings indicated that the courses resulted in greater knowledge, while attitudinal change was less affected, at least as an immediate course outcome. Students seem to see sexuality as a more legitimate nursing concern, some asking for additional training. Keller [16] found that students felt more comfortable in discussing sexuality with clients and were more in touch with their own sexuality after an elective course.

A school faculty's awareness of its feelings, attitudes, and values was also recog-

nized as a necessary before it can understand and help others. Fontaine surveyed 124 instructors in 10 schools of nursing regarding their perceptions of the number of patients who had sexual concerns or problems, frequency of sexuality questions being asked in nursing histories, and the adequacy of their basic education in human sexuality. They were also asked to evaluate their level of understanding of sexuality compared to that of most nurses, their ability to discuss sexual problems with patients, and the adequacy of integration of sexuality in their curriculum and other curricula. Their self-rating in these areas indicated that the ability to discuss sexual concerns with patients falls behind their perceived knowledge. Many did not include sexual needs in taking a nursing history. There was a widespread lack of courses or an indication that sexuality was being integrated into the nursing programs.[17]

This survey provided some objective data that tends to support the observation made in 1974 that nursing education had not done much to prepare health professionals to deal with more than a narrow range of sexual behavior. It also suggests that graduates were poorly prepared to deal with many types of sexual problems.[18]

In a 1976 survey of 218 baccalaureate schools of nursing, the 151 that responded indicated that 98 percent had some aspects of sexuality in the curriculum, but only 15 percent had sexuality as a separate course in the education unit in nursing. Seventy percent indicated that they discussed students' feelings, attitudes, and values, and 67 percent said the students were aware of sexual feelings[19]

In a 1980 survey,[20] questionnaires were sent to all baccalaureate nursing schools in the Western Interstate Council of Higher Education in Nursing (WICHEN). Eighty-three percent of those responding (34 schools) agreed with the statement that "graduates and the public are ill-served by a nursing program which omits study of sexual behavior," but only 91 percent of the schools included content in that area. The majority of the programs integrated content in other courses although five had both integrated content and elective course offerings. The majority of the nursing educators favored integrated course content rather than elective courses.

Progress has been made, however, in increasing the number of nurses doing research on sexual topics. Hott and Ryan-Merritt[21] requested names of faculty and students studying sexually related topics from 75 schools of nursing with graduate programs listed in the NLN "Master's Education in Nursing: Route to Opportunity in Contemporary Nursing, 1978–79." Forty schools responded. The investigators chose to consider studies with sexuality in the title (for example, sex attitudes, education, sexuality related to sex roles, dysfunction, and function) and studies specific to sexual aberration and assault. Responses indicated that the majority of doctoral dissertations and master's theses came from a cluster of programs, especially where there was a faculty member whose research area or teaching specialization was human sexuality. Typically, the subjects were predominantly nursing students, faculty, and administrators, although other students, other health professionals, and clients with specific medical disorders were also popular subjects. Studies in the later 1970s appeared to be more sophisticated about patient-related problems.

Articles about research in sexuality have increased in nursing journals, the majority appearing in *Nursing Research*. Nurses have published research on sexuality in nonnursing journals such as the *Journal of Sex Research*, *Archives of Internal Medicine*, and the *American Journal of Public Health*.

NURSES' ROLE IN PROMOTING AND MAINTAINING SEXUAL HEALTH

Four areas of expertise are needed if the nurse is to be able to promote sexual health:

knowledge of subject matter; skill in assessing and intervening; awareness of beliefs, attitudes, and values; and finally awareness of how these beliefs, attitudes, and values affect practice.

Knowledge of Subject Matter

Knowledge needed by nurses is broad in scope. The subject of sexuality is vast, sensitive, and complex, and more so for nurses, since their goal is not just to learn but also to teach and counsel others. Basic knowledge necessary for understanding the subject includes knowledge about sexual development, reproduction, sexual expression, sexual dysfunction and disease, and sociocultural aspects of sex and marriage and the family. Of equal if not more importance in this area of human relationships is nurses' understanding of the moral, aesthetic, and religious sensitivities of the individuals for whom they care.

Skill in Assessing and Intervening

Skill is needed in assessing, interviewing, teaching, and counseling of individuals and groups. Nurses need to be sensitive in recognizing sexual difficulties in individuals who have not reported the problem in specific terms because of embarrassment or guilt. Depending on the setting, nurses engaged in primary practice need to become adept and comfortable in conducting perineal and pelvic examinations as part of a total physical assessment.

The ability to discuss sexuality in a frank, unembarrassed, objective manner can be attained with practice. Necessary communications skills include the ability to create an environment that is nonthreatening and free of distraction in order to facilitate expression of underlying concerns. Sensitivity in listening for and observing nonverbal cues that indicate sexual concerns increases as the nurse becomes more comfortable with the topic of sexuality.

Skill in the techniques of questioning, reflection, clarification, and validation is essential so that nurses accurately perceive what the patient is expressing and feeling about sexuality. The ability to listen and to use silence constructively is vital for communication about sexuality. When sensitive subjects are brought up, nurses' comfort with silence as patients/clients struggle with the expression of their feelings will facilitate sharing.

How to offer help to a patient, even if the problem is a complex one requiring referral, is a needed skill. This may be nothing more than showing understanding and offering reassurance that help is available. Skill is also needed in using the interdisciplinary team and in making referral to the appropriate source of help.

Awareness of Beliefs, Attitudes, and Values

Awareness of beliefs, attitudes, and values is essential, since these are the major determinants of how one deals with people. Nurses are entitled to their individual feelings, attitudes, beliefs, and standards in relation to sexuality but they must remain objective when caring for people and dealing with their sexuality.

Nurses assess what they believe are normal or abnormal sexual practices. Problems arise, however, because confusion exists about what is normal, since the term may be used in different ways:

1. A pathologic or clinical sense, indicating stress and poor adaptation—people who are anxious or self-defeating are "abnormal."
2. A moralistic model—abnormal equals evil.
3. A cultural model—what one culture sees and defines as normal.
4. A statistical model—if 75 percent of people do something, we are assured of our normality if we do it too.
5. A personal view, by comparison of others to ourselves—if we feel satisfied with ourselves, others are normal, or vice versa.

The difficulty with the personal model is

that many people who feel "OK" about themselves may be sexual chauvinists who are convinced that theirs is the only true way to think, feel, and do. Intolerance may take the form of considering people abnormal and even perverted who are not like oneself and who live by other codes. The sexually sensitive professional will be more tentative in judgments about others' behavior and will try to understand how others are using the term normal at any given time. In analyzing their own beliefs about "normality," nurses review each of the above five ways and consider how they define their beliefs.[22]

Attitudes are formed from birth on and are the result of emotional, social, and intellectual experiences. Six major factors determine attitude toward sex. These include the sexual drive or instinct (libido); the development of personality and behavior patterns; cultural influences; the immediate environment and the people in it (especially home and family); education; and sexual experiences with heavy emotional impact—such as incest, rape, and harsh punishment for normal acts of sexual experimentation.

Assessment of attitudes toward sexuality involves first deciding whether one's attitudes are positive or negative. Negative attitudes can be overcome by self-examination and training experience.[23] The process may take many years before some nurses can be comfortable in discussing all subjects in detail with all persons. Nurses who cannot overcome a negative attitude or who feel extremely uncomfortable in discussing sexuality should allow other nurses to interact with the patient/client, since the negative attitudes will be communicated.

Kempton[24] suggests examination of personal attitudes by evaluating feelings toward giving information about sexual function. She suggests analyzing feelings about reproduction, masturbation, dating, sexual activity such as petting to orgasm, sexual intercourse in marriage, sexual intercourse outside of marriage, childbearing, contraception, sterilization, abortion, venereal disease, and homosexuality. Include your opinion as to where and when such behavior is suitable and how much and what information should be given to others and patients/clients.

Analyzing your feelings about the topic is time consuming but can be invaluable. There are no right or wrong answers. The answers may be discussed, compared and contrasted with those of a colleague or may be used as part of a class or staff development program where the participants can discuss their answers.

Effects of Attitudes and Beliefs on Practice

After beliefs and attitudes are assessed, the nurse looks at how these affect practice—if they deny, inhibit, or allow for the sexuality of the patient. Some questions to consider are: How am I viewed by others? Do patients recognize that I am someone with whom they can discuss problems? Am I comfortable in discussing sexual concerns, or does the idea that "sex is dirty" limit my comfort? Do I send out nonverbal messages that discourage individuals from discussing sexual concerns? Am I sensitive to the nonverbal and subtle verbal requests for help?[25] Do I "penalize" individuals who have sexual beliefs and practices different from mine by giving minimal or hasty, incomplete care?

Becoming open, nonjudgmental, and accepting of others' sexuality and developing comfort in interviewing in the area of sexuality may be an arduous task for some. Before nurses can help others, they must come to terms with their own sexuality. Health professionals may feel insecure about their sexuality, and to cope with this insecurity, they either avoid counseling or teaching situations or intervene without sensitivity, objectivity, and empathy.[26] If the nurse is experiencing difficulties at this level, all energies should be directed to this area. To try to work out one's own sexual problems while helping another is not acceptable nursing practice.[27]

Skill and sensitivity in grasping the patients'/clients' perceptions of their concerns and in relating empathically to them are at least as important as the knowledge that is needed to answer their concerns and, indeed, may be more important.

PROBLEMS RELATING TO NURSING AND SEXUALITY

Sex Discrimination and Harrassment

The nursing profession has not escaped the negative influence of sexism and sexual stereotyping, especially since it is a profession largely made up of women members. Numerically, women dominate the health occupations; 73 percent are women. However, numerical superiority does not mean control of decision making. There are also inequalities in the income earned by men and women in the same profession, males receiving higher salaries than females in all of the major health occupations, including nursing. Sex discrimination is alive and well. Cleland describes four ways to end sex discrimination: by the process of agitation, education, legislation, and negotiation.[28]

Ending sex discrimination is not the only task. The larger goal is to develop the nursing profession so its members effectively utilize their opportunities.[28] Sexual segregation and financial discrimination have negative consequences for health care. Patient care suffers because sex segregation has created communication barriers, partly resulting from what has been termed "the doctor–nurse game."[29]

Some nurses may still believe that the physician is the leader of the health team and that nurses do not diagnose or recommend but instead convey information obliquely. Other nurses are asserting themselves and offering direct suggestions and observations about patient care. The media has begun to recognize that nurses are no longer the doctors' handmaidens.[30] Whether many physicians agree can be debated.[31]

Sexual harrassment is another problem that may confront nurses. It is defined as unwelcome sexual advances, requests for sexual favors, and other verbal and physical conduct of a sexual nature that affects employment decisions or creates an intimidating, hostile, or offensive work environment. It is prohibited under Title VII of the Civil Rights Act and Title IX of the Education Amendment of 1972.[32] Harrassment includes (1) sexist remarks, (2) demeaning, offensive but normally sanctioned behavior such as jokes, suggestive stories *if* the recipient objects to the remarks, (3) promise of reward for sexual favors, and (4) threat of punishment unless the individual agrees to cooperate. Often harrassment is not reported because of fear of "making waves," jeopardizing the career, or belief that "nothing will happen" anyway.[33]

Institutions are taking steps to cope with the problem by developing clear policies prohibiting harrassment, distributing pamphlets giving information about rights of employees, and alerting and training counselors to deal with the problem. Nurses of both sexes must be sensitive to the problem and have the courage to report situations when they occur.

Changing Roles and Relationships

Fortunately, sexual roles and relationships are changing. Along with this change, inevitably, comes conflict. Some nurses still prefer or are at least more comfortable with the culturally defined male–female roles of aggressive leadership versus more passive follower or assistant. Others no longer accept these roles and vigorously, effectively, and consistently assert their right to autonomy and independence in providing health care.

Both female and male nurses are affected by society's stereotyping of what constitutes appropriate female–male role behavior. The female nurse is urged to be independent in decision making and assertive in expressing her beliefs to other health team members. At the same time, she hears about nurturing and tender loving care. For some, the merging of behaviors is accomplished without anxiety, for others, it is a period of stress. Males can feel stress by the expectation that they be tender, gentle, and

loving when they have been reared to be nondemonstrative and assertive.

The stereotypes of "male" and "female" behavior pose problems for both sexes. Fortunately, men are being freed from the pressures of being masculine at the same time women are being freed from the stereotype of "femininity." The issue of whether a male or female nurse should be assigned to certain patients is theoretically irrelevant. The critical factor is not sex but the character, ability, and education of the individual. The ability to give expert care does not come from any gender-endowed innate gifts; it comes from learning and sensitivity to the needs of others.[34]

There is considerable evidence that traditional sex typing is unhealthy. High femininity in females correlates with high anxiety, low self-esteem, and low acceptance. High masculinity in males during adulthood may be accompanied by high anxiety, high neuroticism, and low self-acceptance. Further, greater intellectual development has quite considerably correlated with cross-sex typing, that is, masculinity in girls, femininity in boys.[35] Traditional sex typing restricts behavior, since people learn to suppress any behavior that might be considered inappropriate for their sex. Individuals freed from rigid sex roles, allowing themselves to be androgynous (from *andro,* male, and *gyne,* female), can be more flexible in meeting new situations and less restricted in what they do and how they express themselves.

Keller[36] believes that the late development of nursing theory (in 1950) and the lack of a research emphasis in nursing curriculums are related to female nurses' stereotyping of their sex; a tendency to see themselves as nonintellectual and nontheoretical and to focus instead on practice for practice's sake. She also blames female nurses' need to combine many roles (wife, mother, professional) as the cause of a lack of the leisure time necessary for thinking and theory building.

There are some positive signs, however, that women are beginning to recognize the value of women. Goodwin and Taaffe[37] see the growing preference of female clients for female psychotherapists as evidence of less stereotyped role definitism and expectations.

Persistent stereotyped sexual role identities of women may adversely effect nursing's struggle to become an independent profession. Stromberg investigated the relationship of sex role identity and the image of nursing in 43 female nursing students. Her findings supported the belief that sex role is an important intervening variable in the process of professional socialization. As the student's sex role identity became more masculine, the student's image of nursing was more in harmony with the image advanced by the profession.[38]

In a later study of 92 students, Till[39] also found that the subjects endorsed more feminine characteristics than female college students and did not hold the image of nursing advanced by the profession.

In contrast, Meleis and Dageneis[40] found that 163 soon-to-be graduates of baccalaureate, diploma, and associate degree programs did not differ significantly from the normative groups of female college students in sex role identity and other personality constructs.

Nurse educators and administrators are advocating increased independence and leadership by nurses. However, the prevailing conforming role orientation by many females may preclude acquisition of the traits advocated by the profession. This disharmony may be alleviated by providing time in the curriculum to explore with students the inherent conflicts in the sex role and the professional role and to provide students with time to verbalize how they can deal with the conflicts. The provision of female role models, who exemplify the professional role, may help reduce the stresses involved in conflict over appropriate sex role behavior.

Sexism is a two-edged sword that affects male and female nurses. The male may be perceived more a leader, teacher, or other such authoritarian role than the female. The female who is authoritarian may be labeled a "castrated" or frustrated male, while the male who is able to demonstrate affective behavior may be labeled "homosexual." In addition, sexism is self-confirming. That is, people behave as they are expected by those around them. Hull[41] states that the tragedy of sexism is that it is iatrogenic, self-confirming, and not based on realistic assessment of the potentials and possibilities for human growth and development. Perhaps the real change will come with a new generation, less oriented to the status quo. Until then all nurses will suffer sexism's consequences.

Male Nurses. Male nurses may need to resolve conflicts. They enter into a profession that has emphasized tender, loving care and qualities of gentleness and compassion. Overemphasis on the nurses' affective role to the exclusion of the cognitive and theoretical aspects of nursing can produce conflict. Garvin's investigation[42] of the values of male nursing students showed that males scored higher than females on the theoretical scale of the Allport–Vernon–Lindzey Study of Values Scale, indicating that these male nursing students were more interested in the discovery of truth and a critical and empirical ordering of knowledge than female students.

Fortunately, there is decreased social emphasis on sex-linked occupations. More males are entering nursing, yet data are needed to assist in the development of the image of male nurses. The nursing profession in a changing society needs nurses of both sexes with higher theoretical interests, who value the empirical, critical, and rational orientation, nurses who are at the same time comfortable with and competent in their affective role.

Some male nurses believe policies and procedures have been set up for female nursing students and staff members. Foote[43] sees the major cause of discrimination as female nurses "guarding" certain areas of the hospital.

Acceptance of male nurses into a principally female profession is problematic. Some female nurses hold the negative attitudes that (1) men are acceptable only in specific areas of clinical practice, such as male urology or psychiatric settings, especially units with disturbed patients; (2) male nurses are likely to be homosexuals or very effeminate; (3) male nurses should be used in divisions where physical strength is important, such as orthopedic units; (4) male nurses should not care for female patients; (5) males come into nursing because they could not get into another health profession.

Men will continue to feel that they lose their self-respect and prestige when they enter nursing unless these sex-biased attitudes change. Female nurses who have these attitudes should attempt to change them or assess why they hold them.[44]

Female Nurses. Female nurses are faced with sexual stereotyping of another sort. Society traditionally views them as nurturers, care givers, and part of a hierarchy of health professionals that has tended to place men at the top.

Although nurses place emphasis on health promotion, neither the public nor public decision makers are fully aware of nursing's perspective or what nurses can offer the health care system. Although the profession and its weakness in communication can be faulted, the media must also be indicted. The news media dispenses values and influences sexual behavior. The public often believes that if something matters it will be a focus of media attention, and if something is a focus, it matters.[45] The ways in which nurses are presented, misrepresented, or underrepresented strongly affects the public's image of nursing and nurses as it is or might be.[46]

B. J. Kalisch and P. A. Kalisch analyzed both quantitatively and qualitatively the image of the nurse presented in novels, motion pictures, and television. In analyzing the 207 novels (and this was also true of television and motion pictures), the nurses were almost always female, single, childless, under 35, and white. They were looking for romance and adventure while carrying out the essential job of supporting the "magnificent work" of physicians.[47]

Nurses were at the pinnacle of respectability in the novels of the 1940s and 50s but reached a low point in the 1960s and 70s when they were often associated with sexual promiscuity or depicted as the physician's sexual plaything.[48] Nursing was presented as a technical organization whose members were females and were ultimately submissive to the physician.

A study of 28 television series from 1950 to 1980 indicated that the image of nursing portrayed undermined respect and confidence in the nurse. The one exception to this less than desirable image was the program *The Nurse.*[49,50] The presence of a nurse-consultant during the filming of this series was a concentrated effort to improve nursing's image.[51] A positive change in the treatment of and image of nurses in the television series *M∗A∗S∗H* took place the last several years of its existence. In the early years of the series, nurses slept with officers to keep morale high and were subject to frequent sexual innuendos and advances. Later, *M∗A∗S∗H* offered the most professional view of nurses on prime-time television as essential members of the health team. Unfortunately, no trend was established.[52]

Kalisch and Kalisch also analyzed 204 English-speaking motion pictures released between 1930 and 1979 with similar evidence of peaks and valleys in the image projected.[53] In the 1930s and 40s until the end of World War II, the nurses and the profession were presented as proud and noble. After 1945, women were cast as passive, docile creatures living vicariously through men. The 1960s to 1980 saw a destruction of a proud, noble image. The nurse was a focus of sexual titillation or presented along unflattering and frightening lines. In *One Flew Over the Cuckoo's Nest,* Nurse Ratched was a soul-destroying, castrating mother figure. Nurses were also portrayed as villains in criminal activity.

Although a few pictures portrayed sympathetic, positive nursing characters, the 1970s were the lowest point for nurse characters in rationality, sociability, altruism, warmth, duty, self-sacrifice, integrity, virtue, intellect, and religiousness.[54]

The most blatant sex exploitation of nurses are X- and R-rated movies that feature nurses as female fantasy figures. Titles such as *Nurses Report, Student Nurses,* and *Night Nurse* appear regularly in the local papers. Pornographic films transform nurses into American geishas and reinforce men's longing for a woman to do everything she is told to do—by them. Although it claims to be honest, liberating, and contemporary, the pornographic film is the most rigid movie of all movie forms in its approaches to changing roles and relationships between the sexes.[55]

Sexual fantasy films tend to portray the nurse as knowledgeable about many sophisticated sexual techniques, perhaps because of her dedication to "total care." All the films have two similar themes: obedience to authority and assumption of fundamental dull wittedness.[56]

Redressing Negative Images and Sexism. The image of nursing will not be improved until nurses recognize that the problem exists and become involved in systematic effort toward its eradication. Some collective professional soul-searching may also be in order. Are nurses' own views of self and behavior as much an etiology of the problems as media depiction?

TABLE 2–1.   PROCESS FOR CHANGING THE IMAGE OF NURSING[a]

Get organized:	Establish image of nurse or nurse-in-media committees in hospitals, community agencies, schools of nursing or through local, state, or national nursing groups Establish media-watch committees
Monitor the media:	Evaluate local and national mass communication—television, movies, newspapers, novels, radio for negative stereotyping and for positive portrayal of nurses
React:	Commend or condemn as appropriate —write letters to producers, directors, editors, sponsors, advertisers —develop special media newsletters or news columns in nursing journals —contact top decision makers in media—managers of stations, owner —write letters to the editor —picket theaters showing offensive motion pictures —avoid buying products advertised on programs portraying negative images —picket stores that sell the product —notify manufacturer why product is not being bought
Foster positive image:	Build strong media contacts Plan conferences that bring nurses and media together Offer media consultation Give awards and prizes to those who depict nursing positively Develop health information programs or columns by nurses Seek news coverage of real-life events about nursing Prepare press packages with adequate information for reporters Gain access and appear on talk shows and present a unified stance Air messages and announcements on radio and television through Public Service Announcements (PSAs) Develop campaigns to improve the image of nurses with coverage at all levels

[a]*Adapted from Kalisch BJ, Kalisch PA: Improving the Image of Nursing. American Journal of Nursing 83:48–51, January, 1983.*

There are steps nurses can take to change the professional image in the media. These involve organization of efforts, monitoring the media, reacting when appropriate, and fostering a positive image.[57] (See Table 2-1 for details.)

In order to correct some of the social inequities experienced by the profession, some female nurses have become active in the women's movement. They recognized that when feminists discussed women's position in terms of powerlessness, dependency, and discrimination, this also paralleled nurses' position in the health care system.[58] The number of nurses who are politically aware and are actively espousing women's rights is questionable. In a study involving 28 nurse practitioners, Simmons and Rosenthal[59] found that the nurses had a low sense of political efficacy and that the majority felt overwhelmed by and somewhat at the mercy of the system. The author's conclusion was that although the women's movement has been acknowledged, its impact has been limited.

One early problem in the feminist movement as led by the National Organization for Women (NOW) was the early publicity flyers which denigrated nursing. Nurses did confront the organization and were invited to submit suggested revisions.[60] Whitman[61] believes that nurses have demonstrated to politicians and others that they are a force to be considered and that they are fighting against their second-class citizenship and feeling of powerlessness. Equality is more than equal opportunity for good jobs. Values that are considered feminine must be recognized as important to society. Nurses, instead of seeking more prestigious jobs, should first put the right price tag on their work and improve their workplace.[62]

Pinch[63] suggests nurses need the autonomy and independence to promote the values of caring, gentleness, and responsibility more fully for all the sexes so that in the end we will get a balance of both sets of norms of healthy behavior for men and women.

HUMAN SEXUALITY AND NURSING CARE OF THE FUTURE

What is the role of nursing in helping individuals meet their sexual needs? Masters and Johnson describe nurses as intermediaries between physicians who are uncomfortable with the topic of sexuality and the patients who lack knowledge or who have misconceptions about sexuality. Others see sexual problems remaining in the general province of psychiatry, with physicians dealing with the sexual side of the patients' lives as physicians become more knowledgeable and at ease with the topic.[64]

The World Health Organization sees the physician guiding and supervising other professional colleagues, while the nurse "sets her goals" in terms of supportive relationships with patients who have sexual problems; helping patients in matters such as feminine hygiene, family planning; helping parents deal with the sexual behavior and questions of their children; and assisting teachers with sex education.[65]

Contrary to these rather restrictive views, nursing can be the pivotal profession in the future in promoting and maintaining the sexual health of individuals and groups. Nurses will be comfortable with their own sexuality and in dealing with the sexuality of others. As sex-typed role behavior blurs and eventually disappears, male and female nurses will be assertive, independent, tender, loving, and able to express love irrespective of their biologic sex. Nurses will be knowledgeable about the bio-psycho-social aspects of sexuality throughout the life cycle, about the effects of illness and psychologic and sociocultural deprivations on human sexual functioning.

Although all nurses will not be sex therapists in the narrow sense of the term, all nurses will be able to assess patients in relation to sexuality, just as they now assess other basic needs. Nurses will accurately identify problems and intervene appropriately. Teaching and counseling, if only to relieve the ignorance, misinformation, guilt, shame, and embarrassment manifested by individuals, will be in the province of all nurses.

Nurse sex therapists will use the holistic approach to individuals that their nursing education stressed.[66] They will be able to utilize many therapeutic models to help their clients gain sexual health. Finally, individuals will increasingly turn to nurses for help in achieving sexual health and recognize that nurses are the empathic listeners and counselors with whom they can share their sexual concerns.

NOTES

1. Cook E: The Life of Florence Nightingale, New York, Macmillan, 1942, pp 456–467

2. Jacobson L: Illness and human sexuality. Nurs Outlook 22:50–53, January 1974

3. Baldwin LB: The relation of syphilis and the nursing profession. Am J Nurs 2:103–105, February 1902

4. Harmer B: Textbook of the Principles and Practice of Nursing. New York, Macmillan, 1934

5. Keller MC: Teaching sexuality as a nursing elective. Nursing and Health Care 3:311–313, June 1982

6. Whipple B, Gick R: A holistic view of sexuality—Education for the health professional. Topics in Clinical Nursing 1:91–109, January 1980

7. Solomon J: Human sexuality content: Should this be included in baccalaureate nursing programs. Imprint 27:129–131, December 1980

8. Silbert DT: Human sexuality growth groups. Journal of Psychiatric Nursing and Mental Health Services 19:31–34, February 1981

9. Watts RJ: Dimensions of sexual health. American Journal of Nursing 79:1568–1572, September 1979

10. Hott JR, Ryan-Merritt M: A national study of nursing research in human sexuality. Nursing Clinics North America 17:429–447, September 1982

11. Fisher SG, Levin DL: The sexual knowledge and attitudes of professional nurses caring for oncology patients. Cancer Nursing 6:55–61, February 1983

12. Mace DR, Braverman RHO, Burton J: Teaching Human Sexuality in Schools for Health Professionals. Geneva, World Health Organization, 1974

13. Payne T: Sexuality of nurses: Correlations of knowledge, attitudes, and behavior. Nurs Res 25:286–292, July–August 1976

14. Woods NF, Mandetta A: Changes in students: Knowledge and attitudes following a course in human sexuality. Nurs Res 24:10–15, January–February 1975

15. Mims FH, Brown L, Lubow R: Human sexuality course evaluation. Nurs Res 25:174–176, March 1974

16. Keller MC: Teaching sexuality as a nursing elective, Nursing and Health Care 3:313, 1982

17. Fontaine KL: Human sexuality: Faculty knowledge and attitudes. Nurs Outlook 24:174–176, March 1974

18. Bullough B, Bullough V: Sexuality and the nurse. Imprint 17–18:33, February 1974

19. Woods N, Mandetta AF: Sexuality in the baccalaureate curriculum. Nurs Forum 15:294–297, March 1976

20. Whipple B, Gick R: A holistic view of sexuality—Education for the health professional. Topics in Clinical Nursing 1:34, 1980

21. Hott JR, Ryan-Merritt M: A national study of nursing reserach in human sexuality. Nursing Clinics of North America. 17:430, 1982

22. Malo-Juveva D: Sex therapy and nursing—Do they mix? RN 38:32–33, March 1975

23. Nelson SE: All about sex education for

students. Am J Nurs 77:611–612, April 1977

24. Kempton W: A teacher's guide to sex education. North Scituate, Massachusetts, Duxbury Press, 1974, pp 32–35

25. Krizinofski MT: Human sexuality and nursing practice. Nurs Clin North Am 8:673–679, December 1973

26. Elder M-S: The unmet challenge—Nurse counseling on sexuality, Nurs Outlook 18:39–40, November 1970

27. Mims FH: Sexual health education and counseling, Nurs Clin North Am 10:519–528, September 1975

28. Cleland V: To end sex discrimination. Nurs Clin North Am, 9:563–571, September 1974

29. Bullough B, Bullough VL: Sex discrimination in health care. Nurs Outlook 23:40–45, January 1975

30. Bullough B, Bullough VL: Rebellion Among the "Angels." Time, August 27, 1979, pp 62–63

31. Ibid, p 63

32. Hazel H: Sexual harrassment and nurse anesthetists. AANA Journal 49:277–279, March 1981

33. Ibid, p 278

34. Walker: ML: Do women nurses accept men nurses?. RN 36:25–26, April 1973

35. Bem SL: Androgyny vs. the tight little lives of fluffy women and chesty men. Psychol Today 9:58–62, September 1975

36. Keller MC: The effect of sexual stereotyping on the development of nursing theory. American Journal of Nursing 79:1584–1586, September 1979

37. Goodwin CE, Taaffe CH: Sex-typing and consumer preference for a male or female psychotherapist. Journal of Psychiatric Nursing 18:21–25, April 1980

38. Stromborg MF: Relationship of sex role identity to occupational image of female nursing students. Nurs Res 25:363–369, September–October 1976

39. Till TS: Sex-role identity and image of nursing of females at two levels of baccalaureate nursing education. Nursing Research 29:295–300, September–October 1980

40. Meleis AI, Dagenais F: Sex-role identity and perception of professional self in graduates of three nursing programs. Nursing Research 30:162–167, May/June 1981

41. Hull RT: Dealing with sexism in nursing and medicine. Nursing Outlook 30:89–94, February 1982

42. Garvin BJ: Values of male nursing students. Nurs Res 25:353–357, September–October 1976

43. Foote RH: Double standards: American Journal of Nursing 80:16, September 1980

44. Walker ML: Do women nurses accept men nurses? RN 36:25–26, April 1973

45. Kalisch PA, Kalisch BJ: Prospectives on improving nursing's public image. Nursing and Health Care 1:10–15, July/August 1980

46. Ibid, p 15

47. Kalisch PA, Kalisch BJ: The image of nurses in novels. American Journal of Nursing 82:1220–1224, August 1982

48. Ibid, p 1224

49. Kalisch PA, Kalisch BJ: Nurses on prime-time television. American Journal of Nursing 82:264–270, February 1982

50. Kalisch BJ, Kalisch PA, Scobey M: Reflections on a television image: The nurses. Nursing and Health Care 2:248–255, May 1981

51. Kalisch BJ, Kalisch PA, Scobey M: Behind the scenes on the "Nurse" set. Nursing and Health Care 11:382–384, September 1981

52. Kalisch PA, Kalisch BJ, Scobey M: Nurses on prime-time television. American Journal of Nursing 82:270, 1982

53. Kalisch PA, Kalisch BJ: The image of the nurse in motion pictures. American Journal of Nursing 82:605–611, April 1982

54. Ibid, p 611

55. Wheelock A: The tarnished image. Nurs Outlook 24:509–510, August 1976

56. Ibid, p 510

57. Kalisch BJ, Kalisch PA: Improving the image of nursing. American Journal of Nursing 83:48–52, January 1983

58. Talbott SW, Vance CN: Involving nursing in a feminist group—NOW. Nursing Outlook 29:592–595, October 1981

59. Simmons RS, Rosenthal J: The women's movement and the nurse practitioner's sense of role. Nursing Outlook 29:311–375, June 1981

60. Talbot SW, Vance CN: Involving nursing in a feminist group—NOW. Nursing Outlook 29:593, 1981

61. Whitman M: Toward new psychology for nurses. Nursing Outlook 30:48–53, January 1982

62. Whitman M: Moving into the second stage: An interview with Betty Friedan. Nursing Outlook 29:666—669, November 1981

63. Pinch WJ: Feminine attributes in a masculine world. Nursing Outlook 29:596–599, October 1981

64. Levine SB: Medicine and sexuality. Med Alumni Bull Case Western Reserve Univ, 1:8–11, 1974

65. Mace DR, Braverman RHO, Burton J: Teaching of Human Sexuality in Schools for Health Professionals, Geneva, World Health Organization, 1974, p 16

66. Schuster EA, Unsain IC, Goodwin MH: Nursing practice in human sexuality. Nursing Clinics of North America 17:345–349, September 1982

Chapter 3

Human Sexual Responses

Most of the objective information concerning human sexual response and the problems in achieving satisfying sexual response has been the outcome of the investigations of Dr. William H. Masters and Mrs. Virginia E. Johnson. However, some have criticized their research, alleging that they mechanized and dehumanized sex, ignoring the psychologic components of the sexual experience. Others have pointed out that the subjects were atypical (some were prostitutes) and represented only the midwestern United States. No matter what the criticism, much of which is unfounded, Masters and Johnson were the first to use basic medical research methods to study sexual response in the laboratory and then to apply their findings to clinical medicine. By adding objective measurement of sexual response to the subjective reports that have been obtained in the past, they were able to add to the body of knowledge about sexuality as well as to dispel myths and misconceptions about sexual functioning.

The focus of this chapter will be the normal female and male sexual response cycle as described by Masters and Johnson, as well as the sexual dysfunctions that have a psychologic or sociocultural etiology. Discussion of specific disease processes that affect sexual response is covered in Unit V.

NORMAL SEXUAL RESPONSE

The Sexual Response Cycle—Overview

The sexual response cycle is basically the same for females and males. Four phases have been identified, which, rather than being discrete, overlap each other. The excitement phase is initiated by whatever the individual finds sexually stimulating. If the stimuli are interrupted for any reason or if they become objectionable or uncomfortable, the cycle may stop or be extended a longer period of time. If stimulation is continued, the sexual tension increases. This increase in tension is called the *plateau phase* and may be prolonged and/or decreased if the stimulation is not effective or if it is withdrawn. The third phase, the climactic or orgasmic phase, involves a completely involuntary response. It is at this point the body responds with maximum intensity. During orgasm, the sexual tension is released in a total body reaction, although the most intense sensation is in the pelvic area. The fourth and final phase, resolution, is characterized by decreased sexual tension as the individual returns to the unstimulated state.

There are two physiologic responses in males and females: myotonia, or increased muscle tension, and vasocongestion, especially in the genital organs. Masters and Johnson have shown that these responses are the same whether the stimulation is coital, manipulative, mechanical, or by fantasy, although the intensity and duration of the responses vary with the type of stimulation. In the laboratory, masturbation produced the most intense experiences, partner manipulation next, and intercourse the least.[1]

Criticism of the Masters and Johnson's model of sexual response has arisen because it is based on subjective assessments and interpretations of physiologic and anatomic changes by Masters and Johnson. It has been argued that there was no definitional reliability (interobserver agreement) or sequential reliability.[2]

Kaplan[3] has suggested a biphasic model of sexual arousal consisting of two phases: (1) genital vasocongestion causing erection in the male and vaginal congestion and lubrication in the female, and (2) reflex, clonic striated and nonstriated muscular contractions at orgasm. This model has not been as popular as the Masters and Johnson's model.

Female Response Cycle— Biologic Factors

Excitement Phase. The first physiologic sign of female response to sexual stimulation is vaginal lubrication. In the woman who has not experienced menopause, sexual stimulation results in vaginal lubrication in 10 to 30 seconds. Contrary to what had been believed, lubrication is not provided principally by Bartholin glands in the labia minora or by the cervix. Lubrication results from vasocongestion around and in the vagina causing transudate of fluid to pass through the tissue of the vaginal walls into the lumen— what has been described as a "sweating" reaction.[4,5]

The inner two-thirds of the vagina lengthens and distends, while the front remains closed. The labia minora increase in size and protrude, while the labia majora increase in size, flatten, and extend upward, downward, and outward.[6] The uterus elevates away from the bladder and the vagina.

The vaginal walls, which are purplish red in the unstimulated state, slowly change to a purplish color due to the vasocongestion. The clitoral shaft increases in size two to three times. The end of the clitoris, called the glans, increases in size from a barely discernible diameter to a twofold expansion.[7]

During late excitement, muscles become tensed. The rectal sphincter may be tightened by some women to increase stimulation. Involuntary tensing of the abdominal and intercostal muscles may occur.[8] The nipples of the breasts become erect due to concentration of blood in the tissues, and the breasts of those who have not nursed infants may increase in size. In women who have, size does not increase so markedly, because milk production has altered blood vessels and fibrous tissues.[9] The sex flush described by Masters and Johnson includes a maculopapular, measle-like rash just under the rib cage and spreading over the breasts.[10]

Plateau Phase. The outer third of the vagina, which has only slightly enlarged during the excitement phase, becomes engorged with venous blood so that the opening decreases by at least a third. This distended outer third of the vagina is called the *orgasmic platform.*[11]

In those who have never given birth, the labia minora change from pink to a bright red. For those who have, the color change is to deep wine. This is called the *sex skin reaction,* and when it occurs, orgasm inevitably follows.[12]

The clitoris retracts to a relatively inaccessible place under the clitoral hood,[13] and the tissues around the nipples fill with fluid, decreasing the evidence of nipple erection.[14] The sex flush may spread to all areas of the breast, chest, abdomen, and other body surfaces and reaches its peak of color.[15]

Orgasmic Phase. Immediately before and during orgasm, there is an increase in vital signs. The pulse increases to more than twice its usual rate to 110 to 180 per minute, respirations rise to 3 times the usual rate, and blood pressure rises by one-third, up 30 to 80 mm Hg systolic[16] and 20 to 40 mm Hg diastolic. Muscles tense and rhythmic contractions begin in the orgasmic platform at 0.8-second intervals and occur from 3 to 15 times. Uterine contractions may occur at the same time as those of the vagina but do not occur in a definite pattern.[17] The external rectal sphincter contracts, as do the pelvic floor muscles around the lower third of the vagina, forcing the blood out of the engorged blood vessels. Physiologically, there is release of muscular tension and of the blood vessel engorgement. Subjectively, orgasm is the experience of peak physical pleasure. This is conditioned, however, by a variety of psychologic and social factors. Women reportedly respond to the total person and the total situation, while men are more genitally oriented (Fig. 3-1).

Recently the presence of "female ejaculation" during orgasm has been described after stimulation of a vaginal area named the "Grafenberg Spot" (G-Spot).

Female ejaculation is a term used to denote the emission of fluid from the urethra during orgasm. This fluid differs from urine in taste, odor, and chemical content. The orgasm that results is said to be qualitatively different than orgasm achieved through clitoral stimulation.[18,19] Further research is needed to confirm these findings but they do confirm that fluid emissions during female orgasm are normal and not necessarily due to stress incontinence.

Resolution. The length of resolution parallels the length of the excitement phase. The clitoris, which has been retracted and invisible, returns to its normal position 5 to 10 seconds after orgasm. If there has been any swelling of the clitoris, this disappears.[20] The labia majora return to their usual size in 3 to 4 minutes.[21] The orgasmic platform also disappears, and the vaginal opening is wider. The inner two-thirds of the vagina become less distended and return to the usual size in

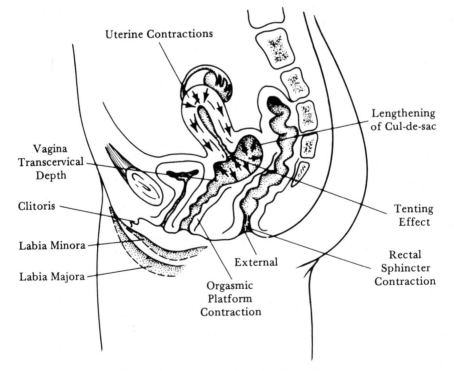

Figure 3-1. Orgasmic phase: female pelvis.

3 to 4 minutes.[22] The uterus returns to its unstimulated position. There may be some irritation of the urinary bladder in women who have not had children, since pelvic structures not yet stretched by delivery hold the penis in a position that may cause irritation.[23]

Male Response Cycle— Biologic Factors

Excitement. The male's first physiologic response to sexual stimulation is penile erection.[24] This is caused by engorgement of blood in spongy tissue as a result of increased arterial blood flow into the organ, contraction of valves that redirect and trap the blood, and consequent decreased venous outflow. Erection can be induced by two stimuli—touching the genitals, which sets off a reflex through the sacral spinal cord like the knee jerk reflex, and through the brain by seeing, feeling, and thinking.

The average penis is about 4 inches long nonerect and 6¼ inches erect, so it increases in length by about 50 percent. Its diameter increases from 1¼ to 1½ inches, or about 20 percent. There is no correlation between body size and penile size, and there is little correlation between the erect penis and the nonerect penis. The small penis gets about as large as larger ones during stimulation. The vagina, which is elastic, can accommodate any size penis.

Changes occur in the scrotum and testes. There is thickening and tensing of the scrotal skin and the entire scrotal sac is elevated toward the body. The spermatic cords shorten so that the testes are pulled further up in the sac.[25] Nipples of the breasts may erect and swell, and the sex flush may occur. There is also a total body response, which includes spasm in the muscles of legs and arms, tension in the muscles of the abdomen, and increased respiratory rate.[26]

Plateau. Erection of the penis is completed in the excitement phase, but during the second stage, there is a slight increase in diameter of the coronal ridge at the base of the glans penis and sometimes a deepening of the reddish purple color of the glans.[27]

The testes are pulled up higher in the scrotum because of shortening of the spermatic cords. Full elevation of the testes indicates that orgasm is imminent. If the testes do not elevate, as happens in older men, the pressure of ejaculation is greatly reduced. There may be emission of a few drops of seminal fluid before true ejaculation. This fluid contains sperm—one reason coitus interruptus (withdrawal of the penis from the vagina before ejaculation) may be an ineffective means of birth control.[28] Vital signs increase to a greater degree than in women. Systolic blood pressure increasing 20 to 80 mm Hg and diastolic 10 to 40 mm Hg.

The same measle-like rash develops in the male as in the female, but it is less frequent and may not develop during each response cycle. In the male, muscular tension may be more evident than in the female. Involuntary spasm of muscles of the face, neck, and abdomen occur. During masturbation, there is an involuntary increase in hand movements and increase in pressure on the genitals. The rectal sphincter may be tightened voluntarily as may the muscles of the buttocks to heighten tension.[29]

Orgasm. Male orgasm, like the female's, is characterized by a series of rhythmic contractions of intervals of four-fifths of a second. Following the first contraction, the interval between contractions becomes greater and then tapers off. The testes, prostate gland, and seminal vesicles are involved as they collect sperm and seminal fluid and expel it into the prostatic urethra. At this stage, there is a feeling of inevitability, that the male cannot hold back from climax. The subjective feeling of orgasm occurs at this stage.

The second stage, ejaculation, is caused by contractions of the urethra and muscles of the penis and the sensation of the pressure of the seminal fluid. A large ejaculate is subjectively more pleasurable for the male. Therefore, the first orgasm of the male is usually more pleasurable, while the opposite is true

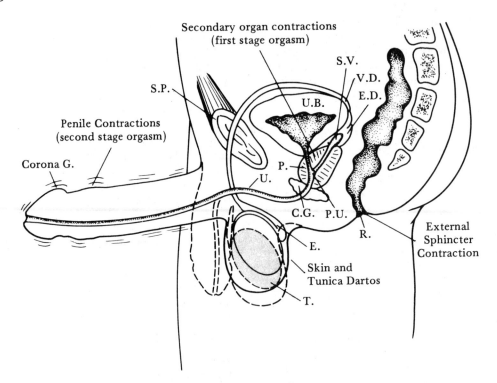

Secondary organ contractions
(first stage orgasm)

Figure 3-2. Orgasmic phase: male pelvis. S. P. = symphysis pubis, U. = urethra, P. = prostate, U.B. = urinary bladder, S. V. = seminal vesicle, V. D. = vas deferens, E.D. = ejaculatory duct, P.U. = prostatic urethra, C.G.= Cowper's glands, R. = rectum, E. = epididymis, T. = testis.

for the females. In the younger male, the semen may be projected under great pressure as much as 2 feet beyond the tip of the penis.[30] (Fig. 3-2).

At ejaculation, the internal bladder sphincter closes to prevent retrograde ejaculation into the bladder.[31] There may be contortion of the face in a grimace and contraction of the muscles of the neck, arms, and legs as well as muscles of the abdomen and buttocks. Men may experience carpopedal (hand and foot) spasm but are usually unaware of the muscular exertion.

The elevation of heart rate is similar to that of the female, between 100 and 175 beats per minute, but the blood pressure is often greater, systolic raising 40 to 100 mm Hg and the diastolic 20 to 50 mm Hg. Respiratory rate may peak at over 40 per minute.[32]

Resolution. After ejaculation, half of the erection is lost rapidly, although this may be delayed if the erection has been present for a long period of time. The second stage of resolution includes further loss of erection. This may be slower if the penis is left in the vagina or if the partner is held close.[33]

The male sex flush disappears, and the scrotum and testes return to their unstimulated state slowly or rapidly. If the male nipples have erected, they return to normal slowly. The vital signs return to normal gradually. Perspiration may be present but it is usually confined to the palms of the hands and the soles of the feet.

A refractory period follows the male resolution period. During this time, unlike the female, the male cannot be sexually aroused or have another erection.[34] In young men it may be brief, a matter of minutes, but in others, it may be longer, gradually increasing in duration as the man grows older.

Recently, some preliminary research has indicated males may have the same multi-orgasmic potential as females.[35] Brauer and Brauer[36] contend that orgasm occurs in a continuum and that both men and women may experience three different types of orgasm depending on the site of stimulation.

Men have also claimed to have multiple orgasms by delaying ejaculation. If so, the concept of absolute refractory period must be reconsidered. It may be more accurate to say that men have an absolute refractory period after ejaculation.[37] rather than after orgasm.

Biochemical Factors Affecting Function. Other factors involved in sexual function have been suggested without conclusive experimental proof as yet. Vasoactive intestinal polypeptide (VIP), a potent vasodilator and smooth muscle contractor, may be a neurotransmitter that causes uterine and vaginal contractions, changes in circulation of the penis and the vagina, and changes in secretion of the endometrium and cervix.[38]

Endorphins, endogenous peptides with morphine-like activity, may play a role in reinforcement mechanisms, sexual drive, and satisfaction. In the male, prostaglandins may be involved in sperm transport, motility, in the vasodilation of erection, and in contraction of musculature during ejaculation. In the female, they may aid fertility by being absorbed across the vagina or cervix from the ejaculate, then passing to the uterus and fallopian tubes, aiding sperm movement.[39] Prolactin secretion in males increases during sexual arousal and may have a role in sperm motility.[40]

Myths and Misconceptions Related to Sexual Response

Role of the Clitoris. Sigmund Freud believed that women can experience two kinds of orgasms, clitoral or vaginal (see Chapter 7). This theory of vaginal orgasm as distinct from clitoral orgasm has raised many questions and criticism in sexual literature. Mas-

ters and Johnson have shown on the basis of direct observations and laboratory measurements that the same events occur following clitoral stimulation, vaginal stimulation, or (in some women) breast stimulation.

During vaginal intercourse, the thrusting of the penis causes motion of the labia minora, which come together above the vagina to form the prepuce of the clitoris. Movement of this hood back and forth over the glans of the clitoris stimulates it effectively even if no direct stimulation is used.[41]

Intensity of female orgasm has also been studied in relation to size, anatomic position, and amount of swelling of the clitoris. Increased size and anatomic position allowing better penile contact are not related to responsiveness or orgasmic ability in women. Because the clitoris retracts, it is relatively inaccessible to hand or penile stimulation, contrary to instructions in many marriage manuals. Manipulation of the clitoris may be painful, especially if it is done too long or too hard.

Simultaneous Orgasm. Many marriage manuals stress that simultaneous orgasm is a mark of superior sexual achievement and capability. However, efforts to coordinate what are basically involuntary responses cause the partners to observe themselves mentally, rather than losing themselves in the feelings of love making, resulting in diminished response. If one partner does not achieve orgasm, the other may manually stimulate him/her until orgasm is attained.

Sexual Response During Menstruation. Sexual intercourse during menstruation is neither painful nor harmful to the woman. There is no physiologic reason for continence, but rather it is a question of individual preference. If for aesthetic reasons one partner does not desire intercourse, the other should agree. Some women report orgasm is effective in relieving dysmenorrhea.

Multiple Orgasm. Women are capable of being stimulated to other orgasms after the first climax. Physiologically, repeated orgasms do not differ from single orgasms and are not less intense experiences. In some individuals, they are considered more intense subjectively. Physiologically, after the first orgasm, the clitoris descends to the usual position and the orgasmic platform and labia majora and minora lose their engorgement. These events may all be reversed with renewal of stimulation. Multiple orgasms are more likely to occur with autostimulation (masturbation), since few men can maintain erection long enough to effect multiple orgasms in their partners.

Phallic Myths. One of the most common fallacies is that the size of the penis is related to the male's virility and his ability to satisfy his sexual partner. Many boys and men are worried about penile size, and negative comparison with others may be a source of anxiety, particularly in adolescence. Penile size, however, has little relationship to a sexual partner's satisfaction in intercourse. A male with a relatively small penis having intercourse with a female with a relatively large vagina can introduce his penis in the vagina earlier in the excitement phase, and the fully erect smaller penis can function as effectively as a dilating agent as a larger penis. If the female has a small vagina, the male with a large penis can delay entry until a more advanced stage of sexual excitation.[42]

Many men also believe that circumcision makes the glans (head of the penis) more sensitive to sexual stimulation and that ejaculatory control is more difficult. However, Masters and Johnson found that there was no difference in the responses of circumcised and uncircumcised men.[43]

Psychosocial Concomitants of Sexual Response

Subjective Feelings. The peak experiences of the male are the feelings of ejaculatory inevitability as sexual fluid collects in the prostatic urethra, and second, the sensations of contractions of the urethral sphincter and the expulsion of seminal fluid through the urethra.

Females have reported three stages of experience. First, there is a sensation of "suspension" or "stoppage," followed by a peak of intense sensation in the clitoris, which then spreads into the pelvis. There are variations in intensity of this stage, which may also include sensations of "falling," "opening up," or of emitting fluid. This is followed by a feeling of warmth spreading through the pelvis to the rest of the body, followed finally, by pelvic throbbing. Women responding to the questionnaire by Hite[44] described arousal as "floating," "exciting," "being alive," "warm." Orgasm was characterized as a "hot rush," "feeling of warmth," "indescribable." Some described sensation focused in the genital area, especially with clitoral stimulation, while with vaginal intercourse, orgasm was described as more diffuse and a total body response. Therefore, some women saw this as a "stronger," more satisfying experience.

After orgasm, women feel "tender," want to be "close," strong, wide awake, alive, while the male feels placid, sleepy, quickly returning to the prearousal state psychologically and physically.[45]

Although there are variations in intensity of orgasm, the male orgasm seems to be physiologically and psychologically more standard. Females experience differences in intensity, and there is the possibility that they experience orgasms that differ in quality and that involve physiologically different mechanisms.[46]

Bardwick[47] describes three types of orgasmic response in the woman. The young and relatively inexperienced woman achieves what might be called a minor orgasm, a pleasant or tingly sensation (Pattern A). Maximal arousal is not reached, and consequently a maximum orgasm is not achieved. Resolution occurs slowly, and gratification is based primarily on the feeling of affection and love. Pattern B is an intermediate level of arousability. The woman attains a physiologically defined orgasm but stops at the plateau level and can have more than one orgasm. Resolution is slow, but less so than in Pattern A. Pattern C orgasm is closest to that of the male. The woman reaches a high plateau state, achieves a maximal orgasm, and then has a rapid and total resolution. Like the male, she will take 15 to 20 minutes to recover from the resolution. Bardwick states that Pattern C is the least frequently reported among women and reflects the most mature and elusive sexual response pattern in women.

In contrast to some descriptions of orgasms that focus on physical sensation, Schaefer[48] stresses that women do not even have to experience orgasm for gratification, which might come instead from feelings of spiritual and physical closeness, from giving pleasure to a loved one, or from feelings of being in control of one's self, the other individual, or the situation.

She argues, too, that the sexual orgasm instead of being an experience has become an achievement or test of competence. How the woman perceives the experience determines what is pleasurable. Some women experience intense orgasms but have cold, detached interpersonal relations, while the opposite is true of others.

SEXUAL DYSFUNCTIONS

Psychologic factors may interfere with satisfactory sexual response. Anxiety and guilt about sexual activity may interfere with orgasmic response. Fear of failure may become a self-fulfilling prophecy. Lack of privacy, fear of detection, etc., may also adversely affect sexual pleasures.

Relational causes, partner rejection, lack of trust, power struggles, sexual sabotage, or failure to communicate have all been indicated in the etiology of dysfunction.[49] Hatch[50] suggests that penile and vaginal vasocongestion may be under some voluntary control rather than under the control of the autonomic nervous system. If this is true, sexual disorders may be a type of learned behavior. Masters and Johnson state, "Sociocultural deprivation and ignorance of sexual physiology, rather than psychiatric or medical illness, constitute the etiologic background for most sexual dysfunction."[51]

Sexual Dysfunction in the Female
Orgasmic Dysfunction (Anorgasmia).

Masters and Johnson have used the term *primary orgasmic dysfunction* to identify women who have never experienced orgasm in any way—by masturbation, love play, or coitus. *Secondary orgasmic dysfunction,* or *situational dysfunction,* refers to conditions in which the woman has experienced at least one orgasm in the past. A term used in the past was *frigidity,* which is sometimes called hyposexuality or sexual anesthesia. (See Chapter 4.) Frigidity may involve combinations of difficulties; the most common and most disturbing form is that in which the woman has sexual drive, desire, and arousal but is unable to reach orgasm.[52]

Different writers define orgasmic problems differently, so incidence varies because of criteria selected. Estimates range from a low of 30 to 40 percent to a high of 70 to 80 percent of all women. In this country of six million wives, about one in four are thought to be dissatisfied with sexual relations, prefer to avoid sex, or else are not gratified in their relations.[53]

Causes. Causes of orgasmic difficulties are complex but usually are based on psychogenic factors. Physiologic factors include inadequate sensory stimulation, weakened perineal musculature, neurologic or vascular damage due to illness or medication, and extreme fatigue (see Unit V).

It is the psyche, however, that has the highest potential for facilitating or inhibiting the total orgasmic experience.[54] Negative sexual experiences while growing up may contribute to sexual repression. Girls may be taught to be afraid of intimacy, to be careful of sexual advances by boys, and that sex is dirty, sinful, and dangerous. The topic of sexuality may not be discussed at home. This is especially true in families with orthodox religious convictions.

The woman's ability to respond sexually, unlike the man's, is based more on the feeling of trust, security, tenderness, intimacy, and affection in regard to the sexual partner. Any negative life events, such as rape or incest, may make her less open to these feelings. Other negative influences include an unpleasant first coital experience, feeling of being rejected by parents, misunderstanding after viewing the sexual activity of parents (sex seen as an act of aggression, threat of injury, loss of control), conflict over being a woman accompanied by strong penis envy, fear of pregnancy and childbirth, or an underlying homosexual tendency with conscious or unconscious hostility toward men. These factors are not mutually exclusive, and a number may operate at the same time in one person.[55]

If the woman is able to have orgasm by other ways than coitus, causes may be related to the partner's premature ejaculation. Inadequate foreplay may be a factor, although Huey, Kline–Graber and Graber[56] found that duration factors had little or no effect in their retrospective study of 619 sexually dysfunctional women. Other factors may be disturbance in the nonsexual relationship with the partner such as feeling neglected and unloved, quarrels over money and children, inadequate personal hygiene, lack of tenderness, and infidelity.

Masters and Johnson have identified as the most frequent cause of orgasmic dysfunction in their patients the inability of the woman to identify with her partner. She may see him as a social bore, financial failure, a "slob," a perfectionist or the "second best man."[57] These psychologic factors operate to halt physiologic response by sending inhibiting impulses from the cerebral cortex acting on the spinal center that controls the final common pathway to orgasmic discharge.

Treatment. Early therapy involved psychoanalysis or psychoanalytically oriented psychotherapy. It was possible to get at the dynamics of the behavior, but the therapeutic results were often unsatisfactory. The behavior modification type of technique used by Masters and Johnson has been one of the most successful to date. (See Chapter 12 for description of various therapies.) Nurse practitioners have become involved in group counseling of women combining techniques of sex therapy and techniques used in group therapy and with women's consciousness raising groups.[58]

Vaginismus. In rare cases, muscular spasms of the walls of the vagina may make penile penetration of the vagina impossible. *Vaginismus* is the term given to this involuntary constriction of the outer one-third of the vagina. The musculature of the pelvis and perineum and thigh area are affected. The condition can be acquired at any stage of the female's life.

Causes. Causes may be physiologic or psychologic. Lesions at the opening of the vagina, cysts, or abscess may cause pain and tensing of the musculature. The individual who has had an episiotomy and has intercourse before complete healing takes place may also be a candidate for the problem. Usually the pattern of fear related to real or anticipated pain causes a voluntary guarding effect to protect from abrupt penile entry, but in these cases, relaxation eventually occurs. This is not considered vaginismus unless it becomes an involuntary response. An intact hymen or irritated hymenal remnants or painful scars may also cause the pain–fear reaction.

Psychologic causes are more frequent: a strict religious upbringing in which sex is considered dirty and taboo, traumatic early experiences with sex, rape, childhood molestations, an incestuous situation, or a first intercourse that was painful. The first pelvic examination by a physician who is tactless, "efficient," and unfeeling may set up a fear reaction. Phobias about pregnancy, venereal disease, or cancer may also be causes.[59]

Treatment. Therapy in the Masters and Johnson approach is directed at showing the sexual partners that the vaginal spasm is real. Illustrations are used to explain vaginismus anatomically and physiologically, and the problem is discussed with the sexual partner who often has been told the problem is in the "woman's head." When it is explained that the condition is not under her voluntary control, the burden is off the woman. Then, with the woman positioned for a pelvic examination on the examining table and with the partner present, the physician inserts a finger into the vaginal canal. The involuntary spasm closes the outlet. The woman is then taught to reverse the reflex by bearing down as hard as she can and then letting go, which results in some relaxation.

Vaginal dilators are then used beginning with one about tampon size and gradually increasing in size. The woman is encouraged to insert and remove the dilator at her own pace, to use it 3 times a day for 20 minutes, and to sleep with it inserted if possible. The emotional problems must also be treated, although with the physical problems relieved and with the cooperation of the sexual partner, therapy has been successful.[60]

Dyspareunia. Painful intercourse is thought of as exclusively a female problem, but males can have this difficulty too.

Causes. Cause may be related to injuries to the vagina or outlet structures. Other causes include Bartholin gland infection, intact hymen, clitoral disorders due to irritation or trauma, vaginal disorders (such as vaginitis, allergies and sensitivity to douches, creams, jellies, or the material in condoms or diaphragms, senile vaginitis with shrinking of the vaginal barrel, radiation vaginitis, scarring of the roof of the vagina after hysterectomy), pelvic infections, endometriosis, tumors, cysts, and laceration of the broad ligaments.[61] (See Chapter 28 for discussion of gynecologic problems.)

However, one of the most common causes of the aching, burning, and itching during intercourse is a failure of adequate vaginal lubrication. Inadequate lubrication may also cause pain for the male during intercourse. Vaginal lubrication is the female response to sexual stimulation that parallels the male erection. Without it, the woman is not physiologically or psychologically ready for intercourse. Inadequate lubrication is most commonly due, in the absence of physiologic causes, to a lack of affection, respect, personal identification with, and understanding for her partner or when he does not evidence any of these things for her. Fear of pregnancy, pain, social retribution, or sexual inadequacy in the man may also result in inadequate lubrication.

Dyspareunia may also occur in males as a result of sensitivity of the penile glans immediately after ejaculation so that he withdraws immediately afterward. Discomfort may be relieved by retracting the foreskin back over the head of the penis. Poor hygiene, phimosis, infections of the penis, downward bowing of the erect penis, spasm of the prostate, and enlargement of the prostate may all cause dyspareunia.[62] (See Chapter 28) for discussion of genitourinary diseases.)

Sexual Dysfunction in the Male

Impotence. This problem is the inability of a male to achieve an erection sufficient to achieve coitus. It may be primary or secondary in both homosexual and heterosexual individuals. In primary impotence, the man has never been able to achieve a satisfactory coital erection, while in secondary impotence, the man has been potent but develops potency problems subsequently. The term does not refer to the occasional erectile failures that all men may have due to fatigue, excess alcohol, or other negative circumstances. Any interruption of parasympathetic fibers, transmission of impulses from the spinal cord to the penis, or of the ability of the corpora cavernosa to fill with blood will cause impotence. Organic causes include vascular or neuromuscular disease, endocrine or metabolic conditions, radical pelvic surgery, trauma, and certain medications.

Impotence has been ascribed to deficiency in E and B complex vitamins, especially niacin and pyridoxine, and minerals manganese and zinc.[63] There has been some shift to investigation of the physical causes of impotence since more cases that were thought to have been psychogenic are now known to be organic or a combination of the two.[64]

References to impotence are found in the Bible, mythology and history, film, and the theater. It has been ascribed to evil spirits, angry gods, demons, and recently to liberated aggressive women. Although it may be due to pathophysiology, it is more likely psychogenic in origin.[65] According to Masters and Johnson, there has never been an impotent woman. With the exception of those with anatomic or psychosomatic problems, women can have intercourse and children by passively accepting the male's advances. "The cultural concept that the male partner must accept full responsibility for establishing full coital connection has placed upon every man the psychological burden for the coital process and has released every woman from any suggestion of similar responsibility for its success."[66]

Impotency and sterility have been frequently confused. The impotent male cannot have intercourse and cannot reproduce, because he is incapable of penile intromission or because he cannot maintain the erection long enough after entry to ejaculate. The man who is sterile does not have enough sperm cells to reproduce but can have an erection and ejaculate. A sterile man can function well sexually.

The incidence of impotence is difficult to evaluate, since males often do not want to admit to the problem. Kinsey[67] (1948) found that it was a rare occurrence before 35 years, increased after 45, with an even more rapid increase after 55 years. By 70 years of age, 27 percent of white males were impotent, by 75 years, 55 percent, and by 80 years, 75 percent. Of 213 males referred to Masters and Johnson for potency problems, only 7 had problems with a physiologic basis.

No correlation between the level of sex hormones (17-ketosteroids) and potency problems have been found. The impotent male may have above average 17-ketosteroid levels or less than average. Testicular castration before puberty usually results in primary impotence, but after puberty, impotence

need not occur, since cortical centers are able to compensate for loss of testicular activity. Generally, the older the male is when castrated the less is the effect on the libido. If a large amount of estrogen is given for therapeutic reasons, there is loss of libido and impotence, but giving testosterone does not cause the opposite effect.[68,69]

Primary Impotence. Primary impotence is indicative of more serious intrapsychic difficulties then secondary or situational impotence. Males presenting with the problem often come from a sexually repressed or religiously orthodox family background, where sex was never discussed or where it was treated as sinful, ugly, or immoral. There is also frequently a history of an abnormally close relationship with a seductive mother and strong unconscious feelings of incest, guilt, and castration anxiety.

Any life experience that makes the male afraid of intimacy, unable to love or be loved, feel unusually immature, inadequate, or deeply distrustful or hostile toward women may also cause problems. Other contributing factors may include a rejecting or derogatory father, dominant older siblings, intense parental quarreling, and rejection by peers.[70]

A traumatic initial failure during the first attempt at intercourse may precipitate the problem. An experience with a prostitute who was amused and derisive in a degrading atmosphere destroys some young males' confidence. An initial experience in the back seat of a car, with fear of detection, guilt, and anxiety, causes initial failure, and once failed, the vicious cycle of fear–failure continues. Finally, some males have a basically homosexual orientation and have never been able to think or feel sexually about women.[71]

Secondary Impotence. Secondary impotence occurs in the male who has had previous successful coitus. In Masters and Johnson's patients, the most frequent antecedents were premature ejaculation and continuous and excessive use of alcohol. The wife of a man who ejaculates prematurely may openly express frustration over his inability to provide her sexual satisfaction. He begins to worry about his performance and is unable to lose himself in the sexual experience.[72] Soon he begins to experience some erective failure, becomes fearful, and the fears are so strong he does fail. Impotency related to ejaculatory problems is partly related to the social milieu. Men from lower socioeconomic groups who ejaculate shortly after intromission often do not feel they have a problem, while those from higher socioeconomic groups are concerned because of greater pressure to satisfy the sexual partner.

Other causes include (1) a drinking pattern that results in occasional failure may set up the same fear–failure cycle; (2) interpersonal problems with the sexual partner not dealt with on a verbal level may result in the problem being experienced sexually; (3) larger psychiatric syndromes, such as depression, grief, or unconscious hostility toward women, may result in the male having the capacity to have intercourse with prostitutes but not with one held in high regard.[73]

Social factors may also operate. Men are expected to be the sex experts but may get performance anxiety if the women do not reach orgasm. It is difficult for men to understand that women may enjoy sex occasionally without orgasm. The male feels disappointed if he did not "give her" one or disturbed if he reaches orgasm too quickly.

As was mentioned earlier, the question of the effects of the Women's Liberation Movement has been raised. Women are assuming a more active, assertive role in sexual activity, and this may be threatening to some men. However, the healthy male is not threatened by an active female. If the man is threatened by his passivity, it usually indicates a character problem that existed before the women's movement started.[74]

Children of dominating parents who set impossible goals for the child may destroy the young male's confidence in his masculinity. Sons of dominant mothers often choose domineering wives who overwhelm their husbands. Sons whose self-confidence is undermined by a domineering father may have anxiety about performance in all areas of life, including the sexual.

Males with early homosexual experiences or with homosexual orientation may marry for social appearances and have little feeling for their wives. Although sexual performance may initially be satisfactory, conflict between homosexual urges and heterosexual demands produce secondary impotence (see Chapter 5). Situational factors such as lack of privacy or interruptions may also contribute to the genesis of potency problems.

Medical and surgical conditions that may cause impotence are discussed in Unit V.

Treatment. Treatment of impotence in antiquity involved magic potions and aphrodisiacs. Later, prostatic massage, irrigation of the bladder, the passage of cold sounds, testicular diathermy, ligation of the dorsal vein of the penis, tightening weak perineal musculature, and administration of male sex hormones have been utilized.[75]

Masters and Johnson have been able to treat impotence by desensitizing the performance anxiety with the help of the female sexual partner (see Chapter 12). They have obtained better results than traditional psychoanalytically oriented therapy. However, regular dynamic psychotherapy is needed if primary impotence exists with underlying feelings of guilt, anxiety, and emotional immaturity.[76]

Premature Ejaculation. Masters and Johnson define premature ejaculation as inability to delay ejaculation long enough for the women to have an orgasm 50 percent of the time. Ejaculation may occur before or immediately after penetration of the female introitus. Others define the problem as any ejaculation that occurs sooner than 30 to 60 seconds after intromission.[77] Definition becomes a problem, since it is relative to the ability to satisfy the sexual partner. Extended foreplay may make the women orgasmic soon after intromission of the penis.

There are few adequate studies to provide incidence figures, but premature ejaculation is probably the most common problem of male sexual function. It is relatively recent in origin. In the Victorian Era, women were not concerned about it but were more anxious to get sex "over with." Now that women are articulating their rights to sexual pleasure, it is becoming a matter for greater concern. This is especially true if the woman has no opportunity to reach climax and is left with resentment and no relief of sexual tension.[78]

Cause. The cause is possibly related to anxiety during the sex act. The first sexual experiences may have been with a prostitute or under furtive conditions when the man had to hurry to ejaculate and "get it over with." In other cases, the male who focuses on orgasm as the essence of the sex act, downgrading the aspects of lovemaking and interpersonal relationship, may get performance anxiety, and the cycle of fear–failure begins.[79] If the condition persists and the woman becomes reproachful, frustrated, and tense, empathy leaves and the outcome may eventually be secondary impotence.

Treatment. Treatment in the past included efforts to decrease anxiety, concentration on nonsexual fantasies, use of cerebral depressants or sedatives, and distractive maneuvers such as tightening the anal sphincter, pinching the skin, or biting the tongue or cheek. To decrease penile sensation, anesthetic ointments were applied, condoms were used, and penile movement in the vagina was minimized.[80] Psychoanalytic therapy was directed toward relieving unconscious incest–guilt or castration anxiety, fear of the vagina, and hostility toward women, all considered etiologic factors. Success rates were not encouraging.

Masters and Johnson's method includes desensitizing sexual guilt, removal of performance anxiety, and techniques to lower penile excitability (see Chapter 12). Unfortunately, many men with premature ejaculation seem unaware of or unable to think about their wives' needs. Masters and Johnson state that they do not consider their partner's involvement, but consider only their own sexual functioning.[81]

Ejaculatory Incompetence. Retarded ejaculation or incompetence is the inability to ejaculate in the vagina. It may be primary or secondary. It is less common than premature ejaculation, but exact incidence figures are not available. It is the equivalent problem to anorgasmia in women.

Cause. The cause involves psychologic precursors much like those of primary impotence. The male may have a rigidly compulsive personality: orgasm means loss of control. Secondary incompetence is usually the result of disturbances in interpersonal relationships with the partner. The wife may want to become pregnant; the husband does not want a child. There may be interpersonal friction and loss of sexual attractiveness of the partner. Among some cultures, fear that ejaculation and loss of semen will impair health may be a factor.[82]

Organic factors include neurologic conditions that interfere with the sympathetic innervations to the genitalia—lumbar sympathectomy, syringomyelia. Parkinson's disease may cause ejaculatory incompetence due to central thalamic disturbances. (See Chapter 25.) Drugs with antiadrenergic action, such as guanethidine and methyldopa, may also be involved in the etiology.

Treatment. Treatment by psychotherapy is necessary if a deep-seated personality disorder is involved. If the problem is situational, these secondary factors must be dealt with.[83] Masters and Johnson have used a combination technique beginning with manual stimulation of the male by his sexual partner in whatever way he finds exciting. She continues to manipulate the penis in as stimulating manner as possible to cause ejaculation and help him see her as a source of pleasure. After this is accomplished, the next step is to have the female insert the penis when the male is near the point of ejaculation. The procedure is continued until the male is able to ejaculate intravaginally.[84]

The important concept pervading Masters and Johnson's therapy for all sexual dysfunctions is the need for communication between partners. If the partners can be brought together and feelings of love and consideration expressed, a favorable climate for correcting sexual problems is created.[85] Building a relationship that is supportive and open, where both partners can share feelings and concerns, and discuss what is pleasurable and not pleasurable, can be the beginning of amelioration of sexual difficulties.[86] Attitudes and ignorance rather than psychopathology or physical illness are the cause of most sexual problems. Attitudes that can be learned can be unlearned. Misconceptions can be corrected and attitudes modified.[87] Other types of sexual therapy and counseling are detailed in Chapter 12.

Penile Implants for Impotence

Although corpora cavernosum revascularization procedures are being investigated,[88] increasingly, impotence may be corrected by the use of penile implants, especially if it is organic in origin (see Unit V). Implants may also be considered for patients with psychogenic impotence when psychotherapies fail.

Two types of devices are available. One consists of two sponge-filled silicone rods, the Small–Carrion device, which are implanted in the corpora cavernosa. These prostheses are encapsulated by silicone, have no movable parts, and provide enough length, width, and girth to stimulate normal penile response and allow vaginal penetration. One disadvantage is that the penis remains in a state of semierection, and this may not be socially acceptable to the patient or his partner.[89]

Variations of the rod prosthesis have been developed. A silicone rubber prosthesis in which silver wires are imbedded allows for voluntary manual bending of the penis for urination and resting position and straightening for intercourse.[90] A flexirod hinged prosthesis allows the penis to move freely and hang in a dependent position. It has a conical tip that conforms to the distal corpus.[91]

Partner–patient satisfaction is much higher with the second type, the inflatable penile prosthesis,[92] a hollow silicone cylinder that is surgically implanted in each corpus cavernosum. A reservoir containing radiopaque solution and a bulb is implanted in one scrotal sac. The cylinders, reservoir, and bulb are connected by silicone tubes. When the patient squeezes the bulb in the scrotum, solution flows from the reservoir to the cylinder in each corpora cavernosum and erection occurs. A one-way valve keeps the solution in the cylinder. When the patient wants the erection to subside, he compresses a release valve in the lower portion of the bulb in the scrotum and the fluid returns to the scrotum[93] (Fig. 3-3).

Criteria for selection of patients are less stringent than before but patients are selected after careful counseling of the man and usually the sexual partner. Criteria that may be used include impotence indicated by sexual history, presence of a strong sexual desire, desire to again satisfy the partner as strong as the need for self-satisfaction, the presence of some penile sensation with the ability to have something resembling an orgasm, and no prostate or genitourinary problems.

A willing sexual partner is important, however. Maddock[94] found that VA patients treated surgically had greater problems in self-esteem and other psychologic disturbances than those treated with psychotherapy. He also indicated that the outcome

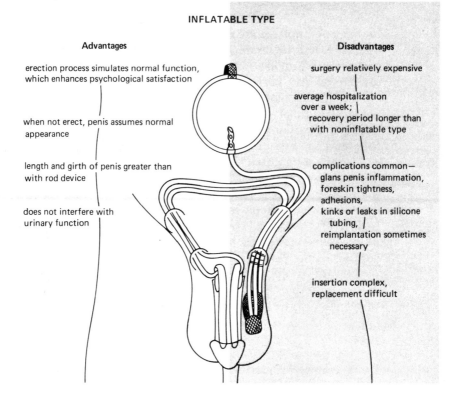

INFLATABLE TYPE

Advantages

erection process simulates normal function, which enhances psychological satisfaction

when not erect, penis assumes normal appearance

length and girth of penis greater than with rod device

does not interfere with urinary function

Disadvantages

surgery relatively expensive

average hospitalization over a week; recovery period longer than with noninflatable type

complications common— glans penis inflammation, foreskin tightness, adhesions, kinks or leaks in silicone tubing, reimplantation sometimes necessary

insertion complex, replacement difficult

Figure 3-3. Penile implant. (From Wood RY and Rose K: Penile implants for impotence. *Am J Nurs* 78(2):236, February 1978. Courtesy of American Medical Systems.)

of and the motivation for surgery is strongly linked to the attitudes and behavior of the female partner.

Mechanical dysfunction of the device is 8 percent and usually occurs within 3 years after implantation.[95] These problems include possible bending of the penis due to unequal filling of the cylinders and cone-shaped penis due to insufficient filling of the distal part of the cylinders.

NURSING IMPLICATIONS: PENILE IMPLANTS

Preoperative Care

The nurse answers any questions or concerns the man has and assesses how the surgery affects his image of himself. Assessment of his and his partner's expectations of the postoperative period and the expected effects on their sexual satisfaction is necessary. It also helps strengthen the nurse's understanding of the patient and his/her ability to help him before and after surgery.

Goals and expectations with regard to device implantation and function are discussed with patient and partner, since level of satisfaction with the procedure is heavily dependent on these factors.[96]

Postoperative Care

Silicone implants are inserted through perineal or penile incisions. Penile edema should be minimal, since the rods are inserted through the corpora and there is little trauma. Inflatable prostheses are usually inserted through perineal incisions. Scrotal edema occurs in the scrotal sac containing the pump mechanism. At the time of the operation, the device is inflated once to check for leaks, to dilate the tissue and break any constricting bands. It is not inflated again until the patient sees the physician usually a week after discharge. Hospitalization is only 3 days. Pain medication is given about one-half hour before the procedure, since the pumping is painful.

A urethral catheter may be inserted during surgery and may be taped to the body so that the penis is kept somewhat perpendicular to the body.

Preventing wound infection is essential. Antibiotics may be given preoperatively and immediately postoperatively, but good medical and surgical asepsis is the best prophylactic measure.

Pain. With newer procedures, an abdominal incision is no longer required and postoperative pain is markedly reduced.[97] It is increased, however, by patient movement or penile manipulation, so medication should be given readily. A cradle to hold covers off the area is helpful to relieve pressure.

Elimination. Elimination is achieved by a urethral catheter, which is removed the day after surgery. Perineal edema and pain may inhibit bladder function, so the nurse observes for urinary retention and infection.

Activity. Activity is resumed on the evening of surgery when the patient dangles and the first postoperative day when he is allowed to walk. Sexual activity is usually resumed in 4 to 8 weeks following either procedure. Sexual intercourse can be resumed sooner by men with a perineal rather than a penile incision, but in either type, if pain and edema exist, intercourse is delayed. The male is instructed to be sure that ample lubrication is used to prevent penile trauma. Both partners are taught to deflate and inflate the inflatable prosthesis before discharge from the hospital. If ejaculation and orgasm were possible before surgery, they will remain intact, but surgery will not restore these functions if they had not been present.

Patients are encouraged to wear street clothes. Underwear of the brief style is recommended to disguise the semierect penis if the silicone implant is used. The penis is placed either in the normal position or flat against the abdomen. Sports, work, or recreational activities should not be limited by the prosthesis, although strenuous activity is contraindicated for about 3 weeks after surgery.

Teaching. Teaching in preparation for discharge from the hospital is facilitated by involving the patient in his care, particularly if he has an inflatable device, so that he and his partner are able to inflate and deflate the prosthesis. Although the device is not inflated during hospitalization, the pump must be pulled to the lowest part of the scrotum daily, a procedure taught to the patient. Starting about 3 weeks after surgery the patient inflates and deflates the prosthesis every day for 6 weeks. This is done to promote the formation of a fibrous tissue sheath around the reservoir and cylinders. The patient is taught to locate the pump and hold it in a fixed position, squeeze the bulb of the pump 10 to 15 times for inflation. The patient presses the release valve on the side of the pump to deflate the device. This takes the most practice since the release valve is small and hard to locate. Patients are reassured that with time the procedure will be easier.[98]

Emotional Support. Emotional support is essential, since impotence, whether of psychogenic or organic origin, is a tremendous assault on the individual's sexual self-esteem. Patients may be embarrassed, hostile, stoical, or aloof. The nurse can gain the patient's self-confidence and trust by acceptance of him and his sexual partner and by openness and willingness to listen to his concerns as well as to promote his physical comfort. Patients and their partners may have had psychiatric counseling before surgery, and this may continue afterward, whatever the cause of the impotence. The opportunity to talk to someone else who has had successful surgery can be of great help, if it can be arranged.

It is essential that nurses examine their feelings about the surgery. If they have negative or derisive thoughts about the surgery or are embarrassed or sarcastically amused about the use of implants, these attitudes will be communicated to the sexual partners.

Use of Aids in the Management of Dysfunction

Rhodes[99] suggests that sex aids such as toys (plastic breasts, life-sized dolls, etc.) may be helpful in initiating sexual arousal. Attachments are also available for the erect penis to increase its length. Devices such as the Blakoe ring which is attached near the base of the penis improve the erection or prevent its disappearance by holding blood in the corpora.[99]

NOTES

1. Masters WH, Johnson VE: Human Sexual Response, Boston, Little, Brown, 1966, pp 3–8
2. Levin RJ: The physiology of sexual function in women. Clin Obstet Gynecol 7:213–250, 1980
3. Kaplan HS: The New Sex Therapy, New York, Brunner/Mazel, 1975
4. Masters WH, Johnson VE: Human Sexual Inadequacy. Boston, Little, Brown, 1970
5. Wagner G, Ottesen B: Vaginal blood flow during sexual stimulation. Obstet Gynecol 56:621–625, 1980
6. Masters WH, Johnson VE: Human Sexual Inadequacy. Boston, Little, Brown, 1970 p 39
7. Ibid, p 49
8. Ibid, p 295
9. Ibid, pp 28–29
10. Ibid, p 31
11. Ibid, p 76
12. Ibid, p 289
13. Ibid, p 51
14. Ibid, p 29
15. Ibid, p 30
16. Ibid, p 34
17. Ibid, p 118
18. Ladas AK, Whipple B, Perry JD: The G-Spot and Other Recent Discoveries about Human Sexuality. New York, Holt, Rinehart and Winston, 1982
19. Female Ejaculation During Orgasm. Jaffrey, New Hampshire, Human Development Educational Foundation, 1983
20. Masters WH, Johnson VE: Human Sexual Inadequacy. Boston, Little, Brown, 1970, pp 52–53
21. Ibid, p 289
22. Ibid, p 79
23. Ibid, p 33
24. Ibid, pp 182–183
25. Ibid, pp 204–205
26. Ibid, p 173
27. Ibid, p 183
28. Ibid, p 207
29. Ibid, pp 172–175
30. Ibid, pp 214–217
31. Ibid, p 282
32. Ibid, p 174
33. Ibid, p 186
34. Ibid, p 283
35. Satterfield SB, Stayton WR: Understanding sexual function and dysfunction. Top Clin Nurs 1:21–37, 1980
36. Brauer AP, Brauer D: ESO: How You and Your Lover Can Give Each Other Hours of Extended Orgasm. New York, Warner Books, 1983
37. Levin RJ: The physiology of sexual function in women. Clin Obstet Gynecol 7:220, 1980
38. Ibid, p 244
39. Ibid, p 245
40. Ibid, p 246
41. Masters WH, Johnson VE: Human Sexual Inadequacy. Boston, Little, Brown, 1970, pp 66–67

42. Ibid, p 191
43. Ibid, p 189
44. Hite S: The Hite Report. New York, Macmillan, 1976, p 65
45. Ibid, p 86
46. Katchadourian HA, Lunde DT: Fundamentals of Human Sexuality, 2nd ed. New York, Holt, Rinehart and Winston, 1975, p 63
47. Bardwick JM: Psychology of Women, New York, Harper & Row, 1971, pp 63–65
48. Schaefer LH: Frigidity. In Goldman GD, Milman DS (eds): Modern Woman. Springfield, Illinois, Thomas, 1969, pp 165–177
49. Coleman E: The relational cause of sexual dysfunction. Top Clin Nurs 1:33–37, 1980
50. Hatch JP: Psychophysiological aspects of sexual dysfunction. Arch Sex Behav 10:49–64, 1981
51. Masters WH, Johnson VE: Human Sexual Inadequacy. Boston, Little, Brown, 1970, p 21
52. Brown DG: Female orgasm and sexual inadequacy. In Brecher R, Brecher E (eds): An Analysis of Human Sexual Response. New York, New American Library, 1966, p 133
53. Brown DG: Female orgasm and sexual inadequacy. In Brecher R, Brecher E (eds): An Analysis of Human Sexual Response. New York, New American Library, 1966, p 135
54. Rosenbaum M-B: Female sexuality or why can't a woman be more like a woman. In Oaks WW, Melchiode GA, Ficher I (eds): Sex and the Life Cycle. New York, Grune and Stratton, 1976, p 93
55. Marmor J: Frigidity, dyspareunia and vaginismus. In Sadock BJ, Kaplan HI, Freedman AM (eds): The Sexual Experience. Baltimore, Williams and Wilkins, 1976, pp 398–401
56. Huey CJ, Kline-Graber G, Graber B: Time factors in orgasmic response. Arch Sex Behav 10:111–118, 1981
57. Belliveau F, Richter L: Understanding

Human Sexual Inadequacy New York, Bantam, 1970, p 165
58. Carlson B Wheeler KA: Group counseling for pre-orgasmic women. Top Clin Nurs 1:9–19, 1980
59. Belleveau F, Richter L: Understanding Human Sexual Inadequacy. New York, Bantam, 1970, pp 186–192
60. Ibid, pp 192–194
61. Marmor J: Frigidity, dyspareunia, and vaginismus. In Sadock BJ, Kaplan HI, Freedman AM (eds): The Sexual Experience. Baltimore, Williams and Wilkins, 1976, p 402
62. Belliveau F, Richter L: Understanding Human Sexual Inadequacy. New York, Bantam, 1970, pp 203–206
63. Parrish L: Finding a solution to sexual impotence. The Body Forum 4:13–16, 1979
64. Brody JE: Sex impotence focus shifts to physical causes. The Plain Dealer May 24, 1982, p D-1
65. Melchiode GA: Sexual dysfunctions in the male. In Oaks WW, Melchiode GA, Ficher I (eds): Sex and the Life Cycle. New York, Grune and Stratton, 1976, pp 97–103
66. Masters WH, Johnson VE: Human Sexual Response. Boston, Little, Brown, 1966, p 159
67. Kinsey AC, Pomeroy WB, Martin CE; Sexual Behavior in the Human Male. Philadelphia, Saunders, 1948, p 236
68. Marmor J: Impotence and ejaculatory disturbance. In Sadock BJ, Kaplan HI, Freedman AM (eds): The Sexual Experience. Baltimore, Williams and Wilkins, 1976, pp 403–411
69. Bancroft J, Wu FCW: Changes in erectile responsiveness during androgen replacement therapy. Arch Sex Behav 12:59–66, 1983
70. Marmor J: Impotence and ejaculatory disturbance. In Sadock BJ, Kaplan HI, Freedman AM (eds): The Sexual Experience. Williams and Wilkins, 1976, p 404
71. Ibid, p 405
72. Belliveau F, Richter L: Understanding

Human Sexual Inadequacy. New York, Bantam, 1970, pp 134–135

73. Melchiode GA: Sexual dysfunctions in the male. In Oaks WW, Melchiode GA, Ficher I (eds): Sex and the Life Cycle, New York, Grune and Stratton, 1976, p 100

74. Ibid, p 101

75. Marmor J: Impotence and ejaculatory disturbance. In Sadock BJ, Kaplan HI, Freedman AM (eds): The Sexual Experience. Baltimore, Williams and Wilkins, 1976, p 407

76. Ibid, p 408

77. Ibid

78. Masters WH, Johnson VE: Human Sexual Inadequacy. Boston, Little, Brown, 1970, p 97

79. Marmor J: Impotence and ejaculatory disturbance. In Sadock BJ, Kaplan HI, Freedman AM (eds): The Sexual Experience. Baltimore, Williams and Wilkins, 1976, p 408

80. Ibid, p 409

81. Masters WH, Johnson VE: Human Sexual Inadequacy, Boston, Little, Brown, 1970, p 113

82. Lieh-Mak F, Ng ML: Ejaculatory incompetence in Chinese men. Am J Psych 138:685–686, 1981

83. Marmor J: Impotence and ejaculatory disturbance. In Sadock BJ, Kaplan HI, Freedman AM (eds): The Sexual Experience. Baltimore, Williams and Wilkins, 1976, p 410

84. Masters WH, Johnson VE: Human Sexual Inadequacy. Boston, Little, Brown, 1970, p 131

85. Belliveau F, Richter L: Understanding Human Sexual Inadequacy. New York, Bantam, 1970, p 128

86. Wabrek CJ, Wabrek AJ: Sexual difficulties and the importance of the relationship. Nurs Digest 3:44–45, November–December 1975

87. Harris GG, Wagner NN: The treatment of sexual dysfunction. In Gottesfeld ML (ed): Modern Sexuality. New York, Behavioral, 1973, pp 244–250

88. Furlow WL: Sexual consequences of male genitourinary cancer: The role of sex prosthetics. Front Rad Ther Oncol 14:104–117, 1980

89. Wood RY, Rose K: Penile implants for impotence. Am J Nurs 78:234–238, 1978

90. Jonas U, Jacobe GH: Silicone 'silver penile prosthesis: Description operative approach and results. J Urol 123:865–867, 1980

91. Finney RB: New hinged silicone penile implant. J Urol 118:585, 1977

92. Furlow, WL: Sexual consequences of male genitourinary cancer: The role of sex prosthetics. Front Rad Ther Oncol 14:106, 1980

93. Wood RY, Rose K: Penile implants for impotence. Am J Nurs 78:236, 1978

94. Maddock JW: Assessment and evaluation protocol for surgical treatment of impotence. Sex Disabil 3:39–49, 1980

95. Furlow WL: Sexual consequences of male genitourinary cancer: The role of sex prosthetics. Front Rad Ther Oncol 14:105, 1980

96. Ibid, 106

97. Googe MCS, Mook TM: The inflatable penile prosthesis: New developments. Am J Nurs 83:1044–1047, 1983

98. Ibid, p 1047

99. Rhodes P: The use of aids in the management of disorders of sexual function. Clin Obstet Gynecol 7:421–432, 1980

Chapter 4

Sexual Drive, Arousal, and Intercourse

Sexual intercourse not only involves an intimate physical encounter, but also an emotional encounter at some level. This is true whether it takes place within or outside a stable relationship. The desire for sexual activity and the level of satisfaction that individuals obtain from sexual activity is predicated on a complex interplay of bio-psycho-social factors.

This chapter will describe the factors that are important in the initiation and continuation of activity that culminates in sexual intercourse. Attention will also be given to the bio-psycho-social factors that serve either to facilitate or to deter sexual arousal and the experience of satisfaction and pleasure that intercourse and orgasm provide. Sexual drive is the most basic of these factors. Arousal techniques, coital positions, and other forms of sexual activity, such as oral–genital, oral–anal, and masturbation, are also discussed in order to acquaint the reader with the wide range of sexual behavior in society.

SEXUAL DRIVE AND BEHAVIOR

Definition

In 1894, Freud first used the term *libido* to connote a psychic sexual desire. Later he changed his definition of libido, describing it as the sexual psychic energy, which in some way was produced by somatic excitation. *Libido, sex drive, urge,* and *motivation* are terms that are often used synonymously. Kirkendall[1] reviewed the literature on the nature of sex drive and its relationship to needs such as hunger and elimination, as well as to age and bodily vigor. He identified three components of drive—sexual capacity, what one can do; performance, what one does do; and drive, how strongly one desires to do.

Capacity is determined by the ability of the hormonal and nervous system to respond orgasmically to sexual stimuli. Performance, although limited by capacity, varies according to physical and psychologic factors, while drive, the strength or intensity with which the individual wishes to perform, seems to be largely psychologically conditioned and varies considerably from individual to individual and from time to time in each individual.[2] The focus of this discussion is on drive as the intensity with which individuals wish to engage in sexual activity and to a lesser degree on their performance.

Biologic Factors Affecting Drive

Sex drive can not be explained in terms of erogenous zones or the genitals, as Freud postulated, although the genitalia play a significant role in sexual arousal and behavior. Genotypic factors may influence drive in that the tendency for low, medium, or high arousability may be controlled by heredity.

Neurohormonal control of drive is believed to be through the hypothalamus. The anterior portion is important for sexual function and has interconnection with the pituitary gland. The hypothalamus may control drive directly or by its influence on the pituitary gland, which in turn affects the activity of other sex glands. Androgens appear to increase responsiveness of certain central nervous system mechanisms to peripheral excitation. Progesterone seems to decrease response. High prolactin levels (hyperprolactinemia) has been found to be a relatively frequent cause of depressed drive and/or impotence in men.[3] Excess androgen during fetal life of the female may alter the direction of the drive in later life.[4]

In the female, the adrenal glands supply the hormone, and there is some evidence that after adrenalectomy, the woman's sexual motivation decreases.[5] However, castration of the adult male and oophorectomy in the adult female do not necessarily destroy drive that has been established. This is not true in the preadolescent male. The increased androgen that accompanies puberty in the male not only brings about secondary sex changes, but with it also comes increased sexual drive.

Psychosocial Factors Affecting Drive

The amount of sexual drive and the capacity for sexual arousal depend more on childhood training than on genetic factors. In societies that restrict premarital sex play, adult women assume an inactive role in initiating sexual activity. Precisely how the learning takes place is not well understood, but it happens.

Many factors in the experience of the individual may operate to alter sex drive. Previous pleasurable experiences lead to more positive reinforcement and increased libido, but negative factors also operate. Cultural influences, such as religious beliefs and legal restrictions, may result in decreased drive. Social interactions that are stressful, embarrassing, or anxiety provoking may also dampen drive.

Izard[6] describes the relation of sex drive and emotion, arguing that it receives its greatest amplification from emotion. It is an interest–excitement interaction that causes the urgency in drive. Sexual symbols and sexually attractive paraphernalia are designed to capture interest and activate sexual arousal. He identifies an interesting person as a sexually attractive person. Emotions may also negatively affect drive. Sex–fear interactions in the male may result in impotence or premature ejaculation. Even if arousal can occur, fear may cause loss of erection. In the male, fear of not bringing the female to orgasm and fear of failure decreases not only drive, but performance.[7] In women, the effects of fear are not so visible but can be equally devastating. Fear of penile intromission, pregnancy, or sexual inadequacy may cause sexual inadequacy. (See Chapter 3.)

Sex–anger interactions may have positive or negative effects on drive. Some of the brain mechanisms involved in both sexual and aggressive behavior are in close proximity. It is postulated that as a carryover from evolutionary ancestry, heated and protracted arguments end up in heated lovemaking. Parasympathetic discharges in anger also increase the blood flow to the vagina. Although there is not enough biologic evidence of a sex–anger or aggression interaction, the possibility that it exists raises some concern. The danger from such relationships is that it may cause sexual activity without mutual affection, respect, or love.[8]

If sex–disgust is present, it may lead to avoidance of all sexual contact, diminish the pleasure of sex, or result in psychologic or physical abuse of the partner. A contributory factor to the sex–disgust interaction is the belief that sex is dirty, an idea generalized from the sex as sinful idea.

Sex–contempt interaction may be relatively unnoticed by either sex partner. If either looks down on the other in any respect, contempt is present.[9]

Female–Male Sex Drive Differences

Freud postulated that a strong sex drive was essentially masculine in nature. He saw women as castrated males, who had a difficult time reaching genital sexuality (see Chapter 7). Rosenbaum[10] describes women as slower to awaken to sexuality than the male. Whether this is due to cultural determinates of lower androgen levels than the male is open to question.

Bancroft[11] believes that androgens activate the female's "appetite" for sex and the inclination to initiate sexual activity. Women's arousal is described as less intense than males and without the same urgency. At puberty, sexual awakening may be a slower, more subtle, and more diffuse process than in the male. Women initiate sex less and appear to handle long periods of sexual abstinence with more equanimity than men. However, in contrast, Zuckerman found that the assumptions that sexual drive and sexual deprivation are more important for men than for women were not true, that the reverse was true in his subjects.[12] More data are needed, and with the changing sociocultural climate, change in female drive may be observed,[13] especially since some see women's drive as more a function of learning and experiencing than men's.[14]

Decrease in sexual drive in women may be attributed to social factors. Women working outside the home may channel their energies toward jobs. If there is resentment toward a husband who does not help in household tasks, lowered drive may be an unconscious way of punishing him.[15]

Sexual drive in some women may be related to the menstrual cycles, increasing during the ovulatory period and decreasing the week prior to menstruation.[16] However, other women have normal sex drives or suffer from frigidity or overexcessive urges for gratification independent of menstrual phases.

The relationship of age and sex drive is less strong and more variable in women than in men. The highest drive and peak of orgasmic experiences is between 36 and 50 years. However, a woman is capable of multiple orgasms in her 50s and 60s.[17] Some women's interest in sex wanes at menopause and

after, especially with the estrogen deficiency that causes vaginal changes. Others, freed from the concern of pregnancy, seek out and enjoy sexual relationships.[18]

The peak of male sex drive (and arousal) is in the late teens, when the adolescent may be alternately proud, delighted, ashamed, or frightened by almost instant erections. The male may have four to eight orgasms a day with a refractory period that is a matter of minutes. This continues through the 20s and then declines. In the 30s, the sexual urge decreases. Similar changes continue through the 40s and 50s, when sexual pleasure is more diffuse and less genitally centered.[19] (See Chapters 16 and 17.)

Purpose of Sex Drive and Behavior

The purpose of sex drive and behavior is influenced by individual value systems and cultural norms. Sex drive and behavior have the fundamental purpose of reproduction; some behavioral scientists believe one of the important functions of sex drive and behavior is to facilitate the mating process by establishing and maintaining bonds between people. Emotions, drive–emotion interactions, affective–cognitive orientation, and unique sensory pleasure all contribute to the bonding power of sexual intercourse. The man and woman, formed as a social unit, provide for each other mutual protection, security, and affection. Their division of the many responsibilities of a social unit, especially child rearing, provides optimal conditions for the survival, growth, and development of the individual.

Another function of drive, and particularly sexual activity, is to facilitate sexual and personal identity. However, assuming that sex drive and sexual activity are of equal importance to men and women, it would follow that it is heterosexual activity rather than the drive per se that serves identity and selfhood and enhances masculinity or femininity.[20]

Variations in Drive Intensity

Problems of low sex drive and arousal are difficult to treat.[21] The low libidinal syndrome has been termed hypoactive sexual desire or inhibited sexual desire (ISD).[22] Individuals may have a long history of low interest in sex or some may acquire the problem after a traumatic event.

Other problems in this phase are hypersexual feelings which may occur during the manic phase of manic-depressive illness and genital anesthesia in which persons feel nothing during a sexual activity.

If there is no organic or other problem and both sexual partners are satisfied with the level of sexual activity, therapy is not indicated.[23] However, some women have been conditioned not to ask for sex and it may be hard for them to take the initiative if the male has a low sex drive.

In a study involving 100 white well-educated couples, however, it was the overall relationship aspect of marriage, the "affective tone" that determined whether the couple viewed the sexual relationship as positive, even when they reported difficulties such as lack of interest or low frequency.[24]

Variation in sexual drive has been noted throughout history. Whether men have a stronger drive than women or whether the opposite is true is not so important as the effect of drive on their lives. Although there is no accurate yardstick to measure amount of sexual drive, Hastings presents a means of comparison by use of the normal distribution curve. This bell-shaped curve shows that 68 percent of the population are in the center of the curve's area, while there are smaller numbers with much lower or higher sexual drive. This does not imply normality or abnormality, only difference from the majority. At the one end of the curve, some individuals have drives that result in three or four episodes of coitus a day; at the other end are people who have coitus once a month or every several months.[25]

Couples may project expectations for sexual performance onto one another that do not match up with what each can live up to.[26] Of special importance is the similarity of drive between sexual partners. In each individual, drive varies in relation to time, place,

circumstance, age, etc. Difficulty between sexual partners and psychologic problems arise when there is an inequality in drive. One partner may consider the other as "undersexed" in relation to himself or herself and vice versa. A person is "oversexed" or "undersexed" only in comparison to a specific sexual partner—with another individual, there may be no difficulty. Hastings states that there is no "normal" or "abnormal," but only differences in strength of drive.[27] However, pathologic variations in drive have been labeled and described. These disorders have been called problems of acception and include hyperphilias, such as nymphomania, satyriasis, and Don Juanism.[28]

Satyriasis. Satyriasis is uncontrollable sexual appetite in males, although "excessive" coitus itself does not constitute satyriasis. This problem is characterized by drive for sexual satisfaction so overpowering that it becomes such a dominant thought in the person's life that he seeks sexual gratification in a promiscuous, impulsive, and insatiable succession of sexual activity. The object(s) may be females, males, children, or animals. These men may have a compulsive neurosis, or the behavior may be a symptom of psychosis. Genetic factors may be involved in some. An XYY chromosomal pattern has been found in markedly aggressive males who have a tendency to commit sex crimes.[29]

Treatment by administration of oral contraceptives every day or every other day has been successful in reducing drive in some of these men. An antiandrogen, cyproterone acetate, is being used in Europe with some promising results. Castration by orchidectomy may result in some relief, but if surgery is performed as a punishment, little change seems to occur.[30] A judge, however, has offered chemical castration to two convicted sex offenders as an alternative to long imprisonment for their crimes.

Nymphomania. Nymphomania in females is characterized by inability to be sexually satisfied and by constant seeking of sexual gratification. Some females are unable to reach orgasm and repeatedly seek another sexual partner. Others have multiple orgasms, but satiation does not occur, and they constantly pursue sexual contact.[31] Nymphomania from adulthood to the late menopausal years is rarely due to excess hormones. Most frequently, it is psychogenic in origin, although occasionally a female with a virilizing tumor of the adrenal glands or ovaries may have excessive sexual drive. Treatment has been tried with progestational drugs and tranquilizers over a long period of time with some relief.

Frigidity. This is the partial or complete inability to be sexually aroused or to achieve orgasm. It is a term that is less frequently used, having been replaced by the term *orgasmic dysfunction.* (See Chapter 3.)

This problem differs from lack of libido or drive. Some individuals may not particularly desire sex but they can be stimulated to arousal.[32] The etiology is usually psychogenic. Drug therapy has been attempted, but there are no safe drugs that can be given to increase libido. Contrary to popular belief, there are no aphrodisiacs: cantharides, or "Spanish fly," a legendary stimulant, is a powerful poison. Administration of androgens is beneficial for some women. Drugs such as alcohol, heroin, cocaine, LSD, and marijuana, contrary to popular opinion, are not aphrodisiacs. These drugs may affect sexual feeling, increasing it in some individuals, but more often decreasing it.[33] (See Chapter 30.)

SEXUAL AROUSAL

Existing information indicates that sexual arousal and activity result from an interaction of heredity, brain processes, hormonal state, external stimuli, and experiential phenomena such as imagery (visual, somesthetic, auditory) and thought processes.[34] Many different stimuli can bring about sexual arousal, and individuals have their own cluster that have particular value and effectiveness for them. The level of arousal, or indeed, whether it occurs at all, is affected by the complex interplay of biologic and physical, psychologic, and sociocultural factors.

The usual outcome of sexual arousal is heterosexual intercourse and orgasm, but arousal may result in homosexual activity for some. (See Chapter 5.) When no sexual partner is available, the outcome may be autoerotic activity; masturbation has been used throughout history as a means of relieving sexual tension. Other individuals may sublimate their desires and refrain from any sexual activity.

Biologic and Physical Factors Affecting Arousal

Arousal Techniques. Sexual arousal preliminary to coitus is initiated by some of the same activity used during masturbation, but usually with a sexual partner. (See information on masturbation on p. 63.) The initial arousal stimuli may be psychologic in nature, but these are later combined with direct touch stimuli to the genitals or other erotic areas. However, arousal can also be brought about by touch without psychologic stimulation.

Foreplay may include kissing, oral–genital stimulation, and tactile stimulation (petting). There is not one way that is "better" than others, since what is pleasurable to the sexual partner will have the most erotic value. Consequently, communication of what is pleasurable or what is not is most important. People learn by experience, and if the experience is negative, sexual learning is compromised. Mutuality is also important, and arousal is greater if both partners are active participants in sexual activity. Passivity indicates disinterest and tends to decrease the sexual pleasure of the partner.

Physical contact is necessary. The skin or any part of the body from which individuals gain sexual pleasure may be considered erogenous zones, which, defined anatomically, are the junctions between the skin and the mucous membranes. Thus, the mouth, male and female breasts, the vulva, the penis, and the anus are traditionally included in this category.

Orality, or the use of the mouth in sex, is universal. Physiologically, this is explained by the fact that the brain centers for sex and oral pleasure are close together and connect directly to each other. Inserting the tongue in the partner's mouth is called "French kissing." This activity may include deep exploration of the mouth as well as light tongue caresses and may continue throughout coitus for some partners.[35] Kissing may not be restricted to the partner's lips; any part of the body may be stimulated. The neck, ear lobes, breasts, insides of the thighs, fingertips, and palms of the hands, as well as the genitals have high erotic potential.[36] Kinsey found that upper-level respondents considered oral eroticism natural, desirable, and a fundamental part of lovemaking. Simple lip kissing was practiced by most of the college educated and was the prime source of erotic arousal. Lower socioeconomic level respondents had a distaste for deep kissing, considering it dirty, filthy, and a source of disease. Mouth–breast contact was also used primarily by upper social level individuals. The male manipulated the female's breasts, rarely the other way around. Lower social level individuals considered it a perversion— what babies do when nursing.[37]

Oral–Genital Stimulation.

Oral stimulation of the penis is called *fellatio,* literally, sucking. Common terms are "getting sucked off," "getting a blow job," "giving head," and "cocksucking." *Cunnilingus* is oral stimulation of the vulva, literally, licking the vulva. Kinsey found that 60 percent of persons with college degrees practiced oral genitality, 20 percent of those of high school level, while fewer than 11 percent with grade school education did. Women participate less frequently.[38] Current information indicates that oral genitality is becoming more prevalent since the Kinsey survey.[39] A couple may also engage in mutual oral–genital contact, or "sixty-nine," with either partner on top.

Oral–genital stimulation can add variety to sexual activity. Some object to it on hygienic grounds. However, if the genitals are clean, their normal flora is no more virulent that that of the mouth. Others consider it repulsive or immoral. Oral–genital relation should always be by mutual agreement of both sexual partners and should be conducted with tenderness and awareness of the partner's responses.

Tactile Stimulation.

Fondling, caressing, or light scratching of the sexual partner's body is a common means of sexual stimulation. Although the erogenous zones are the most frequent areas for attention, every individual has his/her own erotically sensitive areas. The object of the action is to stimulate sensitive areas of the skin. Tactile stimulation is enhanced if the surfaces are moist. Use of lotions that have a pleasant scent increases the sensation and the erotic potential. In addition to physical effects, use of lotions prolongs foreplay, makes it more deliberate and helps the partners stimulate each other more openly than furtively. Even the "messiness" may have an arousing quality, perhaps because of the association with genital fluids.[40]

Tactile stimulation of the woman's breast is used in many cultures. Female stimulation of the male breast is less common, yet the male breast has the same erectile muscles as the female's and responds like the female nipple.

Tactile stimulation of the genitals is also an important part of sexual activity. In the Kinsey sample, 95 percent of males and 86 percent of females reported that they manually stimulated the genitals of their partners.[41,42] The techniques of genital foreplay are similar to those described in the section on masturbation later in this chapter.

Stimulating the anal surface by inserting a finger in the rectum is stimulating to some, but rejected by others for esthetic and other reasons. If a finger or the penis enters the rectum, it should be cleansed before insertion into the vagina to prevent bacterial contamination. Each individual knows what he/she finds most erotically stimulating. Each sexual partner must communicate his/her feelings and desires. It is better to start slowly and gently and become more vigorous as the wants and needs of the sexual partners indicate. Katchadourian and Lunde[43] have identified some useful principles:

1. Sensitive surfaces respond best to gentle stimulation; larger muscle masses require firmer handling.
2. An area singled out for stimulation should be attended to long enough to elicit arousal.
3. Avoid either frantic shifting from one body area to another or monotonous and endless attention to one area.
4. Effective stimulation is steady and persistent, its tempo and intensity varied, but sexual tension should not be allowed to wane.
5. Erotic arousal requires patience, but effective lovers find ways to maintain a sense of novelty and a feeling of excitement as if the sexual interaction were the first time.

Other Factors Affecting Arousal. Pain has erotic potential. For some, mild pain from bites and scratches may be stimulating. Tickling is an activity that is erotic to others. The relationship between sex and smell has been investigated. In some primitive cultures, vegetable juices that smell like genital secretions are supposed to have aphrodisiac effects. Results of study of the impact of smell on human sexual behavior suggests that smelling copulins, substances found in vaginal secretions, may stimulate the desire for intercourse in some couples. Although the findings are tentative, they do give intriguing leads for further research.[44]

The amount of stimulation necessary for sexual arousal varies from person to person. Preference for stimuli also varies, so it is best

for each couple to decide for themselves what is pleasurable.

Psychologic Factors Affecting Arousal

The majority of arousal stimuli are psychologic and individual specific. One person may be stimulated by seeing someone of the opposite sex, another by women with large breasts, another by tone of voice or a glance. Others are aroused by seeing pictures of the other sex undressed and engaging in various types of sexual activity, which some identify as pornography. Sexual fantasy or daydreaming may also serve as a common prelude to sexual excitement.

In a study of 55 women, 27 of whom were married, Heiman[45] found that married women were less responsive than unmarried women to erotic materials on first exposure to these materials and that in the entire group, less physiologic and subjective arousal occurred from fantasies than from erotic materials. Heiman emphasizes that the context in which sexual activity occurs must be considered; that sexual response does not exist isolated from the setting. Physiologic and affective levels of sexual arousal may be enhanced, exaggerated, diminished, or ignored depending on the meanings the person associates with the particular setting.[45]

Fantasies. A sexual fantasy is any mental image or imagination that contains sexual matter and/or is sexually arousing to the person having the fantasy. Fantasies may be the "daydream" type, may be experienced during masturbation, or may be associated with sexual relations, usually leading up to and/or occurring during sexual intercourse.[46]

Efforts have been made to identify gender-specific fantasy patterns or categories with little success. Mednick[47] investigated differences in sexual fantasy patterns of males and females. Results indicated that significantly more females than males fantasized themselves as recipients of sexual activity from persons or inanimate objects, while males fantasize persons or objects as the recipient of the activity from them. It is hypothesized that men are more dependent on vision and visual images while women are more dependent on touch and tactile image.[48]

Fantasies are common at all age levels, and some women are supposedly able to achieve orgasm by fantasy alone. In most fantasies, the dreamer is the central character, while the objects of the fantasies may be acquaintances or others whom the individual knows only from afar. The intensity of feelings involved may range from relatively mild to overwhelming affective responses. Fantasies may involve heterosexual, homosexual, or sadomasochistic encounters and may result in severe guilt to the individual.[49]

Friday[50] found that men generally prefer to fantasize about being subjugated by powerful women. She believes that they function to deal with the frustration, love, and rage men feel toward women.

Fantasies have other functions. They are a source of pleasure. They may serve as substitutes for action and provide temporary satisfactions until concrete ones are available, or they may substitute for unattainable goals, although an individual may not wish the fantasies to come true, no matter how much they are yearned for. Sexual fantasies allow partial expression of forbidden wishes, but do not supply gratification of sexual drives. Fantasies, by easing the pain of past negative experiences, help make them more bearable. Finally, fantasies help prepare for real-life situations when the individual mentally rehearses modes of action and ways to cope with new situations.

For most people, fantasies are pleasurable, even though they include occasional unacceptable thoughts and cause some degree of shame and guilt. In rare cases, a person may lose control and commit a seriously antisocial act. These individuals need psychiatric or other professional help. Unpleasant or disturbing fantasies are not easy to deal with. Conscious attempts to remove them often causes individuals to focus on them more strongly. It is better to take them for what they are, isolated thoughts that do not really mean much. Keeping involved in various activities helps in minimizing the opportunity for fantasizing that is unwanted.[51]

Pornography. Obscenity and pornography are poorly defined, and their consequences in terms of antisocial behavior are also poorly understood. There are moral and legal sanctions against pornography, and many individuals are concerned about its negative effects on sexual behavior and morality in general. There is much disagreement, however, about the dangers of exposure to erotic material. The Commission on Obscenity and Pornography was established by Congress in 1968 and given the charge to study the causal relationship of erotic material to antisocial behavior and to recommend constitutional means to deal effectively with traffic in obscenity and pornography.

Their investigation of erotica and antisocial and criminal behavior did not support the belief that exposure to erotic material was a statistically significant factor in causing sex crimes and delinquency, although it was not possible to state unequivocally that erotic material did not contribute to the likelihood of an individual committing a sex crime.[52]

Although some argue that in adults repeated exposure to pornography leads to satiation and boredom, there is insufficient information about its effect on children. Opinion polls show parents do not wish their children exposed to erotic material, and many religious groups argue that great harm is done by pornography. Organizations such as Morality in Media, founded in 1962 by three clergymen, and Citizen for Decency through Law have been organized to stop traffic in pornography and to inform the public about pornography.[53]

Research on the effects of pornography continues. There is no question that viewing erotic material is sexually exciting. Males have been described as being more sexually aroused by pornography than women, and some argue that this difference stems from the biologic differences between the sexes. However, Zuckerman found that women were as easily aroused and responded to sexually explicit films with a reaction equal to men's.[54]

Fisher and Byrne[55] also found that there was no sex difference in response to erotic films and that romantic interest was not a prerequisite for female arousal. They speculated that past studies showing female disinterest in erotica may reflect culturally imposed expectations of behavior. How much is cultural indoctrination and how much is biologic is unclear. Other changes in response to erotica also seem to be taking place. Pietropinto and Simenauer[56] report that most men are bored by nudity in girlie magazines and find it ineffective as a sexual "turn on," preferring a natural look to the image conveyed by "heavily made up models."

Mood Setting. Sexual activity and coitus must be viewed within the longer emotional context. For those in love, the touch of the beloved can be exciting; for others, there may be little erotic stimulation. Others achieve gratification without emotional involvement. However, even in these latter situations, there is some awareness of the partner as a person. How one sets the mood or the emotional environment for sexual activity varies from individual to individual, but mood is important.

Watson[57] found that marked sexual, marital, and mood problems often coexist. Dim lights or darkness may be preferred by some; full illumination by others. Expressions of affection, a mixture of seriousness and lightheartedness is often an effective mood. Sex can be fun; it covers a variety of feelings and it can be perfectly natural to laugh and tease during sex. Some couples chase each other or wrestle on the floor. Mutual undressing can be exciting and gratifying. What is important is that each couple feel free and comfortable to do whatever

seems interesting and acceptable to them. There is no right or wrong, good, better, or best.

How one approaches the sexual partner is just as variable. The male may be the instigator of sexual activity. In other situations, the female takes the initiative and the male is more passive. In either case, the needs and desires of the sexual partner are considered. There is much to recommend a setting and a mood that is different from the hustle and stress of everyday life. A leisurely approach to sexual activity, a sense of intimacy and awareness of each other fosters pleasure. One couple planned a weekend "trip away from the family" to a nearby motel at least every 6 months.

Attitudes and Behavior that Inhibit Sexual Arousal. Earlier in the chapter, emotions that affect drive were described. These same negative feelings can inhibit sexual arousal. Fear, shame, disgust, or depression may reduce or completely inhibit sex drive and sexual response. The memory of some traumatic event or a feeling that the sexual partner is not really interested in the individual as a person can also destroy sexual excitement. The impact of negative emotion seems especially intense in women and can lead to self-doubt and frigidity.[58]

Ignorance and misinformation about sexual activity and fear that certain kinds of behavior are harmful will also dampen response. Problems may be due to simple sexual misinformation or inadequate knowledge. One of the greatest factors in the etiology of sexual dysfunction is religious belief that identifies sex as sinful or dirty and to be indulged in only for the purpose of procreation.[59]

Some individuals may fear loving and committing themselves to another in the closeness and intimacy of coitus. They desire love, intimacy, and closeness but find them frightening. Freud believed, however, that women on the whole are prepared to abandon themselves to closeness and love with greater ease and less anxiety than men (see Chapter 7).

Anger at the sexual partner, irritating personal habits and practices, rejection, and inconsideration may also limit sexual responsiveness. Paradoxically, however, Stoller[60] argues that qualities of beauty, gracefulness, and ideals of character in the sexual partner actually dampen sexual excitement unless the individual wants to sully them. Although these qualities produce feelings of love, they oppose being able to "lust." He believes that hostility, overt or hidden, is what generates and enhances sexual excitement, and its absence leads to sexual boredom. To sharpen excitement, one introduces elements of risk that must be escaped. Stoller states that he is not saying that love, affection, generosity, and concern cannot contribute to sexual excitement, but they do so only in the rare individual.

In a continuum from more toward less use of hostility, one goes from the bizarre (psychiatric) use, through character disorders such as perversion, into normative behavior where excitation is enhanced by the hostility, but where affection and capacity for closeness also thrive; the individuals at the far end of the continuum are those who enjoy loving, unhostile relationships with someone else and are not frightened by intimacy.[61]

Sociocultural Factors Affecting Arousal

No one is exempt from cultural influences and social mores. These are discussed in Chapters 8 and 9. In a more restricted sense, the immediate environment in which sexual activity takes place can inhibit or enhance sexual expression.

Environment. The cramped back seat of a car along with accompanying fear of detection are calculated to insure an unsatisfying first sexual experience for one or both of the partners. After marriage, the bedroom walls, a crying baby, the ringing phone or doorbell, and fear of interruption may all serve to de-

crease and/or prohibit sexual responsiveness, especially in the woman who depends on continuity of physical stimulation. Men, however, are less distracted by environmental influences and lack of privacy.

The Work Ethic. One contemporary influence on sexual response may be rooted in the work ethic, the belief that performing a task is good in itself and that it demonstrates commitment to the group and responsibility for its welfare. Work is productive, and whoever plays is wasteful. Society is still involved in the ethic and gives only lip service to spiritual emotion and physical pleasure. Work may be substituted for sex; work to the exclusion of playing, doing instead of being. Some individuals have difficulty making the transition from an individual with limited time and place for work to an individual who is spontaneous and free. Others hide behind work to avoid a sexual encounter or are too exhausted from the work to engage in sexual activity. For some persons, sex becomes work and performance is evaluated as good, better, best. They do not see sex as a way of expressing feelings or nourishing commitment, but as an accomplishment. Satisfaction in sex decreases and interest wanes as people lose interest in and warmth for each other.[62]

Social Class. As a rule, persons from higher socioeconomic class levels tend to experiment more than lower-income groups. Kinsey found that upper-class persons were more likely to engage in mouth–breast stimulation, oral–genital stimulation, and masturbation.[63] The differences in black versus white attitudes toward sexual activity are poorly studied and documented but are probably related more to social class than race. However, DeLora and Warren[64] indicate that black lower-class women expect their sexual partners to try to satisfy them sexually and that they achieve orgasm in premarital sexual activities more often than lower-class white women. Black lower-class sex roles and sexuality are similar to lower-class patterns in general: the males try to prove their potency by sexual exploitation of women. Although lower-social-class women may be more sexually open than upper-class women, they are more subservient to men.[65]

Female–Male Arousal Differences

Weinberg[66] describes differences in psychologic factors that affect male and female response. The male responsiveness is influenced by previous experience, objects associated with previous experience, the vicarious sharing of others' experiences, and sympathetic responses of the sexual partner, while females are much less affected by these factors. Males are more aroused than females by observing the opposite sex, observing nude figures in drawings or photographs, and observing genitalia or other parts of the body. They are more likely to initiate sexual activity through genital manipulation, while females prefer tactile stimulation on other parts of the body.

Problems arise because of differences in male–female response to sexual fantasies and psychic stimuli. Males are usually more intensely aroused before the beginning of sexual activity, before any physical contact with the partner, and sometimes have difficulty understanding why females desire more sexual contact. Many women desire a long arousal period and at times arousal for its own sake.[67]

Women often do not understand why men cannot get along without sexual activity and why the male is distressed when he cannot get or must abandon plans for coitus when household duties or social life interfere. In turn, he does not understand why the female is not aroused by anticipation of activity or why she needs more physical contact before achieving sufficient arousal for coitus to be satisfying.[68]

SEXUAL INTERCOURSE

Biologic and Physical Factors Affecting Intercourse

Love manuals detail about 100 positions for sexual intercourse. However, most are a variation of five basic positions. Knowledge of positions is only one facet of coitus. The quality of the emotional union and factors that affect arousal and response may make coitus fulfilling or unsatisfactory to one or both partners.

Basically, all positions can be reduced to these major ones: (1) man on top; (2) woman on top; (3) side positions, lying; (4) rear entry; and (5) sitting, standing positions. The number of positions, however, are limited only by the imagination and dexterity of the sexual partners. Knowledge of positions is helpful to afford variety and avoid monotony. However, experimentation with positions can help the sexual partners achieve the most satisfying sexual experience. Knowledge of different positions is also helpful when physical disability makes "usual" positions painful or impossible to achieve.

Male Superior Position. A position with the man on top can be easily modified, is highly stimulating to the man and only slightly less to the woman. It suggests the psychologic situation of the man initiating and controlling the activity. The woman's legs may be parted and extended or the knees may be slightly bent. The man may support himself on his hands and knees. This allows both partners to look at their genitals and permits the woman more freedom to move. A disadvantage is that the man may tire of supporting his weight. The woman can vary this position by wrapping her legs around his waist and hips. This shortens the vagina and allows deep penetration. The penis can make easy entry into the vagina or the woman can guide entry by her hand.

This position also provides easy opportunity for men and women to kiss each other's mouths, breasts, faces and shoulders. The woman also has her hands free to fondle the scrotum or the base of the penis. The male superior position is sometimes called the "missionary position," since it supposedly was the position missionaries taught to South sea islanders. Most persons have tried it, and most persons use it as the prima-

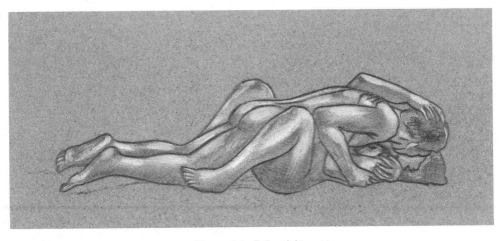

Figure 4-1. Full weight.

ry or exclusive position (Figs. 4-1 through 4-3).

This position is difficult if the male is obese, if the woman is pregnant, if the man has an incomplete erection, or if the woman has lost elasticity of the vaginal barrel.

Female Superior Position. The woman on top of the man provides her freedom to move, set the pace, and determine the course of coitus. In the past, people argued that men on top was the only position that was natural, because males should be in control. However, if the man feels tired or anxious and the woman active, the female superior position is the position of choice. This position is best if the woman is having orgasmic difficulties or the man potency problems. In all cases, it may provide the greatest sexual stimulation for both partners.

The woman paces the movement, and although there is a chance of too deep penetration, the woman can control this factor also. Almost any movements in this position provide for stimulation of both partners, and clitoral stimulation is maximized. The man has his hands free to caress the woman's body, and there is also opportunity for kissing. He is less pinned down by her weight than she is by his.

A variation of this position has the woman lying at a 30 degree angle across the man with one of her legs between his. In this position, they are both free to thrust and make pelvic movements. (Figs. 4-4 and 4-5).

Lateral Positions. Lateral, or side by side, positions do not permit deep insertion of the penis or freedom of movement. The sexual partners can position themselves in a number of ways. Effort must be taken to relieve weight and pressure on his or her thigh. The woman can be half on her side and half on her back with one leg extended. The man rests both thighs on top of her bottom leg, and she raises her upper leg to encircle his top thigh. Positions can be reversed. With his thigh against hers, the man can press against the clitoris, providing greater stimulation.

Couples find this position restful, a good position for fatigue or pregnancy, and pleasant for prolonged sexual activity. If penile entry is difficult, entry can be made in another position first and then the side by side position assumed. Pillows can be used to support body parts (Fig. 4-6).

The only sensation of touch inside the vagina is in two small areas about one-fifth inch in diameter about one inch inside, at the

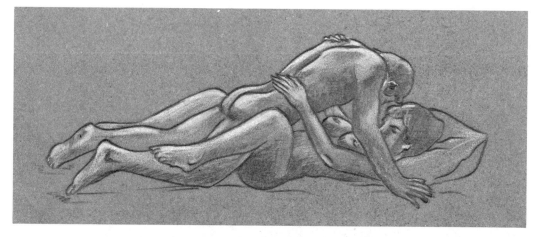

Figure 4-2. Weight supported.

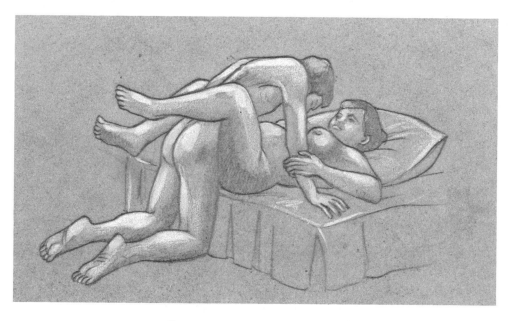

Figure 4-3. Stout or pregnant. Across bed.

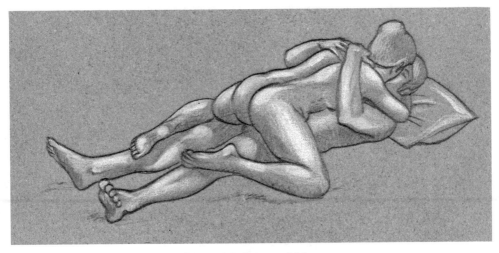

Figure 4-4. Between thighs.

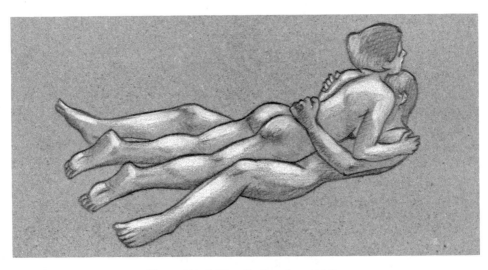

Figure 4-5. Full length. Female superior.

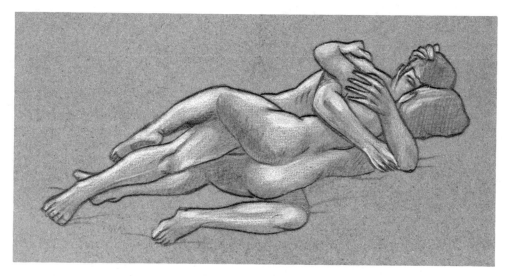

Figure 4-6. On side. On male's thigh.

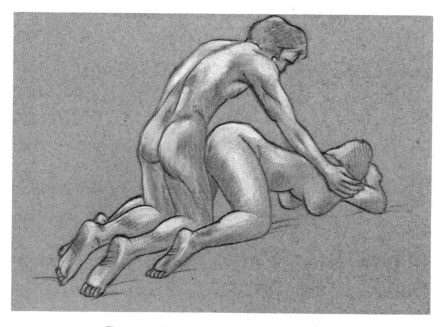

Figure 4-7. Rear entry, knee-chest: dog fashion.

positions of four and eight o'clock. Side by side position provides the most stimulation to these areas in the front of the vagina.[69]

Rear Entry Positions. This position is sometimes referred to as dog fashion. It is the only position used by mammals other than man. Actually, the penis can enter the vagina from the rear in any of the positions. The woman can be on her stomach and raise her pelvic area and arch her back, while the man kneels astride her thighs and inserts his penis between her thighs. She may also kneel on her hands and knees. If she kneels so that her head and breasts touch the bed and her pelvic area is raised higher than in the lying position, he can kneel behind her (Fig. 4-7). In one variation, the woman may also be on her side in a curved position, although in this position the penis may slip out of the vagina. Position can be maintained if the woman can press her thighs together (Fig. 4-8).

Unless the partners are slim, there may be difficulty with rear entry positions. A small amount of air enters the vagina in the kneeling position, expanding the vaginal walls, reducing friction, and sometimes making a noise when it rushes out.[70]

Both partners can move with great freedom in rear entry. Vaginal penetration is medium. The man's hands are free to hold or move his partner's hips or stimulate her breasts or clitoral area, which is some distance from the penis. The woman can reach behind, either between or around her thighs, and stroke the man's testicles.

Sitting and Standing Positions. Sitting positions, face to face, provide close body contact, but opportunity for only a moderate amount of movement. The man may sit on the edge of the bed or a chair with the woman sitting on his thighs (Fig. 4-9). The man keeps his knees apart. The woman lowers herself on the erect penis, and the penis is inserted with downward pressure. The man can press the woman's hips toward him and moves his pelvis forward and upward. The

woman's feet can encircle the man's back or lock them behind the chair to provide more penetration. The woman can also sit on the edge of the bed, spread her thighs, and lean back, while the man stands, bends, or kneels by the side of the bed and inserts his penis.

The man may stand while the woman can raise one leg onto the man's shoulder, or he can pick her up and hold her on his erect penis, while she wraps her legs around his waist and her arms around his neck. He supports her buttocks.

Psychologic Factors Affecting Intercourse

The number of positions for intercourse are not limited to these described here. The couple's imagination and willingness to experiment may enable them to find positions that provide maximum sexual satisfaction for both. Many couples use several different positions for coital activity, starting with one and moving into others until orgasm is attained. The important factor is that the couple communicate to each other what is pleasurable and satisfying and that their activity is mutually acceptable.

The best technique for some may not be satisfying to others. Each sex act has different meanings for people. Some may be anxious about certain sex acts and may choose to avoid certain activity. Other couples may prefer a specific coital activity to the exclusion of others. That is their choice. Many couples, however, wish to experiment and need only some explanation and encouragement about techniques of coitus to proceed.

Sociocultural Factors Affecting Intercourse

The oldest depiction of coitus was found from the Ur excavation in Mesopotamia. The drawings were made from 3200 to 3000 B.C. The art of other civilizations—Peru, India, China, Japan—show many positions and activities during intercourse. Of all cultures, only the Anglo-American has dictated that one position for intercourse, the male superior, is natural and the others perversions.

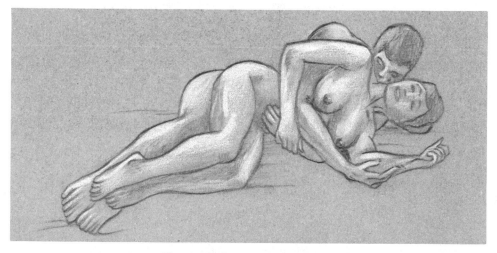

Figure 4-8. Rear entry: side lying.

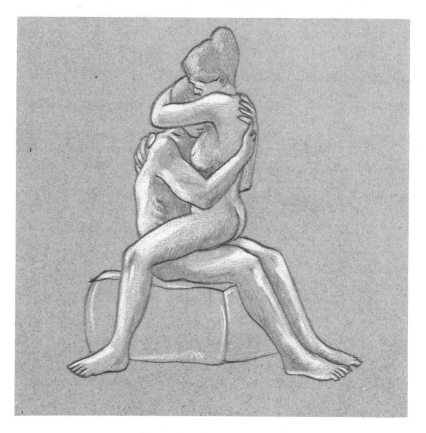

Figure 4-9. Sitting position.

Upper-social-level individuals are more likely to use different positions than the "missionary." Lower-level individuals consider any other an abnormality in which the female becomes masculine and the male effeminate, with destruction of the dignity and authority of the male. An older erroneous belief is that the male who engages in other positions has homosexual tendencies. In studies reported by Weinberg, each level was convinced its pattern was best and rationalized its behavior in its own way. The upper social level rationalizes by what is right or wrong, the lower social level by what is natural or unnatural.[71]

Cultural mores of a specific group exert powerful influences. Whether or not individuals engage in certain sexual activities depends on whether they are encouraged, permitted, or inhibited. However, even if certain practices are condemned, certain individuals may participate, or when encouraged, some will still refrain.

Different cultures have different views of the need for holding and cuddling prior to coitus. The traditional female Chinese woman has less desire to be cuddled and no "decent" Chinese woman shows sex desire and pleasure. They are inactive partners. Sex is for procreation and to satisfy man's sex drive. However, the Americanized Chinese woman expects more from sexual intercourse, much like her Caucasian counterpart.[72]

Various cultures show tremendous variation in frequency of coital activity, ranging from once a week by the males of the semi-nomadic tribe of New Guinea, the Keraki, to ten times a night by the Chagga of Tanganyika. In many primitive societies, adults had daily intercourse during periods when sex was permitted.

In a study of married couples in the United States, Thailand, Belgium, and Japan, it was found that female age not male age was the most important factor in the decrease in the frequency of marital intercourse during childbearing years. The authors believed that decreased androgen levels may be the cause.[73]

Every society had some restrictions on sexual activity. None permits individuals to engage in sex at any time and place, nor gives complete freedom for erotic activity. Some primitive groups believed, as many do now, that frequent sexual activity adversely affected health.[74]

Pretending Pleasure and Orgasm

Pretending orgasm can make sexual pleasure impossible. Any type of deception has the potential to be destructive. A woman's purpose may be to shield the man from feeling inadequate, but once begun, deception can take place on later occasions. Habitual pretense is linked to one or both partners' acceptance of double-standard values, especially the belief that the two sexes are unequal and incapable of understanding each other. "Faking" orgasm may be a means of "getting the business over with."

Other women, who take the traditional passive role in intercourse, are afraid to risk taking the initiative and suggest activity that might be more pleasurable. To do so would be aggressive and not "normal." Because they misperceive the female role, they may not consider it "decent" to admit having desire for greater pleasure. Faking orgasm is easier. Unfortunately, acknowledging the deception may injure the relationship, since the man may wonder if the whole relationship is a show, just as the pretended orgasm was.

Commitment and Sexual Pleasure

Although Stoller[60] indicates that hostility may increase pleasure, others have found that altruistic feelings and engaging in altruistic activity may be related to sexual response. In the hierarchy organizing the phylogenetically old and new structures of the brain, there appears to be a neural connection between elevated sexual feelings and high altruistic service.[75]

Some may argue for sex for gratification only, but commitment, affection, and a loving relationship still seem to be the norm before sexual involvement. Although there has been a gradual increase in the numbers of women particularly who engage in premarital intercourse, indiscriminate, casual sexual activity among young people has not increased. Masters and Johnson,[76] sometimes accused of a mechanistic approach to sex, stress the importance of the commitment, of concern, of caring for, and of being responsible for or wanting to take care of someone else. They stress that it is not simply enough to be admired or desired, but individuals need to be confirmed as sexual persons. A man wants to be reassured that he is like other men, the woman that she is like other women.

In longstanding marriages or permanent sexual relationships, commitment to goals of achievement, rather than to each other, may result in less caring, desire, and valuing. If the couple can preserve these feelings for each other, sex will continue to be a strong force drawing them to each other. Commitment sustains a couple through the years. In the beginning, it forces them to explore the hidden dimensions of their sexuality, engaging in sex as both pastime and passion. In later years, it is the satisfaction of their sexual and emotional bond that individuals find reason enough to be glad they have another day together.[77]

SEXUAL ACTIVITY THAT MAY SUBSTITUTE FOR COITUS

Oral and Anal Genitality

Oral–Genital Activity to Orgasm. Cunnilingus and/or fellatio may be used to stimulate the sexual partner to orgasm. Cunnilingus may be highly satisfying one moment or painful another, so verbal and nonverbal communication is essential. Cunnilingus is particularly productive of multiple orgasm. However, one technique may be hazardous to women, especially during pregnancy. Fatal air embolism can be caused by forceful mouth inflation of the vagina with air. Some women find this distension very pleasurable, but when death occurs, autopsy

reveals air in the uterine veins, trauma to the placenta, and evidence of air embolism. This technique, consequently, should be used with extreme caution and definitely not during pregnancy.[78]

Fellatio may be used to bring the man to orgasm when the sexual partner allows deeper penetration of the penis in the mouth with in-and-out thrusting motion. The hands may be used at the base of the penis to move it up and down. Deeper thrusts bring the penis to the back of the mouth, coming in contact with the throat itself. The gag reflex may be elicited, and effort is made to relax the throat muscles while keeping the mouth firm enough to provide stimulation to the sexual partner. Semen when first ejaculated has little taste but later is salty. Some swallow the semen with pleasure, others choose not to do so.[79]

Increased oral genitality has resulted in some medical problems. Fellatio may cause oral candidiasis or gonorrhea.[80] Traumatic lesions may occur due to surface area denudement by mandibular incisions while the tongue is protruded.[81] Direct trauma by the penis may also cause submucosal hemorrhage in the palate.

Anal–Genital Activity. Heterosexual (or homosexual) activity may involve anal intercourse. Some couples may use it as an occasional alternative or as a preliminary to penile–vaginal intercourse. Used occasionally, it does not appear harmful, although vaginal infections may follow anal intercourse if the penis is not washed carefully before vaginal entry. However, frequent or vigorous anal intercourse may result in injury to the anus or rectum.

Masturbation

Self-manipulation of the genitalia resulting in sexual gratification and usually in orgasm is a frequent practice. Kinsey found that 92 to 96 percent of all males[82] have masturbated at some time in their lives, and 62 percent of all females.[83] Masturbation has no adverse physiologic consequences, but it may be accompanied by guilt and shame resulting in anxiety. It has been and still is condemned as immoral by some religions (see Chapter 9).

Early psychoanalysts were interested in the instinctual aspects of masturbation, focusing their attention on "too little or too much" adversely affecting mental health. Some believed that after puberty, marked masturbatory activity or incomplete "sexual discharge" resulted in an accumulation of noxious substances, causing anxiety and neurasthenia. Freud first believed that excessive masturbation had an effect on mental functioning causing anxiety, but that moderate masturbation was harmless or even helpful.[84] In his book *Three Contributions to the Theory of Sex,* Freud divided masturbatory activities into three phases. Infantile activity is initiated by thumbsucking (pleasure sucking) coupled with rubbing contact with breasts or genitals and lasts only a short while.[85]

Childhood masturbation was believed by Freud to be critical to the development of neurosis. During the second phase, children of about three go through the oedipal stage and are capable of fantasizing incestuous wishes during masturbation and feel guilt and fear punishment. They may also be threatened or punished by parents who may suggest that harm will come to the genitals if the activity continues. The child is beset by unconscious conflicts that shape the psychologic future.

Freud believed that during puberty, masturbation becomes a testing ground for adult behavior, a way to rehearse future sexual behavior with the final conversion to the heterosexual outlet of coitus. Later, masturbation may be resumed when intercourse is not available.[86]

Masturbation during puberty may result in unconscious fantasy about earlier infantile behavior. Frank[87] believes that conflict and guilt is not about masturbation but because of fantasies that are oedipal in origin or may refer to other family members. This guilt may be transferred to adult sexuality or

to the marital partner and lead to further inhibition or guilt.

At the present time, few people have concern about pathophysiologic effects of masturbation. The concerns pertain to psychologic issues, that is, the motivation behind the practice, degrees of dependency as a sexual outlet, and the extent to which the activity excludes development of sociosexual interpersonal relationships.[88] Additional concerns are related to the moral issues involved.

Masturbation may be used to relieve sexual tension, especially when a sexual partner is not available, or may be relied upon as an auxilliary source of gratification, even by the happily married. Others masturbate for nonsexual reasons—to combat feelings of loneliness and to relieve tensions caused by personal or job-related problems.

In spite of the more general approval of masturbation by the medical profession, masturbation, of all sexual practices, elicits the most reticence, defensiveness, and shame,[89] even though it is becoming more socially acceptable.

The incidence of masturbation is lower in females than in males. The reasons are speculative. Some hypothesize that females are not encouraged or expected to be sexual. In addition, the clitoris is not subject to chance stimulation like the penis. With the Women's Liberation Movement, masturbation is more openly advocated as an alternate form of sexual activity, freeing women from worrying about the partner's needs and opinions, a way of enjoying themselves. It has been described as the female's sexual base, since everything done beyond that is how women socialize their sexual lives.[90]

Female Masturbation. Women masturbate by stimulation of the clitoral shaft, the labia minora, or the mons veneris by stroking, tugging, or pressing. Direct stimulation of the clitoral glans is avoided, since contact may be painful. The clitoris is often the primary erotic area, but Masters and Johnson[91] have reported that women usually manipulate the mons area as a whole.

Some women masturbate by using saliva or vaginal secretions to rub around the area of the clitoris. Others masturbate by crossing their legs and exerting rhythmic pressure on the genital area, using a stream of water or an electric vibrator. Insertion of a finger, candle, or peeled cucumber in the vagina may be preferred. The breasts or other parts of the body are erotically sensitive for some.[92]

Male Masturbation. Most males masturbate by gripping the penis and using an up and down motion to stimulate the glans and the shaft. The degree of pressure, speed of movement, and extent of contact with the glans varying with individual preference. Others lightly touch or pull at the skin around the frenulum or lightly flick the penis with the fingers or other objects. Vibrators or artificial vaginas are used by a few men.

Use of Objects. Both males and females may use friction against objects to achieve orgasm. A pillow, towel, nightclothes, or bed covers tucked between the legs or the edge of the mattress may be convenient to rub against, thus achieving orgasm and still obeying the dictum not to touch the genitals. Rubbing the body with creams, lotion, or oil may be used as a means of increasing erotic feelings.

Fantasizing. Fantasizing is an important part of masturbatory activity, particularly for the male. Kinsey found that 72 percent of men and 50 percent of women reported fantasizing during masturbation. Males reported fantasizing about naked women, especially the breast and genitalia and "getting sex" in an impersonal encounter in which they are powerful and aggressive.[93] Females report fantasizing about romance and love and being forced to submit to intercourse.[94] Fantasies may be stimulated by erotic pictures or literature, music, and wine.

Autoerotic Asphyxia. One of the most dangerous sexual activities is autoerotic asphyxia; self-induced erotic pleasure enhanced by near asphyxiation, usually with a noose around the neck. Consciousness may be lost and the individual may die before he/she can restore the oxygen supply. Death may be attributed to suicide at first but the victims are typically described as happy persons, predominently male adolescents or young adults. They are often found hanging by the neck, wearing women's clothing and the presence of semen indicates that they died while masturbating. Pornographic material and equipment to release themselves from the noose are also present.

Parents and health professionals should be alert to signs of the activity: bloodshot eyes, marks on the neck, disoriented behavior, possession of ropes, chains or other methods to induce partial asphyxiation such as plastic bags, gags, or gas inhalation devices.[95]

Sociocultural Factors. Kinsey found that the frequency of masturbation correlated with education among males and was highest among college-educated groups. Among females, social class did not affect the frequency. In Kinsey's sample, masturbation was an important sexual outlet for the better-educated male[96] and nearly two-thirds of the females.[97] It was the chief source of male orgasms before marriage. Even after marriage, more than two-thirds of college-educated men masturbated at least sometimes afterward.

Greater frequency of masturbation among college-educated people than those with less education may result from (1) less fear of masturbation as a health hazard; (2) difference in class attitudes toward coitus (among the less educated there are strong taboos against masturbation, but not coitus); (3) difference in class attitudes toward premarital coitus (the better educated are usually less permissive about premarital intercourse and use masturbation as a substitute).[98]

Masturbation has been found in all societies. In some it is condemned, in others it is encouraged in children but condemned among adults. The Kwoma of New Guinea are extremely prohibitive of masturbation. When a woman sees a boy with an erect penis, she beats it with a stick. In Melanesia, masturbation is regarded as a safe and healthy outlet for young unmarried persons.[99]

NURSING IMPLICATIONS

Nurses come to the patient care situation with their own values, attitudes, and beliefs about the suitability and/or morality of certain arousal techniques, coital positions, and behavior. Imposition of their beliefs and values on the patient/client is especially difficult to avoid in the area of sexuality. They give information under the guise of health promotion, but the amount and kind of information that is shared can be shaped by the nurse's biases.

More subtly, the nurse may nonverbally communicate negative attitudes about sexual activity and practices to the patients/clients when they bring up questions or have concerns about sexual activity. If the nurse has the firm belief that discussion of all sexual activity or of certain types of sexual activity is wrong or inappropriate or if she/he feels extremely uncomfortable or embarrassed, it is preferred that someone else undertake the sexual counseling or teaching. (See Chapters 10 through 12 for information about assessment, teaching, and counseling.)

Assessment
Age, social class, and sex are considered. Values and attitudes about sexual activity are determined. Individuals may have strong beliefs and attitudes that prohibit certain activity, or they may be eager and open for more information and desire to talk about their concerns. The nurse determines what the usual sexual practices are and if they are satisfying.

Are there problems that are longstanding or recent? A longstanding problem usually requires psychotherapy. Is the problem one of relationship? Are one or both partners bothered by guilt, fear, shame, disgust? For some of these persons, clarification of misconceptions and giving of information may be sufficient. Is the problem due only to ignorance? This can easily be remedied by information. (See Chapter 11.)

Planning
Age, sex, social class, sexual drive, male–female differences in response, and preferences in arousal techniques should be considered in planning interventions. However, since sexuality is so variable from individual to individual, from social class to social class and within social class, it is essential that these factors be considered in relation to each individual's unique responses, desires, and values.

Intervention
If an upper-social-class woman complains that her husband is brusque, engages in little foreplay, and is inconsiderate of her feelings, talking with both partners, stressing the importance of communication and consideration and teaching some arousal techniques can be very effective. If the husband comes from an environment where "macho" male behavior is the norm and where women are sex objects, this approach may be futile.

Suggesting arousal techniques may help many individuals. Use of pictures and diagrams of various coital positions can be more helpful than a thousand words. Most important is stressing the importance of open communication, of caring and consideration for the sexual partner, the importance of a loving word or glance, and a nonhurried private environment.

Nurses help individuals understand that no one type of sexual activity is acceptable or provides satisfaction for everyone and that standards of "normality" vary from person to person and group to group. The nurse's role is to help persons feel more in control of their bodies, more in touch to what is pleasurable or not pleasurable, and more comfortable in communicating their needs to their sexual partners. Nurses can also help individuals see that there is nothing wrong in not wanting to engage in sex.

NOTES

1. Kirkendall LA: Sex drive, in Ellis A, Abarbanel A (eds): Encyclopedia of Sexual Behavior. New York, Aronson, 1973, pp 939–948
2. Goldman GD, Milman DS: Modern Woman. Springfield, Illinois, Thomas, 1969, p 6
3. McGregor AM, Scanlon MF, Hall K, Cook DB, Hall R: Reduction in the size of pituitary tumor by bromocriptine therapy. N Eng J Med 300:291–293, 1979
4. Greenblatt RB, McNamara VP: Endocrinology of human sexuality. In Sadock BJ, Kaplan HI, Freedman AM (eds): The Sexual Experience. Baltimore, Williams and Wilkins, 1976, pp 104–118
5. Goldman GD, Milman DS: Modern Woman, Springfield, Illinois, Thomas, 1969, p 8
6. Izard CE: Human Emotions. New York, Plenum, 1977, p 199
7. Ibid, p 179
8. Ibid, p 183
9. Ibid, p 184
10. Rosenbaum M-B: Female sexuality. In Oaks WW, Melchiode GA, Ficher I (eds): Sex and the Life Cycle. New York, Grune and Stratton, 1976, pp 87–95
11. Bancroft J: Endocrinology of sexual function. Clin Obstet Gynecol 7:253–280, 1980
12. Zuckerman M: Research in pornography. In Oaks WW, Melchiode GA, Ficher I (eds): Sex and the Life Cycle. New York, Grune and Stratton, 1976, pp 147–161
13. Rosenbaum M-B: Female sexuality. In Oaks WW, Melchiode GA, Ficher I (eds): Sex and the Life Cycle. New York, Grune and Stratton, 1976, p 89
14. Izard CE: Human Emotions. New York, Plenum, 1977, p 177
15. Scott N: Wear and tear of job shows in love life. The Plain Dealer April 27, 1979, p 5-D
16. Money J: The development of sexuality and eroticism in humankind. Quart Rev Biol 56:379–403, 1981
17. Ibid, p 178
18. Greenblatt RB, McNamara VP: Endocrinology of human sexuality. In Sadock BJ, Kaplan HI, Freedman AM (eds): The Sexual Experience. Baltimore, Williams and Wilkins, 1976, p 116
19. Izard CE: Human Emotions, New York, Plenum, 1977, p 177
20. Ibid, p 177
21. Crown S, D'Ardenne P: Symposium on sexual dysfunction: Controversies, methods, results. Brit J Psych 140:70–77, 1982
22. Leo J, Castronovo V: In search of sexual desire. Time April 4, 1983, p 80
23. Duddle M, Brown ADG: The clinical management of sexual dysfunction. Clin Obstet Gynecol 7:293–323, 1980
24. Crown S, D'Ardenne P: Symposium on sexual dysfunction: Controversies, methods, results. Brit J Psych 140:71, 1982
25. Hastings DW: Sexual Expression in Marriage. Boston, Little, Brown, 1971, pp 33–34
26. Money J: The development of sexuality and eroticism in humankind. Quart Rev Biol 56:375, 1981
27. Hastings DW: Sexual Expression in Marriage. Boston, Little, Brown, 1977 p 35
28. Money J: The development of sexuality and eroticism in humankind. Quart Rev Biol 56:395, 1981
29. Greenblatt RB, McNamara VP: Endocrinology of human sexuality. In Sadock BJ, Kaplan HI, Freedman AM (eds): The Sexual Experience. Baltimore, Williams and Wilkins, 1976, p 113
30. Ibid, p 114

31. Ibid, p 117

32. Duddle M, Brown ADG: The clinical management of sexual dysfunction. Clin Obstet Gynecol 7:297, 1980

33. American Medical Association Committee on Human Sexuality: Human Sexuality. Chicago, AMA, 1972, p 122

34. Izard CE: Human Emotions. New York, Plenum, 1977, p 175

35. Miller PR: Human Sexuality—Its Anatomy, Physiology and Psychology. (Audiovisual slide-tape) Baltimore, Williams and Wilkins, 1974

36. Katchadourian HA, Lunde DT: Fundamentals of Human Sexuality, 2nd ed. New York, Holt, Rinehart and Winston, 1975, p 288

37. Kinsey, AC, Pomeroy WB, Martin CE: Sexual Behavior in the Human Male, Philadelphia, Saunders, 1948, pp 574–575

38. Ibid, pp 576–577

39. Katchadourian HA, Lunde DT: Fundamentals of Human Sexuality, 2nd ed. New York, Holt, Rinehart and Winston, 1975, p 289

40. Ibid, p 291

41. Kinsey AC, Pomeroy WB, Martin CE: Sexual Behavior in the Human Male. Philadelphia, Saunders, 1948, p 575

42. Kinsey AC, Pomeroy WB, Martin CE, Gebhard P: Sexual Behavior in the Human Female. New York, Pocket Books, 1965, p 257

43. Katchadourian HA, Lunde DT: Fundamentals of Human Sexuality, 2nd ed. New York, Holt, Rinehart and Winston, 1975, p 292

44. Hassett J: Sex and smell. Psychol Today 11(10):40–45, 1978

45. Heiman JR: Female sexual response patterns. Arch Gen Psych 37:1311–1316, 1980

46. Mednick RA: Gender—Specific variances in sexual fantasy. J Pers Assess 41:248–254, 1977

47. Ibid, p 252

48. Money J: The development of sexuality and eroticism in humankind. Quart Rev Biol 56:394, 1981

49. Katchadourian HA, Lunde DT: Fundamentals of Human Sexuality, 2nd ed. New York, Holt, Rinehart and Winston, 1975, p 260

50. Friday N: Men in Love. New York, Delacorte, 1980

51. Ibid, p 262

52. Lipton MA: Pornography. In Sadock BJ, Kaplan HI, Freedman AM (eds): The Sexual Experience. Baltimore, Williams and Wilkins, 1976, pp 584–593

53. O'Connor FM: Pornography is sick and doing well. Liquorian, June 1978, pp 24–28

54. Zuckerman M: Research in pornography. In Oaks WW, Melchiode GA, Ficher I (eds): Sex and the Life Cycle. New York, Grune and Stratton, 1976, p 160

55. Fisher WA, Byrne D: Sex differences in response to erotica? Love versus Lust. J Pers Soc Psychol 36:117–125, 1978

56. Pietropinto A, Simenauer J: Beyond the Male Myth. New York, Times Books, 1977, p 27

57. Watson JP, Bamber RWK: Some relationships between sex, marriage and mood. J Internat Med Res 8 (Suppl) 3:14–19, 1980

58. Goldman, GD, Milman DS: Modern Woman. Springfield, Illinois, Thomas, 1969, p 38

59. Stephens GJ: Mind–body continuum in human sexuality. Am J Nurs 70:468–471, 1970

60. Stoller R: Sexual excitement. Arch Gen Psychiatry 33:899–909, 1976

61. Ibid, p 909

62. Johnson VE: Masters WH: Contemporary influences on sexual response: The work ethic. J School Health 46:211–214, April 1976

63. Kinsey AC, Pomeroy WB, Martin CE: Sexual Behavior in the Human Male. Philadelphia, Saunders, 1948, pp 571–576

64. DeLora JS, Warren CAB: Understanding Sexual Interaction. Boston, Houghton Mifflin, 1977, p 125

65. Ibid, p 126

66. Weinberg MS: Sex Research. New York, Oxford, 1976, pp 74–75

67. Hite S: The Hite Report. New York, Macmillan, 1976

68. Weinberg MS: Sex Research. New York, Oxford, 1976, p 83

69. Miller PR: Human Sexuality—Its Anatomy, Physiology and Psychology. (Audiovisual slide-tape) Baltimore, Williams and Wilkins, 1974

70. Sadock BJ, Sadock VA: Techniques of coitus. In Sadock BJ, Kaplan HI, Freedman AM (eds): The Sexual Experience. Baltimore, Williams and Wilkins, 1976, pp 206–215

71. Weinberg MS: Sex Research. New York, Oxford, 1976, p 74

72. Hussey HH: Cuddling: The influence of culture on sex. JAMA 235:417, 1976

73. Udry JR, Deven FR, Coleman SJ: A cross-national comparison of the relative influence of male and female age on the frequency of marital intercourse. J Biosoc Sci 14:1–6, 1982

74. Katchadourian HA, Lunde DT: Fundamentals of Human Sexuality, 2nd ed. New York, Holt, Rinehart and Winston, 1975, p 206

75. MacLean PD: Brain mechanisms of elemental sexual functions. In Sadock BJ, Kaplan HI, Freedman AM (eds): The Sexual Experience, Baltimore, Williams and Wilkins, 1976, pp 119–127

76. Masters WH, Johnson VE: The Pleasure Bond. Toronto, Bantam, 1975, pp 267–283

77. Ibid, p 285

78. Sadock BJ, Sadock VA: Techniques of coitus. In Sadock BJ, Kaplan HI, Freedman AM (eds): The Sexual Experience. Baltimore, Williams and Wilkins, 1976, p 213

79. Ibid, p 214

80. Damm PD, White DK, Brinker CM: Variations of palatal erythema secondary to fellatio. Oral Surg 52:417–421, 1981

81. Mader CL: Lingual frenum ulcer resulting from oral sex. J Am Dent Ass 103:888–890, 1981

82. Kinsey AC, Pomeroy WB, Martin CE: Sexual Behavior in the Human Male. Philadelphia, Saunders, 1948, p 499

83. Kinsey AC, Pomeroy WB, Martin CE, Gebhard P: Sexual Behavior in the Human Female. New York, Pocket Books, 1965, p 175

84. Moore WT: Genital masturbation and adolescent development. In Oaks WW, Melchiode GA, Ficher I (eds): Sex and the Life Cycle. New York, Grune and Stratton, 1976, pp 53–66

85. Freud S: Three Contributions to the Theory of Sex, 4th ed. New York, Nervous and Mental Disease Publishing, 1930, pp 44–49

86. Ibid, pp 76–79

87. Frank OS: The therapy of sexual dysfunction. Brit J Psych 140:78–84, 1982

88. Katchadourian HA, Lunde DT: Fundamentals of Human Sexuality, 2nd ed. New York, Holt, Rinehart and Winston, 1975, p 283

89. Sorensen RC: Adolescent Sexuality in Contemporary America. New York, World, 1973, p 143

90. Boston Women's Health Book Collective: Our Bodies, Ourselves, 2nd ed. New York, Simon and Schuster, 1976, p 47

91. Masters WH, Johnson VE: Human Sexual Response. Boston, Little, Brown, 1966, p 64

92. Boston Women's Health Book Collective: Our Bodies, Ourselves, 2nd ed. New York, Simon and Schuster, 1976, p 47

93. Kinsey AC, Pomeroy WB, Martin CE, Gebhard P: Sexual Behavior in the Human Female. New York, Pocket Books, 1965, pp 164–167

94. DeLora JS, Warren CAB: Understanding Sexual Interaction. Boston, Houghton Mifflin, 1977, p 58

95. Brody JE, Autoerotic asphyxiation. The Plain Dealer, April 8, 1984. p C-1

96. Kinsey AC, Pomeroy WB, Martin CE: Sexual Behavior in the Human Male. Philadelphia, Saunders, 1948, pp 339–343.

97. Kinsey AC, Pomeroy WB, Martin CE, Gebhard P: Sexual Behavior in the

Human Female. New York, Pocket
Books, 1965, p 177

98. Katchadourian HA, Lunde DT: Fundamentals of Human Sexuality, 2nd ed.
New York, Holt, Rinehart and Winston,
1975, p 277

99. Davenport W: Sexual patterns in a
southwest Pacific society. In Brecher R,
Brecher E (eds): An Analysis of Human
Sexual Response. New York, New American Library, 1966, p 199

Chapter 5

Alternative Forms of Sexual Expression

Penile–vaginal intercourse between biologic males and females has been the norm in most societies, although other forms of sexual expression were more or less accepted or tolerated depending on the cultural mores of the times (see Chapter 1).

Instead of or in addition to engaging in heterosexual coitus, individuals may obtain sexual satisfaction in a homosexual relationship or in bisexuality, while some will choose celibacy. As an alternative to engaging in a sexual relationship with others, some persons may obtain sexual gratification through transvestism, voyeurism, exhibitionism, masochism, or sadomasochism. Finally, there are the individuals who are transsexual, believing that by some cruel trick of fate, they are one sex in the anatomic body of the other sex.

This chapter will focus on the bio-psycho-social factors related to these types of sexual expression, the treatment modalities used if indicated, and society's attitudes and response to sexual activity other than heterosexual intercourse.

HOMOSEXUALITY

Homosexuality has occurred in all societies and is as old as humanity. The definition is not clear-cut but operationally includes any behavior involving sexual relations with the same sex. The term also refers to the individual's strong erotic attraction to members of the same sex and the ability to be aroused by one's own sex just as heterosexuality indicates ability to be aroused by the opposite sex. It does not mean that the individuals necessarily act on these feelings to indulge in overt homosexual behavior. Intense social fears or moral prohibition may prevent that.[1]

There may be a wide variety of motivations that underlie homosexual activities. Some enter into a homosexual relationship because heterosexual objects are not available or because of loneliness, boredom, or rebelliousness. Homosexual behavior may be sporadic and transitory, as in preadolescence or adolescence, or it may occur in the disorganized schizophrenic. It may be behavior in which the homosexuality represents sexual curiosity and a wish for diverse sexual experience, or it may be due to hidden but incapacitating fears of the opposite sex (reparative homosexuality).

Difficulty arises because homosexual and heterosexual behavior in humans are points on a continuum that ranges from exclusive heterosexuality to exclusive homosexuality with gradations of bisexuality between. There are as many different kinds of homosexuality as there are heterosexuality, and one cannot judge the nature of the personality, social adjustment, and sexual function on the basis of the sexual orientation.

It is speculated that a large number of individuals are homosexual at certain periods of their lives and that the nature of the activity changes with age, life circumstances, and culture. The feelings are more important than the behavior in defining homosexuality, since the majority of male homosexuals and even a larger number of female homosexuals indicate extensive heterosexual activity but without deep emotional satisfaction or intense sexual arousal.[2]

Kinsey[3] reported on the incidence of homosexuality in a sample of 5000 white males. Ten percent of white males were more or less exclusively homosexual for at least those years between 16 and 55, and 4 percent were exclusively homosexual throughout their lives. Thirteen percent of the same group reacted erotically to men but had no overt sexual contacts.

Among women, Kinsey[4] found that 2 to 6 percent of unmarried but only 1 percent of married women had been more or less exclusively homosexual between 20 and 25 years. Twenty-eight percent reported some homosexual experience, but only 13 percent to the point of orgasm. It must be noted that Kinsey's study suffers from sampling bias, since it did not include racial and ethnic minority groups.

Bell and Weinberg[5] emphasize the diversity of homosexuals, stressing that it is also important to identify those aspects that are universal in human societies. Whitman,[6] on the basis of field research observation and questionnaire data from four societies (United States, Guatemala, Brazil, and the Philippines), identified six *tentative* conclusions about cultural similarity: (1) homosexuals appear in all societies; (2) the percentage seems to be the same and stable over time; (3) social norms neither impede nor facilitate emergence of homosexuality; (4) homosexual subcultures appear in all societies; (5) in different societies homosexuals tend to be alike in certain behavioral interests and occupational choices; (6) all societies have the continua from overtly masculine to overtly feminine homosexuals.

As a conclusion of the study, Whitman indicates that homosexuality is not created by society, but is a universal natural manifestation of human sexuality and is not pathologic.

Homosexuality: Variant Behavior or Illness

In 1973, the American Psychiatric Association voted to remove homosexuality from the list of mental disorders. They defined it as a "sexual orientation disturbance" in the *Diagnostic and Statistical Manual of Mental Disorders,* stating, "This is for people whose sexual interests are directed primarily toward people of the same sex and who are in conflict with or wish to change their sexual orientation. This diagnostic category is distinguished from homosexuality which by itself does not constitute a psychiatric disorder.[7]

By creating a new category, sexual orientation disturbance, a label was applied only to those homosexuals who are bothered by their orientation and not to those who state they are well and who have no impairment in social effectiveness. The members of the association also felt they would be removing one of the justifications for denial of civil rights to homosexuals.[8]

Green[9] questions whether homosexuality should be defined as a "disorder," a "disease" or an "illness." Militant homosexuals tend to see homosexuality as a variant form of sexual expression and many psychiatrists argue that the fact that their life style is not in step with societal conventional sexual behavior is not in itself a basis for a diagnosis of psychopathology. Psychoanalytic theories may apply only to a homosexual subgroup and are not relevant to others.[10]

When a nonclinical sample of homosexuals is compared with an equivalent heterosexual sample, there are few differences in psychologic functioning seen.[11] Bell and Weinberg[12] (1978) found most homosexuals on the whole to be as psychologically well adjusted as heterosexuals.

More homosexuals seek professional

help or have attempted suicide, but this can be laid on the steps of a hostile society that provides little support and that may respond with rancor and hostility.

Some members of the American Psychiatric Association, responding to a mailed questionnaire, still believe "homosexuality is usually a pathologic adaptation, as opposed to normal variation," that homosexuals are less happy than heterosexuals and less capable of mature loving relationships. Seventy percent said homosexual problems have more to do with their inner conflicts than societal stigmatization.[13]

Ruse[14] points out that people differ in their views on homosexuality as a disease because they bring different assumptions about disease, illness, and homosexuality to their arguments and that until there is agreement in these areas there will continue to be conflict of opinion.

Etiology—Bio-psycho-social Variables

In nineteenth century society, homosexuality was believed to be caused by genetic factors or by some degenerative disease of the nervous system. The psychoanalytic explanation combines the concept of organic bisexuality (the apparent hermaphroditic characteristics of the human embryo) with developmental theory based on psychosocial factors.

A hormonal etiology related to decreased levels of testosterone in the male, and increased levels in the female has been postulated. In males there may be lack of fetal hypothalamic exposure to androgens; in females decrease in progesterone in the hypothalamus may result in failure of feminization and loss of protection from the masculizing effects of androgens.[15]

It appears that psychosexual behavior is influenced by prenatal hormones but to a very limited degree. The type of behavior most affected is rough-and-tumble play and rehearsal of parenting behavior (doll, play interest in babies). Evidence, however, is inconclusive and data indicate that hormones do not rigidly determine homosexual or heterosexual orientation.[16,17]

There have not been any well-controlled, adequately designed studies that demonstrate that female homosexuals have different hormonal levels than heterosexual females. Recent studies of hormonal differences in men have been positive in some, negative in others.[18]

A genetic predisposition has been investigated but not confirmed. In a study of 40 monozygotic pairs of twins, all were homosexual, while 45 dizygotic pairs had an incidence of homosexuality only slightly higher than normal. Chromosomal studies have found no characteristic differences in those of homosexuals from heterosexuals. The question of innate genetic differences between homosexuals and heterosexuals is unsettled.[19]

Freud believed that individuals have normal psychic bisexuality, based on human biologic bisexual predisposition. All persons go through a homoerotic phase as children. If homosexuality occurs later in life, Freud believed that in the male it was not an illness but an arrest of normal development. He suggested it could also be a result of pathogenic family relationships characterized by a failure to satisfactorily identify with an adequate father figure and a close but ambivalent relationship with the mother figure. This results in a strong unconscious fear of women.[20] However, he believed that in all individuals, even those without overt homosexuality, latent homosexual tendencies exist as sublimated patterns of affection for members of one's own sex, or else in certain passive tendencies in men and aggressive tendencies in women.[21]

Bieber describes pathologic relationships between the parents and the male child. Typically, mothers of homosexuals are inappropriately close, are seductive, and tend to inhibit aggressiveness in the boys. Fathers are covertly or overtly hostile, expressing the hostility by detachment, cruelty, or brutality. The prehomosexual child suffers rejection and hostility from other significant males, brothers and peers. The mother may dominate and minimize her husband. Homosexuality becomes a substitute adaptation replacing heterosexuality, which fear has made inadequate or unavailable.[22,23]

In females, Bieber describes a mother–daughter relationship that is rejecting, critical, without warmth and affection. The mother may prefer her sons. In other groups, the mother may be possessive, dominating, and controlling, thus interfering with the daughter's heterosexual development and discouraging her romantic attachments.

Fathers may be of two types also. The first is detached and may be perceived as rejecting, neither affectionate nor tender. These fathers are submissive to their wives and fail to support the girl against the mother's negative behavior. In the second group, the father may be overpossessive and seductive and form an alliance with the daughter, excluding the mother. He is jealous of his daughter's interest in males.[24]

In 1974, Siegelman[25] attempted to replicate Bieber's etiologic findings in nonclinical samples and was unable to do so.

In a more recent cross-national study, Siegelman[26] again found few differences in the parental backgrounds of homosexual and heterosexual men. He suggested a need for a more multifactional and developmental theory of sexual orientation to replace explanation involving types of parental behavior.

Some lesbians describe an unexceptional parental background. Others have had strong rivalry with their male siblings, which caused hostility to boys and rejection of the female sex role. Others feel that the parents wanted a boy and feel rejected. Some may desire the pleasure of body love with and from a mothering woman.[27]

Sociologic factors may operate in female homosexuality. Some women choose homosexuality because they feel unattractive, are shy, or fear rejection or, because of the unavailability of men, are closed off from heterosexual relationships. With the Women's Liberation Movement, women's resentment toward males and their sexist attitudes was released, and there was a tendency of some women to reject men sexually and seek women for sexual release. If not homosexual, a bisexual pattern developed among some women.[28] The radical wing of the Women's Liberation Movement views lesbianism as a revolt against the female role of passivity, hypocrisy, and indirect action. It is also a rejection of what some women view as the brutality and mechanicalness of male sexual passion.[29] Bell and Weinberg[30] found that lesbians feel that females are more gentle, more sensitive, and more competent at the art of making love.

Demographic Variables

Weinberg and Williams[31] chose the homosexual population of three societies—the United States, the Netherlands, and Denmark—to investigate the effects of societal reactions on the adaptations the homosexual makes (1) to the heterosexual world, (2) to the homosexual world, and (3) to potential psychologic problems. They provide some demographic data regarding the groups studied and their correlation with homosexual behavior.

Age, occupational status, religion, religiosity, and race correlate with behavior. Older homosexuals were less involved, often lived alone, had less sex and were no worse off on psychologic dimensions than younger homosexuals.[32] Homosexuals in higher-status occupations were less open and more worried about exposure. They had more social involvement with heterosexuals of their own class than with homosexuals of lower classes.

There were no differences in the psychologic problems between homosexuals with higher-status occupations and those with lower-status occupations. The higher-status homosexuals did show more self-acceptance and faith in others. These results seemed to contradict the belief that homosexuals in high-status occupations experience greater psychologic maladjustment.[33]

No general relationship was found between the life styles, psychologic problems, and religious background of the groups. Less is known about religious homosexuals however. They are more concerned with passing as heterosexuals and attach more importance to the opinion of others. They are less likely to be socially involved with other homosexuals and less likely to have been involved in sexual practices common to homosexuals.

The conflict between religiosity and homosexuality did not cause greater psychologic problems after the guilt, shame, and anxiety that followed the first homosexual experience. Many reinterpreted their religion as not violated by homosexuality. Only among the most religious of the respondents did psychologic problems correlate with the perception that homosexuality violates religion.

Black homosexuals differed from whites in that they expected less negative reaction and anticipated less discrimination as a result of their homosexuality. They had earlier first experiences, were more likely to have exclusive homosexual relationships, and when living with a homosexual were more likely to be lovers with the roommate. Blacks were somewhat more self-accepting than whites. Generally, however, race was uncorrelated with the psychologic factors measured.[34]

Sexual Activity

Interest. Homosexuals, like heterosexuals, differ in the amount of attention they give to sexual aspects of their lives. Some live their lives with little awareness of sexual interests, others eroticize all social contacts. Male homosexuals report higher sexual interests than female homosexuals. Homosexuals who have just "come out" and are in the process of defining their homosexual potential are much more apt to consider sex an important aspect of their lives.[35]

Level of Sexual Activity. Some homosexuals are satisfied with their degree of sexual activity, others are not. Those involved in a relatively permanent sexual relationship are usually more satisfied, while individuals without a permanent sexual partner who have to "cruise" (look for a sexual partner) usually are less so. Successful "scoring" is not as frequent as some believe. Some have difficulty initiating an approach and want to be approached, while others enjoy the "chase" even more than the sexual outcome.[36]

Sexual Repertoire. Homosexuals may indulge in all erotic positions that characterize heterosexual activity except those limited by identical anatomy: kissing, tongue play, mutual genital stimulation by hand or body friction, oral–genital relations, breast stimulation and kissing (especially by females), and anal intercourse (by males).

Some males are penile inserters, that is, insert the penis in the mouth or anus. Others perfer being the recipients. However, although there may be a preference for some activity, it is most often modified by the partner's expectations or individual's interest and arousal. Some have a rigid repertoire. The number of different sex roles and activities the homosexual is willing to engage in is directly related to age, length of homosexuality, the degree of acceptance of sexual impulses, and homosexual orientation.

Lesbians may use artificial phalluses (dildoes) to stimulate the partner, but intercourse is rare in females. Some couples are satisfied with mutual embracing and kissing; mutual genital stimulation may be performed, and oral stimulation, cunnilingus, is frequently used. Some may prefer tribadism, body friction that simulates coitus.[37,38]

Contrary to popular belief, homosexuals do not fall into an active or passive role during sexual activity. They may have different preferences but in practice they vary technique. There is no reliable correlation between appearance, social mannerisms, and sex practices. Masculine-appearing individuals may assume passive sex roles, while those with an effeminate appearance may prefer an active role.

Sociocultural Structure of Male Homosexual Relationships

An ethnographic approach to study male homosexual relationships was used by Sonenshein.[39] After living in a homosexual community for 1½ years, he identified six types of sociosexual relationships.

In a permanent social relationship, sexual activity is not involved, but close friendship is maintained over time. In the nonpermanent relationship, the individuals are good friends, but there is no continued contact, sex play is common but genital relations are rare. The permanent sexual relationship is materialistic and includes being "kept." It provides sexual activity but is unstable and contains a factor of infidelity by the "kept" boy.[40]

The nonpermanent sexual relationship ("one night stands," "affairs") is the most frequent type of sexual relationship. These may be liaisons made in gay bars, in public baths, on certain streets, or in public rest rooms. Often they are anonymous and depersonalized, and their sole purpose is sexual activity and orgasm. They are "consummated" in the time it takes to reach orgasm. This is the most popular type of homosexual activity for those with high social rank and those tremendously committed to sexual activity.[41]

Some homosexuals may be involved in many such liaisons. Some report over 500 sexual partners during their homosexual careers. This sexual promiscuity may be due to an underlying psychodynamic factor, the avoidance of an interpersonal commitment of intimacy or responsibility, or it may be due to sociologic factors. If the homosexual relationship is exposed, legal, occupational, and social sanctions occur. There is less chance of this danger in transitory contacts.[42] However, we must be careful not to generalize about sexual behavior. Not all homosexuals are promiscuous. The more mature are likely to want a stable relationship with a permanent love object.

Another type of "affair" may be relatively long in length, lasting weeks or months and possibly involving a love relationship. This involves more of a trial relationship as a prelude to a more committed one.

Two types of permanent sociosexual relationships were found. The first involves some type of ritual (exchange of rings, ceremony) much like a heterosexual ceremony, a "marriage." The value system of the partners was based on a romantic conception of ideally unending love. Social roles may be dichotomized. One partner stays home and takes care of the house, the other works. One may be more effeminate, the other more masculine; but these are a minority. Dichotomization of social role is not as automatic as is commonly thought.

The second type of relationship is less formalized. There may be only an exchange of rings and the setting up of the household. This "cohabitation" was more permanent than the first. It, too, is based on a conception of love, but is not as sexual as the first. Individuals made a conscious effort at congruency of values and interests. The "cohabitation" relationship is more permanent than the first, where the formalized ritual seems to serve less as a reason to cement a relationship than as an excuse for a party. The "marriage" becomes a group event in contrast to the private pairing of the cohabitants.[43]

In the nonpermanent sociosexual relationship there are situational contacts where the individuals identify as "friends" but also as potential sexual partners. Social interactions occur before sexual activity, in contrast to the nonpermanent sexual relationships, where sexual activity occurs first. In the community studied, these were rare.

Sociocultural Structure of Female Homosexual Relationships

Less information is available about the life style of lesbians. Society does not stigmatize sexual intimacy between women as it does between men. Women can kiss, embrace, and walk down the street arm in arm without causing comment. Two women living together is taken for granted, while this is not always true with men. Consequently, women are not so fearful of disclosure and feel more secure and adequate.

A greater proportion of female homosexuals have a stable pattern of social relationships. There is less promiscuity than in males, but there are only one-half the number of females openly committed to homosexuality than there are men. Marmor postulates several reasons. The feminine identity is more easily achieved than the masculine, and a dependency adaptation is more acceptable for women if necessary. In addition, it is easier for women to simulate competence in the heterosexual act. The degree of exclusive homosexuality is much lower in women than in men. More women with fear or aversion to heterosexual activity repress their sociosexual needs so that they never have sociosexual relationships throughout the adult years. The double standard accepts abstinence from sexual activity in women but not in men.

More lesbians marry than do male homosexuals, possibly because it is easier to pretend to enjoy intercourse, because of social pressures to marry, desire for children, and desire for security and companionship.[45]

Lesbianism is becoming more open, however. There are lesbian communities in cities and university towns, lesbian hotels, restaurants, health centers, magazines, radio shows, and music festivals.

Problems Related to Homosexuality

Sociosexual Problems. Some problems are little different than those of heterosexual individuals. Finding a sexual partner may be difficult because of age, attractiveness, and social inhibitions. There may be difficulty in maintaining the affection of the sexual partner or in responding to the partner's sexual interests. There may be concern about sexual adequacy: males who are impotent or who cannot ejaculate, females who are nonorgasmic. Finally, developing understanding of the other is difficult, since the relationships are often impersonal and furtive because of society's attitudes.[46]

Some individuals who have not entirely accepted homosexuality feel they have let down their parents and fear their rejection. The most covert homosexuals ("closet queens") sometimes experience high anxiety because of fear of detection and describe a great deal of tension because of the disparity between their outer behavior and their inner selves. Some are ashamed because they have not been open about their homosexuality.

Sociocultural Attitudes. Societal attitudes are described by many homosexuals as the most problematic, for example, societal sanctions against homosexuals in regard to employment, housing, and public accommodations. Some cities have passed "gay rights" measures prohibiting such discrimination, but others have repealed similar laws. Under the ordinances passed, persons claiming discrimination can file a complaint with the Human Rights Commission and sue for damages. However, much discrimination still exists.

Psychologic Problems. Weinberg and Williams[47] found that the sexual orientation of the groups they studied was not strongly correlated with psychologic problems. However, the homosexuals did score lower on measures of happiness and faith. The more negatively the homosexual perceived the appraisal of others, the greater were the psychologic problems. Being freely accepted by either heterosexuals or homosexuals correlated with psychologic well-being. Infrequent sex, never having an exclusive relationship, loneliness, interpersonal awkwardness, and effeminacy were all related to psychologic problems. The "closet" homosexual worried about exposure and anticipated discrimination. The more known homosexual was seen to be more psychologically comfortable than the covert.[47]

Physiologic Problems. Syphilis, gonorrheal prostatitis, and oral gonorrhea are found in the homosexual population. Gastrointestinal upsets and infectious hepatitis may occur because homosexual activity often involves analingus and anal intercourse.[48] Anal cancer has been associated in one study[49] with anal intercourse. Acquired immune deficiency syndrome (AIDS) is the newest and most feared sexually transmitted disease associated with homosexuality (see Chapter 22).

Anorectal changes occur in those who habitually practice rectal intromission. Flattened perianal folds and an open relaxed anal sphincter may result from continued penile–rectal activity.

Lesbian health problems are underreported since lesbians may avoid gynecologists because of fear of condemnation and disclosure.[50]

Gay Liberation Movement

Homosexuals, or "gays," are increasingly fighting for their rights, and gay organizations are increasing in number. There are gay dances, gay Alcoholic Anonymous groups, a lesbian credit union, and Jewish lesbian groups. There are approximately 800 gay groups in the United States. The *Advocate* is a tabloid for gays.[51] The more political of the homosexuals say there are 20 million of them, most still "in the closet." Political action by gays has resulted in the repeal of antisodomy laws in some states. Several large corporations have announced their willingness to hire gays.

Coming out has been described as important to strengthen the movement. However, the militant gays pose dilemmas for homosexuals who have much to lose if they disclose their sexual orientation. Jobs may be lost and families alienated.[52] The first response of parents may be "What did I do wrong?" often followed by bitterness, anger, and hostility. However, many older homosexuals reveal themselves to avoid the strain of living a lie. Still, there are those who say that coming out made life more difficult.

Politically, young lesbians may be facing an identity crisis. They feel torn between the male-dominated gay liberation movement and the feminist movement, which often seems embarrassed by them. Women who are lesbian, are married, and have children may give up their children for fear of exposure if the marriages break up. Some lesbians fight battles in court to win custody.

Reaction of Society. Reaction of society to the gay liberation movement has been mixed. As a civil rights issue, many agree legal discrimination is wrong. However, many individuals are concerned about the gay goal of full acceptance in society. They fear that their assertion that "gay is good" will result in homosexuality being taught as part of school sex courses and gay love stories being published to go with heterosexual "puppy love" stories for youths. Others fear that homosexuality may spread, especially among the young. Serious analysts are divided on the question and reflect that if some homosexuality comes from faulty child rearing, it makes little sense to "celebrate the results rather than to try and strengthen the family."[53]

The evidence that backlash exists to the gay liberation movement is the success that some groups have had in overturning gay civil rights ordinances by large margins. Some argue against the full acceptance of homosexuals because of religious conviction that homosexual behavior is immoral (see Chapter 9). Others argue that "normalizing" homosexuality—by stating that it is a variation of normality or a transient state of adolescence without severe consequences—has negative implications. Socarides[54] believes that the greatest damage is done to youths who are borderline in their orientation and without guidance gravitate to the homosexual life, undergoing bitterness and disappointment in discovering that, contrary to published accounts, life is unhappy.

Children of Homosexual Parents. Society argues that children raised by homosexuals will be homosexual. This does not appear to be true. Although the study was limited by lack of a control group, nonsystematic data collection, and lack of followups, Green[55] found that 36 of 37 children raised by 20 lesbians, 7 male to female transsexuals and 9 female to male transsexuals were heterosexual in their orientation.

Role modeling by homosexual parents cannot be a sufficient cause in itself to cause homosexual orientation in the child, since more homosexuals come from parents who are heterosexual. Those growing up in an atypical family pattern of sexual identity are also influenced by peer groups, television, books, and movies. The child may be able to label the family as idiosyncratic and develop conventional patterns of behavior.

Some counselors report that children of gay parents share common concerns: fear of becoming gay; a strong desire to move to the home of the straight parent; self-blame for parent's homosexuality; worry about negative effect on younger siblings; ridicule and desertion by friends; emotional denial.[56]

Psychotherapy and Homosexuality

If "gay is good" and a normal variation in sexual behavior, in every way as desirable as heterosexuality, one might argue that prevention and therapy is not indicated. However, society has not accepted homosexuality as such, and certainly some "closet gays" do not lead what could be described as a reasonable happy life, based on their own description. Others are happy with their sexual orientation and do not want to change. However, if the individual is an adolescent, parents need help to prevent rejection of the child. The child, too, must be helped to cope with the social consequences of the sexual orientation.

Some homosexuals come for treatment because they have difficulty attracting partners or after the breakup of a relationship, respond with neurosis and depressive reactions. The treatment is like that given the heterosexual who is depressed or neurotic.

The individual who is unhappy with homosexual orientation may seek help. Therapy is not easy, especially when the sexual activity is highly gratifying to the individual. No specific form of therapy has been

found superior to others, and there must be much motivation to change.[57]

In the male, psychoanalytic treatment is oriented toward uncovering the causes of fear of a sexual relationship with a woman and resolving these fears. In the female, it focuses on the identification and working through of problems such as fears of competition with women for men, of rejection by males, and of having children.[58]

In behavior modification therapy, desensitization is used. There is an active gradual approach to heterosexual activity, including having women in bed. Male responsiveness may be increased by aversion therapy. Electroshock pain or apomorphine is given in conjunction with suggestive homoerotic pictures. Heteroerotic pictures and female nude pictures are sometimes preceded by testosterone injections.[59]

Posthypnotic suggestion may be used for habit correction, assertive training to correct self-deprecation, and all combined with insight therapy to remove reachable early developmental factors.[60] Other methods that have been used in the past include temporal lobectomy, male hormone therapy, and sex surgery, including castration.

Homosexual individuals cannot be directed into heterosexual activity by appealing to their moral sense or good intentions or by shaming, taunting, frightening, or punishing them. It is equally futile to try to stimulate the males' erotic interest in women by encouraging them to attend public dances, watch burlesque shows, read pornographic material, or visit prostitutes. It may be helpful to encourage them to socialize with young women to improve their ability to get along with the opposite sex. The belief that marriage can cure homosexuality is fallacy. Whether the bride is aware of the condition or not, her feminine attraction is not a match for the male's homosexual tendencies.

Lesbians may be wary of psychiatrists and physicians. They are considered reactionary and harmful especially to women, since they may try to change the homosexual orientation instead of treating the problem that has been presented.[61] Urging a lesbian to "find yourself a good man" to take care of homosexual tendency is as fallacious as advising a male homosexual to find a prostitute.

Other Concepts Related to Homosexuality

Facultative or Experimental Homosexuals. These individuals are usually a group of unmatured, impressionable adolescents who are befriended by a masculine-oriented homosexual who dislikes the effeminate gay but finds straight youths exciting. These young adolescents, given a glimpse of the gay world, find it exciting, eroticizing, glamorous, free, and hedonistic. The younger man enjoys the warm attention he receives. He is not coerced, pushed, or bribed, but the mystique of homosexuality seduces him. He represses shame and guilt and lets heterosexuality go. Often, an unsuccessful date or a girl's rejection may confirm the belief that he was gay anyway. These young men are not true homosexuals or bisexuals, but individuals with a personality that rendered them vulnerable to a homosexual advance.

Pseudohomosexual Anxiety. Men with doubts about their masculinity express these doubts in the form of fear that they may be homosexual or will be considered so by others. Reasuring them that everyone has latent homosexual tendencies (as described by Freud) is not therapeutically effective. Since the fears are related to masculine inadequacy, they need help in this area.

Homophobia. Homophobia is a pathologic fear of homosexuals. It usually indicates a deep-seated insecurity that the individual has about his or her own gender identity. It also reflects prejudice against homosexuals. The signs include antagonism and abhorrence of and discomfort with homosexuals, generally cloaked in religious, moral, legal, or pseudoscientific rationalizations.[62]

Homosexual Love. It is difficult for heterosexual individuals, many with ingrained feelings of moral and personal condemnation of homosexuality, to grasp the concept of homosexual love. Yet homosexuals in a committed relationship describe the affection, tenderness, and concern that each has for the other, the depth and meaning in their relationship. Just as in a committed heterosexual relationship, separation from the loved one brings sadness and depression, while closeness, not just in a sexual sense, brings joy and fulfillment.

Research and Homosexuality

Although considerable research has been directed toward the study of male homosexuality, there is a paucity of research on lesbianism. In addition, to a large extent, heterosexual bias has been present in all research into homosexuality, since much of it has been directed toward the questions of diagnoses, cause, and cure.[63] Inherent research difficulties are also present, since there is no such thing as a representative sample of lesbians or homosexual men. The population being sampled is essentially hidden or invisible. There is also difficulty in defining homosexual groups, so no generalizations can be made about homosexuals as a group.[64]

Studies related to homosexuality are often poorly conceived, based on inadequate sampling procedures or on nonsystematic observation of individuals under psychiatric care. Research must be directed in the natural history of homosexuality, its components, and outcomes. Epidemiologic research is especially needed.[65]

NURSING IMPLICATIONS

Nursing care of the ill or hospitalized homosexual individual is discussed in Chapter 14, since homosexuals may be discriminated against by nurses because of ignorance about homosexuality, fear of homosexuals based on that ignorance, or beliefs about the immorality of homosexuality. Nurses must be in touch with their own feelings and must recognize when negative feelings compromise the care that they give. Haphazard and minimal care may be provided by nurses, not out of malice, but because of discomfort with relating to someone with a different sexual orientation. Staff meetings and conferences can do much to reduce nurses' anxiety and, one hopes, some of their prejudices against someone different from themselves.

BISEXUALITY

Bisexuals or ambisexuals, are individuals who will not define themselves in sexually restrictive ways. They can respond to various persons, and different sexes, and do not avoid chances for various types of sexual activity. Bisexuality can refer to sexual behavior or to sexual identity. Bisexuals may experience sexual interaction with both sexes during any time period and during any period of the life cycle. They may alternate between homosexual and heterosexual activity for long periods of time.

Bisexuality in the male may be considered a subgroup within the spectrum of homosexuality and usually implies a high degree of masculine identification. Bisexual marriages differ from the arrangements of exclusive homosexuals who live in a usually sexless marriage of convenience in that there is more commitment to the union. Children may be born. The bisexual individual's heterosexual activity may range from only one woman whom he marries, to a moderate degree of promiscuity. The homosexual component may be continually present or it may appear from time to time. Even with a satisfying marital relationship gay activities occur as "slip-ups" in self-discipline as the husband experiences irrepressible longing for a male companion.

There is a question whether the bisexual person's feelings can be as intense for women as those of exclusive heterosexual orientation. For some it may be, but the intensity of sexual gratification with the female rarely equals that of homosexual relations. In mar-

riage, the male may have to use homosexual imagery or pornography or else use a fetish device to maintain interest and potency.[66]

Many people are moving from exclusive heterosexuality or homosexuality to bisexuality. Gay males linked to the gay movement and some women in gay activist organizations are shifting to bisexuality. Some media idols are openly bisexual and others may indulge in bisexual activities in order to appear sophisticated and cosmopolitan.[67]

TRANSSEXUALISM

Transsexualism is a disorder of gender identity and the most extreme type of gender reversal. It is a belief by an anatomically normal person that he or she is a member of the opposite sex. In this sense, the anatomic male, for example, feels he has a woman's mind trapped in a man's body.[68] Data are sparse in relation to numbers of transsexuals. The prevalence in males has been estimated from 1 in 20,000 to 1 in 40,000, but for females there are no reliable data, although it is thought to be one-third to one-half as common.[69]

In the narrowest sense, the term refers to the most feminine of males and the most masculine of females and those who have been so since any gender behavior occurred. They may have never had any period of masculinity or femininity such as heterosexual activity or marriage.[70] The gender reversal is present as soon as "masculine" or "feminine" behavior begins, as early as 1 year of age. As gender identity develops, there is no behavior noted that is appropriate to the sex; rather the person continues the behavior begun in early childhood. The individual has a continuing sense of incongruity between the assigned sex and the gender identity. These individuals represent only one group of transsexuals. There are other transsexuals who have lived an apparently "normal" life appropriate to their anatomic sex, marrying and having children.

Bio-psycho-social Variables and Etiology

The cause of male transsexualism may be an excessively close symbiotic relationship between mother and child. When signs of femininity appear, the mother defines them as graceful and appealing. The child has no interest in masculine activities and spontaneously takes part in girl's activities. By age 5 or 6 he is committed to his gender identity.[71]

In such a family, the father is usually absent, ineffectual, or hostile. The child perceives the father as a weak and a relatively distant figure but sees the mother as strong and protective. Being a girl seems more natural than being a boy.[72]

Hellman[73] and associates found that the probability of an individual being transsexual is greatest when there was extensive cross-gender behavior as a child.

In female transsexualism, the infant may not be seen as pretty or cuddly, but as strong and vigorous. In some cases, the mother may be absent, depressed or have a severe physical or psychologic illness resulting in inadequate mothering. The father may use the girl to help cope with the wife's problems. He also may encourage masculine behavior—she is like his boy, taking part in hobbies and activities.[74] In both sexes, parents may not be worried about gender dysphoric behavior, do not discourage it, and may even encourage it.[75]

Some experts speculate that transsexualism may be the result of genetic, hormonal, or central nervous system factors or a combination of these factors. The theory of neuroendocrine etiology implies that there are definite inborn psychologic differences in the sexes. In the fetal male, androgen is necessary for masculinization. Without androgen, the male develops along female lines. If for some reason androgenization of sex-specific areas of the hypothalamus does not occur, or in females, if androgenic influences in the fetal hypothalamus are increased, transsexualism may be the result. The fetus may receive enough hormonal stimulation to develop external and internal genitalia, but in the critical period before birth, it does not receive adequate stimulation for neural differentiation, so that a difference exists between biologic gender and perceived gender.[76]

Another theory is that of competitive blocking of the steroid reception cells in the brain by various drugs taken by the mother—actinomycin D, pentobarbital, some phenothiazines. These drugs compete with testosterone for these sites and keep the brain of a male fetus from being masculinized. In laboratory animals, severe stressing of the mother also produces steroids that compete with testosterone for the receptor cells.[77]

Treatment of Transsexualism

The male transsexual is repelled by his male body and everything that reminds him of his masculinity. Some believe that they are a "victim of a cruel joke" and resist efforts to restore masculine identity.

Behavior modification has been attempted as treatment of the feminine boy. Femininity is discouraged and masculine activity and its pleasures are encouraged. The mother is treated so that she will not sabotage the boy's treatment and draw him back to her. Attempts to involve the fathers in treatment have been unsuccessful, since these men usually remove themselves from the families.[78]

Psychotherapy of the adult transsexual boy in mid to late childhood may sometimes be successful, but it is usually fruitless in the adolescent or adult transsexual. No treatment has been reported that will make the adult male transsexual masculine or the female feminine.

Surgery for Sexual Reassignment

The true transsexual wants his/her genitalia and physical appearance changed to conform with his/her sexual identity. A transsexual describes feelings of alienation from society; spouse, children, and friends may desert him or her.

Psychologic Aspects. Transsexuals have deep feelings of loneliness and isolation. Many experience intense anxiety to the point of becoming suicidal. There are now a number of gender dysphoria (basic disturbances of sexual identity such as transsexualism and transvestism) clinics in the country. Some do not offer precounseling or treatment, but others use extensive long-term evaluation before any surgery and long-term followup after surgery. More people are seeking help as the media spread information about surgical techniques to effect structural changes in the external genitalia.

Great care is taken to determine if the individual is a candidate for a sex change operation. Each person has a different personality structure and a different tolerance of stress. The purposes of the observation are (1) to eliminate persons who are psychotic with delusions of sex change, effeminate homosexuals, and fetishistic transvestites; (2) to test the patient's ability to live and pass as a member of the opposite sex; and (3) to administer hormone therapy to affect secondary sex changes.[79] The sex change team must be sure that the desire for sex change is an irreversible behavioral status rather than a reactive and changeable state.

There is an initial interview, with a psychologic and medical examination as well as psychologic evaluation of the patient's siblings and parents. Psychometric testing is done along with chromosomal and endocrine studies. During the 6 to 24 months before surgery, psychologic counseling, cross-gender role training, and legal advice are given.[80]

In some clinics, patients have individual sessions, first with a clinician of one sex, then with one of the opposite sex. Transsexuals often have very stereotyped ideas about sex roles. Females want to become macho-type males, and males desire to stay in and clean house. Part of the preoperative therapy involves helping them overcome sexist attitudes.

Some transsexuals have fantasies about becoming immortal through sex change surgery. These fantasies may relate to their despondent and lonely existence.

Sociologic Aspects—Living the New Sex. Patients are encouraged to move into the new social role while they are undergoing hormonal therapy. Some are already living as the desired sex, while others change jobs, move to different towns, and assume first names appropriate to the sex. In the married transsexual, this may involve breaking up of the family and leaving the significant others. So strong is the drive to change sex that many transsexuals do so. However, the relationship has often deteriorated before the move.

The interval of living as the new sex may be anywhere from 6 months to 2 years, depending on the treatment regimen. The patient is to experience first hand the day-to-day living in the new life. This may involve the social and political consequences of the change. Men living as women may discover that employers treat women differently. The therapist working with the patient helps him meet these challenges.[81]

Biologic Factors

Hormone Treatment. The male patients are femininized by the administration of both estrogen and progesterone. The hormones develop the breast, soften the skin, and reduce body hair. The frequency of erections and libidinous conflict is also decreased by suppressing testicular and androgen production. Beards are removed by electrolysis, and some patients take voice training to raise the pitch of the voice.

The female patient is given testosterone to cause masculinization by deepening the voice, coarsening the skin, and increasing body hair. Hypertrophy of the clitoris and cessation of the menstruation also occur. If hormonal therapy is discontinued, these changes are essentially reversible, except for the voice change and beard growth in the female.

Surgical Treatment for the Anatomic Male.
For the male, the first surgical intervention
was in 1931 in Europe. It involves orchiectomy and vaginoplasty in either a one-step or
two-step procedure. The vagina is formed by
dissecting a plane between the prostate and
the rectum and lining the cavity with penile
and/or scrotal skin after the corpora cavernosa and most of the urethra is removed.[82]

To maintain the shape of the vagina in
the immediate postoperative period, a mold
or vaginal splint is inserted after surgery. It
is worn continuously for several weeks. Once
healing is complete manual dilation or penile
penetration is necessary to prevent narrowing through contraction of scar tissue.

Complications are not common; the more
usual include vaginal stricture or stenosis,
rectovaginal fistula, urethral stenosis, and
pressure necrosis from a rigid splint. Anuria
results from urethral stenosis. Brachial plexus palsy can occur from the position on the
operating room table.

Patients are usually discharged 2 weeks
after surgery. By 6 to 8 weeks, healing is
advanced. In 2 to 3 months, the individual
may have sexual intercourse.

If the patient is not satisfied with the
primary operation, especially if the vagina
does not seem long enough, or if sloughing or
stenosis of the neovagina occur, vaginal reconstruction using parts of the cecum or the
sigmoid is performed. The sigmoid colon
gives the deepest vagina.[83]

Many of the anatomically male patients
also opt for breast augmentation, usually by
the insertion of implants. Some patients seek
surgical reduction of the Adam's apple and
rhinoplasty. When the transsexual male-to-
female has sexual intercourse, she must use
a lubricant, since she has no natural
lubrication.

*Surgical Treatment for the Anatomic Fe-
male.* This treatment involves a reduction
mammoplasty or a mastectomy, hysterectomy, and sometimes oophorectomy. It is possible to construct a penis surgically by rotat-

ing a flap of skin from the left lower
quadrant of the abdomen and closing the vaginal orifice. So the organ can be used for
urination, a urinary conduit from a portion of
the small intestine can be inserted through
the phallus, although most surgeons prefer
to leave the urinary orifice in its original
position. The new penis lacks sensation and
cannot become erect. However, preservation
of clitoris in the base of the penis serves as a
source of stimulation in intercourse. The artificial vagina is more functional than the
artificial penis, but patients in both groups
have reported orgasms postoperatively. To
attain erection, the female-to-male transsexual inserts a rubber rod in the phallus for
intercourse.

The patients continue to receive maintenance hormone therapy postoperatively.
Without it, they would experience symptoms
of climacteric, hot flashes, and decrease in
general body tone. The discomfort and pain is
considered worthwhile, and the patients are
generally delighted with their new bodies
and are indistinguishable from their
neighbors.

Life Style After Surgery. Many transsexuals are very open about their condition,
about surgery when they have it, and about
their life styles. Some live a very conventional life style, others, especially the male-
to-female transsexuals, try to out-do being a
woman, seeking constant attention from
males as prostitutes, showgirls, or strippers.
Some go through a short period of promiscuity right after surgery, others continue for
a longer period of time.

A group of 23 male-to-female transsexuals seemed happier after the operation.
Eighteen reported satisfactory sexual relations and 13 reported multiple orgasms.[84]

The typical pattern of sexual activity
was heterosexual after the operation, as most
male-to-female individuals preferred males
as partners.

Longer-term followup to observe the effects of estrogen therapy is needed. Patients

should have a yearly breast examination, since the gynecomastia is a cancer hazard, and a routine palpation of the prostate.

Legal Status. Legal confirmation of the new sexual status involves getting a legal name change by court order and then applying for changes on official papers and documents, such as social security records, driver's license, and passports. It is more difficult to get changes in the birth certificate. Some states will issue certificates with the new name and sex; in other states, only the name will be changed, not the sex.[85]

Long-term Effects of Surgery. Psychiatrists are questioning whether surgery makes a major improvement in mental health. Studies show that the vast majority of patients do not reject their decisions and are subjectively improved, but there is less objective improvement and the complete picture is still unclear.[86,87]

Fifty percent of a group of male-to-female patients reported phantom penis sensation, ejaculatory sensation, despite removal of all male tissue. This may indicate that the female body image, self-concept, and gender identity continues to be influenced by the prior male identity.

Postsurgery male-to-female transsexuals had episodes of depressed affect, suicidal thoughts and behavior, and insecurity, although they had no regrets about surgery. Female-to-male transsexuals also had depressed affect and psychic conflict and the surgery caused further gender confusion. The major issue of gender role and identity did not seem to be resolved by sex reassignment surgery in this group. Psychotherapy is still an important treatment after surgery.[88]

NURSING IMPLICATIONS

Staff Attitudes
The attitudes of the nursing and medical staff toward the transsexual patient may be negative. The male-to-female transsexuals seem to be the focus of negative comments and jokes in particular. These patients are struggling for acceptance as women, and it is in the immediate postoperative period that they can try out their new identity. They may be viewed as "weirdos" and "freaks" and may be severely troubled by remarks they overhear.

The male-to-female transsexuals arrive at the hospital with suitcases full of toiletries and clothes. They often seem bent on exaggerating femininity, wearing bright makeup, false eyelashes, and extremely feminine-appearing clothes. They may walk up and down the halls in sheer, low-cut, frilly nightgowns and negligees and behave very seductively toward male members of the staff. Much time may be spent curling their hair and putting on makeup. Off-color jokes and expressions may be a prominent part of their conversation. Many of these behaviors may tend to alienate staff members and may result in inadequate nursing care, unless the staff who will be caring for these patients is prepared. Attitudes, feelings, and biases should be examined. Staff may feel that the surgery is unethical or immoral.[89] and that it is not indicated—that the sexual dysphoria is not life threatening and the individuals should be able to live with their feelings.

Group sessions with the psychologist and knowledgeable nurses will help dispel misconceptions about the patients. The nurses soon see that these are patients who need help, who may feel life is not worth living, and for whom surgery is the last hope.

Preoperative Care
A consistent, accepting approach by all the staff members is essential. The male-to-female transsexual is addressed by his woman's name and is placed in a private room unless there are two transsexuals in the same division.

The patient has been told by the physician that the procedure will cause discomfort, that contrary to some popular belief conception is not possible for the male-to-female transsexual, and that the penis in the female-to-male transsexual will not have erectile ability.

Postoperative Care—Meeting Physiologic Needs

Assessment. As with any surgical patient, continual assessment of the patient's ability to meet basic needs is necessary. For the transsexual patients, particular attention should be given to level of comfort, signs of infection, the integrity of the surgical site, adequacy of elimination, and nutrition.

Intervention

Maintaining Comfort. The patients may experience considerable pain after surgery. The nurse should carefully assess for signs of discomfort and give medication regularly. The danger exists that medication may be postponed by nurses who, because of conscious or unconscious disapproval of the procedure, feel that the patient deserves punishment. The values and negative feelings of the staff should not result in medication being withheld.[90]

Preventing Infection. Massive perineal reconstruction is performed. The extensive surgery along with the proximity to the anal area predisposes to infection. Skin care and cleanliness are vital but may be difficult to achieve because of the patient's discomfort. Sitz baths may be prescribed both for cleansing and for promoting comfort. Giving pain medication before any cleansing procedure will make it more tolerable. The perineum is cleansed carefully after bowel movements, and the patient is taught to wipe from the vaginal area toward the anus after bowel movements to prevent bacteria from being carried up to the surgical site.[91]

Preserving Integrity of the Surgical Site. In the male-to-female patient, a mold is inserted immediately after the operation to preserve the vaginal cavity. Constriction can easily develop and make the vagina nonfunc-

tional. The mold is rotated in place several times a day to prevent scar tissue from adhering to it. The nurse rotates the mold the first few days, when the procedure causes more discomfort. Later, the patient is taught to rotate the mold, and she continues to do this until healing is complete.[92]

The patients can usually have sexual intercourse 6 to 8 weeks postoperatively, and this will maintain the vagina's potency. If the patient does not have intercourse regularly, she must insert the mold to maintain the cavity and its elasticity.

Maintaining Elimination. In the male-to-female patient, a catheter is inserted at the time of surgery, and careful assessment must be made of urine output, color, consistency, and amount. Because of the extensive perineal reconstruction and the proximity to the bladder, the bladder or urethra may be traumatized. The catheter is removed 8 to 10 days postoperatively, and the nurse should assist the patient in voiding, since this is the first experience with voiding as a female. The nurse should note the strength and direction of the urinary stream.

Meeting Nutritional Needs. The male-to-female transsexual still has her former appetite. If hospital servings are too small, she may hesitate to ask for extra food, considering a large appetite too masculine a trait. The nurse can decrease this embarrassment by reminding the patient that she will still have the same dietary habits even after her surgery.[93] In addition, for several days postoperatively, some physicians may order a clear liquid diet to delay the first bowel movement and lessen chance of contamination of the surgical site.

Postoperative Care—Meeting Psychosocial Needs

The postoperative transsexual patients are usually delighted with their new bodies, and the surgery is seen by them as the resolution of their identity crises. It may be so, but it also initiates their struggles to live as women or men and to be accepted as women and men by the rest of the community.

Assessment.
The nurse should evaluate the patients' feelings about the surgery postoperatively. Are they satisfied? What are their fears, insecurities, and concerns about relating to others and their future lives? Do they feel, perhaps unrealistically, that "all will be fine"? Are the patients depressed, and do they know the reasons for the feelings? Are they concerned about their appearance—usually whether they look, act, and talk like someone of their sex should?

Have they made realistic plans for the future? Since many of the patients have been living as the desired sex before surgery, this may not present a problem, but others may have concerns about jobs, housing, and family relationships. Is the help of a social worker needed if one is not already involved in the patient's care?

What are their spiritual needs? Does the patient wish to see a clergyman? Do they have some spiritual beliefs from which they draw strength? How can the nurse help them to use these coping means?

Planning.
In planning care, the nurse recognizes that the transsexual patient focuses primarily on self and the new body, that he or she is now a new person mentally and physically. The nurse's goal is to help the individual resolve feelings of doubt and to work toward a positive acceptance of self and a satisfying life.

Intervention
Resolving the Patient's Feelings of Doubt.
Although the surgery has been eagerly anticipated, patients may have doubts about their ability to function in their new role. The male-to-female patient is delighted to have lost a penis that was a source of shame or anxiety, but she may worry that she will not be feminine enough. The female-to-male patient may have similar fears. Acceptance by the staff does much to dispel these fears.[94]

Establishing Relationships. Patients may have difficulty in establishing relationships with their family. If they are married, some have close relationships with their spouse and children and may try to stay with the family. Unfortunately, this may fail. Family members may have to seek therapy. The nurse may have to be a supportive listener.

The body of the transsexual individual is changing and maturing in terms of gender characteristics, and the individual is in the process of developing his or her identity as an adult man or woman. Like adolescents, they are extremely self-conscious of their appearance and search for role models, often an idealized person of the new gender.[95]

Female nurses can act as nonthreatening role models for the female patients, offering the way they dress, use makeup, sit, and walk as a resource for the patient. They can answer questions about how one acts when going out with someone of the opposite sex. A male nurse can be a special source of support for the female-to-male patient, answering questions similar to those addressed to female nurses.

Use of communication and teaching principles is vital (see Chapter 11). Patients may need to be confronted with behavior that is inappropriate and to have limits set if the behavior is disruptive to the division. Nurses who are comfortable in their own feminine or masculine roles can do this without being unduly harsh or punitive.

Evaluation.
The transsexual can best judge if the nurse's intervention was helpful in his or her achieving a satisfactory adjustment to the surgery. Expression of pleasure with the altered body, with appearance, and with self all indicate that the individual is adjusting.

TRANSVESTISM

Transvestism may be confused with homosexuality and transsexuality. Stoller[96] defines it as fetishistic cross-dressing, that is, sexual excitement is caused by wearing the garments of the opposite sex. This behavior is found almost exclusively in males. It usually starts in adolescence but may be first seen in the prepubertal boys and adult men in their 30s or 40s.

Cross-gender dressing may be a feature of all gender disorders, but the clinical features vary. Most transvestites are overtly heterosexual, are married and have children, work in professions that require masculine interests and hobbies, and dress in masculine clothes except when cross-dressed. They do not usually wish to be females, cross-dress intermittently, and spend most of the time as males.

The males obtain intense sexual gratification when in women's clothes and have histories of masculine development, unlike the transsexual male who has had gender identity problems from early life and who does not get sexual gratification when in women's clothes.

Croughan and associates.[97] in an interview study of 70 male members of a cross-dressing club, found that in early development cross-dressing is almost always associated with sexual arousal and behavior, usually masturbation. Later in adult life, it is more frequently associated with heterosexual intercourse. During late adult life there is a trend toward a more asexual nature.

On the basis of a study of 124 subjects at a Gender Identity Clinic, Freund and associates[98] concluded that over time transvestites or borderline transsexuals may develop cross-gender identity and that transsexuality is almost always preceded by transvestism or accompanied by homosexuality or cross-gender fetishism.

The activity is usually secretive. The man may dress in his wife's clothes, wearing something, such as a bra, or everything, including makeup. Others may find other men who share their interest or, if married, involve the wife in the activity. A few end up in later life as women with penises.

Etiology—Bio-psycho-social Factors

No biologic cause has been identified. Some hypogonadal males (those with Klinefelter's syndrome) may have transvestic traits. In about half the cases, the behavior may follow a situation where the young male is forced to wear women's clothes in humiliating circumstances, usually by a mother or other female, as a means of punishment. This may result in an attack on the boy's masculine identity. Later, the boy finds the cross-dressing enjoyable.

Treatment

Psychotherapy or psychoanalysis is not usually successful. Some behavior modification techniques have been used in some cases. These individuals are rarely motivated to change unless compelled to by wife or family. Some wives describe their anxiety that the children might see their father cross-dressed.

DIFFERENTIATION BETWEEN HOMOSEXUALITY, TRANSSEXUALITY, AND TRANSVESTISM

Many homosexuals have cross-gender qualities. These occur in a continuum, so that male homosexuals may have no effeminate qualities while others evidence persistent effeminacy. Lesbians may range from nonmasculine to extremely masculine in appearance and behavior. Homosexuals consider themselves male or female in congruence with their biologic sex and have no wish to change sex. However, they obtain sexual gratification from those of the same sex. They like their genitals and feel their organs are appropriate. The vast majority are not interested in sex change, and rarely is there sexual excitement from wearing clothes of the opposite sex.

Transsexuals have strong psychic identification with the opposite anatomic sex and consider themselves to be the opposite sex trapped in the wrong body. Transsexuals frequently cross-dress, not to obtain sexual gratification per se, but in accordance with their perceived maleness or femaleness. They have sexual relationships with members of the same anatomic sex, but do not consider this activity homosexual. If one believes himself a female, it is natural to have sexual activity with a male or vice versa.

The transvestite considers himself a male, seeks females as sexual partners, but gets intense sexual gratification from wearing female clothes. Benjamin and Ihlenfield[99] describe the transvestite as having some degree of gender identity conflict, which could be in a continuum with the transsexual. The primary distinction from the transsexual is the lesser degree of gender discomfort and the measures necessary to relieve the discomfort, which involve only cross-dressing.

VARIATIONS IN SEXUAL AIM

Stayton[100] argues for the normality of all types of erotic relationships: with same sex, household or farm pets, inanimate objects (autos, bicycles, chairs, banisters). He sees the universe as a potential erotic "turn-on" indicting religion and culture for limiting sexual activity to exert control and power over peoples.

Many vehemently disagree with his arguments, while others turn to and do utilize other methods for achievement of sexual gratification. Activities that provide sexual satisfaction to some are considered abnormal and perverse by others. Some are punishable by law.

Exhibitionism

Exhibitionism is the display of the genitals before one or more strangers, usually in a public place. It occurs in males about 15 times as often as in females, the typical onset being 14 to 17 years of age.

The compulsive male exhibitionist is neither shameless nor aggressive but is usually beset with feelings of masculine inadequacy. He seeks to shock his victims, not to seduce or harm them. Erotic pleasure is not usually sought or desired, but he seeks to reduce a state of inner pressure and tension. The prodromal period of irritability, restlessness, tension, and headache lends some weight to the theory that exhibitionism is linked to abnormal discharges in the temporal lobes.

The legal term *indecent exposure* is not strictly synonymous with the medical term, but all exposure is a punishable offense. Symptomatic exhibitionism occurs in a variety of personality disorders—the pathologic drinker, middle-aged and elderly men with organic brain syndrome, those with psychopathic personalities, the mentally retarded. These are all potentially dangerous sex offenders.

Treatment of the compulsive exhibitionist usually involves psychiatric care. Sometimes discovery sends them to the physician. Fear of prison sentence or public censure will also cause them to seek help. Regular social and recreational interests are encouraged, especially if the individual tends to isolate himself. Alcohol consumption is discouraged. The wife of the married exhibitionist can supply him with sympathetic support, a necessity if treatment is to be successful. Group psychotherapy, use of psychodrama and hypnosis, and behavior modification have been successful.[101]

Voyeurism, or Peeping Tomism

Voyeurism, or peeping tomism, is observation of erotically stimulating sights and especially viewing of another's genitals. Occasional peeping in childhood and adolescence is frequent. If it occurs later, it is an immaturity reaction. Peeping is almost universal, but is more frequent in males. The typical voyeur's interest is focused on women, and the more he is able to see or imagine, the greater is the sexual excitement. These men do not usually accost the women they spot, since they are afraid, passive, and socially inhibited.

Looking must be surreptitious and actually displaces penovaginal intercourse as the stimulus to orgasm. The voyeur who has a partner builds up arousal by prior peeping on a stranger or, during intercourse, replays images of peeping as a coital fantasy. Otherwise, he has no orgasm.[102]

Paul Gebhard and associates[103] found that the most common type of peepers have less heterosexual experience than is customary for their age and socioeconomic status, are shy with females, and have strong feelings of inferiority. They almost never watch females they know well. A substantial number masturbate while peeping.

The compulsive or habitual peepers are driven or obsessed individuals who consistently seek opportunities for peeping and are sexually aroused. A few commit rape, especially those who enter buildings to peep or who deliberately try to attract the woman's attention. Some psychopathic personalities and mental retardates may move from visual excitement into varying degrees of aggressiveness.[104]

Fetishism

Fetishism is erotic excitement by a particular part of the body, frilly underwear, leather, or other clothes. For most, the excitation caused by fetishism is discharged through intercourse or masturbation with the handling of the object as part of foreplay. In others, the fetishistic object becomes the source of both excitement and gratification.[105]

Masochism and Sadomasochism

Masochists obtain sexual gratification if they are hurt or humiliated by the partner as a part of ritualized activity. The true masochist is not just a passive recipient of pain. He arranges and induces the humiliation and may prescribe the amount of physical and psychic suffering he needs.

Sadism is sexual plasure from debasing, tormenting, or hurting of another person. The two terms are sometimes linked to form one word, *sadomasochism,* since individuals stimulated by one activity may be stimulated by the other also.

The term *sadism* is derived from the Marquis de Sade, a novelist who suffered from this anomaly. Sadists often obtain satisfaction even when the activity is an act, the victim usually a prostitute who simulates suffering. They methodically and ritualistically plan their activities. It is believed that the male sadist does not like women, although he is capable of heterosexual intercourse.

Sadomasochism is extremely complex. Some individuals achieve orgasm during the pain; in other cases, sadomasochism is the foreplay and the session ends in conventional sexual behavior. Some masochists dislike the pain while receiving it, but obtain gratification by anticipation of pain or by thinking about it after it has stopped. "Bondage" people do not enjoy pain but are stimulated by constraint, mild discomfort, and a sense of helplessness.

Sadomasochism seems the monopoly of well developed civilizations. There do not seem to have been any de Sades among Plains Indians or Aztecs. Sexual activity of some preliterate societies did involve moderate biting and scratching, but not well developed sadomasochistic activities. Gebhard[106] believes it may be that society must be complex and heavily reliant on symbolism before the repressions and frustrations of life can be expressed symbolically by sadomasochism. Sadomasochism is suited to symbolism. It gives proof of power and status by inflicting humiliation and pain on someone who does not retaliate and proof of love by enduring and seeking such treatment.

Various tools are used in the sadistic–masochistic scene (the S–M scene). In the United States, knife cutting, cigarette burns, and rope tying are the usual types. Enemas, "animal training," handcuffs, paddles, leg irons, and rawhide are frequently used, and leather especially is a frequent symbol.[107]

Other Variations: Therapy

Anal intercourse (buggery) is common in male homosexuals. Sometimes the male insistence on anal intercourse in a heterosexual relationship is intended to degrade or subjugate the partner.

Necrophilia is intercourse with a dead body. Bestiality is sexual activity with an animal. It is rare and often occurs with unavailability of human contact. Pedophilia is sexual activity with children.

Persons who seek sexual gratification through fetishism, transvestism, sadism, masochism, pedophilia, exhibitionism, and voyeurism have been treated with Depo-Provera (medroxyprogesterone acetate) and have had dramatic relief from these behaviors. The drug seems to exert a calming effect on the brain limbic and hypothalamic arousal system. The effects of the drug include decreased sexual drive, decreased ability to have an erection and ultimately orgasm.[108]

CELIBACY

Celibacy is a conscious decision to refrain from sexual activity. The term as used here applies to volitional situations and does not apply to situations in which sexual abstinence is forced on the individual—the death of a spouse, breakup of a heterosexual or homosexual relationship, unavailability of a sexual partner. The celibate is one who makes an ideologic choice, not one who simply refrains from sexual interaction or for whom sexual interaction is unavailable.

Levels and Types

Complete or Partial. De Lora and Warren[109] identify two levels of celibacy: complete and partial. Complete celibacy is refraining from any volitional sexual tension release, including masturbation. Involuntary sexual response, such as orgasm during erotic dreams, cannot be excluded from response and may occur.

Interpersonal or partial celibacy allows masturbation but no other form of sexual activity, such as oral, anal, and manual stimulation with others.

Experiential Celibacy. This type involves practicing celibacy as another sexual option, either before or after experiencing other varieties of sexual activity. It does not involve any particular ideology or community of celibates.

Religious Celibacy. This form is related to a belief system or ideology. Roman Catholic priests, Lutheran deaconesses, Roman Catholic and Anglican sisters, and some members of Eastern sects live in celibate chastity. Others, not in religious communities, practice celibacy by choice for moral or religious reasons.

In an interview for the press, the feelings of Catholic sisters who practice celibacy were shared.[110]

Celibacy is an expression of personal love of God in imitation of Jesus.

The vow is an unique gift, directing a woman's affective life, her sexual activity toward God. . . . Celibacy is experienced as the freedom to love without hope of return, to love the unlovable,

Living out the vow of celibacy joyfully and faithfully speaks out against the negative aspect and excesses of the sexual revolution.

It contradicts attitudes where infidelity and failure to keep commitments is a way of life.

It makes positive contributions to the women's movement since it is an affirming that a person is a person first and not secondary to a sex function.

It provides insight into the sexuality of the woman herself as a total person, not as an individual dichotomized into body, spirit and soul.

The Catholic sisters described celibacy as more freeing than binding, a personal mystery, and releasing them to be "the best me." Others emphasized that marriage was also a beautiful way of life and that celibacy was not a denial or rejection of sex, but a choice of another loving way of life, one that did not use genitality. Some admitted that "it is hard" and that "we can't say that we're happy all the time."[111]

Feminist Celibacy. Political and social ideology is the basis of feminist celibacy. Some women enter freely into periods of temporary celibacy, freeing themselves from a sexual relationship in order to mobilize energy for work, children, or friends. Celibacy is described as giving back integrity, privacy, and pride; freeing and growth-producing; a time to define themselves, not just in terms of another person. Some argue that sexual relationships create anxieties and distractions that keep women from self-awareness.[112]

Some feminists ban not only sexual interaction but all love relationships with men, believing that the romantic mystique of love, perhaps even more than sexual domination, is at the root of male oppression of women.[113]

Celibacy for Health. Complete or partial celibacy may be practiced for medical reasons (although medical indications for celibacy are infrequent). The health–medicine belief systems, such as yoga, stress celibacy as a means of maximizing the energy levels of the body and achieving higher levels of consciousness.[114]

NOTES

1. Marmor J: Homosexuality and sexual orientation disturbances. In Sadock BJ, Kaplan HI, Freedman AM (eds): The Sexual Experience. Baltimore, Williams and Wilkins, 1976, pp 374–390
2. Bell AP: The homosexual as a patient. In Green R (ed): Human Sexuality: A Health Practitioner's Text. Baltimore, Williams and Wilkins, 1975, pp 55–74
3. Kinsey AC, Pomeroy WB, Martin CE: Sexual Behavior in the Human Male. Philadelphia, Saunders, 1948, pp 650–651
4. Kinsey AC, Pomeroy WB, Martin CE, Gebhard PH: Sexual Behavior in the Human Female. New York, Pocket Books, 1965, pp 452–454
5. Bell AP Weinberg MA: Homosexualities: A study of diversity among men and women. New York, Simon and Schuster, 1978
6. Whitman FL: Culturally invariable properties of male homosexuality: Tentative conclusions from cross-cultural research. Arch Sex Behav 12:207–226, 1983
7. Spitzer RL: A proposal about homosexuality and the APA nomenclature: Homosexuality as an irregular from of sexual behavior and sexual orientation disturbance as a psychiatric disorder. Am J. Psychiatry 130:1214–1216, 1973
8. Ibid, p 1208
9. Green R: Homosexuality as a mental illness. In Caplan AL, Engelhardt HT, McCartney JJ (eds): Concepts of Health and Disease. Interdisciplinary Perspectives. Reading MA, Addison-Wesley, 1981, pp 333–352
10. Freedman RC, Green R, Spitzer RL: Reassessment, homosexuality and transsexualism. Annu Rev Med 27:57–62, 1976
11. Bell AP; The homosexual as a patient. In Green R (ed): Human Sexuality: A Health Practitioner's Text. Baltimore, Williams and Wilkins, 1975, p 70
12. Bell AP, Weinberg MS: Homosexualities: A Study of Human Diveristy. New York, Simon and Schuster, 1978, pp 195–216
13. Time, February 20, 1978, p 102
14. Ruse M: Are homosexuals sick: In Caplan AL, Engelhardt HT, McCartney JJ (eds): Concepts of Health and Disease. Interdisciplinary Perspectives. Reading MA, Addison-Wesley, 1981, pp 693–724
15. Macculloch MJ: Male homosexual behavior. Practitioner 225:1635–1641, 1981
16. Ehrhardt AA, Meyer-Bahlburg HFL: Effects of prenatal hormones on gender related behavior. Science 211:1312–1323, 1981
17. Pardridge WM: Androgens and sexual behavior. Ann Int Med 96:488–501, 1982
18. Freedman RC, Green R, Spitzer RL; Reassessment, homosexuality, and transsexualism. Annu Rev Med 27:57–62, 1976

19. Marmor J: Homosexuality and sexual orientation disturbances. In Sadock BJ, Kaplan HI, Freedman AM (eds): The Sexual Experience. Baltimore, Williams and Wilkins, 1976, pp 377–378

20. Freud S: Three Contributions to the Theory of Sex, 4th ed. New York, Nervous and Mental Disease Publishing, 1930, p 85

21. Marmor J: Homosexuality and sexual orientation disturbances. In Sadock BJ, Kaplan HI, Freedman AM (eds): The Sexual Experience. Baltimore, Williams and Wilkins, 1976, p 377

22. Bieber I: Homosexuality—An Adaptive consequence of disorder in psychosexual development, Am J Psychiatry 130:1209–1211, 1973

23. Bieber I: Homosexuality. Am J Nurs 69:2637–2641, 1969

24. Ibid, p 2640

25. Siegelman M: Parental background of male homosexuals and heterosexuals. Arch Sex Behav 3:3–18, 1974

26. Siegelman M: Parental backgrounds of homosexual and heterosexual men: A cross-national replication. Arch Sex Behav 10:505–512, 1981

27. Eisenbud E-J: Female homosexuality: A sweet enfranchisement. In Goldman GG, Milman DS: Modern Woman. Springfield, Illinois, Thomas, 1969, pp 247–271

28. Marmor J: Homosexuality and sexual orientation disturbances. In Sadock BJ, Kaplan HI, Freedman AM (eds): The Sexual Experience. Baltimore, Williams and Wilkins, 1976, p 384

29. Socarides CW: Beyond Sexual Freedom. New York, New York Times Book, 1975, p 33

30. Bell AP, Weinberg MS: Homosexualities: A Study of Human Diversity. New York, Simon and Schuster, 1978, p 78

31. Weinberg MS, Williams CJ: Male homosexuals: Their problems and adaptation. In Weinberg MS (ed): Sex Re-

search. New York, Oxford, 1976, pp 246–257

32. Ibid, p 253

33. Ibid, p 254

34. Weinberg MS, Williams CJ: Male homosexuals: Their problems and adaptation. In Weinberg MS (ed): Sex Research. New York, Oxford, 1976, p 256

35. Bell AP: The homosexual as a patient. In Green R (ed): Human Sexuality: A Health Practitioner's Text. Baltimore, Williams and Wilkins, 1975, p 63

36. Ibid, pp 64–65

37. Katchadourian HA, Lunde DT: Fundamentals of Human Sexuality. New York, Holt, 1975, p 330

38. Kenyon FE: Homosexuality in gynecological practice. Clin Obstet Gynecol 7:363–383, 1980

39. Sonenshein D: Male homosexual relationships. In Weinberg MS (ed): Sex Research. New York, Oxford, 1976, pp 140–155

40. Ibid, p 142

41. Ibid, p 143

42. Marmor J: Homosexuality and sexual orientation disturbances. In Sadock BJ, Kaplan HI, Freedman AM (eds): The Sexual Experience, Baltimore, Williams and Wilkins, 1976, p 381

43. Sonenshein D: Male homosexual relationships. In Weinberg MS (ed): Sex Research. New York, Oxford, 1976, p 152

44. Marmor J: Homosexuality and sexual orientation disturbances. In Sadock BJ, Kaplan HI, Freedman AM (eds): The Sexual Experience. Baltimore, Williams and Wilkins, 1976, p 383

45. Kenyon FE: Homosexuality in gynecological practice. Clin Obstet Gynecol 7:381, 1980

46. Bell AP: The homosexual as a patient. In Green R (ed): Human Sexuality: A Health Practitioner's Text. Baltimore, Williams and Wilkins, 1975, p 65

47. Weinberg MS, Williams CJ: Male homosexuals: Their problems and adaptation. In Weinberg MS (ed): Sex Re-

search. New York, Oxford, 1976, pp 250–251

48. Socarides CW: Beyond Sexual Freedom. New York, New York Times Book, 1975, p 105

49. Daling JR, Weiss NS, Klopfenstein LL, et al: Correlates of homosexual behavior and the incidence of anal cancer. J Am Med Ass 247:1988–1990, 1982

50. Kavanagh J: Lesbians' attitudes toward traditional health care. Unpublished masters thesis. Francis Payne Bolton School of Nursing, Case Western Reserve University, 1979

51. Time, September 8, 1975, pp 32–43

52. Ibid, p 33

53. Ibid, p 45

54. Socarides CW: Beyond Sexual Freedom. New York, New York Times Book, 1975, p 921

55. Green R: Sexual identity of 37 children raised by homosexual or transsexual parents. Am J Psych 135:692–717, 1978

56. Schlatter T: Children need help to accept gay parents. The Plain Dealer, April 3, 1983, pp 14–17

57. Marmor J: Homosexuality and sexual orientation disturbances. In Sadock BJ, Kaplan HI, Freedman AM (eds): The Sexual Experience. Baltimore, Williams and Wilkins, 1976, pp 389–390

58. Bieber I: Homosexuality. Am J Nurs 69:2641, 1969

59. MacCulloch MJ: Waddington JL: Neuroendocrine mechanisms and the aetiology of male and female homosexuality. Brit J Psych 139:341–345, 1981

60. Oliven JF: Clinical Sexuality. Philadelphia, Lippincott, 1974, p 522

61. Boston Women's Health Book Collective: Our Bodies, Ourselves, 2nd ed. New York, Simon and Schuster, 1976, p 89

62. Marmor J: Homosexuality and sexual orientation disturbances. In Sadock BJ, Kaplan HI, Freedman, AM (eds): The Sexual Experience. Baltimore, Williams and Wilkins, 1976, p 388

63. Morin SF: Heterosexual bias in psychological research on lesbianism and male homosexuality. Am Psychologist, August 1977, pp 629–637

64. Ibid, 636

65. Saghir M: Homosexuality. In Green R, Weiner J (eds): Methodology in Sex Research. Rockville Maryland, Alcohol, Drug Abuse and Mental Health Administration, U.S. Department of Health and Human Services. Public Health Services, National Institute of Mental Health, 1982

66. Oliven JF: Clinical Sexuality, Philadelphia, Lippincott, 1974, pp 501–502

67. DeLora JS, Warren CAB: Understanding Sexual Interaction. Boston, Houghton Mifflin, 1977, pp 287–289

68. Benjamin H, Ihlenfield CL: Transsexualism. Am J Nurs 73:461–467, 1973

69. Freedman RC, Green R, Spitzer RL: Reassessment, homosexuality and transsexualism. Annu Rev Med 27:60, 1976

70. Stoller R: Gender identity. In Sadock BJ, Kaplan HI, Freedman AM (eds): The Sexual Experience, Baltimore, Williams and Wilkins, 1976, pp 182–195

71. Zugar B: Effeminate behavior in boys present from early childhood. J Pediatr 69:1098–1107, 1966

72. Stoller R: Gender identity. In Sadock BJ, Kaplan HI, Freedman AM (eds): The Sexual Experience. Baltimore, Williams and Wilkins, 1976, p 188

73. Hellman RE, Green R, Gray JL, Williams K: Childhood sexual identity, childhood religiosity, and "homophobia" as influences in the development of transsexualism, homosexuality, and heterosexuality. Arch Gen Psychiatry 38:910–915, 1981

74. Rowland WD: Surgery for sexual reassignment. AORN J 22:735–740, 1975

75. Jones SL, Tinker D: Transsexualism and the family: An interactional explanation. J Fam Ther 4:1–14, 1982

76. Money J, Ehrhardt AA: Man and Woman, Boy and Girl, Baltimore, Johns Hopkins University Press, 1972

77. Oliven JF: Clinical Sexuality. Philadelphia, Lippincott, 1974, p 489
78. Stoller R: Gender identity. In Sadock BJ, Kaplan HI, Freedman AM (eds): The Sexual Experience. Baltimore, Williams and Wilkins, 1976, p 190
79. Oliven JF: Clinical Sexuality. Philadelphia, Lippincott, 1974, p 490
80. Markland C: Transsexual surgery. Obstet Gynecol Annu, 1975, pp 309–327
81. Benjamin H, Ihlenfield CL: Transsexualism. Am J Nurs 73:460, 1973
82. Markland C: Transsexual surgery. Obstet Gynecol Annu, 1975, pp 311–328
83. Ibid, p 321
84. Ibid, pp 327–328
85. Rowland WD: Surgery for sexual reassignment. AORN J 22:740, 1975
86. Sørenson T: A follow-up study of operated transsexxual males. Acta Psychiat Scand 63:486–503, 1981
87. Sørenson T: A follow-up study of operated female transsexuals. Acta Psychiat Scand 64:50–64, 1981
88. Lothstein LM: The postsurgical transsexual: Empirical and theoretical considerations. Arch Sex Behav 9:547–566, 1980
89. Oles MN: The transsexual client: A discussion of transsexualism and issues in psychiatry. Am. J. Orthopsychiatry 47:66–74, 1977
90. Strait J: The transsexual patient after surgery. Am J Nurs 73:462–463, 1973
91. Faber H: Specifics of physical care. Am J Nurs 73:463, 1973
92. Ibid, p 463
93. Strait J: The transsexual patient after surgery. AM. J Nurs 73:463, 1973
94. Oles MN: The transsexual client: A discussion of transsexualism and issues in psychiatry. Am J Orthopsychiatry 47:67, 1977
95. Ibid, p 69
96. Stoller R: Gender identity. In Sadock BJ, Kaplan HI, Freedman AM (eds): The Sexual Experience Baltimore, Williams and Wilkins, 1976, p 192
97. Croughan JL, Saghir M, Cohen R, Robins E: A comparison of treated and untreated male cross-dressers. Arch Sex Behav 10:515–520, 1981
98. Freund K, Steiner BW, Chan S: Two types of cross-gender identity. Arch Sex Behav 11:49–63, 1982
99. Benjamin H, Ihlenfield CL: Transsexualism. Am J Nurs 73:459, 1973
100. Stayton WR: The theory of sexual orientation: The universe as a turn on. Top Clin Nurs 1:1–8, 1980
101. Oliven JF: Clinical Sexuality, Philadelphia, Lippincott, 1974, p 471
102. Money J: The development of sexuality and eroticism in humankind. Quart Rev Biol 56:379–403, 1981
103. Gebhard PH, Gagnon JH, Pomeroy WB, Christenson CV: Sex offenders: An analysis of types. In Weinberg MS (ed): Sexual Research. New York, Oxford, 1976, p 129
104. Oliven JF: Clinical Sexuality. Philadelphia, Lippincott, 1974, p 492
105. Brandon S: The range of sexual variations. Clin Obstet Gynecol 7:345–361, 1980
106. Gebhard PH, Gagnon JH, Pomeroy WB, Christenson CV: Fetishism and sadomasochism. In Weinberg MS (ed): Sex Research. New York, Oxford, 1974, pp 162–165
107. Oliven JF: Clinical Sexuality, Philadelphia, Lippincott, 1974, p 478
108. Kelly JR, Cavanaugh JL: Treatment of the sexually dangerous patient. Curr Psych Ther 21:101–109, 1982
109. DeLora JS, Warren CAB: Understanding Sexual Interaction. Boston, Houghton Mifflin, 1977, pp 299–303
110. McCormack P: Nuns emphasize the right to live without sexual love. Cleveland Press, July 25, 1978, p B-1
111. Ibid, p B-1
112. Boston Women's Health Book Collective: Our Bodies, Ourselves, 2nd ed.

New York, Simon and Schuster, 1976,
p 77

113. DeLora JS, Warren CAB: Understanding Sexual Interaction. Boston,
Houghton Mifflin, 1977, p 302

114. Ibid, p 302

Chapter 6

Sexual Assault: Rape

Many think of rape as an unjustifiable sex act. However, the sexual aspects are subordinate to aspects of power, anger, and aggression. Rape can be considered the ultimate expression of negative attitudes toward women and an exaggerated acting out of some of society's conventional ideas about women; women belong to men, they "ask for it."[1] In rape, sexuality is in the service of other, nonsexual needs. Izard[2] believes most sexual crimes are probably motivated by interaction of the sex drive with some combination of anger, disgust or contempt toward women. Thus, rape may be seen as having both psychologic and sociologic factors operating in its etiology.

The focus of this chapter is on rape of women by men, the typology of rape, the characteristics and the responses of adult and child victims and of society. Brief mention is made of rape of men by women, which is beginning to gain attention in the literature and the laws.

DEFINITIONS

Heterosexual Rape

Heterosexual rape is hard to define, describe, and prove.

One of the major problems with rape research is isolating definitions of rape that exist and how they systematically differ between the sexes. A working definition of rape is needed.[3]

Definitions have never remained the same. Just as the punishment for rape has changed, so has its definition or description. There are now three major elements that are necessary as defined by law: (1) a penetration of the female organ, though slight, by the male organ; (2) done without consent or with consent induced by terror or by mistake as to the identity of the male or the nature of the act; (3) an act by a male (not under the age of 14 and not the husband of the female) who is aware that his act is or may be without consent or with consent induced by terror or by mistake in the identity of the male or the nature of the act.[4] By this legal definition, the male who cannot have an erection is unable to commit rape, and oral sex or indecent touching is not rape.[5]

A broader definition is given by Sadoff,[6] who includes sexual activity between same-sex persons. He states that rape is sexual intercourse by use of force, fear, or fraud between individuals of the same sex or the opposite sex. Oral and anal penetration is also classified as rape.

The first scientific evidence that men are raped by women was presented at a meeting of the American Association of Sex Educators, Counselors and Therapists. Dr. W.H. Masters and Dr. P.M. Sarrell presented 11 cases of males. These males reacted emotionally and physically as female victims suffering impotence, loss of self-esteem and confidence, and rejecting intimacy.[7]

Thirty-seven states now have "gender-neutral" statutory rape laws covering both males and females under some specified age so that equal protection of the laws is offered to juvenile females and males who have been raped.

Homosexual Rape

Homosexual rape usually occurs in closed institutions, such as prisons. It is more frequent among men and is a reflection of hostile aggression, rather than sexual attitudes. The rapist doesn't usually see himself as a homosexual, but sees the victim as a "punk" or passive homosexual. The one raped often feels ruined and fears that he may become homosexual because of the attack.[8]

Statutory Rape

Statutory rape is unlawful sexual intercourse between a male over 16 and a female under the age of consent (this varies from 14 to 21 years depending on the jurisdiction). If a male of 18 has intercourse with a female of 15 and it was with consent, he may still be held for statutory rape if the girl or her parents wish to press charges. Statutory rape is not considered a sexual deviation, except when a considerable age difference exists; then it is called *pedophilia*. In these cases, the age discrepancy must be greater than 10 years or the girl must be 12 years old or under.[9] Of all sexual assaults, that on a child arouses the most outrage.

THE RAPIST

Six types of rapists have been described by Gebhard and associates.[10] The commonest types are men whose behavior includes unnecessary violence. Sexual activity alone is insufficient, and maximal gratification can only be attained by physical violence or serious threat. These men may be sadistic and often feel hostility toward women. The second most common are the amoral delinquents who pay little attention to social controls and who are characterized by egocentric

hedonism. They wish to have coitus and the female's desires are of no importance. They see women as sexual objects, but are not hostile to them. If the woman objects, they use force, threat, or weapons. The drunken aggressor is about as common as the second type of rapist. His behavior ranges from uncoordinated grappling to hostile and vicious behavior released by intoxication.

Explosive aggressors constitute 10 to 15 percent of the group. They are usually average, law-abiding citizens, sometimes criminals, whose aggression appears suddenly and inexplicably. The double-standard males comprise about 10 percent of rapists. They divide women into good, who are treated with respect, and bad, who are not entitled to consideration. These men are somewhat like the amoral delinquents, but they resort to force only when persuasion fails. The remainder of rapists are mental defectives, psychotics, and a mixture of those described.

Sexual Arrousal

It is difficult to get data in relation to arousal of rapists. The belief that rapists are more easily aroused was supported by studies of Abel[11] and others who measured the erections of rapists and nonrapists during audiovisual description of rape and nonrape sexual scenes. The rapists developed erections to the scenes while nonrapists did not.

As was mentioned earlier, some rapists experience difficulty in sexual arousal during rape. In a study of 170 convicted rapists by Groth and Burgess,[12] erectile inadequacy characterized by partial or complete failure to get an erection was most common. Some experienced "conditional" impotency, being able to erect only after the victim stimulated him manually or orally or put up an acute struggle. Ejaculatory incompetence is not usually reported as a frequent problem, but in this group of rapists it was the second most common problem. Most had no difficulty in the nonassaultive sexual relations. Premature ejaculation was not a common difficulty in this group, although some ejaculated during the assault without intercourse.

Evidence of sexual penetration, especially the presence of sperm in the victim, is needed for legal prosecution of the rapist. However, this study indicates that negative results of the physical and laboratory examination of the victim does not rule out sexual assault and penetration, since many rapists were impotent or ejaculated outside the vagina.

TYPOLOGY OF RAPE

Power, anger, and sexuality operate in rape, but only one of these issues dominates in each case. Sexuality is a less frequent factor. In a study of 133 offenders and 92 victims, Groth and associates[13] did not find any instances when sex was the major issue.

Power Rape

This type of rape involves use of physical aggression, guns, or physical immobilization of the victim. The victim is kidnapped and held helpless. Sexual intercourse is an indication of conquest. The rapist usually has poor interpersonal relationships, feels inadequate in the sexual and nonsexual areas of life, and sexual activity is a means of increasing identity, strength, and potency. He experiences anticipatory pleasure and fantasies along with some anxiety before the rape, but tends to find little satisfaction afterward. The rape never quite lives up to his expectations, so he has to find others. There is no conscious effort to hurt or degrade the victims. Power assertive rapists see rape as a sign of virility and dominance, while the power reassurance rapists need to rape to resolve self-doubts about sexual adequacy and masculinity, so they want to put women in a position of helplessness.[14]

Anger Rape

Some rapists need to express anger, rage, and contempt for their victim by hurting her sexually, assaulting her, and forcing her to submit to the performance of additional degrading acts. He may inflict physical violence by striking, beating, or tearing clothes. He vents his rage for perceived rejection or wronging from females. Subjectively he may react to the sex act with disgust.[15] Acts of anger rape are usually impulsive and episodic.

This type of rapist may have difficulty getting an erection or ejaculating during the assault. His relationship with important women in his life is marked by conflict, irritation, and jealousy, and his motive for revenge and punishment in extreme cases can result in homicide.

THE VICTIM

The victims of rape may be any age, from small infants to elderly women, but the majority are between 15 and 25 years of age. Most come from lower social classes and are unmarried. In rare cases, men have reported that they have been raped by women.[16] No matter what age or social class, victims of rape have been found to resort to specific cognitive, verbal, and physical coping behaviors, before, during, and after the attack.

Before the Attack

Some victims identify danger, a "sixth sense" that something is going to happen. If they cope, they react quickly and attempt to avoid or escape the situation. Much of their ability to react depends on the amount of time between perception of threat and the attack. Their basic strategies include mentally assessing the situation and determining alternatives, for example, how to get out of the room or escape. They may employ verbal tactics and try to talk themselves out of the situation. Physical action includes fighting and fleeing. Some victims have no strategies but are physically paralyzed and totally overpowered. Some may be overcome by surprise because the rapist is known as a friend. Others may be psychologically paralyzed—"blacked out," "could only think of death."[17]

During the Attack

Some victims mentally focus and direct their attention to some specific thought to keep their mind off the event and focus on survival. Some remain calm so as not to provoke additional violence. Others play detective and try to remember the rapist or try to remember what others said to do.

Verbal strategies include screaming and yelling, partly to decrease tension and partly to deter the rapist. Some talk to the rapist and try to calm him in order to avoid further demands. Others try to frighten the rapist by reminding him of the trouble he will be in. Physical action includes fighting and struggling. Some victims recognize that this is what the attackers want and that he only gets more excited by their resistance.

Physiologic responses during the rape include choking, gasping, nausea, vomiting, urinating, hyperventilating, and losing consciousness.[18]

Psychologic reactions during the rape include use of the defense mechanism of denial. "I can't believe it's happening"; dissociative feelings, "I pinched myself to see if I was real"; suppression, "I missed 10 minutes of my life"; and rationalization, "I felt sorry for him, if it was the only way to get sex."

After the Attack

Escaping the rapist was uppermost in the victim's mind in addition to thoughts of how to get help. Bargaining for freedom also takes place. The rapist sometimes apologizes to gain sympathy or tries to persuade the victim not to tell. The victim copes by remaining silent or agreeing to the instruction or by promising not to tell. If the victim frees herself, she often feels mastery, since she has survived.[19]

BIOLOGIC EFFECTS OF RAPE

Genital and other injuries, infection, and pregnancy are the major sequelae to rape.

Injury to the genital area may include bruises and lacerations of the perineum, hymen, vulva, vagina, cervix, and anus. Trauma, such as stab wounds, lacerations, and bruises may occur to other parts of the body. Vaginal bleeding and injury to deeper pelvic tissue may also be sequelae.[20]

The aftermath of rape may leave the woman with vaginismus or dyspareunia. She may have difficulty being orgasmic with her husband, even if the relationship was satisfactory before the rape.[21]

Venereal disease may be acquired from the rapist and is a serious concern of rape victims. Three percent of the patients who are untreated develop gonorrhea, and approximately 0.1 to 0.25 percent contract syphilis. In treating the patients, the physician can wait for cultures and then treat specifically.[22] Other acute vaginal infections may also develop and become chronic, causing adhesions and fixation of pelvic viscera and subsequent sexual dysfunction.

Pregnancy is the most feared sequela. Untreated, only 1 percent of rape victims become pregnant. However, medically, pregnancy control is part of standard treatment for rape victims. Assessment is first made to determine if the woman is too young or too old to conceive, if she has been taking birth control pills, has an intrauterine device in place, or is menstruating. In these cases, she does not need pregnancy prevention. For women who can become pregnant, diethylstilbestrol (DES) is given. This prevents implantation of a fertilized ovum by causing sloughing of the uterine lining.[23]

Any of these biologic sequelae to rape can result in sexual dysfunction, especially when combined with the psychosocial effects of rape.

PSYCHOLOGIC EFFECTS OF RAPE

Notman and Nadelson[24] have described rape as an example of psychologic stress. Rape is a crisis situation in which the balance between the individual and the environment is broken. Like other disasters, it is unexpected, and the coping mechanisms of the victims vary. How the individual responds depends on her age, her life before the rape, the circumstances surrounding the rape, the woman's personality style, and the responses of those from whom she seeks support. The first phase of the rape stress reaction is marked by acute disorganization with behavioral, somatic, and psychologic manifestations. The second phase involves long-term reorganization with variable components, depending on the ego strength, the experience, and the social support of the victim.

Initial Response

The initial response of the rape victim is one of overwhelming fear and terror. After the rape, she may exhibit profound fatigue and exhaustion. She may have delayed reporting the rape and have had little sleep for a protracted period. She may suddenly realize that she may be injured, become pregnant, or contract venereal disease.

Some may respond in an overcontrolled way, by being stoic and exhibiting little emotion. Others may be unable to talk at all or may be angry, tense, crying, or trembling. Still others may inappropriately laugh and smile to cover up the trauma.[25] The victim does not want the attention that accompanies followup care and frequently wishes to just forget the experience as soon as possible. Instead, she is caught in a process of care that she does not understand. Often, someone other than the victim reports the rape, acts as an intermediary for the victim, or persuades the victim to seek help.[26]

Requests for Help

Burgess and Holmstrom[27] investigated the requests of 146 rape victims between the ages of 17 and 73 years. Five categories of crisis requests were identified: medical intervention, "I need a physician"; police intervention, "I need a policeman"; psychological intervention, "I need to talk to someone"; uncertain, "I'm not sure I want anything"; control, "I need control." Telephone followup after the rape experience indicated the re-

quests changed to ones for psychologic support services, and of these, four categories were identified.

Confirmation of the concern of the counselor was sufficient for the largest number of the sample. The women often felt relieved after talking, were positive about the phone calls, and looked forward to them.[28]

A second group of women sought clarification to put the crisis into perspective and settle it psychologically. They wanted to sort out conflicting thoughts and feelings.

The third group explicitly asked the counselor for advice; alternatives; or how to handle legal, social, physical, and psychologic problems associated with the rape. They made good use of psychologic support but also saw the counselor as someone who could help them deal with other concerns.

A final group of women wanted nothing and stated they did not need counseling service or any followup.[29]

Anger

Direct anger is usually repressed, although it may be expressed at the rapist and the act of rape or it may be displaced onto the police interrogation or the hospital system. Later it may be expressed as fear, anxiety, guilt, and shame. The rape experience may resurrect memories of childhood punishment for misdeeds, so that the woman feels that she is being punished and is in some way responsible. These feelings may surface as nightmares or be displaced on others. Anger may be transferred into a pattern of self-blame, since society reinforces the suppression of aggression in females.[30]

Guilt and Shame

Some women feel they should have handled the situation differently, regardless of how appropriate their responses were. They are concerned about their degree of passivity or activity that might have prevented the attack. Victims usually perceive the aggressive, violent aspects of rape, but society views rape as sexual. The old adage when rape cannot be avoided to "relax and enjoy it" illustrates society's attitude. Contrary to this notion, rape is dehumanizing, but the woman feels she ought to have been able to set limits.

Unconscious Fantasies

Rape fantasies are some of the most prevalent of those experienced by women (see Chapter 4), but their prevalence does not make women willing victims. Individual defenses usually prevent individuals from acting out their fantasies, but rape presents confrontation with another's sadism and aggression and one's vulnerability. It threatens the woman's ability to maintain her defenses and her controls.[31]

Other Later Responses

Other later responses of women include an increased sense of helplessness, increased conflict over dependence and independence, anxiety, depression, devaluation of self as a person, and profound interference with trust relationships with men. At this point, problems with the marriage and other relationships become evident. Women may develop phobias of strangers, of dark places, of being alone, or of being outdoors.[32]

Sexual concerns that may be experienced differ if the victim has not had previous sexual activity or has been sexually active. The sexually inexperienced may be forced to confront sexual feelings without opportunity for emotional preparation. Sexually active victims may see themselves as "damaged merchandise" or fear accusations of infidelity. They may be anxious about resuming relations with their husbands or boyfriends.[33]

Religious beliefs may affect response. A scrupulous woman may have more severe trauma, since she may view it as her sin and place greater blame on herself for the rape than one who is more wholesome in her religious attitudes. The nature of the rape itself affects response. A rape that involves multiple assaults and/or assailants is more traumatic than the acts of a single individual.[34]

LIFE CYCLE AND RESPONSE

A small child may not understand what has happened to her and may think that the rape was a "bad thing." Her reactions in a large part may mirror those of people around her. If they are upset, she will be upset. If they express anger toward the rapist, she may feel the anger is directed toward her or that she is somehow at fault.[35]

Rape may be particularly traumatic for the adolescent, who feels embarrassed and guilty. The aftermath is additional trauma. The physical examination may be viewed as another rape, if the physician is insensitive and impatient with her shyness and blunt with his comments.[36]

The 17- to 25-year-old woman, the most frequent victim, is often alone and inexperienced. Her relationship with men may have been only with trusted, caring figures. She may be raped by a date, an old friend, or an ex-husband and may reproach herself for not knowing better. Often she refuses to prosecute the rapist. The rape may color her future relations with men, especially if this experience of violence and degradation was the first sexual experience.[37] Rape may also raise concerns about her sense of adequacy and ability to care for herself. Relatives and friends may offer to care for her, and this fosters her regression.

Divorced or separated women are more likely to be blamed for the rape and their credibility, life style, morality, and character questioned. The victim may see the rape as confirmation of her feelings of inadequacy and her ability to function independently. She may worry about her ability to care for her children and may question her adequacy as a mother. An overriding concern is what, how, and when to tell her children about the rape.

Middle-aged women also have concerns about their independence and sexual adequacy. This period of the life style is fraught with doubt and is a period of reassessment and biologic change. Rape presents an added stress during a stressful time. The husband may be going through his own midlife crisis and is less able to be responsive and supportive.[38]

SOCIOCULTURAL FACTORS

Significant others, physicians and nurses, the law, and the larger society all respond to rape in their own way. This response is colored by their own experiences, psychologic status, and the myths and misconceptions about rape to which they are subject.

Sexual Partner's Response

The husband or male sexual partner feels indignant and identifies with the victim. He may feel that his masculinity is violated by the attack on a woman who belongs to him, by his helplessness and inability to have prevented the attack. Since males also have some feminine identification, they may also view the attack as directed toward self.

The man may become overly protective, partly due to his sense of guilt over not being protective enough. Simultaneously, he is angry at the attacker and at "his woman" for allowing herself to get into this position. He may have complex feelings about his own sexual impulses and therefore is unable to be supportive and helpful to the woman. Because of his own rape fantasies, concern for "used merchandise," and anxiety, the man may withdraw from the woman without even being aware that he is not supportive.[39]

Police Attitudes

Women may be asked by police if they "enjoyed it."[40] Some detectives view rape as woman's revenge: "If she thinks she is pregnant, she'll go for a rape charge." When a woman does not resist, but submits to rape to avoid being beaten, she may be assumed to have consented. Some rape victims report being treated like criminals, being asked questions such as "What were you wearing? Were your pants tight?"[41]

Many rape victims report that their complaints are met by hostile, insensitive police, especially if the victim is of lower social class. Those who have reported good experiences were for the most part older women, children, those accompanied by husbands, and those who had professional and middle-class occupations.[42]

Fortunately, in many areas, police are now being given special training to help them be more knowledgeable about rape, its causes, and how to deal with the victim in a more empathetic and sensitive manner.

The Legal System

The courts may also appear insensitive to the victim. In order to prosecute, physical evidence of rape (penetration) and use of force without consent of the victim is necessary. In the past, the defense tried to show that a woman had a "bad reputation" and to put her character on trial. In addition, the jury has to weigh the oath of a woman who says she is raped against that of a male.[43]

Several states protect the male defendant against the word of a woman by requiring independent corroborative proof in addition to her testimony. This means that the prosecution must prove, apart from the victim's testimony, that there was penetration, that force was applied, or that the man on trial was the true offender. The impossibility of this happening is illustrated by New York's conviction rate. In 1971, in 2415 rape complaints, the police made 1085 arrests. Only 100 cases were presented to the grand jury; 34 resulted in indictments, from which only 18 convictions resulted.[44]

Changes are being made in the laws. Since the mid-70s, Congress and half the states have adopted "rape shield laws" that protect the victim from being unfairly questioned about past sexual activity. The judge hears this evidence in chambers before deciding if the jury should hear it. Other laws are being passed that make rape "sex neutral" containing no assumption that rape is only something done by men to women.

In most states victims do not have to prove that they resisted to the utmost. Sentences are more flexible: the greater degree of violence, the longer the sentence. New laws in Michigan, for example, have resulted in 90 percent more convictions in 1977 than in 1972.

A few states have abolished the old common law rule that a husband cannot be convicted for raping his wife and some states are considering a change.[45]

Disagreement exists over the appropriate penalty for rape. Some judges believe lighter sentences will increase the number of convictions, since juries are less likely to convict if the penalty is severe. Others favor stiffer penalties, mandatory prison terms, or restoration of the death penalty for rape. Others suggest surgical or chemical castration as a penalty.[46] In some states, the severity of the penalty has been related to race. Black males, especially if they raped white women, were more likely to be given the death penalty when it was permitted.[47]

Public Attitudes

Metzger[48] views rape as brutalizing the communal aspect of sex. She views society's underlying attitude toward rape as the rights of men over women. The social custom of "giving" the bride in marriage and the rites and rights of the marriage bed, all enforce the idea of women as property.

She also sees rape as typifying society's attitudes toward power: (1) to be weak is a crime deserving punishment; (2) the weak are accomplices in the crime against them; and (3) the victim has committed the crime.[49] Consequently, the woman is suspect as an accomplice or the instigator rather than the victim of rape.

Public attitudes may be changing. A Harris survey indicated that by a 71 to 16 percent margin, Americans rejected the decisions of judges in California and Wisconsin who let off defendants charged with rape because "the way women act and dress these days, they often provoke men to commit sexual acts." In Wisconsin there was a recall referendum and the judge in question was unseated.[50]

In one survey, a vast majority of those questioned felt that rapists are sick and perverted, that rape is a violent crime that cannot be justified by the way women dress. They rejected the argument that the woman leads the man on, although a majority did believe that women have intercourse, become frightened, and then call it rape.[51]

The relationship of religiousness and extent of devaluation of the rape victim was investigated by Joe and others.[52] They found that the subjects who were intrinsically oriented toward their religion (lived their religious beliefs) devalued the rape victim less than subjects who were extrinsically oriented toward religion (were nonreligious or held "general" religious beliefs). The intrinsically religious person seems to have internalized the religious values of humility, compassion, and love of neighbor.

Amir[53] conducted an empirical study of 646 rape cases to explore and disclose patterns of forcible rape. (Few studies exist that supply systematic and accurate knowledge of the rapist and his victim and the social conditions that encourage rape.) His findings identified and debunked some misconceptions about rape. Rape, contrary to popular belief, is an intraracial act, especially between black men and women. Rape does not usually occur between total strangers. Black intraracial rape involved mainly close neighbors, while white rape occurred among acquaintances who established their relationship before the event.[54]

Contrary to certain misconceptions, the investigator found that rape is not: (1) a hot-season crime, (2) due to sex–marital status imbalance in the community, (3) associated with drinking, (4) an unplanned event, (5) an event that occurs on a deadend street or dark alley, (6) precipitated by the victim's behavior.[55]

REACTIONS OF HEALTH PROFESSIONALS

Professionals' Behavior

Nurses who are uncomfortable with their own sexuality may find caring for the rape victim anxiety provoking. Denying that the patient's problem is real and a tendency to be judgmental may make therapeutic intervention difficult.[56] In addition, nurses working in a busy emergency ward may put the rape victim low on the priority for intervention. Staff members may show their bias and ambivalence by statements such as, "The woman is faking," or "I don't believe all the stories I hear."

Male professionals, nurses and physicians, have to contend with their own biases. In the past, psychiatrists have felt that rape was not a psychiatric issue and shared the view that the victim "asked for it" or that the accusation of rape was false. The image of the rape victim was that of a young, sexually attractive girl who could have avoided the danger or who used the accusation of rape to protect herself from criticism. This view of rape implies that it happens only to marginal people and that it is sexual, not violent, in nature—that the woman and the rapist were only seeking sexual gratification.[57]

Studies of student nurses'[58] and registered nurses'[59] perception of rape victims demonstrated that they may have more negative attitudes toward victims whom they perceive as careless.

Male versus Female Counselors. Clinical evidence indicates that female rape victims relate better to women counselors during the acute phase, although Bassuk and Apsler[60] found no evidence of different attitudes toward or different therapy of 41 female rape victims by either male or female therapists.

The male counselor may feel he will be rejected by virtue of being a man, since the pain and trauma was experienced at the hands of masculine aggression. Change in patterns of care may be indicated so that the male counselor can prove that some men can be gentle, empathetic, and trustworthy. Changes in strategy suggested by Silverman include changes in the use of space, tone of voice, and physical contact.[61] Intervention should be based on assessment of the wom-

an's reponse to a male. Some male counselors find it is effective to sit closer to the woman than they usually would, while others sit farther away. Some hold the woman's hand or pat her shoulder; others feel these gestures are not appropriate. Most counselors talk more softly than usual.[62]

Male biases are evidenced by the tendency of counselors to focus on the sexual aspects of the rape, rather than its violent aspects. Women may sense that the man does not empathetically appreciate the violence she has experienced and find him neither supportive nor understanding. Male counselors may unconsciously identify with the rapist, as well as the husband, boyfriend, or other significant male of the victim.

Silverman believes that women have to confront feelings of vulnerability throughout life, have them more under control, and in general are able to master the attendant anxiety. This may explain why they are more comfortable in the counseling situation than males. If the counselor's anxieties cause him to avoid dealing with the victim's affective responses, he may confirm the client's suspicion that what has happened is so awful it cannot be discussed.[63]

The woman may not seek out help and it is wiser for the male counselor not to expect or ask a firm commitment for return contacts. As much as possible, the plans should be left up to the client. Overzealous and too active attempts to convince the victim to "accept" help may be seen by her as aggressive or "assaultive" communication.[64]

NURSING IMPLICATIONS

Sister Charlotte Van Dyke pinpoints the role of the nurse in caring for the rape victim. "The victim of rape is an individual who presents herself to us for care. The rapist has seen her as a body. The prosecutor sees her as a client; the police classify her as a victim. Someone needs to see her as a person."[65]

Assessment

Because of the legal ramifications of rape the nursing process approach is especially important in the area of assessment.

An accurate and precise initial interview and physical assessment is essential since the victim's hospital record, with or without the testimony from the hospital staff, may be used to corroborate or weaken the victim's claim of rape or sexual assault.[66] (See Table 6-1.)

Physical Evidence. Physical evidence (or trace evidence) is any fragment, particle, or remnant of a substance that can be examined microscopically or chemically to corroborate a crime. It is particularly important to note signs of physical trauma, such as bruises, swelling, lacerations, or teeth marks, especially on the arms, legs, face, neck, breasts, and the inner aspects of the thighs. Gynecologic examination includes inspection of the vulva, perineum, hymenal ring, vagina, and rectum for tenderness, redness, swelling, bruises, and lacerations.[67]

Wherever possible, photographs should be taken of the victim. Laboratory evidence

of the presence of semen is obtained by using a swab on any part of the body that appears to have semen. A swab is taken from any orifice that was penetrated, the vagina, mouth, or rectum and a smear of the specimen is examined for sperm. Presence of acid phosphates in the vaginal pool is indicative of prostatic secretions, so the specimen should be obtained.[68] If tests for sperm are negative, the victim's statement on whether she bathed or douched after the assault is important.

Tears, stains, or soil marks on the victim's clothing, broken fingernails, and dirt under the fingernails are usually indicative of a struggle. Pubic hair combings, along with a sample of the victim's pubic hair in a properly sealed and labeled envelope can become evidence.

Rape cases that involve patients who refuse to have examinations present special problems. This is documented and the patient signs a release indicating her awareness that she is being discharged against medical advice.[69]

Nursing History. The nursing history should include the patient's verbatim statement describing the assault and the types of sex acts demanded and carried out and the order in which the demands were made. Penetration, the crucial element of rape, does not have to be complete. Even the slightest penetration is sufficient.[70] Signs of emotional trauma, such as the assailant's threats and method of force, especially if a weapon, hands, or fists, are noted.

The nurse should avoid subjective impressions. A record that is thoroughly, accurately, precisely, and legibly written is one of the strongest documents of corroborating evidence of the patient's physical and emotional state. Value words such as *normal, satisfactory, negative,* or *positive* should especially be avoided.[71]

Assessment should be made of the victim's coping behavior and strategies,[72] the previous adjustment, stress tolerance, and personal strengths. Identification of signifi-

---

TABLE 6-1. INITIAL ASSESSMENT GUIDE

General observations
  Appearance, verbal style, emotional style

Nursing History
  Circumstances of assault; description of assailant; conversation; sexual details; threats, physical and verbal; weapon

Subjective data indicating trauma
  Statements describing physical trauma, statements describing emotional trauma

Objective data indicating trauma
  Signs of physical and gynecologic trauma: physical evidence: semen specimens, clothing, nails, hair samples, photograph taken; signs of emotional trauma

---

Adapted from Ann W. Burgess and Ann T. Lazlo, Courtroom use of hospital records in sexual assault cases, American Journal of Nursing, 77, No. 1 (January 1977), 65.

cant others is essential so they can be involved.[73]

The nurse as a counselor asks the woman to tell what has happened but does not press her to discuss it if she is reluctant. Forcing her often contributes to her feelings that she is being raped again.[74] Assessment, in addition to providing needed data, can be therapeutic. It serves as a supportive measure, since listening to the victim retell the rape not only helps identify coping behavior but also by acknowledging this information to the patient ("You did well to act as you did.") assures her that her coping behavior, whatever it might have been, was a positive, adaptive mechanism. In addition, by verbally sharing information and receiving positive feedback, the patient's guilt is decreased and a positive sense of self-esteem and worth is fostered. The nurse's feedback also starts a process of giving positive expectation that the victim will be able to regain her previous level of functioning.[75]

Assessment also gives the nurse baseline information to begin crisis intervention. At the same time, the victim begins to analyze the behavior she used and its effectiveness, identifies strategies for future crises, and begins problem solving.[76]

Planning

The nurse considers the age of the woman, coping behavior, and her significant others and the degree of support they supply.[77] It is the legal implications of rape and highly charged emotional situations that the nurse must especially consider in planning her care and which makes care of the rape victim different from that of other persons.

The goal of nursing intervention is to help the patient achieve adaptive coping and to prevent maladjustment. The thrust of counseling is to accept the patient's feelings and manner of expression, to begin to dissipate the power of feelings, and to give the woman a positive picture of herself.

Intervention

Fox and Scherl[80] describe (1) an acute reaction immediately after the rape and lasing

several days, (2) a period of outward adjustment, and (3) final integration and resolution of the experience. The nurse intervenes in all stages.

During the acute phase, time is a high priority, since police may be waiting to see the victim, and medical examination and laboratory tests must be done. Someone stays with the woman—family or friends if a nurse is not available—and provides emotional support.

Biologic Aspects. The nurse prepares the woman for the gynecologic exam. It is important to find out if she has ever had a pelvic examination. For children, especially, it may be the first time, and the victim needs to know what is expected of her, what the physician will be doing, and the reasons.[78]

Promoting physical comfort of the woman may involve giving her small items such as safety pins, a drink of water, a needle and thread to mend tears, cigarettes, and tissues. Some women may be dirty, some have been urinated on, and helping them wash up after the medical examination is completed and evidence has been gathered promotes not only physical comfort but self-esteem. Women who have been forced to have oral sex appreciate mouthwash.[79]

If prophylactic treatment is given for venereal disease, and possible pregnancy, the nurse teaches about the side effects of penicillin and the diethylstilbestrol (nausea, vomiting, vaginal spotting) and reminds her about the followup examination and culture for venereal disease and infection. The nurse also makes sure the woman has a clear understanding of basic sexual functioning and its relationship to what has happened to her. One victim thought that every act of intercourse resulted in pregnancy.[80]

Psychosocial Needs. In some areas, a counselor is called as soon as a rape victim enters the emergency service or health care faclities. In many other areas, it is the admitting nurse who must provide support. The nurse listens carefully as the woman recounts her story. She is encouraged to talk and often wants to share thoughts and feelings. An attitude of warmth, empathy, calmness, and consistency is most helpful. The nurse is personally involved, but professionally objective. If relatives or friends are not with the victim, the nurse can help her to decide who will be told (for example, parents, fiancé, friend, husband, clergyman) and how they will be notified. The woman may want to notify them herself or have someone else do it. As much as possible, the victim should carry through with this notification. If she cannot, she should be present when the call is made by the nurse or others. This helps prevent opportunities for the victim to misunderstand, distort, and fantasize about what the health professional has said or done.[81]

Health education and anticipatory guidance during this first phase is essential. It is helpful to assure the woman that her feelings are similar to those experienced by other women in the same situation, and that after several days or weeks she will be less troubled and be able to return to her usual activities. She can also be told that most women go through a third phase of recovery in which they feel depressed and mentally relive the rape experience.[82]

The victim is anxious, fearful, and often emotionally distraught, so she may misunderstand or fail to hear instruction about medications and followup care given to her by the physician. The nurse emphasizes, restates, and clarifies this information after assessing what the woman does remember. Written information is useful.

Discharge planning includes making sure that the woman has some means of getting home or wherever she is going. She is also given information about the availability of further counseling and help, and legal rights and options, which includes the right to prosecute or not.[83,84] In some states the victim does not have to pay for the collection of medical evidence and there may be crime victims compensation funds available for those who have suffered bodily injury as a result of a criminal act.[85]

OTHER SOURCES OF HELP

Role of the Rape Counselor

The rape counselor begins ideally in the emergency room or other settings where the patient has presented herself. Upon meeting the woman, she explains who she is and what the woman can expect from her. The woman is told that the counselor will stay with her all the time in the emergency room and that the counselor will telephone her at intervals for the next month or two. The counselor answers questions about the procedures to come, allows the woman to talk, and broaches the subject of whether the attack included more than just vaginal intercourse. She helps the woman decide what to tell her family, children, and friends. If requested, she gives information about what the police and court will be like.[86]

The counselor also provides a list of resources for medical and legal problems, giving names and telephone numbers, including her own. She may also be the one to communicate results of diagnostic tests when she does followup calls. Careful documentation of what the patient says and does, and what the counselor observes is valuable, not only if the rape is prosecuted, but as a record for the woman's benefit.

During the second phase of the rape recovery, followup calls are made, usually in 48 hours and then 2 weeks later. The counselor recognizes that during the period of outward adjustment, the victim's interest in seeking help and talking about the situation decreases, while the defense mechanisms of denial, suppression, and rationalization take place. The counselor's role is to provide support and make sure the woman keeps her followup appointments. Many victims consider themselves back to normal but may become depressed when the third phase begins.

Because of this fact, the counselor calls again about 6 weeks after the rape.

The counselor may work with the relatives and friends who may need someone to talk to. If they feel the woman has been ruined or become angry at her, feeling that she was seductive and careless, her self-esteem may be further damaged. The counselor helps these significant others work through these feelings.[87] Anticipatory guidance is important, since most patients do not expect to have further emotional reactions. The worker describes the normal feelings during phase three and assures the patient that health resources are available if she needs them. The victim's relative or friend is also given information about the patient's current status and future reactions and is given opportunity to discuss his feelings.[88]

During the third and integration phase, two central issues to be worked through are the victim's feelings about herself and her feelings about the assailant. It is at this time that feelings of guilt, shame, and self-punishment surface. The counselor does not reassure the victim that the attack was not her fault, but allows her to work through her feelings and reach this conclusion herself. If the patient is partially responsible for the assault, she must be helped to understand her behavior. Feelings of being dirty or despoiled that continue may require psychiatric referral. Her anger for the assailant is distorted into anger toward herself and is expressed as depression. Consequently, it is important that the victim be allowed to express her anger.[89]

Usually, phase three is brief, but if the woman experiences continued problems with eating and sleeping, if she suffers from generalized fears, or if she is involved in compulsive ritualistic behavior, psychiatric consultation is advisable.

The Fabricated Rape. The woman who cries rape without sufficient cause needs help also. These are women who feel helpless and desperate. They may be the victims of social, economic, psychologic, and family problems, which they are unable to handle.[90] Their entry into the health care system may provide the opportunity to direct them to the help they require. Believing the patient is a useful attitude for gathering evidence. It is up to the court and the jury to determine if a story is not true. The emergency room is not the place to ask, "Was she really raped?"

Clergy

Members of the clergy can be important resources for followup, especially if the patient is amenable to spiritual care and can receive support in a long-standing relationship with a pastor or clergy member. However, their help should not be forced on a victim, since it only adds to the abnormality of the episode for those without strong affiliation to a church. This area must be handled sensitively.[91]

The Rape Crisis Center

As the number of rapes have increased, groups of persons are organizing crisis centers to bridge the gap in services between the victim and society's system for dealing with rape. These centers provide 24-hour, 7-days-a-week services to aid victims.[92] The purpose is to provide early intervention, which can help in the prevention of psychologic or psychosomatic disorders subsequent to rape. These volunteer counselors provide emotional support and information to the victim and her significant others under the direction of professionals. The volunteers receive crisis training through staff meetings, use of videotaped interviews with victims, role playing, and discussion to sensitize them to stress of the victim.[93]

After the initial contact with the rape victim, followup phone calls are made in 48 hours and in some centers for 1 year afterward. Centers also conduct extensive educational programs for the community so people will understand what rape is and why it happens.[94] They also provide information about courses of action if a woman is raped (Table

TABLE 6–2. WHAT TO DO IF YOU ARE ATTACKED

1. Find a safe place.

2. If you are alone, call someone to help you: a close friend, a relative, the police, or the Rape Crisis Center.

3. It is important to take care of yourself medically. If you want to go to court, you will need to preserve all the evidence. Bathing, giving yourself a douche, or cleaning up in any way will destroy evidence. The sooner you see a doctor, the better chance there is to find evidence.

4. Immediate medical attention can also take care of any concerns you may have about venereal disease or pregnancy.

5. The decision of whether or not to report a rape to the police is up to you. If you go to an emergency room, you should know that most hospitals notify the police as a matter of policy. Sometimes they will not tell you before they call.

6. If the police come to the hospital and you do not want to file a report, you do not have to. Simply tell them what you want to do. Or you can file an initial report and then decide whether you want to go to court later.

7. After the hospital and police business are finished, find a comfortable, safe place you can go with someone you can talk to.

8. This is a good time to take a bath. It will make you feel better.

9. Be sure to find a friend, relative, or a counselor you can talk to about how you feel about what happened. You will need a good outlet for the hurt, shock, and anger that you feel after an assault.

From Cleveland Rape Crisis Center.

6–2), group sessions, and individual and family counseling.

THE CHILD AS SEX VICTIM

Children may be sexually abused or molested without actual rape taking place (see Chapter 15). Freud believed that the reports of childhood assault were fantasies that the child developed as a defense against her own genital pleasure and her guilty wish to sleep with her father. Generations accepted his beliefs. Psychoanalytic literature on child molestation puts the onus of blame on the child's "seductive behavior." Kinsey, too, seemed unable to imagine that a sexual assault on a child was a devastating shock and insult. Brownmiller states that sexual assaults are barely noticed except in the most violent and sensational cases.[95]

Findings in a study of sex crimes in Brooklyn disclosed that the sexually abused child was more prevalent than the physically abused child. The median age of the children was 11, but infants also have been molested. Ten girls are molested for every boy, and 97 percent of the offenders are male. The majority of offenders are relatives or friends of the family.[96]

Schultz argues that it is not the sexual act per se that creates trauma, but the parents' behavior toward the child after the offense is discovered; that single instances of sexual trauma produce few negative consequences, unless reinforced by court testifying or parental overreaction.[97]

Assessment and Intervention— Childhood Assault

The Child. Saperstein[98] has some specific suggestions for dealing with children. The child's cognitive and life experience age must be assessed so that the nurse can respond to the child in a way she can understand. It is necessary to ascertain what the rape means to the child and deal with it at that level. Rape may mean social ostracism (or acceptance) by peers, and it may arouse fear of the neighborhood or questions about parental reaction. The child who is a victim of a family-related rape will be concerned about her family believing her and/or possible familial repercussions.

The child is told why she is in the hospital and what is going to happen to her. (She is in the hospital because she may be hurt and the doctor is going to examine her.) She will experience less anxiety if the unknown is made known. The counselor must be honest but avoid elaborate explanations that are confusing to the child, using language the child can understand, such as the "doctor will examine your bottom." Watching her expression will determine her understanding. By being calm and treating the examination as a normal process, the child's anxiety is alleviated.[99] The mother should be present if at all possible. A sedative may be given and the vaginal examination may be delayed or done under general anesthesia.[100]

To prevent sexual assault, parents should be told to teach children that some people can cause harm, who is allowed to touch or kiss them, what parts of their body can be touched, who is allowed to undress them, and what is private body space.

The Parents. The rape counselor must also work with the parents. Saperstein[101] states that it is necessary to help parents focus on their child's pain. Their confused feelings and sexual "hang-ups" cloud the issue. Parents will usually be in the state of crisis. The counselor provides positive feedback to assuage their guilt feelings and help them direct their anger toward prosecution of the rapist, not their daughter.

The parents receive information about how to deal with their daughter's stress and about the importance of parental feelings and attitudes for the girl's feelings of self-esteem. The nurse stresses that they should be available to their daughter but neither to force her to talk nor to cut her off. They are reminded that encouraging the child to continue usual routines and activities is beneficial. They are also informed of legal and medical procedures and told that the medical examination is for the child's safety and to provide legal evidence.

PREVENTION OF RAPE

Women are assertively working to prevent rape. Some argue that, from early childhood on, systematic training in self-defense is needed. Brownmiller[102] argues that women must learn to defend themselves when sexual assault occurs.

The predictable pattern of the rapist is to decide whom to assault (target), determine how easily he/she can be intimidated (test), and threaten (usually verbal). The target stage is the best time to fight back, shout or talk. During the test stage, self-confidence, assertiveness, and aggressiveness may cause the rapist to give up. During the threat stage, prevention includes running, yelling or fighting back, going for vulnerable areas: eyes, throat, groin and knees, and using hands, feet, teeth, elbows, head, umbrellas or keys. The point is to inflict pain, confuse or disable the rapist.[103]

Rape crisis centers are seeking to reduce the incidence of rape by educational services to individuals, agencies, and organizations that serve rape victims.

NOTES

1. Boston Women's Health Book Collective: Our Bodies Ourselves, 2nd ed. New York, Simon and Schuster, 1976, pp. 155–166
2. Izard CE: Human Emotions. New York, Plenum, 1977, p. 184
3. Schwartz P: The scientific study of rape. In Green R and Wilner J (eds): Methodology in Sex Research. Rockville, Maryland, Alcohol, Drug Abuse and Mental Health Administrations. U.S. Department of Health and Human Services, Public Health Service, National Institute of Mental Health, 1980, pp 145–192
4. Snelling HA: What is rape? In Schultz LG (ed): Rape Victimology. Springfield, Illinois, Thomas, 1975, pp 145–156
5. Sadoff RL: Sex and the law. In Sadock BJ, Kaplan HI, Freedman AM (eds): The Sexual Experience. Baltimore, Williams and Wilkins, 1976, pp 567–575

6. Ibid, p 570
7. Meeting told of first evidence of female rapists. The Plain Dealer, March 14, 1982, p 22A
8. Sadoff RL: Sex and the law. In Sadock BJ, Kaplan HI, Freedman AM (eds): The Sexual Experience. Baltimore, Williams and Wilkins, 1976, p 570
9. Ibid, p 570
10. Gebhard PH, Gagnon JH, Pomeroy WB, Christenson CV: Sex offenders: An analysis of types. In Weinberg MS (ed): Sex Research. New York, Oxford, 1976, pp 118–134
11. Abel GG, Barlon DH, Blanchard EB, Guild D: The components of rapists' sexual arsenal. Arch Gen Psychiatry 34:395–905, 1977
12. Groth AN, Burgess AW: Sexual dysfunction during rape. N Engl J Med 297:764–766, 1977
13. Groth N, Burgess AW, Holmstrom LL: Rape: power, anger, sexuality. Am J Psychiatry 134:1239–1243, 1977
14. Ibid, p 1240
15. Ibid, p 1241
16. Cleveland Press, May 3, 1978, p 10
17. Burgess AW, Holmstrom LL: Coping behaviors and the rape victim. Am J Orthopsychiatry 133:413–417, 1976
18. Ibid, p 415
19. Ibid, p 417
20. Burgess AW, Holmstrom LL: The rape victim in the emergency ward. Am J Nurs 73:1740–1745, 1973
21. Notman MT, Nadelson CC: The rape victim: Psychodynamic considerations. Am J Orthopsychiatry 133:408–412, 1976
22. Van Dyke C: Why a Catholic hospital provides rape relief. Hosp Prog 58:64–69, 1977
23. Ibid, p 66
24. Notman MT, Nadelson CC: The rape victim: Psychodynamic considerations. Am J Orthopsychiatry 133:409, 1976
25. Van Dyke C: Why a Catholic hospital provides rape relief. Hosp Prog 58:67, 1977
26. Burgess AW, Holmstrom LL: The rape victim in the emergency ward. Am J Nurs 73:1741, 1973
27. Burgess AW, Holmstrom LL: Crises and counseling requests of rape victims. Nurs Res 23(3):196–202, 1974
28. Ibid, p 200
29. Ibid, p 201
30. Notman MT, Nadelson CC: The rape victim: Psychodynamic considerations. Am J Orthopsychiatry 133:409, 1976
31. Ibid, p 410
32. Van Dyke C: Why a Catholic hospital provides rape relief. Hosp Prog 58:68, 1977
33. Silverman D: First do no more harm: Female rape victims and the male counselor. Am J Orthopsychiatry 41:91–96, 1977
34. Van Dyke C: Why a Catholic hospital provides rape relief. Hosp Prog 58:69, 1977
35. Boston Women's Health Book Collective: Our Bodies Ourselves, 2nd ed. New York, Simon and Schuster, 1976, pp 155–166
36. Lieberman F: Sex and the adolescent girl: Liberation or exploitation. In Gottesfeld ML (ed): Modern Sexuality. New York, Behavioral Publications, 1973, pp 224–243
37. Notman MT, Nadelson CC: The rape victim: Psychodynamic considerations. Am J Orthopsychiatry 133:410, 1976
38. Ibid, p 412
39. Ibid, p 411
40. Sadoff RL: Sex and the law. In Sadock BJ, Kaplan HI, Freeman AM (eds): The Sexual Experience. Baltimore, Williams and Wilkins, 1976, p 571
41. Boston Women's Health Book Collective: Our Bodies Ourselves, 2nd ed. New York, Simon and Schuster, 1976, p 157
42. Brownmiller S: Against Our Will. New York, Simon and Schuster, 1975, p 364
43. Ibid, p 369
44. Ibid, p 372

45. A revolution in rape. Time, April 2, 1979, p 50
46. Katchadourian HA, Lunde DT: Fundamentals of Human Sexuality, 2nd ed. New York, Holt, 1975, pp 514–516
47. Wolfgang ME, Riedel M: Rape, race and the death penalty in Georgia. Am J Orthopsychiatry 45:658–667, 1975
48. Metzger D: It is always the woman who is raped. Am J Orthopsychiatry 133:405–408, 1976
49. Ibid, p 406
50. Cleveland Plain Dealer, October 24, 1977, p 18-A
51. Ibid
52. Joe VC, McGee SJ, Dazey D: Religiousness and devaluation of a rape victim. J Clin Psychol 33:64, 1977
53. Amir M: Forcible rape. In Schultz LG (ed): Rape Victimology. Springfield, Illinois, Thomas, 1975, pp 43–58
54. Ibid, p 56
55. Ibid, p 44
56. Clark TP: Counseling victims of rape. Am J Nurs 76:1964–1966, 1976
57. Notman MT, Nadelson CC: The rape victim: Psychodynamic considerations. Am J Orthopsychiatry 133:412, 1976
58. Damrosch SP: How nursing students' reaction to rape victims are affected by a perceived act of carelessness. Nurs Res 30:168–170, 1981
59. Alexander CS: The responsible victim. Nurses' perceptions of victims of rape. Health Soc Behav 21:22–33, 1980
60. Bassuk E, Apsler R: Are there sex biases in rape counseling. Am J Psych 140:305–308, 1983
61. Silverman D: First do no more harm: Female rape victims and the male counselor. Am J Orthopsychiatry 41:92, 1977
62. Ibid, p 92
63. Ibid, p 94
64. Ibid, p 95
65. Van Dyke C: Why a Catholic hospital provides rape relief. Hosp Prog 58:68, 1977
66. Burgess AW, Laszlo AT: Courtroom use of hospital records in sexual assault cases. Am J Nurs 77:64–68, 1977
67. Ibid, p 66
68. Ibid
69. Van Dyke C: Why a Catholic hospital provides rape relief. Hosp Prog 58:68, 1977
70. Ibid, p 67
71. Ibid, p 68
72. Burgess AW, Holmstrom LL: Coping behaviors and the rape victim. Am J Orthopsychiatry 133:416, 1976
73. Notman MT, Nadelson CC: The rape victim: Psychodynamic considerations. Am J Orthopsychiatry 133:412, 1976
74. Clark TP: Counseling victims of rape. Am J Nurs 76:1965, 1976
75. Burgess AW, Holmstrom LL: Coping behaviors and the rape victim. Am J Orthopsychiatry 133:416, 1976
76. Ibid
77. Clark TP: Counseling victims of rape. Am J Nurs 76:1965, 1976
78. Burgess AW, Holmstrom LL: The rape victim in the emergency ward. Am J Nurs 73:1745, 1973
79. Ibid
80. Fox SS, Scherl DJ: Crisis intervention with victims of rape. In Schultz LG (ed): Rape Victimology, Springfield, Illinois, Thomas, 1975, pp 232–241
81. Ibid, p 235
82. Ibid, p 236
83. Smith ED: Victims of violence and abuse (rape). In Smith ED (ed): Women's Health Care: A Guide for Patient Education. New York, Appleton-Century-Crofts, 1981
84. The rape examination. Cleveland Rape Crisis Center, August, 1979
85. Rape resource. Cleveland Rape Crisis Center, 1979
86. Clark TP: Counseling victims of rape. Am J Nurs 76:1965, 1976
87. Fox SS, Scherl DJ: Crisis intervention with victims of rape. In Schultz LG (ed): Rape Victimology, Springfield, Illinois, Thomas, 1975, p 237

88. Ibid, p 238

89. Ibid, p 239

90. Clark TP: Counseling victims of rape. Am J Nurs 76:1966, 1976

91. Van Dyke C: Why a Catholic hospital provides rape relief. Hosp Prog 58:69, 1977

92. Huerd D: How a rape advisory service works. Hosp Prog 58:70–71, 1977

93. McCombie SL, Bassuk E, Savitz R, Pell S: Development of a medical rape crisis intervention center. Am J Orthopsychiatry 133:418–421, 1976

94. Flyer from Cleveland Rape Crisis Center, 3201 Euclid Avenue, Cleveland, Ohio 44115

95. Brownmiller S: Against Our Will. New York, Simon and Schuster, 1975, p 278

96. Ibid

97. Schultz LG: The child as a sex victim: Sociolegal perspectives. In Schultz LG (ed): Rape Victimology, Springfield, Illinois, Thomas, 1975, pp 257–273

98. Saperstein A: Child rape victims and their families. In Schultz LG (ed): Rape Victimology, Springfield, Illinois, Thomas, 1975, pp 274–276

99. Ibid, p 275

100. Woodling BA, Kossoris PD: Sexual misuses: Rape, molestations and incest. Pediat Clin North Am 28:481–497, 1981

101. Saperstein A: Child rape victims and their families. In Schultz LG (ed): Rape Victimology, Springfield, Illinois, Thomas, 1975, pp 274–276

102. Brownmiller S: Against Our Will. New York, Simon and Schuster, 1975, p 404

103. Pope S: Fighting against rape. The Voice of the Nightingale. Newsletter of Cleveland Rape Crisis Center, Cleveland, 1983, p 1

Chapter 7

Psychologic Theory and Sexuality

There is not one comprehensive, generally accepted theory relating to sexuality. Although many theories that are extant attempt to explain the evolution of sexuality in a developmental context, some aspects of sexual development are best explained by one theory, others by another. Despite the many theoretic formulations about the nature of sexuality and its development, there is little disagreement that sexual and psychic processes are intimately related and that it is difficult, if not impossible, to understand one apart from the other.[1]

The scope of this text cannot include a comprehensive exposition of all theories, but those of Freud, Erickson, and some of the behaviorist, existential, and humanistic schools will be presented. Information about body image and self-concept and their relationship to sexuality will also be presented, since disturbance in these areas may have major, adverse effects on sexuality.

PSYCHOANALYTIC THEORIES

Sigmund Freud

Freud's theories were and still are controversial, but his contribution to theory of sexuality cannot be ignored. His major contributions, at a general level, were the identification of sexuality as an acceptable topic of research and analysis and his conception of psychologic determinism (the theory that causes of human behavior are located in psychologic processes that are universal and cross-cultural).[2]

Freud described unconscious forces operating in patients who suffered from conflicts that he believed were rooted in sexual development. If these conflicts were brought to the surface. understood and dealt with, the individual could be helped, if not completely cured.[3] In Freud's view, sexuality began at birth, and he stressed that its manifestation must be studied throughout the life cycle.

Freud described a sex instinct, a psychophysiologic process with physical and mental manifestations. By *libido* (Latin for *lust*), he meant the psychologic manifestations, the erotic longing aspect of the sexual instinct. (See Chapter 4 for further discussion of libido.) Freud revised and altered his theory repeatedly throughout his life, so his definition of "sexual" is difficult to determine. Sexuality included the sense of pleasure through orgasm, but he extended the term to include pleasurable experiences ordinarily considered nonsexual, so in this broader sense. sexuality is the central theme of psychoanalytic theory.[4]

All psychoanalytic theory starts with the assumption that the newborn has libidinal "capital," and psychosexual development is a process by which the sex energy is "invested" in certain pleasure zones of the body (the mouth, anus, genitals) at successive stages of development. If problems of libido occur during development, not only will the individual's sexual functioning be

113

compromised, but also the entire personality, the psychologic. and at times, the physical health.[5]

In his book *Three Essays on the Theory of Sexuality,* Freud wrote of the "normality" of the sexual impulse in the child, stating that the newborn infant has the "germs of sexual feelings," which develop and are then suppressed. He stressed that infantile sexuality was qualitatively different from adult sexuality but was alike in that sources of pain and pleasure caused a specific set of responses. The child has sexual feelings, but they have different meanings to the child and are not the same as adult sexual feelings and impulses.[6]

There are three characteristics of infantile sexuality: (1) at its origin, it attaches itself to one of the vital body functions; (2) it is autoerotic—it has no sexual object; and (3) the sexual aim is dominated in sequence by erotogenic zones. Consequently, the child goes through different stages of psychosexual development—oral, anal, phallic, and genital[7]—interrupted by the latency phase.

Pregenital Sexuality. The first of the developmental phases of sexual organization described by Freud are the pregenital, composed of oral and the sadistic–anal phases.

Oral Stage. The newborn infant depends on sucking for nourishment, but sucking provides more than food, the process itself provides the infant gratification. The mouth is the main source of pleasure, and like all pleasure, it is basically erotic. The first zone of libidinal investment, consequently, is the oral zone, and the mode of gratification is through "taking in" or incorporation.[8] The mouth as a source of pleasure continues and varies in importance at any stage of life. Thumbsucking, for example, may be a transient source of pleasure for the school child, who may revert to it under stress, boredom, rejection. or other unhappiness.[9] The use of the mouth for pleasure continues—kissing, smoking, drinking, and the use of drugs provide gratification and relief through intake (incorporation) of external substances. However, it must be remembered that oral needs are not the only motivation for activities such as smoking or drinking; social pressures also may be operating.

Anal Stage (Sadistic–Anal). Two modes of gratification are described—retention and elimination. If all goes well, the individual obtains pleasure from defecation. The child also develops greater mastery of other muscles to increase ability to function independently. In terms of behavior, the child is able to say yes or no, to love, and to give, but to withhold and be aggressive, if necessary. During the anal stage, the child tends to be stubborn, self-assertive, willful, and cruel, alternating between love and hate. Freud viewed this ambivalence as a result of the conflict between retention and elimination that characterized this period. Contrasts in sexes, which run through the sexual life, are developed at this stage, but cannot be called masculine or feminine, but rather active or passive.[10] Activity is supplied by the musculature of the body through the mastery impulse. The erogenous zone is the mucous membrane of the bowel, which is an organ with a passive sexual aim.[11]

Phallic Stage. At 3 years, the child becomes more keenly aware of the genitals and the pleasure associated with their manipulation. The zones invested with libido are the penis and the clitoris, and behavior is characterized by an "intrusive" mode. Children poke fingers into things and, if allowed, the 3- to 4-year-old makes deliberate sexual exploration. The main psychoanalytic issue is the Oedipus complex in boys and the Electra complex in girls.

In these complexes, the child develops erotic attachment to the parent of the opposite sex and feelings of aggressive rivalry toward the parent of the same sex. These feelings are extremely problematic for the child who does not have the capacity to gratify the genital impulse and who still loves (and fears) the "rival" parent. Inevitably, guilt occurs. The boy thinks he deserves punishment by damage to the genitals (castration) since they are the "offending part." He also discovers that girls do not have penises, so fear of losing his penis is substantiated. The girl's reaction to the fact that boys have penises is that she has lost her own and that she envies the male's advantage.

If development continues without disturbance, the child resolves the oedipal conflict by giving up the parent as an erotic object, while continuing to love the parent, because of fear of disapproval, retaliation, and the loneliness of the desire. The child begins to identify with the parent of the same sex, and the entire conflict is buried in the unconscious so that these unacceptable wishes do not torment the person or will not be fulfilled.[12]

The Latency Phase. The child then passes into the latency phase, hopefully after the successful resolution of the Oedipus complex, a resolution that makes possible genital maturity. The 3- or 4-year-old is not sexually an adult, but the next period, the latency phase of development is, for most children, a period of intellectual and social growth and relatively limited sexual activity.

Genital Sexuality. The major transformation of puberty is the subordination of erogenous zones to the genital zones. The sexual aim of the male is the discharge of sexual products. This is not contradictory to the previous aim of pleasure, but pleasure is not the highest aim, the sexual impulse enters into service of propagation and becomes altruistic.[13] The sexual impulse, which was primarily autoerotic, now finds a sexual object.

Freudian View of Male and Female Sexuality. Freud identified the differences in the sexuality of males and females on the basis of penis envy and castration anxiety. He felt that the male sex was superior, more intelligent, and creative. The female, without the penis, was considered basically a cas-

trated, passive, and inadequate male. The male, having a penis, also possessed active sexuality. However, having a penis brings its own anxieties, because the male must fear losing something little girls do not possess. Freud's theories have caused much argument and discussion. However, the impact of his theory must be viewed in line with the cultural values of the family and society at Freud's time. Freud was a product of Victorian society in which the male was considered superior to the female in almost every way. Some now view the concept of penis envy as being meaningless today, since sexuality is viewed differently than it was 70 years ago.[14]

In Freud's view, two kinds of female orgasms were possible. As long as the girl or woman retains a wish for the penis, she focuses on her clitoris, "the damaged penis" and has only a clitoral orgasm, which is not as healthy or as developmentally mature as vaginal orgasm. Only when the woman has given up her wish for a penis and settled for a feminine role function—to bear children—can the psychic shift take place. Instead of cathecting or fixating on the clitoris, she cathects on the female reproductive organs—the vagina and womb. It is at this point that the woman accepts her sexual role identity and can enjoy the highest level of sexual fulfillment, vaginal orgasm.

The clitoris is the chief erogenous zone. It becomes excited during the sexual act, but its role is to conduct excitement to the vagina and womb.[15] This transference takes time, and during this time, the woman is anesthetic in terms of vaginal orgasm. If the clitoris refuses to give up its excitability, the anesthesia becomes permanent. While the woman must change her zone for sexual activity if she is to "mature" sexually, the man retains his from childhood. This division of female orgasm has given rise to controversy that still continues. Masters and Johnson state that from a biologic point of view, there is no difference between vaginal and clitoral orgasm. The response of the pelvic viscera are the same.[16]

Problems of Psychosexual Development. Problems occur in psychosexual development if needs at a given stage are either excessively or insufficiently gratified. When gratification is excessive, the child is reluctant to give up and move on to another stage of psychosexual development. If it is insufficiently gratified, the libido does not keep pace with physiologic maturation, as it were, and the body zone appropriate to the next phase of development does not become adequately eroticized. In either case, the child is "fixated" at the stage, with hampering of subsequent development. The individual does not mature psychosexually or at least is handicapped by a tendency to "regress" to the fixation point when under stress.[17]

Two major types of adult behavior ensue. In the first, the adult seeks erotic gratification of an infantile stage in an undisguised manner. For example, an anally fixated person may seek actual stimulation of the anus through anal intercourse and becomes a "passive homosexual." Freud considered overt gratification of infantile erotic impulses a "perversion." Therefore, perversions or sexual deviations are a frequent outcome of infantile fixation.[18] In the second and more common adult behavior, the infantile libidinal drive is repressed and permitted expression in highly symbolic form and results in many forms of neuroses. For example, if an individual is fixated at an oral stage, oral traits will be manifested—excessive and chronic preoccupation with food, drink, etc. Or the individual may become an oral character and require constant pampering, eager to receive but not able to reciprocate.[19] Anal fixation may be characterized by the ambivalence or stubborn behavior of a 2-year-old.

Problems of the Phallic Stage. Problems may arise in the phallic stage. Oedipal conflicts may not be resolved, either because the child did not have a sustained relationship with both parents or adequate substitutes or because the individual is still fixated at a pregenital level and never engaged in the oedipal situation. If one parent is seductive toward the child or if both parents are deeply and openly hostile to each other, the child's oedipal hopes are unrealistically increased and the resolution of the conflict is also more difficult. Problems may arise if a parent becomes sick. The child may blame self, ascribing the illness to the hostile feelings and wishes that characterize the period. The presence and number of siblings and the individual's place in the family constellation are also likely to influence the outcome of the oedipal dilemma. The individual's concept of sex roles, pride in gender, respect for the other sex, and moral attitudes toward sexual activity are shaped at this stage.[20]

If an individual enters this phase with conflicts from the pregenital period, serious problems are especially likely to ensue. Males with unresolved conflicts may be sexually inhibited and timid. Sons threatened by punitive fathers may have decided not only to "give up" their mothers, but all women as erotic objects. A mother who is hostile to all men may interact with her son in the same way, causing him to avoid all women. Daughters of aggressive fathers may develop masculine traits or those with punitive mothers may either mimic their behavior or rebel against them and attempt to ally themselves with passive fathers.[21]

The traditional result of unresolved oedipal complex is the male personality with exaggerated sexual traits, the male exhibitionist and narcissistic Don Juan, constantly seeking sexual conquests. He is involved in shallow, unrewarding relationships that serve the sole purpose of demonstrating to himself and the world his potency and daring. His tendency to court women married to other men may be another indication of oedipal longings.

The woman who is exhibitionistic and seductive but also competitive and manipulative (a "castrating" woman), is the female countertype of this type of male. She may delight in humiliating men.[22]

Many persons of both sexes may have less severe manifestations of this trait and are often considered charming. exciting, and attractive by many people.

Problems of the Genital Stage. During the genital stage, the adolescent can initiate adult sexual interactions *if* past conflicts have been resolved. If they have not been, pregenital fixation may make it difficult to invest libido in "normal" sexual objects.

Conflicts from the phallic stage may be manifested. Boys may be narcissistic, daring, and boisterous, while girls are seductive and flirtatious. Gradually, genitality manifests itself, the young man and woman react with their whole selves. The psychoanalytic idea of genitality includes the integration of pregenital stages to result in the reconciliation of genital orgasm with love to facilitate establishment of satisfying life patterns of sex, procreation, and work. Freud's answer to the question of the central purpose of life was "work and love."[23]

Attacks on Freud and his psychoanalytic theory began with the first enunciation of these theories of sexuality. Freud has been blamed for the "obsession" of Americans with psychology, and indeed, his theories continue to influence much of modern psychotherapy. Some feel Freud's influence will begin to wane, that psychotherapy will play a less important place in life and that it can be replaced by untrained but sympathetic laymen who can do as well as psychotherapists in coping with persons who are anxious, shy or withdrawn.[24] Although detractors exist and continue to renounce Freudian concepts, the continued acceptance and viability of his theories, to a lesser or greater degree, attest to their value in explaining sexuality and sexual behavior.

Erik Erikson

Erikson began with basic psychoanalytic concepts and applied them to the entire life cycle, combining the study of psychosexual development with parallel study of psychosocial development. He divided the entire life span into eight phases, defining each by a primary accomplishment of a specific task, which is described as a *crisis,* in the sense that it is a critical period of life rather than a threat or a catastrophe. The phases are labeled according to extreme successful and unsuccessful solutions. However, the actual outcome is a balance between each extreme. How the child meets each crisis is determined to a great extent by solutions offered or permitted by parents or others who care for the child.[25]

Erikson extended basic psychoanalytic concepts. He also assumed the presence of an all-pervasive libidinal force. Sexuality is considered an important task of identity formation. He described biologic features of individuals, which are the primary givens, but stressed that these alone do not necessarily determine the individuals' definition of themselves as masculine or feminine or the way that they are perceived by others. These definitions and the sex-role expectations that are implied with the identity of "masculine" or "feminine" vary from culture to culture, even if biologic givens are constant. It is up to each individual to clarify and establish his own sexual self as a part of the larger task of identity formation. Erikson stressed the role of culture in this formation of identity by "elaborating on biologic givens."[26] Cultures with clear and consistent models and guidelines facilitate this task of identity. Erikson has more to say about society's effect on the person than the person's effect on society.[27]

Erikson's phychosocial phases one, two, and three—trust versus mistrust, autonomy versus shame and doubt, initiative versus guilt—are similar to Freud's oral, anal, and phallic stages of development. During adolescence, in the stage of identity versus identity confusion, the individual may have increased sexual contacts, but Erikson believed that only after identity formation is well consolidated is true intimacy with the opposite sex possible. He considered adolescent sex as an experimental part of the search for identity.

The task of intimacy versus isolation is specific to young adulthood. Persons develop the capacity to establish a workable relationship between the two extremes. Mature genitality is an important component of this stage of psychologic development. Erikson sees genitality as a capacity to develop orgastic potency free of pregenital influences. When this is true, genital libido is expressed in heterosexual mutuality. He describes orgasm as a supreme experience, which takes the edge off hostilities and "potential rages" caused by the oppositeness of the male and female. Satisfactory sexual relations thus make sex less obsessive, overcompensation less necessary, and sadistic control superfluous.[28]

Mutuality in orgasm is more likely and easier to achieve in a class and culture that make it a leisurely institution. In the more complex society, mutuality is interfered with by factors such as health, tradition, opportunity, and temperament. Erikson describes the utopia of genitality. It includes mutuality of orgasm with a loved partner of the opposite sex, with whom one is willing and able to share a mutual trust and with whom one is able to regulate the cycles of work, procreation, and recreation.[29] One would infer then that Erikson does not see homosexual sexual activity or casual sexual encounters as signs of mature genitality, since the first does not meet the criterion of "other sex," while the second does not involve love and mutual trust.

BEHAVIORIST THEORIES

Erikson's theories differ from those of Freud in that Freud emphasizes internal psychologic processes, whereas Erikson, while recognizing the importance of internal processes, also stressed the importance of external factors of culture and society. If one thinks of these theories of sexual development on a continuum, the behaviorists' theories might be considered at the opposite end of those of Freud and the psychoanalytic school, while Erikson is somewhere between.

Freud was concerned almost exclusively with inner psychic processes, while the behaviorists focus only on observable, measurable human and animal behavior. (The behaviorist conceptualizes three levels of human and animal behavior—instinctive, imprinted, and learned.) The behaviorists do not specifically discuss learning of sexual behavior, but certainly there is no reason to indicate that sexual learning does not occur in the same ways as other learning.

Stimulus–response theory was first enunciated by a Russian physiologist, Ivan Pavlov. His theory of learning has come to be known as classic conditioning.[30]

The process of classic conditioning was used to build an objective psychology that deals only with that which can be observed. Stimulus–response theory is a laboratory theory, in contrast to psychoanalytic and other theories, where the role of clinical or naturalistic observation has been more important. Stimulus–response theory is not a single theory, but a cluster of theories.[31] As the result of ideas and studies of Edward L. Thorndike, John B. Watson, Edward C. Tolman, Edwin Guthrie, and others, the theoretic interest of American psychologists was focused toward the learning process. Many major issues in psychology have been debated within the framework of learning theory.[32]

B.F. Skinner

Behaviorism, today, is associated with B.F. Skinner, whose operant reinforcement theory puts heavy emphasis on the study of responses that are not necessarily elicited by any stimulus (operants) but are strongly under the influence of the responses (reinforcement).[33]

Reinforcement is defined as any event the occurrence of which increases the probability that a stimulus will on subsequent occasions evolve a response. Reinforcers may be positive or negative. Skinner's concept of operant reinforcement differs from classic behaviorist psychology in that classic behaviorist psychology focuses on the relationship of stimulus to response. rather than on the consequences of the response.

A positive reinforcer is a stimulus that when *added* to a situation increases the probability of an operant response.[34] Thus, sexual contact is classified as a positive reinforcer. A negative reinforcer is a stimulus that when *removed* from a situation strengthens the probability of an operant response. A loud voice and extreme heat and cold are all negative reinforcers. The effect of either positive or negative reinforcement is always to increase the probability of response. In other words, in positive reinforcement, the animal responds in order to obtain something desirable, while in negative reinforcement, it responds to eliminate something undesirable.[35]

Negative reinforcement is not the same as punishment, even though both involve something unpleasant. In negative reinforcement, the unpleasant event precedes the act; in punishment, it follows. A punishing stimulus has been labeled an *aversive stimulus,* which when occurring after an operant response decreases the future likelihood of the response.

For the behaviorist, the only legitimate data for understanding sexual interaction are observable responses to overt, observable stimuli. Sexual action is not the result of some intricate psychologic processes that are symbolic of some early childhood experience. Sexual behavior, then, is merely a measurable psychologic response to a stimulus[36] or some reinforcements (the consequences of the responses).

Behavior Modification

Behavior modification involves processes to change behavior by direct intervention, rather than by psychotherapy, although both may be combined at times. The main objective is to change behavior, not to identify the etiology or initiate psychoanalysis of the behavior. This technique is being used to help couples and individuals who have sexual difficulties. Aversive therapy is used to treat the rapist or others who exhibit socially stigmatized sexual behavior (see Chapter 12).

EXISTENTIAL PSYCHOLOGY

While Freudian psychology emphasizes inner psychic processes and behaviorists emphasize overt, measurable behavior, humanistic and existentialist psychologists place their emphasis on sexuality as a part of the total personality. Unlike the Freudian view, however, sexuality is not the cause of human personality development; it is one of the results of it and only one facet of it.

The existential movement is rooted in the theories of Kierkegaard, Nietzsche, Dostoyevsky, and Bergson. Martin Heidegger and Karl Jaspers, however, are considered the creators of existential psychology in this century, and after World War II, Jean Paul Sartre and Albert Camus became existentialism's most articulate spokesmen.[37]

The central idea of existential psychology is being-in-the-world *(Dasein)* or the style of being that the person adapts as his or her essential central approach to life. The individual does not exist as a self or a subject in relation to an external world; neither is he/she an object, thing, or body interacting with other things that make up the world. Individuals have their existence by being-in-the-world, and the world has its existence because there is a Being to disclose it. *Dasein* is man's existence, not a property or attribute of man but the whole of man's existence.[38]

Existential psychologists object to carrying the concept of causality from the natural sciences to psychology, arguing that there are no cause–effect relationships in human existence. At most, there are only sequences of behavior, and one cannot derive causality from these sequences. Something that happens to a child is not a cause of adult behavior. Existential psychology rejects other types of psychology and requires its own method—phenomenology—and its own concepts—being-in-the-world, modes of existence, freedom, responsibility, becoming, transcendence, spatiality, temporality, plus many others.[39] The concept of causality is replaced by the concept of motivation, which, along with understanding, is the operative principle in existential analysis of behavior.

Closely related to existentialist objections to causality is the rejection of the division of man into subject (mind) and object (body, environment, or matter). Their beliefs are articulated in the statement, "Man thinks, not the brain." There is unity of the individual-in-the-world. Any view that destroys this unity is considered to fragment and falsify human existence.[40] Existential psychology also rules out explanations of an individual's existence in terms of self—an unconscious psychic or physical energy—or forces such as instincts, drives, or brain waves.[41] Rather than pulling persons apart to understand them, the aim of existential psychology is to make the articulated structure of the human being transparent.

In addition, persons are not to be regarded as things like stones or trees. Such a view dehumanizes man and prevents the psychologist from understanding persons in the full light of their existence in-the-world. Like Erikson, who emphasized the role of society and culture in personality and sexual development, existentialist psychologists recognize the role of society and environment, but argue against estrangement, alienation, and fragmentation of man by technology, bureaucracy, and mechanization. When persons are treated as things that can be managed, controlled, and exploited, they are prevented from living in a truly human manner.[42]

However, existential psychology cannot be seen as particularly hopeful or optimistic about people. The belief that "I am free" means at the same time that "I am completely responsible for my existence." In the existential view, being a human being is difficult and few achieve it. There is also a certain bleakness in their writings; nothingness is nearby, and dread is as large as love.[43]

Existential Psychotherapy

The unique features of existential psychology are brought out in their treatment of dreams. The concept of symbolism, as well as other Freudian mechanisms and interpretations, are rejected. A dream is just another mode of being-in-the-world *(Dasein)*. The contents of the dream must be accepted with their full meaning and content, just as they are felt to be in the experience of the dreamer. Dreaming and waking are not entirely different modes of existence; in fact, dreams duplicate existence in waking life and bring to life areas of the human world that the dreamer is unaware of in waking life.

This can be illustrated in the dreams of one patient who was being treated for depression and impotence. During existential psychotherapy, he progressed, in a 2½ year period, from dreaming about things to dreaming of plants, animals, and finally a passionate woman.[44] As the dreams changed so did his waking life. The depressing meaninglessness of his life changed and sexual potency returned.[45]

May is one of the most ardent American exponents of existentialism, and his books *Existence* and *Existential Psychology* have been important sources of information about existentialism.[46] He is concerned with how contemporary sexuality can block self-actualization. He sees it as mechanized, banalized, and alienated from the experience of passion. He states that Victorians sought love without sex, while modern people are sexy, but repress passion, since they are so preoccupied with such technical aspects of sex as performance. Anxiety and guilt are engendered by inadequate performance, and since, concurrently, people seek for their identity in the sex roles they play, sexual failure generalizes into failure as a person.

May believes that "good" sexuality can provide a sense of personal identity; sexual love can be an affirmation of self. Other values of sexual love are the expansion of the person's awareness by the experience of commingling, the experience of tenderness and togetherness and loss of aloneness. In addition, sexual climax unites a couple in a transcendent consciousness that make them one with nature.[47]

May describes an earlier breakdown in

values, causing an individual to "founder in storm-shaken seas."[48] Therapists avoided any moral judgment, seeing guilt as always neurotic, a feeling that ought to be eliminated. One harmful effect of the "values don't matter" attitude is the implication that sexuality is a matter of "release" on a "sexual object." The acceptance of sexual promiscuity leads to near anxiety and insecurity in the whole area of sexual behavior. "Full freedom" of sexual expression separates and alienates the person from his world, removes structure to act within or against, and leaves no guideposts in a lonely world existence."[49]

May believes that a philosophy of puritanism is not the answer either and has its own dangers. A new puritanism and emphasis on behavior control of the mind and personality is a denial of freedom of the person. Both an exaggerated freedom from values and the moral and social controls of society are inadequate.[50] Freedom can be located only in the self acting as the totality, the "centered self."[51]

HUMANISTIC PSYCHOLOGY

Humanistic psychologists are concerned with the concept of self, and a number of personality theorists consider the self in their formulations. However, the term *self* as used in modern psychology has two meanings. On one hand, it is the person's attitude and feelings and perceptions about himself or herself, as an object. In other words, the self is what the person thinks of himself or herself. The other meaning may be called the *self-as-process* definition—the self as a doer in the sense of a group of processes such as thinking, remembering, and perceiving. Humanistic psychologists do not view the self as a psychic agent that regulates man's actions. *Self* refers to the object of psychologic processes or to those processes themselves.

Sidney Jourard
Jourard states that humanistic psychology seeks to champion a view of man as a free

human being. It seeks to maximize growth and to discover the social conditions that make self-actualization possible for more people.[52] The goal of humanistic psychotherapy is not adjustment, but growth.[53] Healthy personalities grow, find life meaningful with satisfactions, but also in suffering. They love and are loved and have no doubt as to who they are and what their feelings and convictions are. They do not apologize for themselves.[54] Healthy personalities have also fully lived and experienced their bodies, and an important part of this bodily experience is sex, both erotic impulse and feeling. Healthier personalities are able to express erotic feelings without fear and express them in a relationship with a chosen partner without unnecessary inhibition. Unhealthy persons are self-conscious, cannot let sex "happen," and attempt to force sexual activity. This may result in impotence, premature ejaculation, frigidity, and inability to know and to attune oneself to the sexual being of the partner. Jourard states that the cure of sexual difficulties is "made outside the bedroom, but inside the self."[55]

Eric Fromm
Fromm interprets sexuality as a product rather than the cause of the entire personality. He closely links sex with love and believes that the best type of mature adult sexuality is between persons who share intimacy and caring as well as erotic attraction.[56]

Fromm describes the sex act as a prototype of shared enjoyment. However, he also comments that the enjoyment is frequently not shared because partners are so narcissistic, self-involved, and possessive that there may be only simultaneous, not shared pleasure.[57] He believes that the joy in sex is freely experienced only when physical intimacy is experienced along with loving intimacy.[58]

Fromm sees the possible creation of a new society, a "City of Being." If society is to be humanized, women must continue to be liberated from domination by men, since this subjugation of one-half of the human race by the other has done and does harm to both sexes. Changes have already begun. Fromm sees one of the most revolutionary events of the twentieth century as the beginning of women's liberation and the downfall of men's supremacy.[59] He also sees liberation from guilt about sex—sex that will no longer frighten people and that ceases to be unspeakable and sinful.

Carl Rogers

Rogers is identified with a method of psychotherapy that he originated and developed. It is called *nondirective* or *client-centered*. It involves a person-to-person relationship in which the therapist enters into an intensely personal and subjective relationship with the person. From this therapeutic practice evolved Rogers' theory of personality. Rogers brought the "self" back into psychology. His passionate belief in humanistic values, an optimism and implicit faith in the inherent goodness of man, and his belief that troubled people can be helped have attracted many people who consider behaviorism too cold and psychoanalysis too pessimistic.[60]

Rogers describes three effects of his therapy. First, the individual experiences the potential self, not distorted to fit the existing concept of self. Second, the individual can experience affectional relationships. The individual can permit someone to care for him/her and can say he/she cares for and about others. Finally, the individual likes self.[61]

Abraham Maslow

Maslow espouses a holistic—dynamic theory of man. His beliefs fall within the province of humanistic psychology, which he considered a "third force" in American psychology, the other two being behaviorism and psychoanalysis. Like Rogers, Maslow concentrated on the brighter, better half of the whole person, the gaiety, love, and well-being, not only the misery, conflict, and shame.[62] He spoke of enlarging the conception of human personality by reaching to the "highest levels of human nature."[63] Maslow's unique contribution to the organismic viewpoint lies in his focus on healthy people and their sexuality rather than on those who are ill.

The concept of sexuality in Maslow's theory of needs is discussed in Chapter 1. His theory is particularly applicable to nursing, since he assumes that in every human being there is an active will toward health, toward growth, or toward the actualization of human potentials. In his theory, one of his lower-order basic needs is sex, but the concept of sexuality pervades, affects, and is affected by the higher-order needs of security, love—belonging, and esteem. Sexual pleasure in the self-actualized individual is not just a passing pleasure but a kind of basic strengthening and revivifying.

NURSING IMPLICATIONS

Although nursing is developing its own theories, it is also an eclectic profession; it "borrows" theories from other disciplines and applies them to the patient care situation. In the area of sexuality, no one theory has been accepted by all as adequately describing and explaining the motivation for and the psychodynamics of sexual behavior, in health or illness, but some formulations are especially relevant for nurses to consider. Nurses should be knowledgeable about the theories and identify those that seem especially applicable to explain the sexual behavior of patients/clients and to those that contribute to better understanding of the concept of sexuality itself.

There is no one concept that seems to explain adequately the effects of health deviations on sexuality, but there are several concepts that seem to have special significance. Maslow and others discuss sexuality in relation to the self-concept and self-esteem, and these indeed appear to be intimately related. Since the term *self-esteem* will be used throughout this text as it relates to and affects sexuality, a brief discussion of this concept is in order.

SELF-CONCEPT, SELF-ESTEEM

Not all personality theorists introduce the idea of a self concept. For some, however, the most important human attribute is the view or perception that individuals have of themselves. This self-viewing process is often seen as the key to understanding the many puzzling behaviors displayed by any one person.[64] Self-concept may be considered part of the self-system in personality theory.

Allport identified seven aspects of the development of selfhood. During the first 3 years of life, the person develops a sense of bodily self, a sense of continuing self-identity, and self-esteem or pride. Between the ages of 4 and 6, the extension of self and self-image appear, and sometime between 6 and 12, the child develops self-awareness. During adolescence, intentions and long-term purposes appear.[65]

Self or self-concept is one of the central constructs of Carl Rogers' theory. He defines self-concept as "the organized, consistent conceptual gestalt composed of perceptions of the characteristics of the 'I' or 'me' and the perceptions of the relationships of the 'I' or 'me' to others and to various aspects of life, together with the values attached to these perceptions. It is a gestalt which is available to awareness, though not necessarily in awareness. It is a fluid and changing gestalt, a process, but at any given moment, it is a specific entity."[66]

Schain[67] describes four components of self-esteem: (1) the bodily self with functional (what can I do) and esthetic (how do I look) subparts; (2) the interpersonal self with social relations and intimate sexual interactions; (3) the achieving self with elements of work or competitive efforts; (4) the identification self with attitudes and behavior related to spiritual or ethical matters.

Self-esteem might be described as the kinds of pictures that individuals have of themselves. It is based largely on the nature of experiences that children have with their bodies and their worlds. If life has been, on the whole, satisfying, persons perceive themselves as being loved and lovable, as being able to do what others expect and what they expect of themselves.[68] If children grow in a harsh, cold, inconsistent, or deprived atmosphere, they may develop a confused, conflicted, or negative view of self.

Self-concept and level of esteem are also affected by sociocultural factors. Persons who grow up in a minority group often learn that they are living in a world alien and hostile to the group. The initial effect of membership in an ethnic or class group is an increased awareness of self as different, followed by initiation of defenses for interpreting this vicissitude of birth. Children learn to expect unequal treatment and develop concepts of self that tend to reinforce this stereotype.[69] Understanding of what it means to be a member of a particular culture can only be imagined by a nonmember, but such an attempt is necessary if individuals are to understand behavior and its meaning to individuals.

Level of self-esteem grows as children see that they are held in high esteem by teachers and peers and if they develop proficiency in control of their bodies. To a larger degree, the way the children see themselves is related to their physical skills.[70] For example, the preadolescent boy's concept is influenced by his changing body[71] and his ability or inability to compete with other boys in athletic events. Activities such as Little League or class athletic activity may adversely affect his view of self if he is unsuccessful in achievement.

The early adolescent peer group also profoundly affects level of self-esteem, for better or for worse. Early adolescent peer groups value physical adequacy for boys, and for both sexes, group-oriented behavior, high energy rate, good looks, and social skills. Any one who cannot measure up is ignored or forgotten.[72]

For many individuals, self-concept begins at puberty, since they view childhood as a preparation—the true self begins when childhood is over. Gordon found that most adolescent boys report favorably on themselves; male sex-role identification seems to be a potent source of self-esteem,[73] appearing to have a greater value as a basis of self-esteem than female role, regardless if the role is accepted or not. Girls generally view themselves as more inadequate than boys. This is unfortunate, since central to self-concept is the identification with and acceptance of sex role. Although cultural shifts in role are occurring, individuals assess themselves against some standard and measure their adequacy against it.[74]

Many families and indeed entire societies value male children above female. This may account for the differences in self-esteem between male and female adolescents mentioned earlier.

Although the individual's level of self-esteem is established in early life, under certain conditions it can be changed. In one experiment, subjects first made self-ratings of their masculinity. Then they were informed that their masculinity was viewed by others differently than their self-evaluation. When the discrepant view was from a highly credible source, the subjects changed their self-ratings to make them closer to that of others. When the other opinion communicated could be discredited, their self-evaluation did not change substantially.[75]

Some individuals who have a secure, high level of self-esteem will be able to cope with threats posed by life events such as loss of job or illness. For others with a less positive or well-developed view of self, illness, its effects, or its therapy may initiate feelings of worthlessness and failure. Those who place high value on sexual function as a source of esteem and whose function is compromised may be especially disturbed. In addition, body image, a part of the self-concept, may also be threatened or changed by change in function or loss of body parts, posing further threat to self.

Body Image

The human mind is able to regard the self as an object just as it regards objects in the outer world. Body image, or feelings about the bodily self, is central to the concept of self. Ego integration depends in part on keeping a realistic perception of one's body. Several components of body image have been identified. The first, body perception, is the individual's concept of the shape, size, and mass of the body and its parts—the internalized picture the person has of the body's physical appearance. It is the total of conscious and unconscious information, and perceptions about the body in space as different and apart from others.

The second component, body attitude, is the individual's general overall feeling about the form and appearance of the body. These two components are two distinct dimensions of body image.[76]

In addition to appearance, body image also includes the ability to function with control for time and for place—the ability to use oneself to achieve what is intended at precisely the right time and place.[77] Body image influences ability to perform and helps the individual evaluate the space the body occupies.

Those who have a normal body image experience feelings of joy, pride, power, pleasure, and confidence, all of which foster self-esteem and feelings of worth. If a poor body image exists, or when disturbances of body image occur, individuals experience feelings of helplessness, pain, inadequacy, doubt, and guilt.

Body image includes more than the physical body alone. It includes objects in daily use—a cane, jewelry, a policeman's gun. Objects that regularly come in contact with the body may become incorporated into the body image. So loss or removal of these items may result in threat or disturbance.

Developmental Aspects. Body image is not present at birth, but develops gradually. The first components are the sensations the infant experiences in relation to the inner workings of the body and the way these communicate to the total organism. The child begins to explore self.[78] What is experienced is affected by sensory, kinesthetic, and sociocultural variables. The child works at gaining mastery and control of the body and its functions. When this is accomplished, the child begins to explore the environment and works at mastering it. This involves not only learning to manipulate self and the environment, but learning to relate to others. At adolescence, especially, the young person also receives comparative and competitive appraisal of the body and its functions from peer groups and begins to decide whether the body is attractive and normal or not. It is at this stage of the life cycle that "normality" is equated with a physical appearance that mimics that of peers.

After gaining this impression of sensation, mastery, and normality, the individual is ready to move to the third phase of body image development, integration of body image with the psychic components of the self. Intellectual and emotional development becomes more important, and when maturity is reached, the individual values the self and personality as a whole, with less emphasis on the physical self and more on the inner psychic self. Not all persons reach this stage of maturity, and some continue to value body appearance and function over the psychic self.

NURSING IMPLICATIONS

Body image is constantly changing. Illness, injury, or medical or surgical treatment that result in change of appearance or function may cause alteration in body image. In addition, a person's feelings about changes in one part of the body "spread" to alter the entire concept of self[79] with adverse changes in self-esteem and feelings of shame. Body image disturbances may adversely affect recovery from illness and the individual's sexual relationships, so the nurse has the responsibility to identify changes in body image and to intervene appropriately. (See Chapter 13 for discussion of the effects of illness and body image.)

NOTES

1. Katchadourian HA, Lunde DT: Fundamentals of Human Sexuality, 2nd ed. New York, Holt, 1975, p 230
2. DeLora JS, Warren CAB: Understanding Sexual Interaction. Boston, Houghton Mifflin, 1977, p 77
3. Offer D, Simon W: Sexual development. In Sadock BJ, Kaplan HI, Freedman AM (eds): The Sexual Experience. Baltimore, Williams and Wilkins, 1976, pp 128–141
4. Katchadourian HA, Lunde DT: Fundamentals of Human Sexuality, 2nd ed. New York, Holt, 1975, p 234
5. Ibid, p 235
6. Freud S: Three Contributions to the Theory of Sex, 4th ed. New York, Nervous and Mental Disease Publishing, 1930, pp 35–45
7. Offer D, Simon W: Sexual development. In Sadock BJ, Kaplan HI, Freedman AM (eds): The Sexual Experience. Baltimore, Williams and Wilkins, 1976, p 129
8. Freud S: Three Contributions to the Theory of Sex, 4th ed. New York, Nervous and Mental Disease Publishing, 1930, p 57
9. Ibid, pp 44–45
10. Ibid, p 58
11. Ibid
12. Ibid, p 82
13. Ibid, p 66
14. Offer D, Simon W: Sexual development. In Sadock BJ, Kaplan HI, Freedman AM (eds): The Sexual Experience. Baltimore, Williams and Wilkins, 1976, p 130
15. Freud S: Three Contributions to the Theory of Sex, 4th ed. New York, Nervous and Mental Disease Publishing, 1930, p 78
16. Masters WH, Johnson VE: Human Sexual Response. Boston, Little, Brown, 1966, p 66
17. Katchadourian HA, Lunde DT: Fundamentals of Human Sexuality, 2nd ed. New York, Holt, 1975, p 237
18. Ibid
19. Ibid

20. Ibid, p 238
21. Ibid
22. Ibid
23. Ibid, p 239
24. The Sunday Plain Dealer, July 2, 1978, Sec 1, p 38
25. Hall CS, Lindzey G: Theories of Personality, 2nd ed. New York, Wiley, 1970
26. Erikson EH: Childhood and Society, 2nd ed. New York, Norton, 1963, p 91
27. Hall CS, Lindzey G: Theories of Personality, 2nd ed. New York, Wiley, 1970
28. Erikson EH: Childhood and Society, 2nd ed. New York, Norton, 1963, p 265
29. Ibid
30. Hall CS, Lindzey G: Theories of Personality, 2nd ed. New York, Wiley, 1970, p 418
31. Ibid, p 417
32. Ibid, p 418
33. Ibid, p 476
34. Hilgard ER, Bower GH: Theories of Learning, 3rd ed. New York, Appleton, 1966, p 113
35. Ibid
36. DeLora JS, Warren CAB: Understanding Sexual Interaction. Boston, Houghton Mifflin, 1977, p 93
37. Hall CS, Lindzey G: Theories of Personality, 2nd ed. New York, Wiley, 1970, p 552
38. Ibid, p 559
39. Ibid, p 556
40. Ibid, p 557
41. Ibid
42. Ibid, p 558
43. Ibid
44. Ibid, p 575
45. Ibid
46. Ibid, p 555
47. May R: Existential Psychology, 2nd ed. New York, Norton, 1969
48. May R: Psychology of the Human Dilemma. Princeton, New Jersey, Van Nostrand, 1967, p 169
49. Ibid, p 169
50. Ibid, p 170
51. Ibid, p 177
52. Jourard SM: Disclosing Man to Himself. Princeton, New Jersey, Van Nostrand, 1968, p 43
53. Ibid, p 43
54. Ibid, p 45
55. Ibid, p 50
56. DeLora JS, Warren CAB: Understanding Sexual Interaction. Boston, Houghton Mifflin, 1977, p 100
57. Fromm E: To Have or to Be. New York, Harper & Row, 1976, p 115
58. Ibid, p 117
59. Ibid, p 193
60. Hall CS, Lindzey, G: Theories of Personality, 2nd ed. New York, Wiley, 1970, p 544
61. Rogers CR: A theory of therapy, personality and interpersonal relationships, as developed in the client-centered framework. In Koch S (ed): Psychology: A Study of Science. New York, McGraw-Hill, 1959, Vol 3, pp 184–256
62. Hall CS, Lindzey G: Theories of Personality, 2nd ed. New York, Wiley, 1970, p 327
63. Maslow AH: Motivation and Personality. New York, Harper & Row, 1970, p ix
64. Hall CS, Lindzey G: Theories of Personality, 2nd ed. New York, Wiley, 1970, p 25
65. Ibid, p 269
66. Rogers CR: A theory of therapy, personality and interpersonal relationships, as developed in the client-centered framework. In Koch S (ed): Psychology: A Study of Science. New York, McGraw-Hill, 1959, Vol 3, p 200
67. Schain WS: Sexual functioning, self-esteem, and cancer care. Front in Radiat Thera and Oncol 14:12–19, 1980
68. Grodon IJ: Human Development: A Transactional Perspective. New York, Harper & Row, 1975, p 84
69. Ibid, p 144
70. Ibid, p 189
71. Ibid, p 225
72. Ibid, p 313
73. Ibid, p 337
74. Ibid, p 388
75. Hall CS, Lindzey G: Theories of Person-

ality, 2nd ed. New York, Wiley, 1970, p 543

76. Fawcett J, Fryer S: An exploratory study of body image dimensionality. Nurs Research 29:324–327, 1980

77. Rubin R: Body image and self-esteem. Nurs Outlook 16(6):20–23, 1968

78. Selekman J: The development of body image in the child: A learned response. Top Clin Nurs 5:12–21, 1983

79. McCloskey JC: How to make the most of body image theory. Nursing 76:68–72, 1976

Chapter 8

Society, Culture, and Sexuality

Sexuality is a term associated with the individual rather than any society. However, the individual's review of self as a sexual being as well as sexual behavior is largely shaped by the society and the sexual milieu in which he or she grows and lives. Certainly biologic and psychologic factors contribute much toward shaping people's sexual "destiny," as we have seen in previous chapters, but sociocultural factors are of equal, if not greater, importance. The argument of heredity versus environment in shaping a person's personality does not stop when sexuality is being discussed.

The major topics of this chapter include the role of society in the development of sexual attitudes and behavior, methods of research into sexual behavior and attitudes, sexual roles and relationships and variables that may affect them, changing roles and relations in the United States and in other cultures, the Women's Liberation Movement and its part in changing roles and relationships, and finally, alternate sexual life styles that reflect different views of what is appropriate sexual behavior.

ATTITUDES, BEHAVIOR, AND SOCIETY

Attitudes toward sexuality and sexual behavior are closely linked. *Sexual behavior* may be defined as any activity that ends in orgasm. This is a narrow definition, since some behavior that may seem asexual may be filled with sexual meaning for those who engage in it. The terms *romantic, erotic,* or *sensual,* can describe behavior and differentiate it from the sexual. However, the distinction may not always be clear.[1]

In this text, *sexual behavior* is used in a broader sense. It includes not only sexual activity, which has as its goal orgasm, but it also includes all behavior that individuals identify as disclosing themselves as male or female or that they consider a necessary part of their masculine or feminine role. Thus, the men who believe that as males they must assume the aggressor role during coitus and who do so are exhibiting sexual behavior, but the way in which it is expressed is related to sexual role beliefs or attitudes about what is appropriate for their sex.

Attitudes may be defined as the way individuals link feelings and thoughts about sex. They are a result of socialization and the attitudes and behavior demonstrated by parents and can be changed by the influence of peers, education, and counseling. It is important to remember that attitudes toward sexual behavior vary with age, perhaps much as sexual drives vary. Thoughts and feelings about sex are often very different in adolescence and middle age.[2] Attitudes have been further defined as the opinions individuals have about certain behavior, in this case sexual. One may express an attitude about sexual activity but behave in an entirely different way.[3] Both attitudes and sexual behavior must be considered, since they are interdependent. Sexual role behavior has been rigidly defined by society for each sex, but some of the traditional attitudes and behaviors are changing as individuals learn new roles and relationships.

The way in which sexuality is expressed in any society is learned through culture. Individuals are born and raised in a certain cultural context that includes sexual and other norms, ideals, and ideology. Norms are the learned rules that guide behavior, but ideal norms and real norms may differ. Ideal norms are what people say about their sexuality; real norms are inferred from actual behavior.

Social Class, Attitudes, and Behavior

Education and socioeconomic class are related to sexual behavior and attitudes. Kinsey found, for example, that people with college education had different attitudes toward activity such as masturbation and premarital intercourse and exhibited different behavior in these and other areas.[4]

Each social level is convinced its pattern of sexual behavior is the best of all patterns, but each rationalizes its behavior in its own way. The upper level rationalizes by what is right and wrong; sociosexual behavior is a morality issue. Many persons at this level believe that there are few types of immorality more heinous than sexual immorality. Honor, fidelity, and success in marriage involve individuals directing sexual urges to coitus with wives or husbands.

Lower social levels, in contrast, rationalize their pattern of sexual behavior on the basis of what seems natural or unnatural. Premarital intercourse is natural and therefore acceptable. Masturbation is not natural nor is it fitting before intercourse. There is evidence that some individuals at lower levels do see moral issues in sexual behavior but they recognize that nature may triumph over morals.[5]

Other Societies: Attitudes and Behavior

What is "normal" sexual behavior? Studies of the sexual behavior of primitive and modern societies show that there is not a single, stereotyped pattern of behavior but many patterns and tremendous variability in sexual behavior among various cultures and subcultures.

Primitive Societies. Heterosexual and homosexual activity are viewed differently, and norms are variable in primitive societies. Homosexual activity in many societies is viewed negatively, as it is in the United States. In other societies, it is tolerated in childhood but not adulthood. In other societies, homosexual activity is required of all males. Keraki bachelors of New Guinea practice homosexual anal intercourse as part of puberty rites.[6]

Different societies have different views about extramarital and premarital relationships. In many, both are forbidden, but the Toda of India permit women to have several husbands and several lovers, and their language does not have a word for adultery. In contrast, Hopi Indians keep boys and girls aged 10 to 20 apart, and an older woman accompanies girls wherever they go.[7]

Polynesians see love as the life force, the "essence of existence." There are no words in the language for *"sexually obscene," "indecent,"* or *"impure,"* nor are there words for *"illegitimate," "adultery," "bigamy,"* and *"divorce."* Liaisons are lighthearted and can be broken off by saying "I am tired of it."[8]

In contrast to these practices, Messenger describes the sexual attitudes of an Irish folk community, in which lack of sexual knowledge and misconceptions about sex make it one of the most sexually naive of the world's societies. Sex is never discussed when children are around. Menstruation and menopause cause consternation, since little is known about their physiologic significance. The people share their belief (with many western people) that men have greater sexual drive than women, who are taught that sexual relations are a "duty." There is much evidence that female orgasm is unknown, doubted, or considered a deviant response. Sexual intercourse is considered debilitating and nudity abhorrent.[9]

Margaret Mead described three primitive societies. The Arapesh men and women have what has been considered feminine behavior. They are cooperative, unaggressive, and responsive to the needs of the other. Sex is not a driving force. In contrast, the male and female members of the Mundugumer tribe are ruthless, aggressive, and positively sexed individuals. Undisciplined, violent males are married to females with like behavior. The Tchambuli reverse the traditional sex behavior of our culture. The women are dominant and managing, while the men are less responsible and emotionally dependent. The contrasting behaviors of these three groups of people provide some of the data to support the idea that masculine and feminine behavior is the result of social conditioning.[10]

Modern Societies. Sexual behavior and attitudes also vary in modern societies. Although Israel has had a woman as a prime minister, women in Israel are at least a generation behind those in America in terms of social equality. In 1948, they fought in the war of independence but since then have largely returned to homemaker status. Women are expected not only to have jobs but to be homemakers as well. Only the brightest and toughest women rise to the top of the male-dominated society. Women in the work force earn less than males and hold only few of the country's leading government posts. Only half of Israel's women have completed elementary school, and most have little more than 3 years of formal schooling. A cause of the change in status is believed due to the increase in the number of Sephardic Jewish immigrants from Arab countries such as Egypt, Syria, and Yemen. They now constitute the majority in Israel, are less educated but more religious, and hold to the tra-

dition of male dominance associated with Orthodox Jewish beliefs.[11]

In Latin America, women do not seem to want to change their traditional status in a society that is male dominated. Many are protective of their roles and have little interest in changing a situation that is mutually supportive. The cult of male machismo and a female counterpart labeled *marianismo* is prevalent. Marianismo is a belief of feminine spiritual superiority, which holds that women are semidivine, morally superior, and spiritually stronger than men. The man is forced to act or pretend to act aggressively at all times. Males feel the need to prove that they are free with respect to women and that women are submissive to men. However, men's wickedness is a necessary precondition for the women to attain spiritual stature through male-inflicted suffering.

The revolutionary activity in Central America is bringing change in the female role. In Nicaragua, a semi-official Women's Association and a decree of sexual equality has sometimes undermined traditional male domination, although machismo still exists and women hold few senior government positions.[12]

Stevens argues that *male chauvinism* is not an appropriate synonym for *machismo* and that this male–female behavior is not confined to the most sexually deprived groups. There is no rule against women participating in political affairs, but when they do, they adopt a style that reassures others of their respect for stereotypes.[13]

Sexual values of western and non-western societies may produce fundamental conflict. Excision of the clitoris (clitoridectomy) still exists principally in Africa and the Middle East, apparently to enforce chastity by depriving women of the organs needed for sexual pleasure. In Europe, excision has occurred as cheap labor is imported from Africa. Some Third World delegates at the World Conference of the United Nations Decade of Women in 1980 left the meeting rather than support a resolution condemning this mutilation.[14]

The American Navajo Indian family is matrilineal, that is the mother has the power, raises the children, and runs the family. The first menstrual period, signalling the onset of puberty is celebrated but there are no like celebrations for the adolescent male.[15]

Other modern societies show various forms of role behavior. Switzerland has a patriarchal society in which women are to play a submissive role. Not until 1971 did women obtain the right to vote in federal elections and to hold federal office. The Soviet Union has emphasized chastity and deemphasized sex, stressing that sexual activity should be within marriage.

Soviet leadership has regarded sex as virtually nonexistent. Sexual activity exists for the male's pleasure. Women are afforded second-class status although the Soviet constitution guarantees equality of the sexes. Women are an important part of the work force, but top jobs go to men. Mathematics and sciences are masculine occupations, and no women occupy positions of power in the Communist Party. In addition, women have the major responsibility of home and family. Divorce is rising rapidly, one in three marriages failing.[16] The government's concern about marital breakups and declining birthrate may have been the impetus for the announcement in *Pravda* that compulsory sex education is coming to the Soviet Union.[17]

In contrast to these more traditional societies, Sweden has had a much more permissive attitude toward sexual activity. Approximately 98 percent of married Swedish couples have premarital intercourse. Sexual intercourse is widely accepted as important for the unmarried and married. Despite instruction regarding contraception, premarital pregnancies are apparently common. Induced abortion may be used, but illegitimate births account for 10 percent of total births. Neither the unmarried mothers nor

the children are ostracized but are considered "one-parent families."[18]

RESEARCH AND SEXUALITY

Sexual attitudes and behavior may be based on myths and misconceptions, folklore, and folkways that are handed down from generation to generation. There has been a paucity of objective information about sexual attitudes, response, and sexual behavior in general, partly due to the sensitive and personal nature of sexuality but also to the belief that investigation of sexuality was in some way wrong or immoral. When Kinsey published *Sexual Behavior in the Human Male,* it was hailed by some as a break in the barriers of ignorance and by others as an attack on Judeo-Christian morality.

There are inherent problems in any research, but they are especially prevalent in sexual research. Sex researchers must be aware of hidden biases and the danger of focusing on "social desirability"—the tendency to answer questions in a way that is socially acceptable.[19] Investigators must be careful not to overstate their results and jump to premature conclusions.[20] Self-reported sexual behavior needs to be verified.

Surveys of Sexual Behavior
Questions on tools or scales must be specific, not global, and behaviors must be clearly defined so that subjects are responding as much as possible to the same criteria. Valid measures that have the greatest reliability and validity are needed for surveys.[21] Two major methodologic goals exist with surveys: to obtain high proportion of a proper sample from a defined and appropriate population that will answer the questions, and to insure that respondents will tell the truth.[22]

One of the difficulties in doing investigations of sexuality is that respondents to questionnaires may report their attitudes but not what they really think. In addition, they may report certain behavior but because of societal taboos may have forgotten what actually happened or may actually falsify events to conform to societal expectations.

Early research on sexuality was primarily medical, focusing on physiology of sexuality. Sigmund Freud and Havelock Ellis were interested in sexuality as a basic human drive, but the focus of others was on the dynamics of the neurotic or sexually maladjusted individual. Kinsey and his associates investigated the social factors that influence sexuality. The whole purpose of their program was to dispel the myths and lack of knowledge about the subject.[23]

Kinsey was unable to obtain a random sample, and consequently, some groups were either underrepresented or overrepresented in the sample. College students, young people, better-educated people, Protestants, urban residents, and residents of Indiana and the northeast were overrepresented, while manual workers, less-educated people, older people, Roman Catholics, Jews, rural people, and those living west of the Mississippi were underrepresented. The sampling methods were poor, so inferences to entire populations of white men and women must be made with caution. However, good interviewing techniques were used, and much of the data, especially vital statistics and incidence of activity, seem to be reliable, valid, and complete.[24]

Other surveys of sexual behavior have been commissioned by the Playboy Foundation. Research Guild Inc. surveyed sexual behavior, and Morton Hunt analyzed the data and presented his findings in *Sexual Behavior in the 1970s*. The questionnaire was long, raising the question whether the respondents would give thoughtful answers.[25]

Robert C. Sorensen collected information on adolescent sexuality for his book *Adolescent Sexuality in America*. Although the sample size was small, through a complex process, the sample approximated a true probability sample. However, the small size could produce a significant error in statistical inferences. The length of the questionnaire, 38 pages, was another unresolved

problem. It is probable that few adolescents gave thoughtful attention to the last page, despite the presence of interviewers and administrators during the completion of the questionnaire.[26]

Surveys and questionnaires published in popular periodicals, such as *Redbook, Cosmopolitan,* and *Playboy,* are another means of obtaining data about sexual attitudes and behavior. Two difficulties arise with this type of survey. First, only those who read the magazine are exposed to the questionnaire, and this does not constitute a random sample. It is a sample of individuals who read the magazine and as such is of interest but it is limited for scholarly purposes. In addition, those who return a questionnaire are motivated to return it for different purposes than those who chose not to. They may be more comfortable with and have more positive feelings about sex.[27]

Direct Observation or Ethnographic Approach

An ethnographic approach to gathering information involves participant observation. This may involve living with a group, joining in and/or observing their activities. Martin S. Weinberg and Colin J. Williams used this approach in studying male homosexuals in three countries (see Chapter 5).

In the ethnographic approach, the data gathered by field observation tends to be valid, reliable, and interesting, depending on the researcher's training and personal abilities.[28]

Laboratory Studies—Physiologic Measures

There are obvious advantages to using direct observations of sexual behavior. The problems of inaccurate information from respondents is eliminated, and use of tape and film provides data that can be reanalyzed. An additional problem, however, arises, since many individuals do not wish sexual activity to be observed. In addition, the presence of observers may very well alter the behavior being observed. Masters and Johnson used direct observation to gather data about the physiologic changes that occur in men and women during sexual stimulation and the causes of these changes.[29]

Use of volunteers for sex research has been criticized since it is argued that normal people do not undertake such activities in public. Privacy, it is argued, is necessary for normal sexual response. Study of characteristics of some subjects indicated that they were better educated, more intelligent, or higher social class, had need for social approval, and were more sociable than nonvolunteers. Although sex in the laboratory is different from usual sexual encounters, it does not necessarily mean that the physiologic responses are different. The difference from a heterosexual relationship with a loved one may be quantitative rather than qualitative.[30]

Physiologic processes are recorded by use of direct observation, film, and standard medical equipment to record blood pressure and cardiac rates. An artificial coition machine equipped with an artificial penis and equipment that recorded changes in the vagina and lower uterus during sexual response was used by Masters and Johnson.

Research on sexual function in women has involved use of pressure transducers and other objective measures of physiologic response. Vaginal hemodynamic changes during sexual arousal can be assessed by several noninvasive methods. Photoplethysmography involves shining red or infrared light into the vaginal wall; the amount scattered or reflected back is measured and recorded.[31] The thermal clearance method measures tissue blood perfusion by measuring its cooling of a heated metal disc held against the epithelium.[32] A heated oxygen electrode, a third method, measures power consumption as an index of vaginal blood flow.[33]

Quantitative analysis of circumvaginal musculature, especially the pubococcygeus muscle, is done by the use of a perineometer, a pressure sensitive device inserted into the vagina. It is an inexpensive, simple device and is valuable for evaluating female sexual dysfunction.[34]

Other studies of female sexual arousal include measurement of vaginal surface oxygen tension (PO_2) during and after orgasm by use of an oxygen electrode (radiometer) attached to the vaginal wall. Circulatory changes during rapid eye movement (REM) sleep have also been studied. Findings indicate that females undergo phasic shifts in blood flow similar to the nocturnal erections that men experience during REM sleep.

These objective measurements of vaginal changes will be increasingly used in the diagnosis and treatment of sexual dysfunctions. For example, a woman who states that she cannot reach orgasm can have her genital blood flow monitored to see if there is increased blood flow with stimulation. The diagnosis of whether arousal, which is claimed to exist in the brain, is actually occurring in the vagina can be made and therapy for psychogenic or organic anorgasmia can be initiated as appropriate.[35]

Research on sexual function in the male involve measures of penile circumference, blood volume changes, and perineal muscle activity. Nocturnal penile tumescence (NPT) is also measured.[36]

The sexual behavior of laboratory animals is also studied, but there is the problem of generalizability from nonhuman species to human. The complex social system in which sexual behavior and sexual differentiation takes place in human society is not taken into account when making comparisons with animals.[37]

Case Study

Study of a single person, group, or community provides in-depth information about a particular case, insight into an interaction, and the meanings ascribed to the interaction. Generalizations, however, cannot be made to the larger population.

Ethical Considerations

Protection from harm to human subjects involved in any research and provision for their informed consent is an important legal and moral issue in any research. The sensitive and intimate nature of sexuality poses even greater constraints to protect individuals from harm.[38] Anonymity protects individuals from social stigma. Protection from psychologic harm or emotional distress is more difficult, since any type of questioning or interviewing produces emotional responses, even more so when the topic is sexuality. Respondents may bring up past painful emotional experiences that may be reevaluated and redefined.

There may be an element of exploitation of the subject, since except in written surveys or questionnaires, the interviewer strives to develop a trust relationship based on openness and rapport. The respondent may see a personal relationship, but when the investigator finishes, the relationship is ended. This can be harmful to unstable or naive subjects who seek friendship or professional help by revealing inner thoughts and feelings.[39]

Informed consent insures that the subjects are aware of the projected use of their information. Misrepresentation of the purposes of the investigation and covert research involving concealment of the purposes of the investigation from the respondents may involve serious breaches of ethical behavior.[40]

NURSING IMPLICATIONS

Nurses are increasingly interested in research related to sexuality. A review of published studies in *Nursing Research* provides some evidence of this fact. In addition, nurses are increasingly applying the findings of research. No single method is best for sexual research. Different methods provide different insights and conclusions and are necessary to investigate the myriad facets of sexuality. However, nurses must be careful about drawing conclusions from studies about sexuality.

In an area as personal as sexuality, individuals tend to measure their life experiences against the conclusions of the study. If they are the same, one tends to have greater faith in the conclusions. If they differ, doubts arise, and rightly so. However, in either case, nurses evaluate the methodology used by the researcher as well as the representativeness of their life experiences. Care must be taken to avoid generalizations from both when such generalizations are not valid. It must be remembered that there is much more risk of error in generalizing from personal experiences to a whole population than generalizing from a well-designed study.[41]

Since attitudes and behavior are so much of one's identity, it is difficult for nurses to avoid judging others' sexuality in terms of the norms by which they judge their own. Sexual practices and beliefs held by patients/clients may differ radically from those of nurses who may feel that others' behavior is immoral, illegal, or unhealthy. By the others' standards, it is none of these things, however.

Nurses may be tempted to intervene to try to change an individuals' attitudes and behavior. Not only is this difficult or in some cases impossible in a short-term relationship, but also, if these beliefs and attitudes are part of a person's cultural inheritance, anger and hostility toward the care giver and noncompliance with any proposed regimen will result. This is not to suggest that nurses should not do health teaching to change sexual practices that have been shown to cause health deviations, but this should be done only after careful assessment of the sociocultural backgrounds of the individuals and how they are related to their sexuality.

SEXUAL ROLES AND RELATIONSHIPS

Role Behavior
Many argue that sex role norms and sextyped behavior are acquired from "significant others" (parents and others important to the individual) and not primarily by biologic factors. Learning begins in early childhood

and before adolescence is firmly fixed in the makeup of individuals. This early learning about gender role is highly resistant to change even when changes occur in the social milieu and can produce much conflict and distress for the individual.

Many stress that male sex roles and female sex roles are the outcome of this learning. Traditionally, masculinity involves dominance, aggressiveness, and instrumentality, while femininity is defined in terms of submissiveness, passivity, conformity, modesty, emotional lability, and nurturance. In the past, with few exceptions, society has been structured, and to a large extent is still structured, so that men have greater opportunity for economic success, occupational achievement, and political power.[42]

Sexual role norms are to a large extent controlled by society, which sets limits to what is considered appropriate role behavior. Those who choose to defy these norms face the risk of being labeled "deviant," with the negative sanctions the term implies, while conformity is rewarded by positive sanctions.

These facts have implications for nurses not only in relation to their own behavior but also in relation to that of their patients/clients. A review of Chapter 2 will indicate its relevance for nurses and nursing.

Scanzoni[43] identified five key sociologic variables that the literature indicates are associated with role behavior and with the attitude toward male–female roles: sex, age, education, race, and religion. The nurse considers these variables when planning care to meet individual's sexual needs.

Sex. Bardwick sees women as conforming to four types of role behavior: (1) women who are content with the traditional role; (2) women who enter the work force at some time but are not committed to professional achievement and who perceive the job as an extension of their traditional role; (3) women who, having gained success in the traditional role, maintain a core commitment to achievement in a vocation; and (4) women who are not motivated to achieve the traditional role responsibilities and do not desire children or marriage.[44]

It is suggested that men can be expected to be more traditional and women more modern in their sex role orientation. Because women are the subordinate group, it is to their benefit to change the status quo and seek change, while men, for their own best interests, maintain the status quo.[45]

Age. Younger persons might be expected to be more modern in their views of sex roles than older persons. Feminism is becoming more powerful since Ellis wrote of the women's movement in 1900.[46] Each new generation has seen greater female autonomy and independence.

Education. Education, if it is effective, tends to have a liberalizing or modernizing effect on beliefs and behavior: those with more years of schooling will be less role traditional than those with less. Children from higher-status homes are socialized to attain still higher levels of education[47] and the liberalization continues.

Race: Blacks and Sexuality. Although much is written about black sexuality, most of the information is based on folklore. There is little scientific material available on blacks and sex. The Kinsey report and the studies of Masters and Johnson scarcely mention blacks. In the 1948 *Sexual Behavior in the Human Male*, Kinsey stated that there was not enough information about the black male to make an analysis. He did point out that preliminary findings showed as many patterns of behavior among blacks of different social levels as among whites, and that black and white patterns for similar social levels were close if not identical.[48] Kinsey did not include blacks in his study of female sexual behavior. Masters and Johnson did not include black subjects in their final report and clearly stated that their research was weighted to examine white behavior.[49]

Poussaint and Comer state that any differences in black and white sexual behavior in America are minimal, and beliefs in differences between the black and white races are due to sexual stereotyping that can be psychologically damaging to both races and to their interpersonal relations.[50]

There is literature to suggest that black marriages may be more egalitarian than white marriages. This may be due to long-standing discrimination against black men and women. Black men and women were often torn from their homes during slavery. Although slaves had a family life, it was neither socially sanctioned nor protected by society. Since "bodies" were an important socioeconomic asset, encouragement of reproduction was important, but if the father was sold, the black mother might have to raise the children alone. To some extent this is still true; a large proportion of black families are headed by females, although this is changing.

In addition, black women were forced into the labor market because black men had so little opportunity for education and meaningful occupations. As a result, there may be a much greater feeling of equality between black males and females than among whites.[51] The call for sexual equality is met with less interest by black lower-class women, who have experienced substantial female power, chiefly because the male had no resources with which to bargain for status and power. Some blacks feel that anything that takes energy and interest away from improving the position of the black man (and subsequently their women) should get low priority.[52] Black women may not see that the role of equal provider is a privilege to be sought vigorously.

Blacks have their share of sexual difficulties and dysfunction, and the myth of black sexual prowess is just that. Blacks also seem to have the same incidence of homosexual behavior as the rest of the population.[53] Until carefully designed, objective studies of black sexual practices at all socioeconomic levels are done, definitive conclusions about black sexuality are suspect.

Religion.   Throughout history, religion has had a profound effect on sex role behavior and on the broader area of sexuality itself. Kinsey and associates found that the incidence of all types of sexual behavior except marital coitus was lower among more devout females and males and higher among the less devout.[54]

A traditional belief among some religions is that marriage is considered a career in itself, and having a family is of intrinsic importance. Career roles in the world for married women, especially those with young children, may be regarded as incompatible. The biblical teaching that women are subject to their husbands, if followed, literally leaves little room for idiosyncratic role behavior.

Few deny the relationship between religion and religious beliefs and sexuality. Whether the union is a positive or negative one has been and probably will continue to be debated by many. That it may have a profound effect on sexuality is denied by none. (See Chapter 9 for discussion of teaching of various religions and sexuality.)

Changing Roles and Relationships

Historical Overview.   There have been two periods when rapid changes in sexual relationships and behavior have taken place. Around World War I, between 1915 and 1920 and from 1965 to 1975, there were notable increases in divorce and nonvirginity rates.

There was also a change in basic life styles and in the relationship between men and women; sex roles in business, politics, and education changed as women became more involved in these occupations. At the present time, there seems to be another period of consolidation, when after identifying alternatives to traditional roles, society is codifying, ranking, ordering, and deciding what is to be preferred among all the new things.[55]

In the past, nevertheless, different behavior and attitudes have been expected from males and females, and this stereotyping has negatively affected both growth and change in roles and relationships.

Sexual Stereotyping. Sigmund Freud contributed to the belief that males are superior to females and that anatomy is destiny. He stressed that the male's penis makes him feel superior to the female, who, noting her lack, feels inferior. The subsequent character and personality resulting from the oedipal and castration stages of psychosexual development confirms this superiority, since most traits defined as male have more value in society than those designated as female. Women must accept their secondary status and compensate for a lack of a penis by having babies and a husband. If the male can overcome his castration fear, he emerges as a complete human, while the women can never do this (see Chapter 7). Freud gave biologic foundation for the "feminine' traits of "narcissism, jealousy, vanity and competition and all types of defensive behavior."[56]

Ellis stressed that boys and girls should be educated together so that there would be a "foundation of genuine comradeship" laid in youth. He suggested it was the duty of society to provide for the childbearer so she can exercise her social functions. He also indicated that every woman should have not only a sexual relationship with a man but at least one "supreme function of maternity."[57] Others supported this teaching. Erikson felt that women want to be "womanly" companions to men and were destined to be mothers.[58] Margaret Mead was one who was most challenging of the notion of what is masculine or feminine, admitting that there were biologic givens, but stressing that cultural conditions were responsible for sex-linked traits.

Whatever its origin, sexual stereotyping begins in infancy. The parents' physical and verbal approach is different for boys and girls, and the roles that are learned in the home are often reinforced by movies, books, and television.[59]

Mature love can develop only between those who consider themselves equals, and this is difficult with the dominant–submissive, male–female sex roles. We have seen that comparative studies of men and women in different cultures give evidence that there is no pattern of behavior peculiar to one sex that cannot be observed in the other. Many believe that roles are culturally determined. Early teachings of major religions about women and their status have also contributed to the idea that, even if valued and loved by men, women were subject, if not inferior, to them.

Roles have been changing, if too slowly and imperceptibly for some. That is evident when one reviews the history of humankind. In the forefront of those struggling to obliterate sexual role stereotyping has been the Women's Liberation Movement.

The Women's Liberation Movement. Women may be considered a minority group, if not by actual number, by their deprivation when their economic and social status is compared to men's. Some argue, however, that in many ways they are a privileged group and that men carry the heavier burden in society. Whatever differences of opinion exist, the view of many women that they are regarded as second-class citizens is not a new one.

In 1848, the "Declaration of Sentiment" presented by the Abolitionist Movement became the first public statement against the status of women in the United States. After that meeting, others were held under the leadership of feminists such as Susan B. Anthony. At first, women stressed their exploitation, enslavement, and depersonalization, but later in the century, their central issue became the granting of political rights through suffrage. Social and economic deprivation was deemphasized, since it was difficult to persuade some married women that their life was one of oppression and that the prescribed role should be changed.[60]

After 1920, the women's movement declined drastically. Franklin Roosevelt's New Deal took the issues raised by the women's movement into account. Eleanor Roosevelt and Frances Perkins, the first female cabinet member, were concerned about the status of women. Efforts were focused on wages and working conditions of all workers, and women benefited from social security measures, minimum wage laws, and encouragement to get "useful education."

World War II put women into jobs formerly held by men. Women's restiveness in the 1950s and early 1960s may have been caused by the war years' experiences, the increased social mobility of the middle class family, the expansion of education, or the steady number of working women who encountered male prejudice face to face. Intellectual ferment followed. Simone de Beauvoir in *The Second Sex* and Betty Friedan in *The Feminine Mystique* described the effects of a male-dominated society and women's deprivation.[61]

The Commission on the Status of Women was established by President John Kennedy in 1961. In 1963, the commission released a report that stressed the right of all Americans to make basic choices and suggested that women were deprived of as full an opportunity to do so as men, that in many respects women were second-class citizens. Even in the Civil Rights Movement struggling to gain a place for the black in American society, women encountered discrimination. The Black Panthers stated, "Power to the brothers and love to the sisters."

Women continued to protest against sexist institutions through marches, demonstrations, picket lines, and sit-ins at publishers of men's magazines. The National Organization for Women (NOW) focused its attention on economics, aiming to enforce anti-discrimination laws in colleges and businesses. Organizations in various cities were aimed at "consciousness raising," making women aware of their subordinate status and imbuing them with a sense of sisterhood.[62]

Although a large part of the movement is concerned with equality of employment, its early aims were more diverse:

1. Free day care centers for children so that women may work without having to surrender the choice of motherhood
2. Reexamination of marriage as an institution and of the superior–subordinate roles

that culture establishes in the context of marriage
3. Revision of child-raising practices so that women are not programmed to present social roles
4. Revision of educational practices to the same end
5. Political organization to achieve the program

Underlying the program is the goal of a major cultural change: the elimination of prescribing roles on the basis of sex.[63]

Progress has been made, but like all groups, women are divided by age; marital, social, and economic status; and life experiences. The number of women who are organized or who agree with the goals is questionable.

The Equal Rights Amendment to the Constitution was not ratified in 1982 despite a time extension. Equally dedicated and militant women worked against the ERA arguing that rather than benefitting women, it would work to their detriment and to that of society. Betty Friedan[64] stated that the women's movement has come as far as it can in terms of women alone and must move into a second stage. NOW began focusing on the family by recognizing that many women desire husbands and children and that equality in the workplace brings its own conflict between the demands of a position, success, and the demands of a family. Friedan questions why women should replace the glorification of domesticity with the glorification of work as life and identity.[65] The challenge of the 80s has been to create new family patterns based on equality and full human identity for both sexes. The image of the women's liberation movement as opposed to the family is denied and feminists who disparage the family are described as woefully out of step with women.

Friedan has been attacked by other feminists who have accused her of trimming her feminism to suit more conservative times. Other feminists agree that some of them were "beating their heads" against a wall to deny the importance to most women of nurturing, childbearing, and warm familial relationships.[66]

NOW also began diverting its attention toward political action and support of candidates who support laws that solve problems such as the sexist wage gap, sex discrimination, and child care.[67]

Some women are not prepared for their different, more responsible social roles. Some men are threatened by the idea of women gaining more power and independence. Many men will not give up rights, privileges, and powers within the occupational and domestic spheres unless women choose to express the conflict.[68] Not everyone agrees that these changes are beneficial. Some psychologists argue that without clear-cut sex differences, heterosexual ties will be weakened and there will be confusion over sexual identity, while others disagree, arguing that what is taking place is a healthy phenomenon, multidetermined and different for each person.[69]

Sexual Individuality. One can speculate about the effects of sexual role behavior that is freed from the stereotyping of the past so that each person expresses his or her sexual individuality. The result will be vitality, vigor, and excitement in sexual roles and relationships. (See Chapter 2 for discussion of nursing and sexual roles.)

If sex roles are to be changed, the socialization of the child needs to be consciously directed away from traditional sex role stereotypes and toward emphasis of men and women primarily as persons, not as masculine or feminine beings. School curriculum should be organized so that children face sex role questions and consider a variety of possible role gratifications. In addition, they must have the options open to them.[70]

Alternative Sexual Life Styles

The traditional norms of society dictate that the ideal sexual relationship is permanent, monogamous, and legitimized by marriage. Some persons advocate alternate sexual life styles that they consider more satisfying and fulfilling. These may involve extramarital sexual relationships or may involve sexual relationships without marriage.

Open Marriage. Extramarital activity may take place for numerous reasons—illness of the partner, boredom, disinterest of the partner—but there are some couples who engage in extramarital activity who neither lack sex nor express dissatisfaction with their partners. They feel that their sexual drives will be enriched by sexual liaisons with others. In an open marriage, both spouses mutually agree that extramarital activity is permissable and desired, at least in theory, and relinquish their claim on each other's fidelity. Some couples state that it has resulted in a marital relationship that is closer and more caring, while others have had negative experiences, finding the open construct more palatable in theory than in practice. Problems arise because there is more than sex involved in most marriage relationships. Intellectually, individuals may feel that these extramarital liaisons will enrich the sexual life, but on an interpersonal level, spouses may feel threatened, jealous, inadequate, and betrayed, in spite of the belief that they are liberated from such feelings.[71]

Swinging and Group Sex. Sexual avant-garde relationships, such as swinging, involve mutual exchange of spouses between married couples with the consent of all involved. This differs from the open marriage, because it involves a sexual encounter in which the husband and wife are participating simultaneously at the same place, although usually in different rooms. Mate swapping parties may involve discreet sexual activity in which a couple wanders off to a bedroom and returns to continue socializing or "open" parties or "orgies" in which nudity is the rule and where naked bodies engage in sexual activity with whomever comes within reach.[72]

Motivation for swapping may include obtaining sexual variety, expanding one's social life by a new form of recreation, or enhancing one's ego by having sexual attractiveness reaffirmed.[73] The ego may be shattered, however, by the swinging experience, especially for the male who discovers that he cannot always become sexually aroused and responsive to every woman. A woman is faced with less threat, since she can have many orgasms or, if she is not sexually aroused, it is not as visible or culturally defined as failure.[74] Other problems that may arise include jealousy and the possibility of discovery and social ostracism.[75]

Polyfidelity involves individuals living in nonmonogamous groups where they have a fixed sleeping schedule described as "nonpreferential" and rotational. Sexual intimacy occurs equally between all members of the opposite sex. There is no sexual involvement outside the group and there is an intention of lifetime involvement.[76]

Premarital Relationships. Males and females may experiment with premarital intercourse, sometimes recreationally, but often with mutual affection and respect. A more or less permanent commitment to each other may be involved.[77] In some cases, the expectations of one or both partners may be that marriage is in the future; in others, there is no commitment to legalization of the relationship. Even if children are born, some couples feel that a love relationship does not need a marriage contract. These couples are not bothered by any social stigma that may be attached to the relationship, although some may introduce each other as husband or wife. Problems arise when they desire legal guarantees of their *rights*.

Other couples live together to test their compatibility with the expectation that marriage will take place in the future. Problems arise when one individual desires to terminate the relationship while the other is committed to continuing it.[78]

Free Sex. Proponents of new or "liberated" sexuality argue that living together or having coitus with whomever and whenever is desired is a more natural and fulfilling view of sexuality than obeying the constraints society has traditionally placed on sexual activity outside of marriage. Just as avantgarde marital relationships have become less popular, some individuals have turned away from "free sex," discovering "free" sex hurts, and that is is difficult to separate feelings from sexual relationships. Secondary virginity is being practiced by persons who are withdrawing from "meaningless" sexual encounters.

Authorities on psychosexual adjustment disagree about the values of the current changes in sexual attitudes and behavior and their ultimate effect on society. Some make a case for sex without love, going even beyond the norms of many of today's young persons. Others argue that substantial changes in attitudes and behaviors can lead to considerable individual and social problems, that it may be a new form of Puritanism. Like the old, moralistic Puritanism, the new Puritanism results in alienation from the body and from feeling and emotion from reason. The body is conceptualized as a sexual machine, and modern man's principle of full freedom may demand just as rigid conformity of behavior as did the old.[79]

Changing Behaviors. As was mentioned in Chapter 1, the sexual revolution that resulted in alternative sexual life styles and the national preoccupation with sex, appears to be changing. Individuals are rediscovering fidelity, obligation, marriage and commitment, and are moving away from extremes of behavior and developing a sense of cautiousness and greater commitment to careers. College students may be more sexually sophistocated but they also seem to want long-term commitments. In addition to a focus on social and economic security, fear of herpes (Chapter 22), and women's reassertion of traditionalist values may also be factors in the conservative trend.[80] Those involved in studying the psychologic damage suffered by those living an avant-garde life style suggest that some of the glowing reports of this life style may have resulted from reports of researchers who were missionary swingers themselves.[81]

NURSING IMPLICATIONS

Sexual role behavior and relationships depend on complex interrelationship of age, sex, and sociocultural factors. There is no conformity nor unanimity of attitude and behavior, since each individual's sexuality represents a unique blend of these factors. What is more, there is variation within each factor. For example, not all older persons are sexually conservative. Some individuals accept the traditional norms of the church regarding sexuality, while others may not. Not all women are passive and compliant.

Consequently, it is important that nurses be aware of various attitudes and behavior that exist and then determine how these operate in their patient/client. Some questions that nurses need to have answered include:

1. What are an individual's attitudes about sexuality and what do they consider appropriate for themselves?
2. Are they satisfied with their sexual roles, relationships, and behavior or do they desire change?
3. Are they committed to the roles, relationships, and behavior because of strong religious beliefs and commitment and/or other cultural ties?
4. How have life events, illness, therapy, affected ability to carry out role behavior?

Based on the answers to these questions, the nurse can plan interventions. Nurses work within the framework of persons' strong beliefs about sexuality and what is appropriate sexual behavior for them.

Nurses also need to consider the research methods they utilize. MacPherson[82] argues for a new paradigm for nursing research, using a feminist approach, one that is concerned not only with making women visible, but with problems of sexual divisions in the research team. She stresses utilizing feminist theories in order to get beyond sex biases.

Nurses must continue to generate researchable questions about sexuality as part of the nursing process.[83]

NOTES

1. Katchadourian HA, Lunde DT: Fundamentals of Human Sexuality, 2nd ed. New York, Holt, 1975, p 176
2. Izard CE: Human Emotions. New York, Plenum, 1977, p 184
3. DeLora JS, Warren CAB: Understanding Sexual Interaction. Boston, Houghton Mifflin, 1977, pp 566–567
4. Kinsey AC, Pomeroy WB, Martin CE: Sexual Behavior in the Human Male. Philadelphia, Saunders, 1948, pp 327–417
5. Weinberg MS (ed): Sex Research. New York, Oxford, 1976, p 75
6. Johnson WR, Belzer ED: Human Sexual Behavior and Sex Education. Philadelphia, Lea and Febiger, 1973, pp 213–214
7. Ibid, p 215
8. Ibid, p 218–219
9. Messenger JC: Sex and repression in an Irish folk community. In Weinberg MS (ed): Sex Research. New York, Oxford, 1976, pp 273–279
10. Ellis A: The folklore of sex. In Schur EA (ed): The Family and the Sexual Revolution. Bloomington, Indiana, Indiana University Press, 1964, pp 31–50
11. Tergerson D: Women's liberation still

under wraps in Israel. Cleveland Plain Dealer, May 7, 1978, Sec 4, p 26

12. Riding A: Revolution changes female role in Nicaragua. The Plain Dealer, December 4, 1980, sec AA, p 19

13. Stevens EP: Scholar analyzes Latin American sex roles. Images (Case Western Reserve University), December 1976, p 11

14. Cullen RD, Nater T: A sexual rite on trial. Time, November 1, 1982, p 55

15. Rosenblum EH: Conversation with a Navajo nurse. Am J Nurs 80:1459–1462, 1980

16. Rosenblum EH: Frustrated wives, lazy husbands and signs of change. Time, June 23, 1980, p 65

17. Rosenblum EH: Discovering the birds and bees. Time, March 7, 1983, p 87

18. Johnson WR, Belzer ED: Human Sexual Behavior and Sex Education. Philadelphia, Lea and Febiger, 1973, pp 227–235

19. Reiss IL, Walsh, HR, Zey-Ferrell M, et al: Research in heterosexual relationships. In Green R, Wilner J (eds): Methodology in Sex Research. Rockville, Maryland, Alcohol, Drug Abuse and Mental Health Administration, U.S. Department of Health and Human Services, Public Health Services, National Institutes of Mental Health, 1980, pp 80–166

20. Green R: Methodologic problems in research in psychosexual differentiation. In Green R, Wilner J (eds): Methodology in Sex Research. Rockville, Maryland, Alcohol, Drug Abuse and Mental Health Administration, U.S. Department of Mental Health and Human Services, Public Health Services, National Institutes of Mental Health, 1980, pp 252–278

21. Reiss IL, Walsh, HR, Zey-Ferrell M, et al: Research in heterosexual relationships. In Green R, Wilner J (eds): Methodology in Sex Research. Rockville, Maryland, Alcohol, Drug Abuse and Mental Health Administration, U.S. De-

partment of Health and Human Services, Public Health Services, National Institutes of Mental Health, 1980, p 45

22. Ibid, p 62

23. Weinberg MS (ed): Sex Research. New York, Oxford, 1976, p 10

24. Kirby D: Methods and methodological problems of sex research. In DeLora JS, Warren CAB (eds): Understanding Sexual Interaction. Boston, Houghton Mifflin, 1977, p 563–586

25. Ibid, p 571

26. Ibid, p 572

27. Ibid, p 574

28. Ibid, p 582

29. Masters WH, Johnson VE: Human Sexual Response. Boston, Little, Brown, 1966, pp 9–23

30. Levin RJ: The physiology of sexual function in women. Clin Obstet Gynecol 7:213–250, 1980

31. Ibid, p 231

32. Ibid, p 234

33. Ibid, p 236

34. Graber B, Kline-Graber G, Golden CJ: A circumvaginal muscle nomogram: A new diagnostic tool for evaluation of female sexual dysfunction. J Clin Psych 42:157–161, 1981

35. Levin RJ: The physiology of sexual function in women. Clin Obstet Gynecol 7:239, 1980

36. Hatch JP: Psychophysiological aspects of sexual dysfunction. Arch Sex Behav 10:49–64, 1981

37. Herbert J: Neurobiological concepts and methods in the study of sexual behavior. In Green R, Wilner J (eds): Methodology in Sex Research. Rockville, Maryland, Alcohol, Drug Abuse and Mental Health Administration, U.S. Department of Health and Human Services, Public Health Services, National Institutes of Mental Health, 1980, pp 207–251

38. Bentter PM, Abramson PR: Methodological issues in sex research: An overview. In Green R, Wiener J (eds): Methodology in Sex Research, Rockville, Maryland, Alcohol, Drug Abuse and

Mental Health Administration, U.S. Department of Health and Human Services, Public Health Services, National Institutes of Mental Health, 1980, pp 308–313

39. Kirby D: Methods and methodological problems in sex research. In DeLora JS, Warren CAB (eds): Understanding Sexual Interaction. Boston, Houghton Mifflin, 1977, p 584

40. Ibid, p 585

41. Ibid, p 586

42. Bardwick JM: Psychology of Women. New York, Harper & Row, 1971, p 19

43. Scanzoni JH: Sex Roles, Life Styles and Childbearing. New York, Free Press, 1975, pp 19–63

44. Bardwick JM: Psychology of Women. New York, Harper & Row, 1971, pp 161–162

45. Scanzoni JH: Sex Roles, Life Styles and Childbearing. New York, Free Press, 1975, p 21

46. Ellis H: The Task of Social Hygiene. Boston, Houghton Mifflin, 1912, pp 1–59

47. Scanzoni JH: Sex Roles, Life Styles and Childbearing. New York, Free Press, 1975, p 27

48. Kinsey AC, Pomeroy WB, Martin CE: Sexual Behavior in the Human Male. Philadelphia, Saunders, 1948, pp 6–7

49. Masters WH, Johnson VE: Human Sexual Response. Boston, Little, Brown, 1966, p 15

50. Poussaint AF, Comer JP: Sexual studies do not show blacks differ. Cleveland Plain Dealer, June 18, 1978, Sec 4, p 25

51. Makielski SJ Jr: Beleaguered Minorities. San Francisco, Freeman, 1973, pp 41–50

52. Scanzoni J: Sexual Bargaining. Englewood Cliffs, New Jersey, Prentice-Hall, 1972, pp 121–123

53. Poussaint AF, Comer JP: Sexual studies do not show blacks differ. Cleveland Plain Dealer, June 18, 1978, Sec 4, p 25

54. Kinsey AC, Pomeroy WB, Martin CE, Gebbard PW: Sexual Behavior in the Human Female. New York, Pocket Books, 1965, pp 686–687

55. Reiss I: Adolescent sexuality. In Oaks WW, Melchiode GA, Ficher I (eds): Sex and the Life Cycle. New York, Grune and Stratton, 1976, p 51

56. Gruber S: Sex roles and the feminine personality. In Goldman GD, Milman D (eds): Modern Woman. Springfield, Illinois, Thomas, 1969, pp 75–89

57. Ellis H: The Task of Social Hygiene. Boston, Houghton Mifflin, 1912, p 65

58. Erikson EH: Identity, Youth, and Crisis. New York, Norton, 1968, pp 261–294

59. Gould RE: Socio-cultural roles of male and female. In Sadock BJ, Kaplan HI, Freedman AM (eds): The Sexual Experience. Baltimore, Williams and Wilkins, 1976, pp 280–289

60. Makielski SJ Jr: Beleaguered Minorities. San Francisco, Freeman, 1973, p 88

61. Ibid

62. Ibid, p 91

63. Ibid, p 94

64. Makielski SJ Jr: Moving into the second stage: An interview with Betty Friedan. Nurs Outlook 29:666–669, 1981

65. Friedan B: NOW faces a new frontier. The Plain Dealer, November 18, 1979, p 17C

66. Leo J: New frontier for feminism. Time, October 21, 1981, p 118

67. Stainer H: ERA's time to come, NOW president says. The Plain Dealer, March 12, 1983, p 5A

68. Scanzoni J: Sexual Bargaining. Englewood Cliffs, New Jersey, Prentice-Hall, 1972, p 164

69. Gould RE: Socio-cultural roles of male and female. In Sadock BJ, Kaplan HI, Freedman AM (eds): The Sexual Experience. Baltimore, Williams and Wilkins, 1976, p 288

70. Scanzoni JH: Sex Roles, Life Styles and Childbearing. New York, Free Press, 1975, p 187

71. DeLora JS, Warren CAB (eds): Understanding Sexual Interaction. Boston, Houghton Mifflin, 1977, p 259

72. Ibid, p 257
73. "Avant-Garde Retreat?" Time, November 25, 1974, pp 100–103
74. DeLora JS, Warren CAB (eds): Understanding Sexual Interaction. Boston, Houghton Mifflin, 1977, p 259
75. Ibid, p 260
76. Adams V: Polyfidelity: The Kerista village ideal. Psych Today 13:42–43, 1980
77. Izard CE: Human Emotions. New York, Plenum, 1977, p 185
78. Schlatter T: Living together: No key to freedom. The Plain Dealer, October 12, 1980, Sec C, p 13
79. Izard CE: Human Emotions. New York, Plenum, 1977, p 185
80. Leo J: Sex in the 80's: The revolution is over. Time, April 9, 1984, p 74–83
81. Time, November 25, 1974, p 1032.
82. MacPherson KI: Feminist Methods: A new paradigm for nursing research. Adv Nurs Sci 5:17–26, 1983
83. Hott JR, Ryan-Merritt M: A national study of nursing research in human sexuality. Nurs Clin North Am 17:429–447, 1982

Chapter 9

Religion and Sexuality

As we saw in Chapter 1, sex has played a major role in human affairs and has been an important facet of customs, art, laws, and religion. Our standards are largely derived from Old Testament Jewish patterns and the teachings of the early Christian fathers. This Judeo-Christian sexual tradition was brought to America by the Puritans, whose highly regulated and antisexual pattern became the official sexual morality and legal structure. Even though many disagree with these traditions, their influence cannot be denied.[1]

Most religions are alike in more ways than they are different in their attitudes toward sexuality. Most major religions believe in the importance of a good and lasting marriage and the need for mother's loving arms and the father's protective strength. They believe that the development of a strong value system in children with a strong but nonpunitive and realistic conscience as its safeguard is indispensable. They also agree that a stable home is necessary for children to grow to maturity and to relinquish dependency and move to responsible adulthood. The differences arise in specific sexual principles and practices.[2]

Religion has been accused of distorting a proper view of sex, of being behind the times, and of not knowing "what is happening." Some believe more realistic sex laws and a more workable and humane pattern of sexual behavior are necessary.[3] However, Carswell[4] argues that although distortions have

occurred in the name of religion, Judeo-Christian traditions have something meaningful to say, and the task is to separate distortions from truth. When this is done, one can find a concept of sex that is pure and wholesome.

Comfort[5] argues the opposite, that the restrictions and negative attitudes toward sexuality fostered by early Christian teaching still exist, even if these beliefs no longer present the teaching of Christians in most communities. He complains that these attitudes prevent any changes to more modern ideas of sexuality. Depending on the point of view, others may argue that it is religion whose teachings preserve and elevate sexuality beyond mere copulation, whose only goal is orgasm.

There has been a decline in religious orthodoxy, especially among the young. Recently there has been a resurgence of evangelic Christianity with strong emphasis on literal biblical teaching as the source of moral guidance.[6]

The focus of this chapter will be on the teachings of Jewish, Catholic, and Protestant faiths with the recognition that there are other denominations that might have dissimilar beliefs about what constitutes sexual morality.

JEWISH BIBLICAL BELIEFS

The religious teaching of Judaism is that sexuality is God's creation. Sexual inter-

145

course is not a sin, despite the misbelief that the sin of Adam and Eve was sexual intercourse. There should be no guilt attendant to sexual intercourse, since sex is not something dirty and shameful; God commanded Eve to be "fruitful and multiply." Although sex is not a sin, traditional Jewish teaching emphasizes that the appropriate place for sex is between the husband and wife, acknowledging that people are people and that many exceptions are to be found; people do not always live up to the norm. Sexual activity outside of marriage is strongly condemned, however. In the past, there were strong penalties for adultery, ranging up to death by starvation (as it is today, social mores dictated that the penalties were more severe for women).

In Judaism, the sexual relationship is the highest expression of love possible among humans. The word used in the scriptures was *to know*. Adam knew his wife Eve and she conceived (Genesis 4:1). To know a person sexually is both a physical and emotional sharing in its greatest intensity. It is a discovering of the personhood of the other.[7]

Sex was not meant to be joyless, but pleasurable. Sex could coexist with passion and affection. The Talmud tells wives to use cosmetics and ornaments to be attractive to their husband, both in youth and old age. It also encourages all forms of sex play between husband and wife, with emphasis on mutual gratification and orgasm of husband and wife. However, the dominating factor was a belief in procreation as the primary reason for sexual function. Celibacy was sinful, and marriage was encouraged during the childbearing years. Masturbation was considered a form of contraception and was contrary to the ideal of procreation. Sterility and failure to marry meant exclusion from the religious and social community. Homosexuality and bestiality, nonprocreative sexual activities, were forbidden. As a rule, sexual relations between unmarried persons was forbidden as both a religious and secular transgression.

Although women were accorded great respect as wives and mothers, women were held inferior to men. If they bore sons, they had to wait 33 days to purify themselves, if daughters, 55 days before they could engage in sexual intercourse. A daughter belonged to her father, and if she was used by a man sexually he had to marry her or give compensation to the father.[8] Jews were forbidden intercourse during the woman's menstrual period.

By Mosaic law, childlessness after 10 years of marriage was cause for obligatory divorce. Contraceptive use was not forbidden for women, but their use was not allowed for men.[9]

EARLY CHRISTIAN TEACHING

Carswell[10] stresses that nowhere in the teachings of Jesus was marriage or sex depicted as evil or unbecoming and that classical Judaism's high concept of sex was continued and deepened. Jesus affirmed the Jewish law that said the only basis for divorce was adultery, but stressed that it was not God's intention that man and woman separate, "What therefore God has joined together, let no man put asunder" (Matthew 22:1–10). His concepts of marriage and sex were the same as classical Judaism.

In the early Church, a change occurred in the concept of marriage and especially in the attitude toward sex. The apostle Paul, a bachelor, for the first time deprecated sex and marriage. Normal sexual relations were suspect. He justified marriage only for those who could not contain themselves. His stated reason for the negative attitude was that the end of the world and the second coming of Christ were coming soon, and he felt somehow that people would be more fit to greet the lord if they were untainted by sex. He also believed that one could serve God more completely without domestic concerns. He considered the celibate life higher and better than the married state and had a rather poor estimate of women. From the year 50 A.D. and for 350 years, the Church denounced sexual relations as evil, especially for priests and those involved in the ministry of the Church.[11]

With the rise of monasticism, men and women withdrew from the world to live in the shelter of monasteries, taking vows of poverty, chastity, and obedience. Men who renounced secular life in monastic vows were considered more pure and holy before God. Women became the devil's worst temptation.[12]

In the year 375, this attitude of the Church toward sex was pronounced, and it was to continue for centuries to come. St. Ambrose of Rome and St. John Chrysostom of Constantinople both condemned women. St. Augustine of Hippo went further and came to conclusions that have affected much of Christendom to this day. He stated that the continuation of the race is necessary until God has made up His number of the elect, so procreation is a duty. Adam and Eve, before the fall, did not enjoy sex, but part of the penalty of the fall was the enjoyment of sex. Since it was not possible to engage in sexual intercourse without enjoying it and since it was for procreation, man could go ahead and enjoy it without sin.[13]

Later, discussion went beyond Augustine's negative view with the recognition that marriage involved a contract for mutual comfort and help as well as a means of reproduction, but there was little understanding of intercourse as an expression of love between husband and wife. The teachings of Paul and Augustine (that virginity was a better state than marriage) were partly instrumental for the imposition of celibacy by the Church upon priests.[14] St. Thomas Aquinas urged that marriage without sex is more holy than marriage with sexual intercourse, and during the Middle Ages, Roman Catholicism emphasized virtue, compassion, charity, and love, but also asceticism and chastity. Sex was separated from other spiritual and social virtues.

Early Protestantism

Martin Luther challenged the sexual ethics of the Church and attacked the belief that set virginity above marriage. From the sixteenth century on, there has been a Catholic doctrine and a Protestant doctrine. One of the first changes was allowing marriage of pastors. In addition, marriage and sexual intercourse were considered for more than procreation. However, changes occurred under the influence of Puritanism in America and, later, Victorianism; the sex act was considered base and evil and was wrapped in silence as unfitting for decent people to think about, much less discuss.[15] The Puritan influence is still felt, for many people still believe that the churches should not discuss sex.

No word about sex was heard from the Protestant churches in the eighteenth and nineteenth centuries. In 1930, one of the earliest formed affirmations of the positive value of sex came from the Lambeth Conferences of Anglican Bishops, who stated that sex is a God-given factor in human life and is noble and creative. Coitus was identified as a means whereby marital love is enhanced.[16]

THE TWENTIETH CENTURY

A summary of present-day teachings of the major religions about sexuality is fraught with hazards. There is not only a lack of unanimity of opinion between major religious faiths but also within them. In detailing the tenets of the major faiths, the additional problem arises that many of the avowed members of various religious groups may in theory espouse certain beliefs but in practice behave differently. Kinsey found that religious affiliation was not so strongly correlated with sexual behavior as was religiosity and that there is a difference between the religiously devout persons and the religiously inactive persons of the same faith.[17] There are also differences in the teachings of Judaism, Catholicism, and Protestantism from the liberal and conservative viewpoints.

Judaism

In the Jewish point of view, sex and marriage are exemplified in Ecclesiastes: "Enjoy life with the wife that you lovest." The sexual relationship is to be a robust and open one. Jews still have a high regard for marriage and are encouraged to give a great deal of thought to the selection of a partner. Children are desired and loved.

The family is the fountainhead of Jewish worship.[18] In ancient Israel, men were the political, social, and religious leaders. In modern Judaism, women have risen to greater equality. Women, as wives and mothers, have always enjoyed a position of reverence and esteem, but in religious affairs, the change has been slower. However, women are now ordained as rabbis, and the number is likely to increase. Reform and conservative synagogues have abolished separation of men and women in different pews.[19]

The Jewish religion has been traditionally opposed to birth control and abortion when practiced for purely selfish reasons. Abortion is especially opposed as an elective device to limit family size. The exception is to save the mother's life.[20] The life of the mother is considered more important than that of the unborn child, and the most important consideration is what is best for the family.[21]

Birth control is sanctioned if pregnancy presents a hazard to the mother's health or if the children may be born defective. Modern Judaism has extended the concept to include poverty, inadequate living conditions, and threats to the welfare of existing children and the family. Most reform and conservative rabbis support the program of planned parenthood.[22]

Divorce is rare, but if living together is intolerable, Judaism permits divorce and even encourages it. A love-filled home is considered a sanctuary, and a loveless home a sacrilege. Every effort is made for reconciliation. However, if divorce does take place, the divorced persons are encouraged to remarry, since Jewish tradition is against the unwed state.[23]

Adultery is forbidden. The laws against unchastity are second in importance only to those related to theft. "It is forbidden to touch any woman except one's wife and whoever touches a woman, not his wife, may bring death upon himself."[24]

Masturbation is frowned upon in official Jewish doctrine. However, there is a relaxation in parental attitudes toward masturbation under the influence of modern psychosexual theory and practice.[25]

Roman Catholicism

Traditional Catholic teaching emphasizes the sanctity of marriage and the importance of sex within the marriage. Therefore, sex by oneself, premarital sex, or extramarital sex is prohibited. Contrary to the beliefs of early teaching, sex is considered good, human, and meaningful. It involves togetherness, tenderness, and lasting promises.[26]

Healthy sexuality involves an appreciation of sex and of male–female differences. Sex has a dynamic influence on life, but individuals must neither "starve" themselves of sex awareness nor "gorge" their imagination with sex. Sexual attraction is good. It draws individuals together to reach out and touch each other. Sex is seen as seeking a love relationship and then helping to reveal the fullness of the love relationship. Sex acts that are an expression of shared feelings and mutual will and sentiments are real ecstasy.[27]

Sex is seen as good and a part of each human. Few things in life are seen as more intense than sex and its release and rewards. The Catholic view is that sex enhances love and vice versa. Sex is meant to be enjoyable and to bind a couple together.[28]

The views of the Catholic Church on marriage were promulgated by Pope Pius XI in the "Encyclical on Christian Marriage." The need for a stable family unit, the home roles of women, and the prohibition of any contraception, except the rhythm method, were emphasized, and the close attachment of love and marriage were stressed. Pius XI stressed the primacy of the husband with regard to the wife and children and the wife's willing obedience. He stated that the subjection does not take away the dignity of the wife, nor does it mean that she must obey her husband's every request if it is not reasonable. Marriage and intercourse are primarily for begetting of children, and the secondary ends are mutual aid, love, and quieting of sexual desires. Abortion is direct murder of the innocent and against the commandment "Thou shalt not kill," while divorce is against the law of God that was confirmed by Christ.[29]

In "Humanae Vitae," Pope Paul VI reaffirmed the Church's belief in the permanence of marriage, but focused on condemning abortion and birth control. Sterilization and other forms of birth control, except the rhythm method, are illicit. In several passages, Pope Paul put more emphasis on the mutuality of marital love rather than the "submission" mentioned by Pius XI.[30] In 1980, the World Synod of Bishops reaffirmed this teaching.[31]

Pope Paul VI also argued that artificial birth control may open the way to conjugal infidelity and the general lowering of morality—that the man accustomed to contraceptive measures may lose respect for women and consider them instruments of selfish enjoyment.

Although condemning birth control, he refrained from labeling it a mortal (serious) sin and from insisting that confessors refuse offering the sacraments to those practicing contraception in good faith. In general, confessors are encouraging couples using contraception to come to the sacraments and many sincere Catholics no longer confess it.[32]

Pope John Paul II reaffirmed the Church's earlier teachings, also emphasizing that there should be no married priests and no women priests. He urged nuns to return to a "religious garb." Traditionally oriented Catholics were pleased, but liberals felt it was a return to an older orthodoxy, driving many out of the Church.[33]

Although artificial insemination even with the husband's sperm has been condemned on the grounds that the action is immoral, some Catholic theologians accept its morality with the husband's sperm and some argue that even this is not an absolute requirement.[34]

Homosexual acts are considered intrinsically disordered and are in no way approved. However, homosexual individuals are to be treated with understanding. Acknowledgment is made that they are not always personally responsible for their condition.[35] Masturbation may be considered by some to be a normal phenomenon of sexual development, but the Church still rejects this idea, stressing that it is an intrinsically disordered act, since it lacks the sexual relationship.[36]

The Catholic Church's teaching regarding sexual acts is based on the natural law theory, which holds that immutable laws of God are part of human nature. The Catholic Church considers these principles timeless and continues to transmit them, even if the opinions and morals of the world are opposed. However, there may be some opposition within the Church itself. Although the Catholic Church is described as doctrinally conservative, many confessors, theologians, and pastoral counselors, if not condemning some types of sexual behavior, take a sympathetic view of individuals' personal problems; others question if some sexual activities are morally wrong at all.

Springer[37] details another, though unofficial, Roman Catholic view. He holds that new circumstances of life in today's world demand updated sexual ethics, especially for young people. He believes this ethic would allow for psychosexual growth and better interpersonal relations in preparation for later life. His ethic allows sex before marriage, contraception, and masturbation if not carried to excess. Springer argues that neither the Old nor New Testament contain clear teaching against masturbation or premarital petting or sex play.

Springer sees Catholic sexual ethics moving from concentration on sex in marriage for procreation toward sexual expression of love in a deep and stable interpersonal relationship, which is characterized by sharing life in all areas.[38] He also sees women being elevated to their rightful status of equality with man. He believes that the decision for abortion is primarily the woman's, although the father does have a say and the fetus's welfare must remain of paramount importance.[39]

Other sexual behavior is also being examined. The ethical question is whether any act increases irresponsible sexual conduct. In June of 1977, *Human Sexuality: New Directions in American Catholic Thought* was published. It was written by five members of the Catholic Theological Society and commissioned by the society. The principle underlying the ideas presented was that there are no intrinsically immoral acts nor unchanging moral laws. In place of traditional morality based on the laws of God, Church, or civil authority, it sets up a system of values according to which moral conduct should be measured. Among the values as they apply to sexuality is included an assessment of sexual behavior. Seven characteristic attitudes should be present in Christian sexual behavior: (1) self-liberating, (2) other-enriching, (3) honest, (4) faithful, (5) socially responsible, (6) life-serving, and (7) joyous.[40]

The book has been praised by some and attacked by other theologians who hold that the views pay only lip service to the Bible and the Church. The Roman Catholic Bishops' Committee on Doctrine attacked the book, saying the theologians overstepped their bounds by setting guidelines for sexual behavior for Catholics. Some charged that the theologians overemphasized intrapersonal growth and personal relationships in coming to their conclusion, forgetting that good intentions and proper motives do not make sex outside of marriage morally right.

The book is praised for putting in print what has been an actual trend in the thought of many Catholic teachers. In addition, the research done by the authors was careful and worthwhile. For the first time, sexuality was recognized as a part of life not to be wished away.[41]

One theologian pinpoints a major concern about the Catholic Church and its teaching about sexual morality—the widening gap between what the Church is officially teaching and what Catholic theologians are more and more frequently writing. He feels the gap must be bridged or it could lead to tragedy in the American Church.[42]

Protestantism

Considerable differences exist between Protestant sects and even greater differences exist in interpretation of sexual morality among clergymen of the same sect. The more traditional and literal (in terms of biblical teaching) groups have sexual beliefs close to that of the Talmud and Catholic natural law, but more liberal Protestant clergy are more inclined to reinterpret all types of sexual behavior in terms of the total social adjustment of the individual.[43]

Liberal Protestant Beliefs. People are viewed as whole or total beings, and sex is good if it serves their fulfillment as total beings, that is, if it serves God's will for humankind. Hiltner[44] describes the individual as a total personal spirit (which includes the body), so the sex life cannot be totally animal in nature. God seeks fulfillment and realization of his creatures according to his will for them, and he blesses sex so that it may be used for his fulfillment. Sex cannot be confined to one or another aspect or dimension of a person.

Along with other aspects of relationships, sex is to promote love, which is the goal of all relationships. With sex, individuals' personhood is opened up and they look at life with an expanded awareness. There is no guarantee that the choice of the best partner, however, will solve all the wants and needs of either individual.

The developmental aim of sex in human life is toward an integration of the several levels of sexual purpose or function:

1. Biologically, sex reduces tension.
2. Psychologically, sex helps persons find unsuspected depths of selfhood.
3. Socially, individuals discover depth in an-

other and, by implication, potential depth in all other persons.

4. Ethically, individuals find the relationship between fulfillment and responsibility.

5. Theologically, sex is seen as a mystery, but a mystery that is partly revealed.

In the mature adult, the result of the integration of these factors is one whose sex life releases biologic tensions, moves him/her toward self-discovery and ever deeper love for a partner and beyond to the depth of every person. It convinces him/her that personal fulfillment and social responsibility go together and reveals the mystery of sex so that it is at the same time serious, radical, and joyful.[45]

Hiltner emphasizes that sex requires steadfastness and intensity. Steadfastness demands biophysical fidelity, a sense of movement toward depth in the relationship, a constant recognition of new depth in each other, and a growing conviction that faithfulness is its own reward. This is more than just refraining from sex with someone other than the spouse.

The meaning and goal of any sex act or relationship is dependent in some measure on the inner meaning of the persons involved, but the ultimate standards for meaning or good is the judgment and love of God. Although the individual may know God's judgment, the Christian community is likely to have better ideas than individuals about what God's judgment and love imply.

Protestants cannot be sure if they are right just because they do or do not do what their church tells them is right or wrong, especially in the area of sexuality. Legalism, to get a black and white definition, to pigeonhole sex acts without ambiguity is not possible. Some generalizations can be made and are likely to be relevant to most similar situations. Since good of the sex act rests partly on the meaning to the individual, he or she is obligated to consider the meaning of the act as he/she is and wishes to become and the meaning to God. There is no infallible guar-

antee as to the extent to which one is acting according to God's will. The church is likely to think its view of sex is closer to the will of God than that of individuals. However, its attitudes are as much under God's judgment as those of any individual.[46]

Hiltner's view emphasizes the individual responsibility for decisions about sex acts and morality, with the church's beliefs having some validity but taking a secondary role in sexual ethics. Implicit in his words is the notion that there are no acts that are intrinsically evil, but their merit depends on the inner meaning to the individual, with the final standard being God's judgment and love. He seems to be close to the beliefs of a small group of clergymen whom Johnson calls liberal humanists, who believe that sexual morality depends on the particular circumstances and the meaning that the particular sexual behavior has for the persons involved.[47]

Traditionalist and Neotraditionalist Protestant Beliefs.

The Protestant traditionalists believe that the rules laid down in the Old Testament and the New Testament are and always will be the only true rules and that their observance represents sexual morality. The teaching of the Bible is to be followed literally in regard to sexual activities. In the view of the traditionalists, masturbation is wrong, but as among Jews, there is a relaxation of attitudes by parents.[48]

Protestant belief may also take a position somewhere between that of the liberal teaching and that of the traditionalist belief in the biblical standard of sexual morality. Johnson and Belzer call them neotraditionalists. They are loyal to the rules of the church but do not espouse a sex–sin ethic or at least minimize it.[49] Marriage is universally regarded as an optional condition for a good life. Sexuality is seen as an act of sanctification, expressing all that is good and holy in life. Extramarital coitus, for the traditionalist, is sinful and illegal. To the neotraditionalist, coitus out of marriage may be wrong, but under certain conditions, especially with engaged couples whose marriage has to be postponed, they do not see much to condemn. Contraception is accepted for ethical purposes such as family planning and protection of the health of the mother and child. The decision for abortion is a right of the persons involved in consultation with medical authorities.

Protestantism is attempting to deal with promiscuity among young people, but because of its past history of silence and negativism, it may not be sought out for answers by them. Unfortunately, most people look at what was said in the past. What is being said now is described by Carswell as being as different as night and day. He sums up one view of Protestantism and sexuality by stressing that churches are becoming more involved in sex education and that sex is no longer a taboo subject. Religion is teaching children that there is nothing dirty or nasty about sex, not throwing out the biblical concept of sex but emphasizing a concept that has always been there. "It is saying that sex is God's creation, good and holy. Sexual intercourse is for those who within marriage are prepared to risk a high adventure into the mystery and joys of the personhoods of each other in integrity and in love."[50]

HUMANISTIC SEXUALITY

Some individuals argue that what is needed is to restructure the situation—to evolve a more realistic kind of sex education, more realistic sex laws and sexual morality, and a more workable and humane pattern of sexual behavior.[51] Humanistic morality is suggested as having the solution to the problem outside the bounds of religious codes. In *Humanist,* published by the American Humanist Association and Ethical Culture Movement, 34 sexologists published their "New Bill of Sexual Rights and Responsibilities." The humanists celebrate "responsible freedom" after centuries of "bondage to church or state." They state that marriage is a cher-

ished human relationship but other sexual relationships are also significant.

They predict a growing acceptance of premarital, homosexual, and bisexual relationships. Prostitution, sadomasochism and fetishism are "limiting" but should be controlled through education, not laws. Children's genital explorations are considered learning experiences, and masturbation is accepted as a viable mode of satisfaction for young and old. They believe that, for the first time, individuals own their bodies. Stressing that responsibility and mutuality are important, they preach the doctrine that "actualizing" pleasures are among the highest moral goods.[52]

RELIGION AND HOMOSEXUALITY

Religions have had a punitive and rejecting attitude and most have taught that homosexuality is unnatural and its practice sinful.[53] However, some dissenting voices are being heard. Although all the major churches have become sensitive to the gays' need for pastoral care and understanding, gays are still not usually accepted in the mainstream of religious life. In many denominations, small groups are pressing for full acceptance of gays. A group called Dignity is an organization of Catholic gays and their sympathizers.[54] Several Roman Catholic bishops have come out against gay rights, however, and other churches are divided on this issue.

Religious homosexuals are adopting a positive approach, insisting that since God made them as they are, they have every right to share in the life of the church and synagogue.[55]

The Christian case against homosexuality is founded on the concept of natural order. The great Swiss Protestant theologian Karl Barth, wrote of the homosexual: "The command of God shows him irrefutably—in clear contradiction of his own theories—that as a man he can only be genuinely human with a woman, or as a woman, with a man."

Over 20 centuries, all branches of Christianity have barred openly committed homosexuals from the clergy and lay offices. The organized and vocal campaign by homosexuals to be treated as everyone else is treated, however, and the question of the ordination of homosexuals into the clergy have caused dissension and disagreement in various denominations. The United Church of Christ was one of the first to ordain an openly gay minister. The Presbyterian Church designated a task force to study the question of gay clergy, and it did one of the most thorough studies of the issue ever undertaken by a major church. A majority and the minority based their cases on the Bible, Leviticus 18:22 and Romans 1:18–32, which state that homosexual acts are sinful. There was disagreement about the interpretation of the passages, the majority deciding that the passages were opinions of Jewish writers conditioned by time and place so that the teachings were not direct revelations from God. The minority dissented, arguing that homosexual ordination would seriously contradict the will of Christ.[56]

In May of 1978, the General Assembly of the United Presbyterian Church received the report, and by a vote of 12 to 1 refused to accept openly homosexual clergy and lay officers. The decree states that homosexual behavior is always wrong but denounces homophobia (hatred and fear of homosexuals) and stresses that homosexuality should not be singled out as any worse sin than pride, greed, or adultery. The policy also admits the possibility of ordination for people with homosexual orientation as long as they are repentent and committed to celibacy.[57] Other Protestant denominations are confronting the problem.

The National Coucil of Churches has considered an application for membership by a church most of whose 27,000 members are gay. The Universal Fellowship of Metropolitan Community Churches teaches that homosexuality is a "gift from God" and that there is nothing immoral about homosexual relationships. Some denominations threatened to quit the Council if the gay church was admitted.[58]

THE INDIVIDUAL

Some individuals with a firm belief in the tenets of their faith related to sexuality may be confused if not dismayed by what they perceive as a weakening of and a turning away from the established teaching of their church. Others may see the changing attitudes as freeing them from restrictions, regulations that they either followed with difficulty or disobeyed with guilt as an aftermath. Whether one accepts the beliefs of secular humanists or conscientiously follows the teachings of the specific religious faith regarding sexuality, few will disagree that there have been changes in sexual roles and relationships, behavior, and attitudes. Some vehemently reject any "modernizations" of sexual beliefs, and these include lay people as well as clergy.

A more recent study indicates that religion does make a difference in one's beliefs about sexuality. The Glenmary Research Center of Washington, D.C., released the results of a recent survey of 7600 persons. The findings indicate that for some churchgoers the traditional teaching about the role of women, homosexuality, and adultery are still held. In other areas, change is evident. About 80 percent of Protestants and Catholics, as opposed to 93 percent of nonreligious people, believe birth control information should be available to teenagers who want it. Abortions should be legal if there is strong chance of serious defect in the baby according to 81 percent of churchgoing Protestants and 73 percent of churchgoing Catholics. If there is danger to life of the mother by pregnancy, 87 percent of Protestants and 81 percent of Catholics approve abortion, but only a majority of the nonreligious (73 percent) would give an abortion to a married woman who simply does not want any more children.[59]

The sexual revolution ushered in what some called the "new morality," a belief by some that pleasure is the principle and that between consenting adults almost anything is moral. The question is now raised if many Americans watched the new morality without abandoning the old. *Time* magazine commissioned a special survey of what Americans really think about sex morality. The poll did not ask people about their sexual practices but just what they thought (attitudes).[60]

Their findings indicate that although Americans are talking more about sex, they are increasingly confused about the moral values involved. Eighty-six percent felt that it was better that there was more openness about sex, but 61 percent felt that it is harder to know right from wrong. The highest incidence of those "morally confused" occurred among those over 50 (65 percent) and among those under 25 (66 percent).

The people were asked to make judgments on a series of sexual behaviors and to indicate whether they were morally wrong or not. Adultery, exchanging of sexual partners, teenage sex, and cohabitation without marriage were disapproved of by a majority of respondents. There were differences in responses by age groups, sex, and area of the country.

Although teenage sex was disapproved by the majority, those under 25 disapproved of sexual activity by a vote of 60 to 34 percent. However, among those 35 to 49 years old, 72 percent condemned teenage sex, and among those over 50 years old, 80 percent did. About three-quarters of parents approve of classroom discussions of sex relations before high school, and more than three-quarters think parents are doing the right thing in instructing their teenage children about the use of contraceptives.

The only category in which the majority accepted "liberated sexual behavior" was the question of the morality of unmarried couples living together, and that because of the large approval among men and the young. This, however, does not indicate acceptance of illegitimate children, as 70 percent disap-

proved of having children without formal marriage.

The issue of homosexuality, which has created much public controversy, sees people more evenly divided. The issue of abortion seems to have a similar response. The majority of respondents said it was not morally wrong, but the proabortion majority comes from men, while women still oppose it. A large majority, 64 percent, believe that regardless of morality, a woman should be legally free to have an abortion if she wants it. Americans are against government laws that prohibit sexual behavior. The one exception is pornography. People dislike it, and views seem to be becoming more negative.[61]

The survey indicated that there was widespread support for the traditional moral system. It is difficult to measure changes, and even though 41 percent thought they had become more liberal, the majority seemed to be, in general, quite conservative. For example, 76 percent of the respondents agreed that "permissiveness has led to a lot of things that are wrong with this country these days."[62]

Surveys of sexual mores are contradictory, and at times their validity is open to question. The "liberated" change in attitudes toward sexual morality that has been reported in the past may have occurred mainly in the white, middle class, urban areas, which are constantly being examined and surveyed. They do not necessarily reflect the beliefs of the country at large.[63]

It appears, however, that a sizable majority of Americans still hold belief in the many values of family life learned in their own homes.[64]

Religious beliefs may or may not be an integral part of an individual's decision about sexual behavior. Some may abstain from certain sexual practices and behavior because of religious beliefs, while others may engage in certain practices contrary to their beliefs. A third group may not have or may not use religious beliefs as a basis for sexual decision making.

NURSING IMPLICATIONS

Since beliefs about the morality or immorality of certain sexual practices vary between and even within particular religious denominations and between members of any specific denomination, it is essential that the nurse assess what belief systems operate in any particular individual. He or she must respect these beliefs when counseling about sexuality or making suggestions about sexual practices. To ignore these factors is to get people in "trouble with their God" and to foster guilt if the individual sees these practices as immoral. In addition, the patient/client will develop distrust of nurses who, instead of helping them solve problems and come to their own decisions, attempt to impose their beliefs and biases.

Questions to be answered about the patient include moral objections to specific sexual practices, religious life style of the client, and reliance on religion as an important support system.[65]

Nurses' goal in counseling is to help clients make their own choices within the framework of their morality. Oppenheimer stresses, "think clearly and distinguish carefully," that only by sorting matters out in our minds can we avoid harming clients and bring them comfort.[66]

Nurses can help individuals sort out their feelings about their sexual behavior, remembering that crises may occur if overwhelming guilt is the consequence of sexual behavior. (See Chapter 13 for a discussion of guilt.)

When making referrals for sex therapy, the nurse should consider religious beliefs and try to refer clients to a growing number of Christian sex therapists who counsel Bible-believing individuals. In addition, Christian sex manuals are available at religious book stores and may be more acceptable to some clients than secular books.[67]

Nurses may experience negative feelings toward patients/clients who have sexual life styles that they consider immoral. It is difficult to have a nonjudgmental attitude and to accept others as they are. Travelbee[68] believes that a nonjudgmental attitude is a myth, since we all tend to judge others. Travelbee urges that nurses should strive to be aware of the judgments that they make about all people, and after that, they can evaluate the effects on the interpersonal encounter. Acceptance is seen as selective forgiveness in which nurses acknowledge the "undesirable" aspects of the other, gloss over them, and focus on the characteristics most pleasing to the self.

NOTES

1. Katchadourian HA, Lunde DT: Fundamentals of Human Sexuality, 2nd ed. New York, Holt, 1975, p 528
2. Franzblau A: Religion and sexuality. In Sadock BJ, Kaplan HI, Freedman AM (eds): The Sexual Experience. Baltimore, Williams and Wilkins, 1976, pp. 611–626
3. Johnson WR, Belzer ED: Human Sexual Behavior and Sex Education. Philadelphia, Lea and Febiger, 1973
4. Carswell RW: Historical analysis of religion and sex. J School Health 39:673–684, 1969
5. Comfort A: Sex in Society. Secaucus, New Jersey, Citadel, 1963, p 67
6. Hogan R: Influences of culture on sexuality. Nurs Clin North Am 17:365–376, 1982
7. Carswell RW: Historical analysis of religion and sex. J School Health 39:674, 1969
8. Sussman J: Sex and sexuality in history. In Sadock BJ, Kaplan HI, Freedman, AM (eds): The Sexual Experience. Baltimore, Williams and Wilkins, 1976, p 10
9. Franzblau A: Religion and sexuality. In Sadock BJ, Kaplan HI, Freedman AM (eds): The Sexual Experience. Baltimore, Williams and Wilkins, 1976, p 618
10. Carswell RW: Historical analysis of re-

ligion and sex. J School Health 39:676, 1969

11. Ibid, p 677

12. Johnson WR, Belzer ED: Human Sexual Behavior and Sex Education. Philadelphia, Lea and Febiger, 1973, p 135

13. Carswell RW: Historical analysis of religion and sex. J School Health 39:678, 1969

14. Taylor GR: Sex in History. New York, Vanguard, 1954, p 52

15. Carswell RW: Historical analysis of religion and sex. J School Health 39:680, 1969

16. Ibid, p 680

17. Kinsey AC, Pomeroy WB, Martin CE: Sexual Behavior in the Human Male. Philadelphia, Saunders, 1948, pp 465–472

18. Bash DM: Jewish religious practices related to childbearing. J Nurse Midwifery 25:39–41, 1980

19. Kertzer MN: What is a Jew. New York, Bloch, 1973, p 32

20. Franzblau A: Religion and sexuality. In Sadock BJ, Kaplan HI, Freedman AM (eds): The Sexual Experience. Baltimore, Williams and Wilkins, 1976, p 618

21. Kertzer MN: What is a Jew. New York, Bloch, 1973, pp 58–59

22. Ibid, p 59

23. Ibid, p 66

24. Luzzato MH: Cleanness. In Neusner J(ed): Understanding Jewish Theology. New York, KTAV, 1973, pp 126–127

25. Franzblau A: Religion and sexuality. In Sadock BJ, Kaplan HI, Freedman AM (eds): The Sexual Experience. Baltimore, Williams and Wilkins, 1976, p 618

26. Abata R: Sexual Morality: Guidelines for Today's Catholic. Liguori, Missouri, Liguorian Publications, 1975, pp 9–13

27. Ibid, pp. 38–44

28. Kenny J, Kenny M: Sex enhances married love. Catholic Universe Bulletin, Cleveland, Ohio, February 10, 1978, p 22

29. Pope Pius XI: Encyclical on christian marriage. In Schur EM (ed): The Family

and the Sexual Revolution. Bloomington, Indiana, Indiana University Press, 1964, pp 350–360

30. Pope Paul VI: Of Human Life. Boston, Daughters of St. Paul, 1968, pp 3–22

31. Cleveland, Ohio, Synod upholds bond of marriage. Catholic Universe Bulletin. October 31, 1980, p 1:2

32. Ashley BM: From *Humanae Vitae* to human sexuality: New directions? Hosp Prog 59:78, 1978

33. Aftershock from Papal visit. Time, October 22, 1979, pp 67–69

34. Curran CE: After *Humanae Vitae*. A decade of lively debate. Hosp Prog 59:84–89, 1978

35. At bay in San Francisco. Time, October 11, 1982, p 67

36. Kaler P: The gift of sexuality: The Catholic view on masturbation. Liguorian 70:42–47, 1982

37. Springer RE: Marriage, the family and sex—A Roman Catholic view. Perspect Biol Med, Winter 1976, pp 187–197

38. Ibid, p 192

39. Ibid, p 194

40. Muckerman NJ, et al: The human sexuality report: Four theologians react. Liguorian, October 1977, pp 2–8

41. Ibid, p 7

42. Ibid

43. Kinsey AC, Pomeroy WB, Martin CE: Sexual Behavior in the Human Male. Philadelphia, Saunders, 1948, p 485

44. Hiltner S: A modern christian view. In Schur EM (ed): The Family and the Sexual Revolution. Bloomington, Indiana, Indiana University Press, 1964, pp 156–167

45. Ibid, pp 161–162

46. Ibid, pp 163–165

47. Johnson WR, Belzer ED: Human Sexual Behavior and Sex Education. Philadelphia, Lea and Febiger, 1973, p 187

48. Franzblau A: Religion and sexuality. In Sadock BJ, Kaplan HI, Freedman, AM (eds): The Sexual Experience. Baltimore, Williams and Wilkins, 1976, p 618

49. Johnson WR, Belzer ED: Human Sexual Behavior and Sex Education. Philadelphia, Lea and Febiger, 1973, p 187

50. Carswell RW: Historical analysis of religion and sex. J School Health 39:683, 1969

51. Johnson WR, Belzer ED: Human Sexual Behavior and Sex Education. Philadelphia, Lea and Febiger, 1973, p 145

52. Thou shalt not—and shall. Time, January 26, 1976, p 41

53. Katz RL: Notes on religious history, attitudes and laws pertaining to homosexuality. In Livingood JM (ed): National Institute of Mental Health Task Force on Homosexuality: Final Report and Papers. Rockville, Maryland, National Institute of Mental Health, 1974, pp 58–62

54. Gays on the march. Time, September 8, 1975, p 37

55. Woodward KL, Gates D: Homosexuals in the Church. Time, October 11, 1983, pp 113–114

56. Homosexuality and the clergy. Time, January 30, 1978, p 85

57. Homosexuality as sin. Time, June 5, 1978, p 53

58. Time, Debate about homosexuality. May 23, 1983, p 58

59. Survey finds—Churchgoers are different. Cleveland Press, May 6, 1978, p 8

60. The new morality. Time, November 21, 1977 pp 111–119

61. Ibid, p 115

62. Ibid

63. Ibid

64. Ibid, p 119

65. Hogan R: Influences of culture on sexuality. Nurs Clin North Am 17:373, 1982

66. Oppenheimer C, Catalon J: Counseling for sexual problems: Ethical issues and decision making. Practitioner 225:1623–1633, 1981

67. Chandler R: Christian sex therapists base message on the Bible. The Plain Dealer, February 12, 1983, Sec C, p 1

68. Travelbee J: Interpersonal Aspects of Nursing, 2nd ed. Philadelphia, Davis, 1971, pp 140–141

Assisting the Patient/Client to Maintain or Attain Sexual Health

Chapter 10

Assessment of Sexuality

Nurses obtain subjective information from a general nursing history containing questions devoted to sexuality, or they may utilize a longer, more detailed sexual history, depending on the patient's problems, developmental stage, and the practice area. In addition, objective information from the physical assessment and from the observation of patient/client's behavior is obtained. Consultation with other members of the health team, family members, and friends provide other sources of needed information,[1] but the information obtained from the patient interview is the most essential.

The purpose of this chapter is to present practical guidelines for obtaining information about sexuality from the patient/client or, when indicated, the significant others. The basic data to be collected by the nursing history and the rationale for its collection are discussed. A brief overview of relevant aspects of the interview, the interviewer, the setting, and the climate is presented to help nurses conduct assessment interviews that are productive of complete data and that are psychologically comfortable for both nurses and their patients/clients.

THE SEXUAL HISTORY

The sexual history is not taken out of the context of the individual's total being and his environment.[2] Obtaining an isolated sexual history is as meaningless as taking a "heart history" or a "stomach history."[3]

Why obtain a sexual history? A history is essential to insure systematic collection of data related to the patient/client's perceptions of his health status. The data also increase our understanding of the patient/client. A history defines needs, expectations, and behavior and identifies problems, misconceptions, and areas for education, counseling, and reassurance in relation to sexuality. It allows the patient an opportunity to ventilate and ask questions. In addition, by identifying the area of sexuality as one appropriate for discussion, it gives the individual permission to bring up concerns in the future. It indicates that the topic is not a taboo one.[4] The history is also essential in order for the nurse to plan, carry out, and evaluate a comprehensive plan of care, recognize deviations from normal, and refer patients to appropriate persons or agencies.[5]

The information is obtained at the initial encounter, since it communicates the health care provider's appreciation of the importance of sexual health and comfort in meeting these health needs.[6] Whether any significant information is elicited at the first contact is not of major importance, since it may require the establishment of a trust relationship before the individual is comfortable in confiding a long-standing problem.

Certain populations of individuals should definitely have a more extensive history taken: those who have medical or surgical conditions that affect their sexuality; patients who complain of infertility, sexual inadequacy, or venereal disease; pregnant, abortion, gynecologic, or family planning patients; and those individuals in premarital, marital, and psychiatric counseling.

Content of the History

Comprehensive outlines of sexual history information are available but they should not be a questionnaire to which all clients are subjected. The outline prepared by the Group for Advancement of Psychiatry based on the sexual performance evaluation questionnaire of the Marriage Council of Philadelphia is such a questionnaire.[7]

Comprehensive histories contain information about early sexual training and experience, family attitudes toward sex, the degree of family affection, personal attitudes toward sex, and the degree of personal regard for the sexual partner.[8]

If a comprehensive history is not indicated, certain minimal data should be obtained from the patients/clients in all settings. (See Table 10–1 for a list of data to be collected, its significance, and questions to elicit the information.) Other data about sexual function are also collected (Table 10–2).

TABLE 10-1. DATA TO BE COLLECTED BY NURSING HISTORY FOR ALL PATIENTS/CLIENTS

Data	Significance of Data	Nursing History Question
Age	Identifies period in life cycle.	In what year were you born; month, day?
Sex	Each sex may react differently to life events. Highlight gender identity problems.	[Usually is evident by dress, otherwise:] What sex do you consider yourself to be?
Education, occupation	Sexual practices may be related to education–socioeconomic class; change in occupation may contribute to role disturbances.	How far did you go in school? What do you do for a living? What change has there been in your ability to do your job?
Significant others	Other sources of support, stable or otherwise.	What persons do you consider most helpful right now? In what way? Are they available?
Quality of relationship with significant others	Relationship may be supportive, negative, or punitive, and these affect ability to cope with sexual problems.	Are there any differences in the way you get along with these people since you have been ill or hospitalized (or recently)?
Interests, hobbies	Indicates other support systems and avocational interest that contribute to self-esteem.	What do you do with your free time? What leisure and work activities are important to you? How are these being affected now?
Spiritual/religious/philosophical beliefs	Sexual practices may be related to beliefs. Guilt may occur if religious beliefs are compromised. Conflict and anxiety may be experienced by patient if different practices are suggested by nurse.	With what religious denomination are you affiliated? Can you describe any spiritual or other beliefs that are helpful to you now? Do you have or want the support of a clergyman (minister, priest, rabbi)?

TABLE 10-1. (cont.)

Data	Significance of Data	Nursing History Question
Health problems, medical conditions, surgical procedures in past and anticipated in the future; medication therapy	Some medical problems, surgical treatment, or medications result in sexual dysfunction (physiologic changes). Anxiety over outcome or change in body image may lead to functional problems.	What illness and/or surgery have you had in the past? Did they affect your usual way of living or work? Did they affect sexual function? Do you expect this illness/hospitalization will have effects on your usual way of living or work? In what ways? What medications do you take?
Changes in role relationships and ability to carry out the usual sexual role	Change in ability to carry out what is perceived as the usual sexual role may cause anxiety, depression, and/or sexual dysfunction.	What difference has there been in your functioning in the family? Describe. Can you do your usual tasks or jobs? Describe. Have there been any changes in your relationship (with the way you get along) with others (male, female, significant others)?
Potential changes in ability to carry out usual sexual role	Expectations of problems may cause problems (self-fulfilling prophecy).	What changes do you expect after you get home (or in the future)?
Change in perception of self as male or female due to illness or life events	Anxiety and sexual dysfunction may result from threat to gender identity.	How do you expect this illness (or life event) to affect how you see yourself as a man/woman?
Existing or potential sexual dysfunction	Elicits problems (sexual dysfunction).	Has there been or do you expect to have any changes in sexual functioning (sex life) because of (illness, life events)? Describe.

Note: Wording of the questions is changed depending on educational level of the patient/client. See Table 10-3, which gives suggestions for methods of introducing questions in the sexual history.

The Interview

Role of the Interviewer. The interviewer's role is to clarify the purpose and to set the focus for the health history as well as to maintain the momentum of the discussion. Patients/clients may stray from the topic, especially when emotionally laden information is being given, or they may dwell on topics that have particular relevance to them. Some control of the momentum and the direction of the interview must be maintained if the basic data are to be collected in the time frame available. At the same time, the nurse must strive for an unhurried atmosphere. Tapping of a foot or a pencil or glancing at the clock may indicate to the patient/client that time is limited and the information is unimportant. Several interviews may be necessary to complete the history. The interviewer should be comfortable in discussing sexuality and demonstrate interest in the patient/client's information.

TABLE 10–2.   DATA TO BE COLLECTED ABOUT SEXUAL FUNCTION

Female	Male
1. Menstrual history (onset duration, pain, number of pads, intermenstrual bleeding discharge, Pregnancies: number of children, miscarriages, contraception, satisfaction with method.	1. Genitourinary problems: infections, penile discharge, pain with urination, difficulty initiating or nocturnal urination.
2. Sexual response: sufficient vaginal lubrication, pain with intercourse, frequency of coitus, achieve orgasm with intercourse or masturbation.	2. Sexual response: early morning erections, difficulty achieving or maintaining firm erection, change in sexual desire, volume of ejaculate.
3. Satisfaction with sexual response, partner's satisfaction.	3. Satisfaction with sexual response, partner's satisfaction.
4. Infections or venereal disease.	4. Infections or venereal disease.
5. Questions or problems they would like to discuss.	5. Questions or problems they would like to discuss.

Setting and Climate.   These are important for client comfort. The setting should be private, and the nurse must assure the patient/client of confidentiality. This may require taking a hospitalized patient to another area if relatives, friends, or roommates are present. Doors should be closed and note taking avoided.

To maintain a "safe" climate for the patient/client to share information the nurse must be frank, warm, objective, and open, as well as nonmoralistic, reassuring, and empathetic. If the nurse is not embarrassed, the client will not be embarrassed. When the counselor maintains an aura of comfort with the topic and creates an atmosphere free of discernible prejudice toward the individual's sexual values and practices, the patient/client will be free to share concerns and problems.[9]

Structure of the Interview.   The structure of the interview may be directive or nondirective (permissive). The directive interview is the most efficient method for getting information, since the interviewer controls the direction and the momentum of the subject to be covered. However, it is not an effective method of getting at feelings, values, concerns, or problems. The nondirective, or permissive, interview is more effective, although more time consuming. Its use also reduces the chance that the patient will feel threatened by direct factual questions regarding sexual activities. In practice, most histories are a combination of both types. (See any basic text on interviewing for further information about the structure of the interview.)

Conduct of the Interview.   The interview should be guided by three basic principles:

1. The history progresses from topics that are easier to discuss to those that are more difficult—from less sensitive to more sensitive areas. Questions about menstruation, for example, are less anxiety provok-

ing than questions about unusual sexual practices. The latter should be discussed after greater rapport is developed.

2. The patient is asked first how he acquired sexual information before he is asked about sexual experience; for example, he may be asked what sex information he has learned in school before asking about sexual activity.

3. When direct questioning is used, the question is prefaced with a statement about the "universality" or "normality" of the topic being discussed, for example, "most people are hesitant to discuss" or "many people worry over feelings."

Be sure to have a prepared introductory statement that is personally comfortable. For example, "As a nurse I am concerned about all aspects of your health. However, we often neglect helping clients in what may be a very important part of their lives—their sexual needs. I'm going to ask you some questions in this area." If the patient/client inquires about the reason for questions, an appropriate answer is "Many patients/clients have concerns about their sexuality when they are having other health problems and I may be able to help" (Table 10–3).

Communication. There are many steps that may be taken to increase the ability to communicate. One of the greatest concerns of the nurse is the vocabulary that should be used. Klemer[10] urges use of accurate terminology while at the same time understanding the words the patient/client uses. It may be necessary to clarify the vocabulary to have

TABLE 10–3. STATEMENTS BY INTERVIEWER TO FACILITATE COMMUNICATION

Purpose	Facilitating Statement
Giving rationale for question	As a nurse, I'm concerned about all aspects of your health. Many individuals have concern about sexual matters, especially when they are sick or when they are having other health problems.
Giving statements of "generality" or "normality"	Most people are hesitant to discuss . . . Many people worry about feelings . . . Many people have concerns about . . .
Identifying sexual dysfunction	Most people have difficulties some time during their sexual relationships. What have yours been?
Obtaining information from an unmarried individual	The degree to which unmarried persons have sexual outlets varies considerably. Some have sexual partners, others have none, some relieve sexual tension through masturbation, others need no outlet at all. What has been your pattern?

(continued)

TABLE 10–3. *(cont.)*

Purpose	Facilitating Statement
Identifying sexual myths	While growing up, most of us have heard some sexual myths or half-truths that continue to puzzle us. Are there any that come to mind?
Identifying feelings about masturbation	Many of us grown-ups have heard a variety of stories about masturbation and what problems it supposedly causes. This can cause worry even into adulthood. What have you heard?
Determining if homosexuality is a source of conflict	Some say homosexuality is a mental disorder, others an emotional block, others a crime or sin. What is your attitude toward your homosexual orientation?
Identifying older individuals' concerns about sexual functioning	Many people, as they get older, believe or worry that this signals the end of their sex life. Much misinformation continues this myth. What is your understanding about sexuality during the later years? How has the passage of time affected your sexuality (sex life)?
Obtaining and giving information (miscellaneous areas)	Frequently people have questions about . . . What questions do you have about . . . What would you like to know about . . .
Closing the history	Is there anything further in the area of sexuality that you would like to bring up now? I hope that if questions or concerns do come to mind in the future we'll be able to discuss them.

Adapted from Green, Richard: Human Sexuality: A Health Practitioner's Text. *Baltimore, Williams and Wilkins, 1975.*

the person describe his or her sexual life accurately. Note the choice of words. (See Table 10–4 for lay terms commonly used for sexual organs or functions.) Avoid slang words yourself, since the patient wonders about your competence if you use "street" expressions. These have a highly emotionalized connotation for the patient, regardless of how glibly

TABLE 10–4. SLANG EXPRESSIONS FOR SEXUAL TERMS

Formal Term	Slang Expression
Breasts	Tits, sacks, front, headlights, knockers, boobs, bosom, bonkers, bust, jugs, buds
Climax	Come, go off, shoot, cream, blast off
Clitoris	Bad fellow, little gem, badge of shame, gaiety, madness, narrow strip
Cunnilingus	Eating it, going down, eating pussy
Erection	Hard on, stiff, bone, boner, hot rocks, lover's nuts
Fellatio	Going down, sucking, blowing, getting a blow job, giving head, cocksucking
Homosexual	Fairy, fag, faggot, gay, queen, nellie, homo, swish, pervert, pansy, back door artist, lez, sister, lesbo, dyke, bull dyke
Hymen	Cherry, membrane, maidenhead
Impotence	Couldn't get it up, couldn't get a hard on
Intercourse ⎰ Coitus ⎱	Make love, screw, fuck, get down, ball, make it, get laid, mess around, score, bang, jive, frig, get a piece, sleep with, get some tail
Masturbation	Jack off, jerk off, pocket pod, hand fuck, circle jerk, beat the meat, hand job
Menstruation	Curse, monthly period, devil's making ketchup, red-bearded cousin from the south, the flag's up, on the rag
Mutual oral–genital stimulation	Sixty-nine
Orgasm	Come, climax
Penis	Joystick, worm, dick, prick, stick, peter, rod, john, third leg, middle leg, joint, glans, cock, organ, thing
Pubic hair	Beaver, bush, pubes
Semen	Come, juice, egg white, gizzum
Sexual choice	Straight (heterosexual), gay (homosexual), AC–DC (bisexual)
Sexual desire	Horny, cold fish (decreased libido), nympho (increased libido)
Testes	Balls, nuts
Vagina	Pussy, hole, cunt, cat, pocketbook, treasure, twat, furburger, box, beaver, snatch, tunnel

they are used. If you return the word, it adds to the emotional value, and the patient is shocked by the professional's use of "street" language. Some counselors do not agree with this rationale and suggest using the patient's terminology. However, most patients are very eager to learn "the right words" and are grateful for the health professional's desire to teach them when the information is presented in a nonjudgmental manner. It is not necessary that the patient/client use the nurse's choice of words. Be sure, however, to "check out" words to make sure you are talking about the same things.

Consider the patient/client and the sexual partner as a unit. Masters and Johnson[11] emphasize that there is no such thing as an uninvolved partner. Although initially the nurse is interacting with one individual, if problems exist, both partners must eventually be involved if the teaching and/or counseling sessions are to be successful. More important than detailed accounts of the patient's problems are histories that bring out significant feelings and attitudes and expectations toward sexual activities or sexual relationships. It is also important to develop an accurate idea of the patient's/client's life style and philosophy, because any desired change in the individual's behavior must fit into his way of living.[12]

If a detailed sexual history is being obtained, do not follow a rigid format or a predetermined order. Allow the order to be determined by the needs of the individual. The interviewer, however, must be knowledgeable about the baseline information that is required but then proceed from the least to the most emotionally laden areas.[13]

Give the client time to think and to answer your questions. Be attentive for cues that the patient is uncomfortable, but do not answer for the individual. Assume that the patient is anxious. Anxiety may be manifested by inappropriate silence, joking, covert complaints, testing, distortions, or trying to please.[14] Decreased eye contact, rapid speech, increased motor activity (pacing, restlessness, hand movements), diaphoresis,

and facial flushing may also be observable signs that the individual is anxious.

Do not probe deeply into intimate details[15]; wait until rapport has been developed. When barriers are encountered, they are best handled by dropping the topic at the moment and returning to it at a later time if the information becomes essential for treatment.[16]

The nurse does not take anything for granted and does not judge what is right or wrong, normal or abnormal. The patients are helped to arrive at their own answers when exploring moral issues; the individual decides what is normal for himself. Do not judge sexual practices by your own norms. Help the patient/client describe sexual life accurately. At the same time do not have preconceived ideas about the individual's sex life before you begin the interview. Remember, not everyone engages in premarital sex; not all 70-year-olds have stopped sexual activity; not all teenagers are sexually active. It may be very important that the nurse give the client permission not to do something; for example, assuring an adolescent that although many of her friends are sexually active it is perfectly normal to decide to wait until marriage before engaging in coitus.

Just listening or giving validation is an important tool. Letting clients know that it is perfectly understandable that they have difficulties in a given situation lowers anxiety in talking about sex and helps them focus on the problem.[17]

The Interviewer

Up to this point, the focus has been on things to do to facilitate the data collection. One obstacle to accurate assessment regarding sexuality is the perceptual screen that results from the nurse's biases or discomfort with the topic of sexuality. Recognition that these biases exist is the first step in increasing the ability to communicate, and this ability can be acquired.[18] The patient sees the nurse as informed and is very perceptive of her/his attitudes. Any overreaction or under-reaction during the interview will set up a negative climate.[19] Nurses identify their attitudes, feelings, beliefs, and values regarding sexuality; then what they consider normal and abnormal for themselves and others; and finally, how these attitudes may affect or do affect interactions with patients. Nonemotional, objective interest and tolerance of practices and values that are different from the professional's are vital. Most important, the nurse's problems should not be projected on to the patient (Table 10–5).

Comfort in dealing with client's sexual concerns varies from nurse to nurse. Not all nurses are skillful at counseling and teaching about sexuality. However, assessment of

TABLE 10–5. INTERVIEWING TO OBTAIN SEXUAL INFORMATION— SOME DOS AND DON'TS

Do	Don't
1. Obtain information about all need areas.	1. Focus only on sexuality.
2. Provide privacy.	2. Obtain information when others are present or take copious notes.
3. Strive for an unhurried atmosphere.	3. Check your watch, tap your foot.
4. Maintain an attitude that is frank, open, warm, objective, empathetic.	4. Project discomfort, become defensive.
5. Use nondirective techniques when possible.	5. Ask many direct questions.
6. Have a prepared introduction to state purpose of interview.	6. Be vague about the purpose of the interview.
7. Use appropriate vocabulary.	7. Use street terms.
8. "Check out" words to ensure patient understands.	8. Assume the patient understands what you're saying.
9. Adjust the order of questions according to client's needs.	9. Follow a rigid format.
10. Give the client time to think and answer questions.	10. Answer questions for the client.
11. Recognize signs of anxiety.	11. Focus on getting information without recognizing patient feeling.
12. Give permission not to do something.	12. Have preset expectations of the patient's sexual activity.
13. Listen in an interested but matter-of-fact way.	13. Overreact or underreact.
14. Identify your attitudes, values, beliefs, and feelings.	14. Project your concerns or problems on to the patient.
15. Identify significant others.	15. Assume that no one else is involved in the patient's/client's sexual concerns.
16. Identify philosophical religious beliefs of patient/client.	16. Inflict your moral judgments on the patient.
17. Acknowledge when you don't have an answer to a question.	17. Pretend you know when you don't.

the patient's ability to meet sexuality needs provides the baseline information with which to plan, give, and evaluate care. All nurses must be able to contribute to this baseline.

FURTHER ASSESSMENT

If a problem or problems are identified, further information is collected to determine the nature of the problem. The following information should be obtained:[20]

1. Has the patient talked about the problem to anyone or sought other help?
2. What is the marital history of the patient/client?
3. What caused the onset or the beginning of the problem and what were the circumstances leading to the problem?
4. Is the other partner aware of the problem? What is his/her point of view and proposed remedies?
5. What is the patient's/client's impression of the problem? What is his/her point of view and proposed remedies?
6. What are the patient's individual needs for optimal sexual function?
7. How does the problem affect the patient's life style or the rest of a relationship?
8. How does the patient meet needs for intimacy?
9. Is the problem relational or sexual in nature?

In addition, the nurse should evaluate ways the history or background of the patient/client (or partner) enters into the problem. The personality assets and strengths of the patient/client and partner must also be identified so that these assets may be utilized as the basis of intervention.[21]

ADDITIONAL DATA COLLECTION

Biologic Data

The medical or surgical conditions that the patient/client has experienced or will experi-ence may have significant impact on sexuality, either physiologically or psychologically. Certain conditions or procedures may negatively affect sexual function (see Unit V).

The physical assessment provides significant information. The nurse notes any deformity or functional disability in any part of the body, since these may affect body image and sexuality (see Chapter 13). The appearance of the genitalia, the presence of lesions or unusual discharge or inflammation is noted. The patient/client may make negative comments about the appearance of his/her body during the examination. These comments are significant, since they may indicate decreased self-esteem as a sexual being.

Watch for body language and listen to comments during the physical examination. Clients who apologize for not washing or who complain of discharge may mean that they think their sex organs need apology, or "cleaning up." When the examining finger is inserted in the vagina, withdrawal or adducting thighs, difficulty in finding a comfortable position or expressions of fear or disgust may give clues to difficulties the patient may have with intercourse.[22]

Letting the client put a finger in her vagina, providing a mirror to see, and encouraging self-examination gives permission to touch and explore and substitutes reassuring fact for fantasies.

Physical examination of young adolescent males by female health care providers may evoke difficulties. In a study of 45 male adolescents, Mitchell found that the younger adolescents were more concerned about the females touching their body, than looking. They were also concerned about their peers' attitudes when they found out about examination by a female. Mitchell feels that the young male should be given the choice of being examined by a male or female.[23]

Sociocultural Data

Life events such as job loss, change in socioeconomic level, change in the usual role of the sexual partners, which is productive of anxiety and anger, may compromise sexuality. Identification of significant others is important. Equally important is the nature of the relationship—supportive, punitive, or minimal. The nurse gathers data by observing the interactions with others. The patient/client may make comment about the sexual partner's lack of support, disinterest, or the partner's understanding and willingness to help solve any problems.

Data related to religious preference, spiritual and philosophical beliefs, and the degree of reliance on these beliefs as a means of coping are vitally important. The patient/client may be committed to the tenets of the religious denomination. The nurse recognizes this and does not urge sexual practices that may conflict with these beliefs and potentially cause guilt. Other patients may only nominally conform to the rules laid down by their religion. (See Chapter 9 for information about religion and sexuality.)

The socioeconomic background, including level of education, financial status, and social class, is significant, since these factors may affect views about sexuality, and acceptance of various sexual practices (see Chapter 8).

Psychologic Data

The presence of anxiety, hostility, or change in body image may be identified by careful observation of the patient's/client's behavior and that of significant others. Level of self-esteem and the ability to relate to others are assessed. (See any basic text for information regarding reaction to stressful life events.) Chapter 13 gives assessment parameters for self-esteem, body image, and other psychologic reactions.

Consultation

Discussions with other members of the health team may result in other significant information being obtained. The physician caring for the patient/client may be able to add insights and data about pathophysiology that may affect sexuality. He or she may also have knowledge of the quality of support that exists between the patient and significant others.

The social worker may have knowledge of socioeconomic problems that exist and the steps that are being taken to solve them. Significant others provide the nurse with data related to their perception of a problem or, for that matter, whether they perceive a problem at all. As appropriate, the minister, priest, or rabbi may provide valuable information without violating boundaries of their confidential relationship with the individual.

ANALYSIS OF DATA

Collaboration with the patient/client is an important part of any process directed toward health. The nurse recognizes that a trust relationship must develop in order that there be a freedom for both the nurse and client to express themselves freely without fear of negative reactions. They mutually influence each other and their responses. Ideally, data are analyzed with the client for the purpose of identifying abilities, disabilities, problems, and possible bases of the problems.

The bio-psycho-social information obtained from the history, physical assessment, consultations, and the literature is reviewed. Gaps in data are identified. Information relating to basic needs is also considered, as it may affect sexuality.

Data are compared with the "norms." However, sexual "norms" vary from culture to culture and between individuals and are affected by social and biologic variables. Nurses are careful not to impose their norms and to relate objective norms to the patient's/client's definition of what is normal for herself/himself. Chez[24] states that "whatever is pleasurable and gratifying for both participants is normal for that couple as long as there is communication and mutual participation without coercion."

If the nurse and the patient/client have

the same norms, they can arrive at a diagnosis together. If they have different norms, they may disagree regarding the nature of the problem or even whether a problem exists.[25] When the nurse tries to impose her norms on the patient/client, the potential for coming to a satisfactory solution to problems is virtually nonexistent.

NURSING DIAGNOSIS RELATED TO SEXUALITY

Analysis of the data may lead to identification of various problems related to sexuality in addition to the recognition of a specific sexual dysfunction as defined by Masters and Johnson (see Chapter 3). Patients may have decreased self-esteem as sexual beings related to a threat to or change in their sexual roles. Illness or its physiologic or psychologic effects may also decrease sexual self-esteem. Another problem identified may be a decreased ability to carry out the sexual role, related to the effects of illness, therapy, or change in economic status.

Guilt is a frequent problem. It may be related to past or present sexual practices and events. Patients/clients may also experience anxiety, depression, anger, shame, or disturbances in body image. Problems related to sexuality may make it difficult to meet love–belonging needs by affecting the individual's ability to form satisfying relationships with those of the same or the opposite sex (see Chapter 13).

REFERRAL TO OTHER HEALTH CARE PROVIDERS

Certain factors should be considered in making referrals. There is a trend away from making referrals to sex clinics. Management by the primary nurse or the physician may be indicated since clients may be embarrassed or feel "brushed off." Women accept referral better than men whose self-concept may be threatened; younger clients accept it better than older.[26,27]

General indications for referral include:

1. Long history of marital or partner discord
2. Multiple relationship problems
3. Health care provider has similar problems
4. Health care provider lacks the resources, training or comfort in the area
5. Health care provider has inadequate time for counseling.

Referral to a psychiatrist may be indicated with certain problems.[28] These include:

1. Patients who have concerns about sexual orientation or sexual activity
2. Patients with paraphilias
3. Patients with sexual problems accompanied by severe depression or anxiety
4. Patients with problems complicated by alcohol or drug abuse.

NOTES

1. Mitchell PH: Concepts Basic to Nursing, 2nd ed. New York, McGraw-Hill, 1977, p 84
2. Masters WH, Johnson VE: Human Sexual Response. Boston, Little, Brown, 1966
3. Belliveau F, Richter L: Understanding Human Sexual Inadequacy. New York, Bantam, 1970, p 95
4. Roznoy MS: Taking a sexual history. Am J Nurs 76:1279–1281, 1976
5. Elder M-S: The unmet challenge, nurse counseling on sexuality. Nurs Outlook 18(11):38–40, 1970
6. Green R: Taking a sexual history. In Green R (ed): Human Sexuality: A Health Practitioner's Text. Baltimore, Williams and Wilkins, 1975, pp 9–20
7. Sadock BJ, Kaplan HI: The physician's role in sex therapy. In Sadock BJ, Kaplan HI, Freedman AM (eds): The Sexual Experience. Baltimore, Williams and Wilkins, 1976, pp 507–517
8. Brecher R, Brecher E: An Analysis of Human Sexual Response. Boston, Little, Brown, 1966, pp 208–209

9. Masters WH, Johnson VE: Human Sexual Response. Boston, Little, Brown, 1966, p 22

10. Klemer R: Talking about patients' sexual problems. In Klemer R (ed): Counseling in Marital and Sexual Problems. Baltimore, Williams and Wilkins, 1965, pp 118–125

11. Masters WH, Johnson VE: Human Sexual Inadequacy. Boston, Little, Brown, 1970, p 2

12. Belliveau F, Richter L: Understanding Human Sexual Inadequacy. New York, Bantam, 1970, p 101

13. Wahl CW: Psychiatric techniques in the taking of a sexual history. In Wahl CW (ed): Sexual Problems: Diagnosis and Treatment in Medical Practice. New York, Free Press, 1967, pp 13–21

14. Elder M-S: The unmet challenge, nurse counseling on sexuality. Nurs Outlook 18(11):38, 1970

15. Duddle M, Brown ADG: The clinical management of sexual dysfunction. Clin Obstet Gynecol 7:293–325, 1980

16. Elmassian BJ, Wilson RW: Assessment and diagnosis of sexual problems. Nurse Pract 7:13–22, 1982

17. Stoklosa JM, Bullard DG: Talking about sex: Suggestions for the health professional. Front Rad Ther Oncol 14:79–82, 1980

18. Krizinofski MT: Human sexuality and nursing practice. N Clin North Am 8:673–681, 1973

19. Mims FH: Sexual health education and counseling. Nurs Clin North Am 10:519–528, 1975

20. Alexander B: Taking the sexual history. Am Family Phys 23:147–153, 1981

21. Otto HA: Evaluating in-patients' problems for counseling or referral. In Klemer RH (ed): Counseling in Marital and Sexual Problems. Baltimore, Williams and Wilkins, 1965, pp 79–90

22. Tunnadine P: The role of genital examination in psychosexual medicine. Clin Obstet Gynecol 7:283–291, 1980

23. Mitchell JR: Male adolescents concern about physical examination conducted by a female. Nurs Res 29:165–169, 1980

24. Chez R: The female patient's sexual history. In Wahl CW (ed): Sexual Problems: Diagnosis and Treatment in Medical Practice. New York, Free Press, 1967, pp 1–12

25. Mitchell PH: Concepts Basic to Nursing, 2nd ed. New York, McGraw-Hill, 1977, p 109

26. Rosen RC, Gendel ES: Sexual problems: Current approaches in primary care practice. Postgrad Med 69:127–129, 132–134, 1981

27. Ibid, p 132

28. Myerscough PR, Blum A: Referring patients to a gynecologist or psychiatrist and to a marriage guidance counselor. Brit Med J 282:1589–1590, 1981

Chapter 11

Teaching—Learning and Sexuality

Of many health professionals, the nurse has the most opportunity to teach about human sexuality. The busy physician does not usually have the time or often the inclination or comfort to do so. Formally or informally, in outpatient or inpatient settings, the nurse has the opportunity to develop rapport and gain the trust and confidence of patients/clients who have questions about sexuality.

In its broadest definition, teaching is described as activities by which the teacher helps the student learn. An equally broad definition is the view that teaching is any interpersonal influence aimed at changing the way other persons can and will behave.[1] There is an element of control in these definitions with a goal of change in behavior (the broadest definition of learning).

How much change in behavior, i.e., learning, results from teaching is difficult to measure at best, and for those already influenced by negative life experiences in the sexual sphere, one might be especially pessimistic about change in this area. Still, humans are in the process of being and becoming; they change and at some level seek change, and teaching can add to their growth.

The focus of this chapter is on the role of parents, peers, and the school in the sexual learning of individuals. The role of nurses in teaching about sexuality is also explored, and specific information is given to help the nurse plan and/or conduct classes in schools

and in the other care settings. Suggestions are given regarding content, and a nursing process approach is used to identify and apply teaching–learning principles to education about sexuality. A brief description of teaching strategies that have been found successful in teaching about sexuality is also included.

TEACHING VERSUS COUNSELING

For purposes of presentation, teaching is separated from counseling in this text, but there is considerable overlap. Counseling involves provision of emotional, intellectual, and psychologic support. Some believe the nurse functions in a combination of roles—teacher and counselor. Guidance and counseling focus on attitudes and feelings, while the most traditional focus of teaching is on intellectual growth. In the area of human sexuality, the nurses' role of teacher–counselor is especially evident, since it is difficult, if not impossible, to dichotomize learning about sexuality from the attitudes and feelings about sexuality.

Planned or unplanned, nurses teach each time they are with patients/clients, and nurses who are comfortable with their sexuality, who are willing to share information, can communicate both nonverbally and verbally, not only information, but the appropriateness and the importance of sexual health.

Teaching is more than facts about sexual activity. It takes into account not only what an individual does but also what he or she is.

Individuals are increasingly interested in learning about sexuality and sexual functioning.[2] The popularity of books such as Alex Comfort's *Joy of Sex,* and William H. Masters and Virginia E. Johnson's texts *Human Sexual Response* and *Human Sexual Inadequacy* give evidence of this interest. The continuing popularity of "sex hotlines," which seek to reassure the sexually anxious, debunk myths, and disseminate accurate information, also attests to the public's desire for knowledge about sexuality and perhaps to the inadequacy of the education about sexuality they received as children and adolescents. Attitudes about formal sex education for children vary, however, from group to group, although adolescents themselves overwhelmingly endorsed sex education in the school in a Gallup Youth Survey.[3] Eighty percent of all parents wanted such teaching for their children according to a study done by SIECUS, the Sex Information Council of the United States. Yet fewer than 10 percent of all people get a comprehensive sex education course.[4]

ROLE OF PARENTS, PEERS, AND SCHOOLS IN SEXUAL LEARNING

Parents versus Schools

Opponents of sex education such as the John Birch Society, MOTOREDE Parents Opposed to Sex Education, Christian Crusade, The Moral Majority, and others attack sex education courses as invasions of privacy, a danger to society and to morality[5] and argue that it should be provided by parents.[6] Others argue that many parents do not know enough about sexuality and are uncomfortable talking about sexuality with their children. From a religious point of view, the issue focuses on who is responsible for sex education—the school or the home and church. The question arises whether sexual ethics and moral values can be taught in school, since we are a pluralistic society of many races, religions, and socioeconomic groups. Some point out that there is a general lack of adequate sex education of the public, while others believe the present sex education is adequate, that children know about their bodies and that teaching about sexuality is courting promiscuity and sexual experimentation.

Support for sex education has come from churches. The Interfaith Statement on Sex Education released by the National Council of Churches, the Synagogue Council of America, and the United States Catholic Conference Family Life Bureau made a strong positive statement in the schools. The statement stressed, however, that sex education should be based on moral and ethical values and must respect the cultural, familial, and religious backgrounds and beliefs of the individual.[7]

Those who argue for formal sex education stress that it is not to be confused with sex behavior, pointing out that no studies have demonstrated greater sexual activity among students who have taken sex education courses. There is little disagreement that the greatest influence upon children's sexuality comes from the parents and that sex education starts in the family.[8–10]

Parents and Peers

Sexual learning in children may be haphazard, and the primary source of sex information is often peers.[11] Among males, information usually involves stories of sexual prowess in heterosexual exploits. Among females, a small amount of sexual information is exchanged, but most stories revolve around love and affection. The male is cast in the role of technical expert and the female is presumed unknowledgeable about the sex act.

Attitudes Toward Sexuality. If peers are a primary source of information, the parents are the prime agents in developing, promoting, or repressing the sexual attitudes of the child. There is convincing evidence that the child's early experiences have lasting influence on the conduct of later sexual life.[12] Certainly the development of gender identity and role behavior is related to parents' belief that the child is either male or female and their subsequent behavior toward the child. Indirect learning is probably more important in sexual learning than in any other area of development.[13]

Sexual learning of children begins at the moment of birth, when parental attitudes and behavior begin to shape feelings about their maleness or femaleness. As children grow and mature, they more likely obtain information by casual, unplanned methods, rather than by formal teaching.[14] By the time children begin school, whether the parents are aware of it or not, children have a store of information and/or misinformation about sexuality.

The meaning of love, tenderness, and consideration does not come from purposeful instruction. It is learned in the course of years mainly as the child watches the parents treat each other with affection. Teaching the older child, for example, that genital activity is reserved for people when they have grown up and love each other has little meaning in the child's mind if he lives in a home with a discordant marriage.[15]

Moreover, parents can negatively affect sexual learning by their own response to children's sexual behavior. When parents observe this behavior, two responses may occur. The first is to tell the child the behavior is wrong; the second is to nonlabel or mislabel the behavior. This is done by attempting to distract the child with suggestions of other activities or by pointing out negative affects of the behavior not related to its sexual aspects, for example, giving hygienic reasons against kissing. Further mislabeling includes use of infantile nomenclature for the genitals and excretory functions.

Two consequences of this mislabeling occur. First, children get negative and inconsistent information about sexuality, and second, there is spillover of training in control of aggression into that of sexuality, since the child does not clearly identify what behavior

is aggressive and what is sexual. The result is that aggression and sexuality are associated.[16]

Information about Sexuality. Parents contribute little factual information. In studies by Ramsey (1943) and by Gebhard (1965), peers were the primary source of knowledge. In the Ramsey[17] study, 60 percent of the mothers and 82 percent of the fathers had given no sexual information. In the study by Gebhard,[18] approximately three-quarters of the parents of both sexes failed to give any sexual information, or when given, mothers primarily focused on facts about menstruation and pregnancy. The myth of a heart-to-heart talk between father and son is exactly that. The father was even less of a source of sexual information than the mother. There was nothing in the learning process of these children that suggested that they had an integrated body of sexual knowledge.

Unfortunately, information is obtained by clandestine and secretive exchanges between children. Too often, parents attempt to teach their children by general and diffuse admonitions that do not result in cessation of interest or of sexual behaviors by the children, but in concealment and subsequent guilt. Guilty knowledge develops quickly, and the children soon develop the capacity and need to keep sexuality a secret, especially from those they love.

GOALS OF SEX EDUCATION

Realistically, one can not expect sex education per se to change sexual behavior. There is general agreement that it is easier to give information than to change attitudes and values. In fact students who took one sex education course had attitudes less accepting of masturbation. It also appears that it is easier to change attitudes toward others than toward one's own sexual behavior, and it is even more difficult to evaluate changes in behavior as a result of sex education.[19]

Adult sexual orientation is the result of

events that began in infancy and that are still only poorly understood. Gagnon[20] believes that even Erickson's *Childhood and Society* provides only a set of useful labels but does not give definite explanation of process and change. There are so many unplanned and unplannable elements in the development of sexuality that it is difficult to discuss the role of sex education, although many educators believe that information should be given as part of the general curriculum. The age at which the child is given information and the facts given are less important than the child's life experiences that may have traumatized him in relation to sexuality. Gagnon sees sex education in schools playing only a minor role in setting patterns of sexual life. Others disagree with Gagnon's rather pessimistic view of the role of formal education in shaping sexuality and see sex education directed toward not only imparting facts but also providing children with a sense of values by which they can judge the opinions and the behavior with which they come in contact.[21]

Education should enhance the children's self-esteem, prepare them for marriage and parenthood, help them understand love as a basic component of sexuality, and prepare them for responsible decision making. It should also help them increase their understanding of the sexual dimension of their lives and an appreciation and tolerance of those who do not conform to traditional mores.

More research is needed on the import of sex education on attitudes and behavior, using a research design that compares those who have taken and those who have not taken a sex education course.[22]

SIECUS

In May of 1964, the Sex Information and Education Council of the United States (SIECUS) was established. Its purpose was to "establish man's sexuality as a healthy entity." Its board of directors includes representatives from the fields of public health, family life education, religion, sociology, psychiatry, obstetrics, education, law, and home economics. Its focus is on sex education from preschool through graduate school and in adult life.

Dr. Mary S. Calderone, its first executive director, believes that sex education should be part of all education. She stresses that distorted and inadequate information from the literature, television, radio, and peers cannot be in any way counterbalanced by talks about the "facts of life"; that sex education must be more than what is now called "sex education"—a little information of where babies come from, menstruation, and venereal disease, with little ethical information.[23] Calderone[24] states in regard to the ethical facet of sexuality, that the idea of responsibility can and must be taught in the schools.

The Planned Parenthood Federation of America, Inc.

The Planned Parenthood Federation of America, Inc., has been in the forefront of private agencies that are committed to education about sexuality, with special emphasis on responsible parenthood through family planning. Founded by Margaret Sanger in 1916, it has spread throughout the world and is the largest private community-based reproductive health service in the United States. In addition to providing contraceptive services, diagnostic examinations, counseling programs, and referrals to other sources of health care are part of their programs. Booklets are available related to teaching of sexuality.[25] The organization is stressing the need for sex education courses that will teach students sexual responsibility.

EDUCATIONAL PROGRAMS

Nurses may be consulted about the content of educational programs and may also be involved in their initiation. They also have the opportunity to teach and counsel parents and children.[26] It is not only school nurses who

TABLE 11–1. TEACHING CHILDREN ABOUT SEXUALITY

The following suggestions are helpful for parents who have questions about the "hows" of teaching their children about sexuality:

1. Answer questions in a straightforward way.
2. Give the information the child requests.
3. Give the information at the time the child requests it—don't put off answering.
4. Avoid giving more information than the child requests at the time—the child will not be interested.
5. Don't worry about correct timing as to when to give information, for if the child is not psychologically or intellectually ready for the information, he/she won't be interested. Hearing it won't do any harm.
6. *Don't wait to give all information in one dose.*
7. Bring up the topic of sexuality casually and briefly when a child does not ask questions. (For example, when a pregnant woman is seen.)
8. Tell the truth—false stories about the stork or physician bringing babies more often confuses or frightens the child.

may be involved, but nurses in other outpatient and inpatient settings.

Planning Sex Education Programs

Any educational program about sexuality directed toward children and adolescents involves parents, clergy, and the whole community.[27] The question of whether schools should institute a program in sex education presents complex problems. Strawn[28] gives five suggestions the nurse should consider in helping parents and in setting up a formal sex education program:

1. Hold conferences with parents before the children reach the fifth grade (before age 10) to inform them about current data related to sexual activity of children and community services available that can assist with ordinary problems of child-rearing.

2. Encourage teachers to obtain additional training in health and sex education so they can answer questions wisely on an individual basis.

3. Explore the values held by the community and the school. In instances where the values of community and school are incompatible, avoid sex education in classes, since it is more essential that children in primary and intermediate grades maintain trust and have confidence in their parents. They should not be pawns in disagreements among adults.

4. Be candid to parents about the implications of any new programs.

5. Set realistic expectations for sex education. No assurance is possible that the knowledge gained will decrease promiscuity and illegitimacy. It may or may not result in more rational marriages in the future. Sex education should be initiated because the community believes knowledge is better than ignorance and hopes that the future will reflect the knowledge in a positive way.

Content of Education about Sexuality

The teacher of sexuality must take into account the family background and life situation of the students. Some may come from one-parent families, so that content must be altered to fit their conception of "family." Talking about "father" to children who have never known a father will be meaningless and confusing for them.

Parents may turn to nurses for guidelines about the information that should be given children at various age levels and how to teach about sexuality (Table 11-1). The school nurse may be involved in setting up or answering questions about a sex education program, and nurses dealing with children in any setting can help clarify myths and misconceptions about sexuality. The following information provides general guidelines about sexual knowledge that children and adolescents should have at various ages and grade levels in school, but it can be used by parents in the home also. Burt and Brower[29] provide more detailed teaching guidelines in their excellent book (Table 11-2).

Sex education is a continuing process that begins soon after infancy and does not end until late adolescence, if ever. When children's questions are not answered, when the subject is ended abruptly, or when disapproval is shown, children quickly recognize that something is wrong with the subject or may think that they themselves are bad.[30]

Education starts when children start to ask questions, often at 2½ years of age when children begin to see differences in the bodies of boys and girls. At about 3½ years, they may ask where babies come from, and at 4 to 4½, how they get out of the mothers. How the baby gets into the mother becomes of interest before the age of 5. Interest grows in the father's role in greater detail at about 6½ to 8 years. Girls ask questions earlier than boys, but children's individual variation in temperament, alertness, and articulateness and the parents' permissiveness also play a part.[31]

As was mentioned earlier, prohibitions from school or families may exist against

---

TABLE 11–2. CONTENT OF EDUCATION ABOUT SEXUALITY BY GRADES

First grade	Names of body parts; stories of animal families; concepts of father, mother, male, female; discussion of human family; concept of home and happiness working together.
Second grade	Life, growth, living things and how life is reproduced (but not reproduction in sexual terms); life coming from life; different eggs growing into different kinds of animals; living things needing parents to make them; babies made by joining egg with sperm; and mammals' eggs growing in the uterus.
Third grade	Exploration in depth of new life; enhancing and evaluating interpersonal relationships; developing appreciation of self.
Fourth grade	Specific details of the male and female body; roles of male and female in reproduction and heredity.
Fifth grade	Information about growth and changes in body and reasons for changes; reproduction cells; anatomy and physiology of male and female reproductive systems; feminine hygiene (girls only, boys may be uncomfortable with details of menstruation and girls may feel uncomfortable about changes in femininity).
Sixth grade	Male and female sexual cycles; fertilization; pregnancy; married and family love. Emphasis that sexuality exists and that it is basis for family life.
Junior and senior high school	Units in biologic male and female sexual response; pregnancy; childbirth; lactation; population explosion; venereal disease; masturbation; homosexuality; making a choice of sexual conduct.

Adapted from Burt JJ, Brower LA: Education for Sexuality. Philadelphia, Saunders, 1970.

teaching about contraception. Many argue that it may have undesirable effects on those whose basic decisions for abstinence are based on parents' trust. It is like someone saying, "I know you wouldn't do it, but here is a prophylactic just in case." Some believe that to the labile and suggestible adolescent, information may mean license to indulge in sexual activity. The teacher, in a parental role, may appear permissive, confusing the adolescent by seemingly opposing a belief to which the parents are committed. This may tend to pervert the parent image.[32]

The institution of marriage in society should be completely presented and should include factors that negatively affect family life, such as depersonalization, social and economic mobility, industrialization, overcrowding, prostitution, and abortion. Changing roles and relationships should be discussed. Children must be grounded in knowledge and attitudes that allow sound sexual decision making. If responsible parenthood is the ultimate goal, then they must learn responsible attitudes toward sex.

Education must be more than facts. One group of students was more concerned how to tell if someone loved them after a course than they had been before it. Questions about values and decision making were more central than physical aspects.[33] The curriculum must deal with feelings and behavior to be effective.[34]

Role of Teachers

Teachers must help children to regulate their sexual impulses, remembering that norms related to proper sexual behavior are specific to particular cultures, subcultures, and social classes. Teachers have a tendency to stress facts instead of feelings when teaching about sexuality. A humanistic approach stresses the greater importance of students' self-discovery as sexual beings than knowledge acquisition. Students share feelings and beliefs, and this involves risk taking on the part of students, since to express their own feelings about sexual issues can be extremely threatening. Consequently, an important part of this approach to teaching is trust and confidence of the students in themselves, in others, and in their teacher. The outcome can be an awakening to self as a sexual being.[35] A "traditional" class cannot be taken and expected to respond overnight, and much of the success of this approach depends on the real human feelings that are present within the teaching–learning situation.

A major obstacle exists to the formation of sound programs. Just as parents are uncomfortable discussing sexuality, teachers have difficulty teaching about sexuality without fear and embarrassment.

NURSING IMPLICATIONS

To effectively teach about sexuality, nurses must be aware of and accept their own sexuality. They must be knowledgeable about the subject, be comfortable in its presentation, and of equal importance, be knowledgeable about the characteristics of their students and perceptive of how to reach them effectively. They must be tolerant and accepting of the sexual behavior, feelings, and attitudes of others. Their approach to the subject matter should be honest, open, and direct, imaginative, and flexible.

It is also helpful to have a sense of humor. Students may joke about sex since some can only talk about sexuality if they joke about it. "Dirty jokes" have been one means of communicating about sex. The nurse may not approve of these stories, but taking advantage of opportunities for laughter is helpful, especially if there is tension, discomfort, or anxiety.[36]

Two cardinal rules for teaching are to begin as early as possible and to find out what the individual knows before planning the teaching approach. Age 13 is too late for teaching about menstruation and the changes that accompany puberty. Perhaps the individual or group already knows about menstruation but is interested in pregnancy and how it comes about. Valuable time may be wasted in needless repetition of known material.

Assessment

Assess the previous knowledge by group discussion or having individuals explain what they know about the aspect of sexuality you intend to explore. What life experiences have they had in this area? Also assess the level of understanding, education, and vocabulary— is it sophisticated, with correct terminology related to sexual function already part of the repertoire? If not, the teacher may have to use "street" language along with the correct terms as part of the teaching strategy in order to communicate (see Table 10-4 for street terms).

It is important to assess the health beliefs of individuals and socioeconomic status, which seems to be one of the major variables in sexual and all health behavior, knowledge, and attitudes. Those in lower socioeconomic groups are less likely than others to recognize problems or, if they do, are less likely to seek help.

Readiness for learning must be assessed.[37] If individuals do not feel a need to learn more about sexuality, if they are an embarrassed, anxious, or hostile audience, the best teaching will be ineffectual. Even if they are psychologically ready for learning, is their physiologic status optimal? The woman suffering pain after a hysterectomy is not ready to hear information about the procedure's effect on her sexuality. Is the individual motivated to learn?[38] The adolescent girl who believes that using birth control measures will detract from her enjoyment of sexual intercourse will not benefit from the most organized and factually complete classes on contraceptive methods, since she has no desire to change her behavior.

Planning

Identification of and sharing objectives with patients/families is essential. Too often, nurses plan the instruction, get little or no input from their patients/clients, and then wonder why so little interest is evidenced. Objectives must be realistic and reachable. It is doubtful that nurses can teach unwed mothers not be become involved in extramarital intercourse, given the psychologic depth of the problem (see Chapter 16). A more realistic goal might be to help them develop added awareness of reality.[39]

Plan content that is based on the individuals' understanding and readiness to learn. The principles of simple to complex, familiar to new, and concrete to abstract should be applied. Building on what the individual already knows and proceeding from simple facts about sexuality to discussion of changing roles and relationships is more likely to engage the learner's attention than starting with sexual role theory.

When teaching about sexuality, it is especially important that the time and place for teaching be carefully planned. Interruptions or lack of privacy in a busy ward or clinic will distract persons and will also decrease free exchange of ideas because of potential embarrassment. Short periods of time are more effective than longer periods.

Choosing Teaching Strategies

Selection of the proper strategies for presentation of content is essential. Seeing, hearing, and sharing of ideas will help insure retention of content. If possible, plan for active participation of the learners. Group discussion is an especially effective way to get individuals involved in the learning situation.

Use of Audiovisual Aids.

Use of audiovisual aids is essential. Pictures, charts, and diagrams help clarify misconceptions about sexual anatomy and physiology. For small children, dolls and models that have realistic male and female anatomy can be helpful. Asking children to draw a picture of a man or woman with and then without clothes is an effective way to find out what the children know and also how they feel about their bodies.

The use of comic books for sex education of 12- to 18-year-olds has been effective. The content "pulls no punches," including information about venereal disease, sexuality, pregnancy, and drugs. The reader is not "talked down to." Comics are also available for the fourth to sixth grader, but for all ages, the need is to do more with these books than pass them out. After the children read them, the content is used for a starting point for discussion that should move to the areas of feelings, relationships, marriage, and society. The value of the books is in their forthright approach that can be used as a take-off point.[40] Films, filmstrips, and slides can also be helpful for all ages.

Desensitization. One approach to sex education of adults and especially health professionals is a process that aims at desensitizing individuals to sexual behavior. Sexual behavior is demythologized by showing explicit movies of heterosexual and homosexual sexual activity. The viewer is also desensitized from stressful and emotional overreaction to sexual stimuli. Group discussion that follows focuses on sensitization (or resensitization) toward humanistic and professional understanding of the sexuality of oneself and others.

There should be no in-depth probing of thoughts and feeling of students.[41] The ultimate goal is the incorporation of this understanding into the individual's helping behavior, which will be characterized by a more tolerant attitude toward sexual beliefs, attitudes, and practices of others.[42]

Explicit films should not be used as an initial presentation since they may upset some members of the audience. More research is needed to see if sexually explicit material is of value to teachers and students.[43] Students should be given an option to see the material. Start with more neutral films and progress to the more explicit so the student is not shocked or overwhelmed.

Desensitization with words can help break down barriers to talking about sexual topics as well as provide information. Medical terms indicating genital anatomy and types of sexual activity are put on the blackboard. The students are then asked to give verbally or in writing all the street terms they know for the technical terms. The teacher writes the synonyms on the board. This process is especially helpful when teaching student nurses who express concern that they will not understand the sexual terms patients/clients use. (See Table 10-4 for a list of terms and common street synonyms.)

Role Playing. Role playing can be an effective strategy. It is the learning process by which life situations or problems are acted out. Role playing helps the students deal with sensitive subject areas. It is especially helpful in high anxiety areas such as sexuality. It is not a carefully scripted play but the on-the-spot reaction to a real situation. Ideally, use of videotape allows the students to see themselves and critique their behavior, making suggestions for improvement. Use of role playing with or without videotape is especially effective in helping nurses to teach patients/clients. It also can provide them with insight into their own and others' feelings and attitudes about such anxiety.[44]

Value Clarification. There is no question that sex education has been ineffective if the near-epidemic problem of teenage pregnancies is used as a criterion of effectiveness. One method to help individuals and especially adolescents develop sexual values by which to live is a program called Values Clarification in Sex Education. The program is designed to help teenagers examine their existing sexual beliefs and shape a final set of values that will more likely be followed, since they come from within. The program stimulates the adolescents to think, and can include written and oral exercises and group discussion to help one examine and shape values. A true value is prized and publicly affirmed by individuals, is chosen freely from alternatives after serious thought, and is acted upon consistently in life.[45]

Group Discussion. Talking to individuals in a formal classroom setting is a much less effective method of teaching about sexuality than is small groups where ideas and information can be freely shared. Special skills are needed by the leader in order to lead a successful discussion, and Kempton[46] provides valuable guidelines for the group leader. A warm, relaxed atmosphere is important. A helpful technique is to have the persons talk to their neighbors and later introduce each other to the group. (Table 11-3).

When the topic has been chosen, the leader must also recognize when the discussion is dragging and must be moved on. The leader does not control but stimulates discussion and guides by summarizing ideas or raising questions.[47] Facts are given if misinformation occurs, but the leader does not embarrass the group members by asking for information they may not have. Discussion is confidential but does not center on personal problems, which must be reserved for individual conferences. However, if the same problem is shared by all group members, it may be discussed.[48]

Techniques to promote discussion include distributing cards and asking the group to write down topics for discussion, showing and discussing a film, and present-

---

TABLE 11–3. SOME DO'S AND DON'TS IN LEADING GROUP DISCUSSIONS

Do	Don't
1. Provide an environment conducive to discussion: comfortable temperature, chairs arranged in circle.	1. Separate males and females.
2. Limit participants to 10 to 20.	2. Allow "observers" in the group.
3. Provide name tags, food, and drink.	3. Assume everyone knows eveything.
4. Greet the participants.	4. Insist that "proper" language be used.
5. Plan for participants to get to know each other.	5. Moralize.
6. Start where the group is or wants to be.	6. Be upset by giggling and silliness (ignore it or set limits if necessary).
7. Move the discussion if it starts to drag.	7. Be upset by shock intenders who try to put the leader on the spot.
8. Remind the group to respect one another's opinions, feelings, and right to be heard.	8. Allow airing of personal problems.
9. Encourage contribution by praising comments.	9. Omit discussion of attitudes.
10. Ask quiet members' opinions.	10. Embarrass members by asking for direct information.
11. Relieve anxieties based on misinformation.	11. Monopolize the discussion, but guide by summarizing and questioning.
12. Be imaginative and keep the group involved.	

Adapted from Kempton, Winifred: Techniques for Leading Group Discussion on Human Sexuality. Philadelphia: Planned Parenthood of Southeastern Pennsylvania, 1973.

ing situations or information related to sexuality. Discussion of a film seen in a theater also promotes group interest. Playing a popular record and discussing the words and their effects or reading a newspaper or magazine article, column, or editorial on the subject of sexuality will all promote interest and give stimulus to expression of ideas and feelings.[49]

The leader also relieves anxieties based on misinformation and tries to help the group focus on issues that involve values (goals for expressing sexuality, expression of sexuality in relationships, male and female sexual roles, characteristics of sexually responsible behavior).

All members of the group are kept involved by encouraging less responsive members.[50] The leader helps the group realize that almost everyone has had some lack of sex education coupled with negative or guilt-provoking attitudes of parents and teachers. At all times, attitudes about sexual topics must be dealt with, since it is almost impossible to separate them from facts.

Intervention

Implementation of the teaching plan involves controlling the environment to enhance learning. The teacher's openness and comfort with others' ideas and feelings and willingness to listen will help provide an environment conducive to learning. Learning is facilitated by clarifying ideas that seem to be unclear and giving feedback that indicates to students that their ideas or feelings are valuable and are valued even if correction of misinformation is necessary. The leader gives positive, not negative reinforcement, praise instead of criticism, so that the student of whatever age feels safe to express ideas and feelings. When possible, the leader encourages and guides the students in discovering answers to their own questions rather than providing pat answers (see Table 11-3).

Two teachers in a class may be helpful—one can challenge while the other provides support; one can observe the other's presentation, and each can present different or opposing views.[51]

Evaluation

Evaluate what the individuals have learned at the end of each teaching session. Have the individuals describe in their own words what they have learned. Not only does this provide data to indicate if the teaching objectives have been met, but the students' repetition of ideas and facts reinforces the material. The most important indication of successful health teaching is whether there has been a change in behavior. This can be assessed only by careful observation in the future.

Gaining Comfort in Teaching about Sexuality

Formal courses, conferences, and classes on sexuality presented in schools and universities are valid and valuable sources of information and may help to decrease discomfort when talking about sexuality. Reading about sexuality from a wide variety of sources can increase sexual knowledge, but becoming comfortable talking about and teaching sexuality requires "doing." In all settings, nurses interested in increasing their ability to communicate about sexuality and in decreasing their emotional discomfort and embarrassment when doing so will find peer discussion groups helpful. Topics can be chosen by the members depending on their clinical interest. As nurses become desensitized to the subject and are better able to express themselves with each other, it becomes easier for them to talk to patients/clients.

NOTES

1. Redman BK: The Process of Patient Teaching in Nursing, 2nd ed. St. Louis, Mosby, 1972
2. Sexline, films are legacies of group. The Plain Dealer, March 15, 1983, Sec a, p 8
3. Gallup G: Family, sex courses are

favored. The Plain Dealer, December 28, 1980, Sec c, p 3

4. Hechinger F: New ammunition in fight to educate teens on sex. The Plain Dealer, October 17, 1982, Sec c, p 22

5. Scales P: The new opposition to sex education. School Health 51:300–303, 1981

6. Penland LR: Sex education in 1900, 1940, 1980: An historical sketch. J School Health 51:305–308, 1981

7. Gordon S: The case for a moral sex education in the schools. J School Health 51:214–218, 1981

8. Osofsky HJ, Osofsky JD: Let's be sensible about sex education. Am J Nurs 71:532–535, 1971

9. SIECUS, New York University. Principles basic to education for sexuality. J School Health 51:315–316, 1981

10. Lewis HR, Lewis ME: Sex Education Begins at Home. Norwalk, Appleton-Century-Crofts, 1983

11. Thornbury HD: Adolescent sources of information on sex. J School Health 51:274–277, 1981

12. DeLora JS, Warren CAB: Understanding Sexual Interaction. Boston, Houghton Mifflin, 1977, pp. 154–156.

13. Gagnon JH: Sexuality and sexual learning in the child. Psychiatry 28:212–228, 1965

14. NC News Service: Parents flunk in teaching their children about sex. Catholic Universe Bulletin, August 3, 1979, p 19

15. Oliven JF: Clinical Sexuality. Philadelphia, Lippincott, 1974, pp. 23–36

16. Gagnon JH: Sexuality and sexual learning in the child. Psychiatry 28:220, 1965

17. Ramsey G: The sex information of younger boys. Am J Orthopsychiatry 13:347–352, 1943

18. Gebhard P. Gagnon JH, Pomeroy WB, Christenson C: Sex Offenders, An Analysis of Types. New York, Harper & Row, 1965

19. Kilmann PR, Wanlass RL, Sahalis RF, Sullivan B: Sex education: A review of its effects. Arch Sex Behav 10:177–205, 1981

20. Gagnon JH: Sexuality and sexual learning in the child. Psychiatry 28:225, 1965

21. Haughton R: Religious Education and Sex Education. New York, Paulist Press, 1973

22. Philliber SG, Tatum ML: Sex education and the double standard in high school. Adolescence 17:273–284, 1982

23. Calderone MS: Sex education for young people—and for their parents and teachers. In Brecher R, Brecher E: An Analysis of Human Sexual Response. New York, New American Library, 1966, pp 267–274

24. Ibid, p 271

25. How to talk to your teenagers about something that's not easy to talk about. New York, Planned Parenthood Federation of America, Inc., 1975

26. Johnson W: Sex education and the nurse. Nurs Outlook 18(11):26–29, 1970

27. Cassell C: Putting sex education in its place. J School Health 51:211–213, 1981

28. Strawn A: Sex education and the school or whatever you do is wrong. National Elementary School Principal 57(2):23–28, 1978

29. Burt JJ, Brower LA: Education for Sexuality. Philadelphia, Saunders, 1970, pp 179–182

30. Oliven JF: Clinical Sexuality. Philadelphia, Lippincott, 1974, p 24

31. Ibid, p 25

32. Oliven JF: Clinical Sexuality. Philadelphia, Lippincott, 1974, p 112

33. Parcel G: Sex concerns of young adolescents. Birth Fam J 6:43–47, 1979

34. Hacker SS: It isn't sex education unless. J School Health 51:206–210, 1981

35. Read OA: Developing sexual awareness: A humanistic approach. J School Health 42:330–333, 1972

36. Kempton W: A Teacher's Guide to Sex Education for Persons with Disabilities that Hinder Learning. Belmont, California, Wadsworth, 1974

37. Redman BK: The Process of Patient Teaching in Nursing, 2nd ed. St. Louis, Mosby, 1972, p 42

38. Ibid, p 36

39. Ibid, p 51

40. Zalichin O: Clap, claptrap and comics. In Gottesfeld M (ed): Modern Sexuality. New York, Behavioral Publications, 1973, pp 268–272

41. Whipple B, Gick R: A holistic view of sexuality–education for the health professional. Top Clin Nurs 1:91–109, 1980

42. Mims FH, Brown L, Lubow R: Human sexuality course evaluation. Nurs Res 25(3):187–191, 1976

43. Dennis KJ, Elstein M: Education on sexuality in medical curriculum. Clin Obstet Gynecol 7:183–191, 1980

44. Malo-Juvera D: Seeing is believing. Nurs Outlook 21:583–585, 1973

45. Simon SB, Howe LW, Kirschenbaum H: Values Clarification. New York, Hart, 1972

46. Kempton W: Techniques for Leading Group Discussion on Human Sexuality, 2nd ed. Philadelphia, Planned Parenthood of Southeastern Pennsylvania, 1973

47. Ibid, p 4

48. Ibid, p 33

49. Ibid, p 6

50. Ibid, p 5

51. Silbert DT: Human sexuality growth groups. JPN Ment Health Serv 19 February:31–34, 1981

Chapter 12

Therapeutic Approaches to Counseling

Myron G. Eisenberg

Since all acute illnesses and chronic diseases exact their toll on sexual performance, sexual problems are to be routinely found among patients cared for by the nurse in the hospital, rehabilitation facility, and home setting. Nurses, because of their close and continuous contact with the patient and because of the many intimate functions they provide, are often the health care professional to whom the patient may choose to first raise the issue of sexual concerns. Additionally, nurses may be able to identify sexual problems on the basis of behavioral observations or hints dropped in conversations. Nursing personnel, then, are uniquely qualified to identify problems of a sexual nature and, in many cases, because of their close and continuous contact with the patient, to treat or assist in the treatment of sexual problems.

Some forms of treatment require specialized and extensive training that would normally be acquired only by nurses in specialized fields. However, often, the required intervention is much less involved, being supportive in nature, e.g., allowing the patient an opportunity to affirm or reaffirm his or her masculinity or femininity.[1-5] Also, the nurse is often in a position to prevent minor problems from intensifying to crisis proportions requiring intensive treatment. Nurses can provide the proper supportive

backdrop against which the patient's self-esteem can be enhanced; they can assist in remediating life factors that may be disrupting sexual activity and can help alleviate anxiety that may be interfering with sexual performance.

The purpose of this chapter is to acquaint the reader with the various therapies used for treatment of sexual disorders. These include simple information giving, the rational–emotive approach, Masters and Johnson's approach, behavior therapy, general relaxation training, biofeedback training, the Lobitz–LoPiccolo treatment of anorgasmia, sexual assertion rehearsal, Kaplan's approach, multimodal orientation, and finally, group counseling. Precautions that should be observed in sexual counseling are also presented to guide nurses in their approach to the individual.

NECESSARY SKILLS AND ATTITUDES IN DEALING WITH SEXUAL DISORDERS

A nurse who chooses to deal with sexual problems should conscientiously strive to ensure that certain prerequisites of information, skill, and attitude are met. Necessary information includes a knowledge of the physical factors in sexual function—anatomic, hormonal, and neurologic—in normal and pathologic conditions; knowledge of surgical or medical procedures likely to present complications of sexual performance; and an awareness of those diseases which themselves affect functioning, e.g., diabetes, chronic debilitating diseases, and emotional disorders.[6-10]

In terms of skill, the nature of the therapeutic modality to be used dictates the type and extent of training needed. If, for example, group therapy is to be employed, a knowledge of group process is essential; if, on the other hand, biofeedback is the treatment of choice, a thorough understanding of and familiarity with biofeedback methodology and instrumentation are indicated. The American Association of Educators, Counselors and Therapists* (AASECT) offers a wide variety of courses to those interested in providing sex counseling as well as certification as a sex educator or therapist. Guidelines provided by AASECT should be carefully examined and certification sought if nurses are to be properly prepared.

Lastly, one's attitude regarding sexual disabilities plays an important role in the counseling process. It is necessary that nurses can look upon sexual disorders as a legitimate concern, as a dysfunctional state with premorbid influence. Included in this attitude is tolerance of a patient's frailties, regardless of one's own moral or philosophic position and state of function or dysfunction.[11]

ASSESSMENT OF SEXUAL DISABILITIES

There are no absolutes when defining sexual adequacy. One definition posited by Lazarus[12] suggests adequacy is "having the abil-

*American Association of Sex Educators, Counselors and Therapists, Suite 304, 5010 Wisconsin Avenue N.W., Washington, D.C. 20016.

ity to obtain and maintain a sufficient degree of sexual arousal so as to derive pleasure from the sexual act and contribute to the enjoyment of one's partner, finally leading to orgasmic release." This definition, however, limits sexuality to include only those sexual acts that culminate in orgasm. Examining sexuality from a broader perspective to include all those activities that involve caring and concern, such as kissing, holding hands, and mutual pleasuring without orgasm would probably be a more accurate view of sexuality—a *weltanschauung* of how one views himself and others. What can be stated with some certainty, regardless of how one defines sexuality, is that adequate performance for one individual with one partner may be inadequate with another.[13-19]

Presentation of Sexual Problems

Persons with sexual problems often present with such symptoms as headache, fatigability, back pain, being "run down," dysmenorrhea, and a wide range of other nonspecific complaints. For some it is easier to experience physical discomfort than acknowledge sexual dysfunction. Many patients hope the sexual problem is organic in nature, believing or hoping a pill or surgical procedure can be prescribed and thus avoid any personal investment of energy that may be required to correct their dysfunctional status.[20-22]

Only by taking a detailed history can a clue be provided as to the sexual underpinnings of the complaint.[23,24] Much meaningful historical material overlooked by the physician can be gathered by the nurse through daily contacts with the patient. A sexual problem, once uncovered by the nurse, may, for example, represent little more than unrealistic romantic expectations or concerns about sexual propriety. Through unobtrusive intervention, the nurse may be able to resolve such conflicts relatively easily.

The nature and extent of a sexual problem must be carefully delineated prior to constructing a treatment plan. A thorough understanding of the problem requires that certain basic questions be answered.

What is the problem as perceived by the patient? A statement such as "I don't enjoy sex!" from a female patient may represent anything from fear of pregnancy, to primary anorgasmia, to severe neurosis. A woman's complaint of not enjoying sex may also serve as an entrée into treatment for an impotent husband.

What is the duration of the problem? Were impotency problems, for example, intermittent occurrences from when the individual first became sexually active or have they developed after previously satisfactory performance? Has the problem been consistently present since it began, or has it been intermittent?

What are the concurrent events? What other significant events were occurring when the difficulties started? Birth of children, debts, affairs, career failures, drinking, or death of a family member may be precipitating events. It is often profitable to discuss seemingly unrelated events that coincide with disability onset.

What, if anything, has the patient found that will temporarily improve functioning? Temporary improvements can be occasioned by such occurrences as a fight with the spouse, getting the children out of the house, being taken out for dinner, or using a tranquilizer. All these modes of improvement will tend to help focus on the pathogenic agent.

What does the patient feel has caused the problem and how serious does he or she feel it is? Patients often have a clear perception of the etiology and seriousness of their difficulty. This information may be of great help in the ultimate recommendation for treatment.

What are the patient's expectations in terms of treatment? Suggestions from patients may run from hormones, to counseling, to psychotherapy. Such information may

be extremely helpful in selecting the appropriate introduction to the preferred treatment mode.

PLANNING

Nurses should be aware of the variety of approaches to sexual counseling available to the therapist, using those techniques they feel to be appropriate to meet the needs of the patient and only those approaches they feel capable of carrying out. Counseling a patient on his or her sexuality, if done properly, can result in improved functioning. Counseling without the proper training or attitude can be destructive. It is important that nurses hoping to do sexual therapy be thoroughly acquainted with and knowledgeable about a variety of these therapeutic modalities so they will be able to select and offer the correct therapeutic approach to and for the patient rather than fit the patient into the only modality about which they are knowledgeable.

INTERVENTION: TECHNIQUES FOR TREATMENT OF SEXUAL DISORDERS

Approaches to the treatment of sexual dysfunction discussed in this chapter are by no means to be considered comprehensive, nor is each approach described in detail. The purpose of the discussion is to provide suggestions of what the nurse is able to do, when it is time to refer patients, and the wide variety of therapeutic modalities available to the trained counselor. Most of the techniques discussed require extensive training, which can be obtained through reading, workshops, formalized classroom work, internships, and/or practice.

Education/Information Giving
Some sexual problems or concerns can be resolved merely by providing the patient de-

tailed, accurate information couched in understandable language.[25-28] Patients may be selected for brief educational intervention when the history indicates the patient lacks information and experience or has factual misconceptions. Most important, interventions should be offered to patients who, directly or indirectly, express interest in having more data. This technique is usually appropriate in individuals who are just beginning sexual activity. When the partnership has more longevity, there must be some question raised regarding the couple's ability to communicate. Such cases might indicate deep-seated problems in the relationship. The primary effect of providing information in an understanding but matter-of-fact way is to take sexual functioning out of the realm of the mysterious and forbidden.

The Rational–Emotive Approach to Sex Therapy

The rational–emotive therapy (RET) practitioner initially provides corrective information to the client.[29-38] In accordance with RET theory, this information is provided to dispel irrational ideas, e.g., that couples must engage in conventional coitus to have successful and enjoyable sex; that all "normal" men and women constantly desire sex and are aroused and satisfied easily; that spontaneous arousal by both partners must occur if the couple is to have a satisfactory sexual relationship; that loving partners are automatically aroused by their mates; that variety is unimportant in sex relations; that foreplay, to seem proper, must terminate in penile–vaginal copulation; that any knowledgeable individual can easily become aroused and provide many orgasms to his or her partner.[39,40]

Rational–emotive therapists provide not only information to sexually dysfunctional individuals but attempt to help the couple achieve an open, experimenting, individualistic attitude toward sex, love, and marriage. RET also purports to assist individuals in surrendering self-defeating myths, superstitions, and dogmas.

RET evokes the imagination in the treatment process. Males and females who have experienced difficulty in feeling aroused or reaching orgasm are taught how to fantasize. The RET therapist assists the client in learning how to use sex fantasies, various kinds of "pornographic" images, and romantic fantasies regularly.

An integral part of RET deals with bibliotherapy, and recorded therapy. Following an educational model, RET uses a variety of audiovisual modalities, including pamphlets, books, recordings, films, oral presentations, and workshops. Patients are, for example, encouraged to record their own sex therapy sessions and listen to the recordings several times between sessions.

Other examples of various techniques utilized by the RET therapist include "risk-taking" exercises and "shame-attacking" exercises.[41] Risk-taking exercises encourage the client to practice emotive risk taking. For example, the RET group therapist may tell the patient to "Do something that is risky or dangerous right now in this room" or "Take the risk of asking your regular partner to engage in a sex act that you feel afraid that he or she would not like to perform."

Another technique commonly used by the RET therapist is that of shame-attacking exercises.[42] According to RET, shame or "self-downing" contributes heavily to many human disturbances. These exercises are used to demonstrate to the client that if they actually performed so-called shameful or foolish acts, their world would not come to an end. When given such "shameful" acts to perform, either individually or in group RET sessions, the therapist does not suggest that the patient engage in behaviors that might lead to serious problems, such as getting fired or being thrown into jail. Patients are, however, encouraged to perform nonharmful "shameful" behaviors such as wearing sexy clothes or acting in highly assertive ways with members of the opposite sex. Use of these treatment modalities requires extensive training and should not be used by those unskilled or untrained in their execution.

As a general system of therapy, RET envisions most serious sexual problems within a framework of general emotional upset and strives to reduce general levels of disturbability. By so doing, specific sexual problems are also resolved. Use of the rational–emotive approach is most appropriate for people with entrenched cognitive blocks. It is a relatively short-term treatment.

Sexual Therapy of Masters and Johnson

Techniques developed by Masters and Johnson[43] are a functional combination of directive, educational, and behavioral therapies, stemming from research discussed in *Human Sexual Response*. Many assume that the Masters and Johnson approach to therapy is mechanistic, teaching a couple physical techniques. There is, however, a portion of their program that is based upon attitudinal changes. Therefore, before beginning sexual therapy with a couple, it is important to determine whether their attitudes are amenable to change.

Therapy Procedure. The basis of the success of Masters and Johnson sexual therapy is that a man and wife or regular sex partner are treated as a unit. A sexual problem is never just his problem or her problem, it is a shared problem. A second principle of the Masters and Johnson therapy is that the couple be treated by a male–female therapy team. This is done for the purpose of having someone of the same sex available with whom both husband and wife can identify.

The first step in therapy is usually for the male therapist to take a thorough medical and sex history from the male and for the female therapist to take the history from the female. On the second appointment, this process is reversed, with the female therapist taking the male's history and the male therapist taking the female's. This is done in part not only to insure that nothing has been omitted from the data-gathering interview, but also to identify attitudes that may be expressed differently in the presence of one sex

or another. It is felt that this technique is important in recognizing the often unrecognized or unspoken attitudes operating between the husband and wife. Examples of various techniques advocated by Masters and Johnson in alleviating specific types of sexual disorders are given below.

Nonorgasmic Response. If the presenting problem is one of nonorgasmic response, Masters and Johnson propose a step-by-step process be followed by the couple. The most important instruction provided is that the female take the superior mounting position. The reason this is done is that most women have traditionally assumed the opposite position and have never really learned what is most pleasurable or satisfying for their body. In the female superior position, the man is instructed not to thrust until directed to do so by his partner.

In the female superior mounting position, in which the woman is responsible for the insertion of the penis, the female is instructed to lie with her head almost touching her mate's head. Many females take the superior position by squatting down on the penis with the body held upright or tilted slightly backward. In this position, it is possible for the penis to be bent, which may damage the spongy tissue. According to Masters and Johnson, it is the female who should have control over the insertion at all times, because she knows when she is ready for insertion and where the entrance is. A man may find his erection has subsided as he tries to gain entrance if he controls the act of penetration. If communication between partners is developed, they will have no hesitation in instructing one another when each is ready and in receiving assistance from one another regarding timing and method of penetration.

Impotence. In treating impotence, Masters and Johnson suggest there are a series of techniques that can be used by the female to stimulate the penis. When her partner does get an erection, it is the female who makes the insertion. The male is *not* to attempt intercourse. It is the woman who learns when to initiate insertion and movement. Relieving the male from some of the responsibility for the sex act releases him from performance pressure and enables him to relax, enjoy, and perform successfully.

Squeeze Technique.   For males experiencing the problem of premature ejaculation, the squeeze technique is advocated by Masters and Johnson. This technique requires communication and cooperation between partners. Once the man achieves an erection, there comes a point called "ejaculatory inevitability" at which time he knows ejaculation is imminent. Ejaculation takes place only seconds after he has felt that sensation; he has no control over it. The squeeze technique is used just prior to the moment of ejaculatory inevitability. The male must let his partner know when he wants her to perform this act. The squeeze technique is accomplished by the female placing the index finger of her left hand on the glans just above the coronal ridge; the middle finger is placed just below the coronal ridge and the thumb is placed on the frenulum. In this position she squeezes the penis hard for about 3 to 4 seconds until the male feels the urge to ejaculate has subsided. There is no discomfort or pain associated with squeezing as long as the penis is erect. This process can be repeated as many times as desired.

When the technique has been mastered without penetration, the female assumes the superior position and the couple practice its use with penetration. The squeeze technique is a reconditioning process and, over a period of time, can be effective in controlling premature ejaculation about 100 percent of the time.

The Masters and Johnson treatment is particularly well suited to single-behavior problems, such as premature ejaculation or impotence. It is short-term and especially appropriate for individuals who are reluctant to enter therapy. As can be seen from this brief review of the Masters and Johnson sexual therapy, their approach to sexual dysfunction is pragmatic, directive, and authoritative. In the process of learning Masters and Johnson have helped therapists accept the role of being the authority who instructs people that it is not only all right but physically and psychologically good to pursue   pleasure   in   their   sexual relationships.

Behavior Therapy Techniques Used in the Treatment of Sexual Dysfunction

The conceptual framework on which behavior therapy rests is known as "social learning theory."[44-55] The basic tenet of this approach is that behavior is a function of its consequences. A fundamental assumption of behavior therapy techniques is that most persistent behavior patterns are maintained by positive and negative reinforcers (see Chapter 7). Behaviors endure because at one time they promoted pleasure and/or avoided pain, but these behaviors are now interfering with sexual activities. Consistent with the principles of social learning, specific treatment procedures are viewed as reeducative experiences that call for active participation. Thus, written materials, audio tape cassettes, films, and especially homework assignments are all important elements of the educational and behavioral retraining. The main emphasis of such techniques is upon unlearning negative habits and acquiring a repertoire of adaptive feelings and responses more adaptive for the present.

In accounting for the development of sexual dysfunction, psychogenic factors are thought by behaviorists to be predominant etiologically. A basic premise of the behavioral approach is that dysfunctions that have been learned and maintained by environmental references can be overcome through the appropriate reeducative experiences. Sexual dysfunctions often seem to be the result of learned inhibitions, especially anxiety. Interpersonal conflict is another major source of dysfunction. Behavioral techniques are designed to diminish anxiety and interpersonal conflicts that result in sexual problems.

Following are various types of behaviorally-oriented approaches commonly used in the treatment of sexual disorders. They are short-term, goal-specific approaches to treatment and offer the therapist a variety of techniques. Much of the therapeutic intervention formulated by Masters and Johnson, as well as that postulated by Ellis, have strong behavioral components.

General Relaxation Training. General relaxation training in the treatment of sexual dysfunction involves a graded series of therapeutic sessions beginning with touching exercises.[56,57] The theoretic basis for this was the notion that anxiety inhibited sexual behavior and that anxiety and relaxation could not coexist. The most commonly used relaxation techniques include breathing exercises, imagery exercises, and progressive muscular relaxation exercises.

Biofeedback Training. Biofeedback has been used to help the patient learn to control autonomic responses.[58] Generally, these techniques are most often used to help reduce anxiety levels. They can also be used to voluntarily control penile volume through use of penile plethysmographs and other biofeedback apparatus.

Recently, researchers have used biofeedback to assist in the treatment of pedophiliacs. The most important result of this work suggests that continuous feedback to both patient and therapist results in systematic shifting of arousal to more appropriate cues.

Research does indicate that autonomic responses can be influenced by voluntary control if the autonomic events can be recognized by the patient. For a number of patients with secondary impotence, researchers have been attempting to develop and maintain the arousal state through the use of feedback.

Lobitz–LoPiccolo Treatment of Anorgasmia. A problem for nonorgasmic women is often fear of loss of control with orgasm or embarrassment. The "exaggerated orgasm" procedures described by Lobitz and LoPiccolo are useful in effectively dealing with the problem.[59] This technique involves asking the woman to pretend to reach orgasm with her partner present and exaggerate screams and thrashes. The partner is aware of the staged responses and the procedure is repeated several times, passing through three stages—embarrassment, humor, boredom. It has been reported that after having gone through this exercise, a woman will experience her first orgasm.

Remediation of Environmental Factors Influencing Sexual Responsiveness.
Some behavioral therapists will systematically assess those aspects of the environment that produce either sexual arousal responses or responses inhibiting arousal.[60] Paper and pencil surveys are completed by the patient. Interviews follow to clarify the important environmental cues. Research has indicated the importance of these cues for the female sexual response. Couples are then encouraged to use those cues that elicit sexual arousal as a regular procedure prior to the sexual experiences planned in the therapy program.

Sexual Assertion Rehearsal. Some sexually dysfunctional patients have had unpleasant sexual experiences partly because they have been reluctant to discuss ways of modifying the sexual behavior of their partner.[61,62] As a result, the pattern of sexual activity for the couple may involve the dysfunctional member engaging in intercourse when exhausted at the end of the day, being caressed in a way that is uncomfortable, having the sexual interaction occur at too fast a pace, or being deprived of cues needed for arousal. In general, this may result in the unconscious association of unpleasantness or discomfort with sexual activity. To facilitate sexual assertiveness, or direct requests or feedback, some therapists have had patients rehearse assertions. Specific assertive responses generally follow guidelines set forth by Lange and Jakubowski[63] and others.[64,65]

The New Sex Therapy: Helen Singer Kaplan

Kaplan[66] in her text *The New Sex Therapy* succinctly describes new methods for the treatment of sexual disorders, many of which have been described in this chapter, and clarifies some basic underlying concepts by relating the technical material to the theory of psychopathology and psychiatric treatment. The popular text describes the process of sex therapy.

The treatments for sexual problems discussed by Kaplan are admittedly not original; rather, they represent the confluence of multiple theoretic influences—analysis, behavior therapy, psychosomatic medicine, and group therapy. She relies heavily upon short, time-limited interventions and on prescribing tasks for the patient to carry out at home. When spouses are available, the couple is treated as a unit.

The contribution Kaplan has made lies in her accurate, complete, and readable discussion of the active sex therapies within a multicausal, eclectic orientation. Basic strategies and tactics of sex therapy are described as are their underlying rationales. In addition, controversial issues, such as the effectiveness of cotherapists and the significance of transference and countertransference, are discussed lucidly and knowledgeably. The Kaplan text is highly recommended as supplemental reading.

The Multimodal Orientation

It is essential that the therapist dealing with sexual concerns be knowledgeable and flexible enough to use elements of various therapeutic modalities to address seven separate but interrelated elements in the counseling processes that can produce change.[67-69] These seven elements are:

1. Behavior—diminishing maladaptive responses and implementing the patient's social reportoire;
2. Affect—reducing the occurrence of unpleasant feeling states and cultivating positive emotions;
3. Sensation—teaching patients to experience the here and now by enhancing visual and auditory perception and promoting a positive range of tactile, kinesthetic, and olfactory pleasures;
4. Imagery—examining the fantasies that diminish the well-being of the individual as well as those images that can be used to increase adaptive functioning;
5. Cognition—dispelling emotional and irrational notions;
6. Interrelationships—recognizing the interdependence of emotional states and person-to-person interactions;
7. Drugs—recognizing the efficacy of medication in certain anxious, depressed or psychotic individuals.

The clinical consequences of attending to each of these seven factors ensures comprehensive and thorough therapeutic intervention.

The multimodal rationale underscores the importance of correcting irrational beliefs, unpleasant feelings, deviant images, negative sensations, and possible biochemical imbalances. Instead of searching for a single cause of the sexual dysfunction or "the" correct therapeutic modality, the multimodal approach emphasizes that the patient is usually troubled by a host of specific problems that need to be corrected by a similar multitude of specific treatments.

Group Counseling

Group therapies have been criticized for dealing with vague and/or questionable goals[70] and failure to focus on observable interpersonal difficulties that foster maladaptive modes of functioning.[71,72] Critics complain that persons often spend time in groups that are not goal-directed, dealing with internalized problems that often lack objective referents.[73] Problems associated with altered sexual functioning that accompany a variety of physical impairments offer the rehabilitation counselor a unique opportunity to utilize a group format to deal with this highly specific and concrete issue. In dealing with problems of sexual functioning, goals can be specified unambiguously in advance, and results can be empirically measured.

Group therapy as a format within which to conduct sexual therapy does have some advantages over individual interaction. It is necessary, however, to assess the needs of the individual patient to determine if, in fact, a group approach is most appropriate for him or her. In some cases, a combination of individual and group experience may be most effective.[74–76]

PHYSICAL DISABILITY: A SPECIAL PROBLEM

Following the onset of chronic illness or disability, the individual is vulnerable to a variety of factors that can indirectly affect his ability to function sexually.[77] Devaluation and desexualization of the patient by himself and others occur frequently.[78] The person who suffers a physical disability may tend to devalue himself because of the change in his or her physical attractiveness or physical ability. This sense of devaluation may be communicated to others he meets.[79] Society places high value on attractiveness, youth, and physical ability. Thus, the patient's devaluation of himself may be confirmed by the reaction of others.

Devaluation is often correlated with desexualization; the community may not recognize the physically disabled person as a suitable sex partner and may believe that, because the person is disabled, sex is no longer important in his life. All the patient's premorbid social experiences and self-confidence are required to combat the devaluation and desexualization phenomena, and therapists should be aware of these influences on sexual functioning. Specific techniques and precau-

tions to be observed, presented elsewhere in this text, should be discussed with the patient.

NOTES

1. Ard BN: Treating Psychosexual Dysfunction, New York, Aronson, 1974
2. Gebhard P: Situational factors affecting human sexual behavior. In Beach FA (ed): Sex and Behavior. New York, Wiley, 1965
3. Hartman WE, Fithian MA: The Treatment of the Sexual Dysfunctions. Long Beach, California, Center for Marital and Sexual Studies, 1974
4. Lazarus AA: Modes of treatment for sexual inadequacies. Med Aspects Hum Sexuality 3(5):53–58, 1969
5. Wahl CW (ed): Sexual Problems: Diagnosis and Treatment in Medical Practice. New York, Free Press, 1967
6. Cooper AJ: Treatment of male potency disorders. Psychosomatics 12:235–244, 1971
7. Eisenberg M: Group sex counseling for the physically impaired. In Sha'K-d A (ed): Human Sexuality and Rehabilitation. Baltimore, Williams and Wilkins, 1981
8. Katchadourian HA, Lunde DT: Fundamentals of Human Sexuality. New York, Holt, 1972
9. Kinsey AC, Pomeroy WB, Martin CE: Sexual Behavior in the Human Male. Philadelphia, Saunders, 1948
10. Lazarus AA: Multimodal behavior therapy. J Nerv Ment Dis 156:404–411, 1973
11. Hohmann G: Considerations in management of psychosexual adjustment in the spinal cord injured male. Rehab Psychol 19(2):50–57, 1972
12. Lazarus AA: Modes of treatment for sexual inadequacies. Med Aspects Hum Sexuality 3(5):56, 1969
13. Anthansiou R: A review of public attitudes on sexual issues. In Zubin J, Money J (eds): Contemporary Sexual Be-

havior. Baltimore, Johns Hopkins University Press, 1973

14. Eisenberg M, Falconer J: Current trends in sex education programming for the physically disabled: Some guidelines for implementation and evaluation. Sexuality Disab 1:6, 1978

15. Ford A. Orfirer A: Sexual behavior and the chronically ill patient. Med Aspects Hum Sexuality 1(2):57–61, 1967

16. Green BL: Sexual dissatisfaction. In Green BL (ed): Clinical Approach to Mental Problems. Springfield, Illinois, Thomas, 1970

17. Hohmann G: Considerations in management of psychosexual adjustment in the spinal cord injured male. Rehab Psychol 19(2):55, 1972

18. Ince LF: Behavior modification of sexual disorders. Am J Psychother 27:446–451, 1973

19. Kaplan HS: The New Sex Therapy. New York, Brunner/Mazel, 1975

20. Belt BG: Some organic causes of impotence. Med Aspects Hum Sexuality 7(1):152–161, 1973

21. Cooper AJ: Factors in male sexual inadequacy. J Nerv Ment Dis 149:337–359, 1969

22. Lewis JM: Impotence as a reflection of marital conflict. Med Aspects Hum Sexuality 3(6):73–75, 1969

23. Masserman JH (ed): Current Psychiatric Therapies. New York, Grune and Stratton, 1961

24. Meyer JK: Individual treatment of sexual disorders. In Freedman AM, Kaplan HI, Sadock BJ (eds): Comprehensive Textbook of Psychiatry, 2nd ed. Baltimore, Williams and Wilkins, 1975, p. 1544

25. Ard BN: Treating Psychosexual Dysfunction. New York, Aronson, 1974

26. Ellis A: Sex without Guilt. Hollywood, California, Wilshire Books, 1970

27. Ellis A: Humanistic Psychotherapy. The Rational–Emotive Approach. New York, Julian, 1973

28. Ellis A: Disputing Irrational Beliefs. New York, Institute for Rational Living, 1974

29. Ellis A: Reason and Emotion in Psychotherapy. New York, Stuart, 1962

30. Ellis A: The Art and Science of Love. New York, Bantam, 1969

31. Ellis A: Sex without Guilt. Hollywood, California, Wilshire Books, 1970

32. Ellis A: The American Sexual Tragedy. Hollywood, California, Wilshire Books, 1970

33. Ellis A: The Sensuous Person. New York, Stuart, 1972

34. Ellis A: Humanistic Psychotherapy. The Rational–Emotive Approach. New York, Julian, 1973

35. Ellis A: Disputing Irrational Beliefs. New York, Institute for Rational Living, 1974

36. Ellis A: The rational–emotive approach to sex therapy. Counseling Psychologist 5(1):14–21, 1975

37. Maultsby MG, Ellis A: Techniques for Using Rational–Emotive Imagery (REI). New York. Institute for Rational Living, 1974

38. Tosi DJ: Youth: Toward Personal Growth, A Rational–Emotive Approach. Columbus, Ohio, Merrill, 1974

39. Ard BN: Treating Psychosexual Dysfunction. New York, Aronson, 1974

40. Ellis A: The Sensuous Person. New York, Stuart, 1972

41. Ellis A: The rational–emotive approach to sex therapy. Counseling Psychologist 5(1):14–21, 1975

42. Ibid, p 18

43. Masters WH, Johnson VE: Human Sexual Response. Boston, Little, Brown, 1966

44. Bandura A: Principles of Behavior Modification. New York, Holt, 1969

45. Bandura A, Blanchard EB, Ritter B: The relative efficacy of desensitization and modeling approaches for inducing behavioral, affective, and attitudinal changes. J Pers Soc Psychol 13:173–199, 1969

46. Bednar RL, Lawlis GF: Empirical research in group psychotherapy. In Bergin AE, Garfield SL (eds): Handbook

of Psychotherapy and Behavior Change: An Empirical Analysis. New York, Wiley, 1971

47. Fischer J, Gochros HL: Handbook of Behavior Therapy with Sexual Problems. Vol I: General Procedures. Vol II: Approach to Specific Problems. Elmsford, New York, Pergamon, 1977

48. Ince LF: Behavior modification of sexual disorders. Am J Psychother 27:446, 1972

49. Kish RS, Shrivastava DC: Behavior therapy for sex problems. Lancet 1:1295, 1973

50. Lazarus AA: Behavior therapy in groups. In Gazada G: Basic Approach to Group Psychotherapy and Group Counseling. Springfield, Illinois, Thomas, 1968

51. Lazarus AA: Behavior Therapy and Beyond. New York, McGraw-Hill, 1971

52. Lobitz CW, LoPiccolo J: New methods in the behavioral treatment of sexual dysfunction. J Behav Ther Exp Psychiatry 3:265–270, 1972

53. Ullman LP, Krasner L: Case Studies in Behavioral Modification. New York, Holt, 1965

54. Wolpe J, Lazarus AA: Behavior Therapy Techniques. New York, Pergamon, 1966

55. Yates AJ: Behavior Therapy. New York, Wiley, 1970

56. Jacobson E: Progressive Relaxation. Chicago, University of Chicago Press, 1938

57. Jacobson E: Anxiety and Tension Control: A Physiobiologic Approach. Philadelphia, Lippincott, 1964

58. Fischer J, Gochros HL: Handbook of Behavior Therapy with Sexual Problems. Vol I: General Procedures. Vol II: Approach to Specific Problems. Elmsford, New York, Pergamon, 1977

59. Lobitz CW, LoPiccolo J: New methods in the behavioral treatment of sexual dysfunction. J Behav Ther Exp Psychiatry 3:268–269, 1972

60. Gebhard P: Situational factors affecting human sexual behavior. In Beach FA (ed): Sex and Behavior. New York, Wiley, 1965

61. Bandura A, Blanchard EB, Ritter B: The relative efficacy of desensitization and modeling approaches for inducing behavioral, affective, and attitudinal changes. J Pers Soc Psychol 13:173–199, 1969

62. Obler M: Systematic desensitization in sexual therapy. J Behav Ther Exp Psychiatry 4(2):93, 1973

63. Lange AJ, Jakubowski P: Responsible Assertion Training. Champaign, Illinois, Research Press, 1976

64. Alberti RE, Emmons ML: Your Perfect Right. A Guide to Assertive Behavior. San Luis Obispo. California, Impact, 1970

65. Lobitz CW, LoPiccolo J: New methods in the behavioral treatment of sexual dysfunction. J Behav Ther Exp Psychiatry 3:265–270, 1972

66. Kaplan HS: The New Sex Therapy. New York, Brunner/Mazel, 1975

67. Lazarus AA: Behavior therapy in groups. In Gazda G: Basic Approach to Group Psychotherapy and Group Counseling. Springfield, Illinois, Thomas, 1968

68. Lazarus AA: Modes of treatment for sexual inadequacies. Med Aspects Hum Sexuality 3(5):53–58, 1969

69. Lazarus AA: Behavior Therapy and Beyond. New York, McGraw-Hill, 1971

70. Walker DE, Pfeiffer HC: The goals of counseling. J Counseling Psychol 4(3):204–209, 1957

71. Lazarus AA: Behavior therapy in groups. In Gazda G: Basic Approach to Group Psychotherapy and Group Counseling. Springfield, Illinois, Thomas, 1968

72. Ullman LP, Krasner L: Case Studies in Behavioral Modification. New York, Holt, 1965

73. Bednar RL, Lawlis GF: Empirical research in group psychotherapy. In Bergin AE, Garfield SL (eds): Handbook of Psychotherapy and Behavior Change: An Empirical Analysis. New York, Wiley, 1971

74. Bednar RL, Lawlis GF: Empirical re-

search in group psychotherapy. In Bergin AE, Garfield SL (eds): Handbook of Psychotherapy and Behavior Change: An Empirical Analysis. New York, Wiley, 1971

75. Bandura A: Principles of Behavior Modification. New York, Holt, 1969

76. Walker DE, Pfeiffer HC: The goals of counseling. J Counseling Psychol 4(3):204–209, 1957

77. Sha'Ked A: Human Sexuality in Physical and Mental Disabilities. Bloomington, Indiana, University of Indiana Press, 1978

78. Wright BA: Physical Disability: A Psychological Approach. New York, Harper & Row, 1960

79. Ford A. Orfirer A: Sexual behavior and the chronically ill patient. Med Aspects Hum Sexuality 1(2):57–61, 1967

Chapter 13

Effects of Illness or Hospitalization on Sexuality

Healthy sexuality is a product of both physiologic and psychosocial factors. Intact nervous, hormonal, and vascular systems are needed for optimal male and female sexual response. Illness may compromise one or more of these systems. Of equal impact on sexuality is the adverse effect of body image changes, decreased self-esteem, and altered sexual role identity that may accompany illness and/or hospitalization.

High self-esteem, especially, is necessary for good sexual relationships, because it allows individuals to be comfortable seeking pleasure, searching for individual tastes and pleasures, and in asking another to help satisfy sexual needs. Decreased physical capacity causes decreased self-esteem.[1] Surgical procedures can also have profound effect on sexual self-concept and may adversely affect sexual performance.[2]

Nurses intervene to maintain or help individuals attain sexual integrity when it is threatened by illness and/or hospitalization. For some, the ability to carry out their usual patterns of sexual activity may be permanently lost by illness, so nurses help them develop new acceptable role activities and patterns of sexual activity that can substitute for those lost or help them adjust to permanent loss.

Nurses have an even greater responsibility to help individuals maintain optimal sexual self-concept. They can do this by avoiding practices that contribute to shame, by helping alleviate guilt, by providing privacy, and by helping individuals overcome body image disturbances.

The focus of this chapter is on decreased sexual self-esteem as a consequence of illness and/or hospitalization. Biologic factors are discussed breifly, since Unit V contains information about the effects of specific pathologies. Greater attention is given to the concepts of shame, guilt, privacy, and body image, as well as to the effects of sociocultural factors, on individual's response to illness.

BIO-PSYCHO-SOCIAL FACTORS RELATED TO DECREASED SEXUAL SELF-ESTEEM

Biologic Factors

The effects of specific disease conditions on sexuality are discussed in Unit V. Some disease processes may directly compromise the physiologic response to sexual stimuli. In others, the pain and discomfort association with the disease process limits sexual response.

However, even without these problems, any illness itself can compromise sexual performance. As one patient remarked, "All my energy is directed toward getting well. I have

199

no sexual function." Some may have no interest in sexual activity and little concern about their loss of responsiveness to sexual stimuli, either because it was not an important facet of their lives or because their energies are directed to recovery from the physical disability. Others may suffer from anxiety and depression, feeling that a source of pleasure and/or of interpersonal closeness and support has been lost. The sexual partner and the patient suffer this loss at a time when both are experiencing the stress that illness and/or hospitalization can produce.

Sexual problems may be related to other factors; for example, (1) fear of causing, precipitating, or aggravating physical problems by sexual activity may halt sexual activity, often unnecessarily; (2) some persons may use medical illness as an excuse to avoid feared or undesired sexual experiences.[3]

The sexual partner may wish sexual activity but fear requesting or demanding sex, fearful that by becoming sexually aroused the patient may die. One or both may become tense and irritable; guilt, resentment, hostility, and problems with self-esteem occur. Poor communication may further aggravate the situation.

Couples with latent or overt sexual problems may use illness as a protection against sexual activity. Illness may mask a primary sexual problem. The individual may report difficulties that are not supported by objective observation of the physical condition. These chronic sexual problems usually require sex therapy or psychiatric counseling.

Sexual problems may be transient, permanent, or irreversible. Even with irreversible physical changes, individuals can make adaptations in sexual behavior and cope satisfactorily. Tyler[4] states that the concept of irreversible sexual incapacities applies only to the individuals whose total interest, energy, and attention are focused on a painful, debilitating, and terminal illness. In fact, sexual incapacity may occur and go untreated and neglected because of patient's/client's ignorance, naiveté, guilt, and embarrassment and from the professional's similar embarrassment, naiveté, and lack of training.

Psychologic Factors

Admission to the hospital, the information-gathering process, and the treatment of the illness may be more devastating to the individual's sexual self-esteem than the disease itself. The individual is separated from the significant others, who may be quickly shunted aside as the admission process begins. Individuals who value their independence and decision making as part of their sexual self-identity are stripped of this function in regard to the basic activities of daily living; when they eat, when they sleep, who shares their room, what degree of activity they are allowed, in some cases even when they eliminate.

Their sexual identity is further blurred by the removal of clothes and the frequent substitution of an asexual hospital gown— one size and design fits all sexes and sizes. Further control is lost when patients are warned not to keep money, jewelry, or valuables, all or some of which may contribute to sexual identity. Loss of control may be threatening not only to men with the "machismo" belief that is prevalent in some cultures, but also to women who value their autonomy and decision-making ability associated with the mother and homemaker role or with the work world outside the home.

The assessments and treatments are intrusive. History questions focus on areas that have been considered private and that in some cases are embarrassing to discuss. The procedures carried out for diagnosis or therapy and the hospital routines are assaults on sexual privacy, although there may be a deemphasizing of the bounds of propriety during hospitalization.[5]

Privacy. Privacy is defined as the right of individuals to exclude others from certain knowledge about themselves and the awareness that others have this same privilege. Inherent in the term are also the factors of time, place, manner, and amount of information involved. Privacy also involves the exclusion of oneself from others by either physical or psychologic means.[6] It is interactional. When individuals seek distances or closeness, another is involved.[7]

Privacy serves first to insure personal autonomy, the uniqueness of humans, and their worth as individuals. Interpersonal relationships have been described in terms of zones or circles of privacy leading to the inner self. Potential threat is imposed on one's autonomy and one's privacy in situations where a person seeks to enter the inner core and learns secrets. Sexual information is culturally a taboo subject for many individuals. In addition, it is information that may involve feelings of guilt and unworthiness. Yet this information is sought and needs to be sought by health professionals as part of total care.[8]

Emotional release is a second function of privacy. Sexual functions and emotional expression in time of loss or sorrow usually need privacy for their release. These sexual patterns of release are not possible for the individual who usually shares his room, is subject to unexpected interruptions, and who is culturally indoctrinated with the idea that certain environments, such as the hospital, are inappropriate for sexual behavior.

Self-evaluation, whereby individuals integrate experiences and identity their meaning, assess data, consider choices, and take moral inventory, is also done in private. The hospital does little to facilitate either of these aspects of privacy. Limited and protected communication is the fourth aspect of privacy. This involves the opportunity for sharing confidences because of the privileged communication that exists between the patient and professional. This aspect is especially important when individuals give highly charged information of a sexual nature. Privacy is suspended when patients/clients share fears and problems about sexuality. This speaks to the trust that they have in health professionals to use the information for the patient's interests and well being.[9]

The need for privacy is universal to all life. Privacy of space has been described by Hall[10] in relation to described distance zones, which he called *proxemics*. The zones range from intimate distance (0 to 18 inches), personal distance (1½ to 4 feet), social distance (4 to 12 feet), and public distance (12 feet and beyond). The distance individuals maintain between themselves and others speaks to the relationship between them. Anxiety reactions to intrusion into personal space has been observed in animals and humans.

Although the sample was limited in number, Allekian[11] found that patients had some feelings of uneasiness when nurses administer treatment to personal areas of the body. People are usually able to set the degree of distance when they feel protection is needed, but after admission to the hospital, they lose control of this limit setting. Patients must submit to care of an intimate nature by persons of the opposite sex, as well as care given by nurses of the same sex. Invasion into personal space may be a threat and source of anxiety.[12]

Shame. Shame is a psychologic reaction closely allied to invasions of privacy. It can be mixed with other emotions, such as guilt and feelings of inferiority. Webster's dictionary defines *shame* as "a painful emotion caused by consciousness of guilt, shortcoming, or impropriety."[13] Threat of exposure is also part of shame. The early psychoanalytic definition indicated that shame is a defense against exhibitionism and voyeurism: "I feel ashamed" means "I do not want to be seen." The word *shame* is derived from a compound German word relating to the genitals.[14] Shame involves much more than sexual exposure; uncovering of weakness, failure, physical defect, or lack of recognition may all be experienced as shameful. For many people, the experience of illness itself is shameful.

Shame results from tension between the ego and the ego ideal (standards, aspirations, and goals that are internalized through identification with the culture, specifically the parents). There is a discrepancy between the idealized self and the self as actually perceived.[15]

Disgust is connected with the development of shame. To be disgusted with someone else is to see him as unclean and unacceptable. Nurses and others may be disgusted by obesity, disfigurement, sexual deviations, lice, body odors, etc.[16]

Shame for children is first experienced in relation to body image and function. The child feels ashamed of his weakness, smallness, and nakedness. Adults' shame involves abstract concepts such as the values of physical and mental health, beauty, and vocational, monetary, and sexual success.[17]

Shame has a developmental aspect. The child struggles for muscular control during the second to fourth year. Illness may reactivate conflict over body control, especially illness that changes body image and functioning. During the latency or juvenile period, the child looks to the peer group for recognition and hopes to become part of this group. Ostracism becomes a powerful weapon. The child who does not fit because his mannerisms are too feminine, for example, is subject to disparagement and ridicule and experiences shame. During adolescence, physical appearance, conflict about masculine or feminine identity, poor achievement in school, and negative comparisons with peers may all provoke shame. The adolescent who is sick may bring his shame and his search for sexual identity with him. The individual in the middle years and old age may experience shame for what has not been accomplished and for social uselessness.[18]

The cause and feelings of shame may be known only to the person experiencing this reaction, but usually other people are part of the experience of being shamed. Anxiety is present when one is alone, while others are included in social threat and fear of ridicule. Lack of privacy in the hospital forces the patient to deal with the threat of social disapproval. Shame and embarrassment may result.

Two methods of handling shame situations are avoidance and correction. Individuals will conceal parts of themselves that they think are unacceptable, conform socially, and keep away from "loaded" topics. Correction may take the form of maintaining a facade, denying that one is shamed, anger, or joking.[19]

Shame and sex seem to be closely associated. The intimacy and emotional character of the sexual relationship make it a fertile ground for shame. The use of privacy for sexual intercourse gives testimony to its intimate and self-revealing character.[20]

Illness and/or hospitalization that threaten sexuality may be shame provoking. Shame-provoking situations include venereal disease; illegitimate pregnancy; lack of privacy and exposure of the body during procedures, the need to be dependent when the sexual identity is based on independence and self-sufficiency; bodily changes in adolescence and aging; disease or treatment that changes body image, especially that which disfigures the appearance and secondary sex organs; loss of control of bodily functions, especially bowel and bladder control; and loss of sexual function itself.[21]

Guilt. Guilt is closely allied to shame, overlapping rather than identical emotions. Guilt is the feeling related to transgression of a specific code of ethical, moral, and religious standards, while shame can result from actions not related to these codes.[22]

The experience of guilt is unlearned, but there seem to be some innate activators for guilt. In addition to these innate factors, family and religious institutions concerned with human ethics and morals prescribe standards of conduct and teach them to growing children. These moral and ethical principles are the cognitive part of conscience. They are joined with emotions in the mature conscience to form the structures that direct moral and ethical behavior. If these standards of conduct are breached, guilt may ensue. Since guilt is associated with different moral, religious, and ethical views, the causes vary from individual to individual, from group to group. Some people may feel guilty about masturbation, others may not. Some may feel guilty about premarital sex, others feel guilty because they do not satisfy their sexual partner, in or out of marital union.

Guilt is not necessarily dependent on the patient's belief in a written or explicit moral, ethical, or religious code. The codes may be implicit and accepted on the intuitive level. There is a strong relationship between one's sense of personal responsibility and guilt, while shame is frequently caused by the actions of others.

There are many causes of guilt and consequences of guilt, and these vary from individual to individual, culture to culture. There are some spheres, however, in which misconduct and guilt are virtually pancultural. Violation of strictly held sexual taboos elicit guilt in almost all cultures that have some moral and ethical standards relating to sexual acts. For this reason, guilt is probably more prevalent within this area of feeling, thought, and action than others.[23]

The development of guilt can be conceptualized from a religious, psychoanalytic, existential, or learning theory perspective. Most of these theories associate punishment or threat of punishment in some form with guilt. Learning theorists closely link guilt with the use of punishment. Guilt develops as a part of the learning process. As children are rewarded for doing things that are good and punished for doing things that are bad or wrong, they gradually develop their own sense of proper or improper behavior.

Guilt is internalized by various types of social learning. Parental attitudes play an important role. A warm, accepting relationship with a parent figure is the best background for the development of a healthy conscience and an appropriate guilt threshold.[24]

The experience of guilt consists of the gnawing feeling that one is "in the wrong." .Distress and fear accompany this feeling along with a high degree of tension, moderate impulsiveness, and relatively little self-assurance. However, guilt has positive aspects. It compliments shame in fostering social responsibility and serves as a check on sexual exploitation. The development of guilt and conscience fosters growth toward greater psychologic maturity. However, if there is an overdeveloped conscience or if guilt is experienced too easily, serious adjustment problems or psychopathology can result.[25]

The close association of guilt with punishment may explain why some individuals may view their illness as a punishment for recent or past sexual practices that have aroused guilt. Masturbation, homosexual experience, sexual practices such as oral–genital stimulation, etc. may all stimulate guilt if individuals believe they violate their moral or ethical code (see Chapter 9). Other persons who feel that illness is punishment for wrong-doing may try to pretend health rather than appear with the stigma of immorality.[26]

Guilt and sexual behavior has been investigated. On the basis of studies of guilt of college students after visualizing pictures of sexual intercourse, Izard reports that in the case of females, the more sexually experienced they were, the less guilt was evoked. The males who had only one or very few sexual experiences reported more guilt than did men who were virgins or men who were sexually more experienced. The data seem to indicate that for males, the period when first obtaining a sexual experience is likely to be more guilt laden than periods of virginity or sexual sophistication.

Using the Mosher Forced Choice Guilt Scale and the Heterosexual Behavior Assessment Scale, Di Vasto[27] found that guilt and sexual behavior were highly correlated and that guilt was important as a detriment of heterosexual behavior. Guilt also increased as age increased.

Sexual standards also affected guilt. Those who reported they did not believe in premarital intercourse reported greater guilt as a result of visualizing intercourse than did individuals who accepted premarital coitus. In general, the more liberal the participants' sexual attitudes as measured by a sexual standards scale, the less guilt they felt when they visualized sexual intercourse.[28]

Body Image Disturbance. Body image disturbance is a frequent result of illness, therapy, and even the diagnostic procedures that accompany illness. Patients come with their ideas of their body, their own unique way of perceiving their physical self. As seen in Chapter 7, these perceptions are closely related to the personality, the level of self-esteem and of self-identity. During illness, different messages are sent about the body. The individuals interpret and may accept and integrate the message into the body image.

Individuals' response to change in body image is determined by their personal, psychologic, and social interpretation of the disturbance, which may be loss of control,[29] a change in appearance, in function or a loss of a major and valued body part.[30] Loss of body parts and functions that contribute to sexual self-esteem and identity are particularly devastating because of the high psychic investment in these areas. Consequently, diseases and treatments of the genital organs, either external or internal, can be especially difficult to accept and to integrate into the self-concept in a positive way. This is not to limit problem areas to the genital zones. Since changes are interpreted individually, a change in any body part or function may be interpreted as a threat to sexual self-esteem.[31] Because body image changes represent a threat to identity the patient feels "different" than before and may feel that he or she is less of a man or woman.

The nature of the threat perceived by the individual is related to the stage of development of body image. For a young child, a disfiguring illness would not be such a threat to sexual self-esteem and identity as one that would immobilize or take away self-mastery. Adolescents can be devastated by disfigurement, because they are concerned with attractiveness and normality. In adults, threat to body image may be balanced by satisfactions attained in intellectual, spiritual, and social spheres.

One's pattern of adaptation to the environment also plays a role in the perception of the threat. It is more severe if patterns of adaptation are severely interrupted. Thus, the woman who believes that menstruation helps keep the body clean will be more threatened by a hysterectomy than one who does not share this belief.

The extent or degree of change and the rapidity of the change also influence the degree of threat.[32] A woman who has a small benign tumor removed from her breast will usually suffer much less threat than a woman who discovers a "lump," is quickly admitted to the hospital, and has a radical mastectomy.

The value individuals place on the body part or function also influences perceived threat. The breast in American culture, for example, is viewed as an important sexual accessory with erotic meaning beyond its use to provide nourishment to infants. Psychologic responses of individuals to loss of a valued part may include denial, depression, anxiety, and especially shame. Just as with any loss, mourning and grief work must take place. Any of these responses may compromise sexual function.

Sociocultural Factors

Inability to carry out the usual sexual role activities as a consequence of illness and/or hospitalization may result in decreased self-esteem. Sexual role behavior has been described in earlier chapters. It can be considered to have two major components, either or both of which may be compromised: (1) the usual behavior of individuals to obtain the amount and type of sexual satisfaction they need—this may be through hetero- or homosexual activities, masturbation, etc.; (2) other behaviors and the activities that individuals consider an integral part of their sexual identity, for example, breadwinner, homemaker, decision maker, father, mother, lover. Since individuals define and carry out their roles in their own way, these components may differ both between and within the two sexes.

Biologic and psychologic effects of illness may require individuals to change their usual type and amount of sexual activity temporarily or permanently. They may also be unable to carry out other essential aspects of their sexual role. Both aspects of role are interrelated, and one affects the other. The man whose illness takes away his ability to make decisions may develop sexual dysfunction if decision making is an integral part of his masculinity, while the man who becomes impotent because of illness may feel he is also less capable of carrying out his other roles.

Hospitalization may further compromise role performance. Even if pathology has not compromised sexual capabilities, the expectation is that sexual activity is to be suspended in the inpatient setting. Other aspects of the sick role are not always spelled out, but the usual expectation is that the patient be cooperative and nonquestioning. Patients themselves may be concerned with proper behavior and the results of improper demands. They are aware of their dependency on hospital personnel for care and desire to conform.[33] (See Chapter 8 for discussion of sexual role.) The sexuality of males whose concept of their sexual role involves independent decision making and authority over women may be threatened by the female-dominated structure and environment of the hospital division. To certain men, masculinity depends on being active and on ignoring physical discomfort; passivity is equated with femininity. Yet illness may demand passivity, rest, and care by others to meet intimate needs.

Individuals from different cultures and subcultures have additional burdens, since they may have far different beliefs and practices associated with illness and sexual roles than those of the largely middle class health professionals. Leininger[34] stresses the importance of transcultural nursing.

Nowhere in the world is there the diversity of cultural groups with their values, beliefs, and life styles as in the United States. Yet nurses tend to be ethnocentric in their approach; that is, they have a tendency to believe that their own beliefs, values, and life styles are better or more desirable than the life styles of others. Nowhere is this more true

than in the area of sexuality. Cultural shock (being stunned by what one sees) and cultural conflict (between the different set of rules of nurse and patient/client) may make the nurse critical of the patients'/clients' behavior. Nurses may impose their own views and values on the individual or the group (cultural imposition).[35]

These terms can be illustrated by the following situation. A young Appalachian woman who had two children in close succession informed the nurse that she believed that God had "put a certain number of babies" in her and that it was wrong to use any methods to prevent conception (cultural belief). The young nurse of middle class background who believed in women's control of their bodies and the importance of planned and adequately spaced children was dismayed by this idea (cultural shock). She decided that she would still teach about and urge the use of contraceptives for the woman's "best interests" (cultural imposition).

Unfortunately, little investigation has centered on sexual beliefs of European subcultures. Information is available about other cultural groups, although much more research is needed.

Mexican Americans. Mexican American males are extremely embarrassed if a female nurse asks them to undress or give a urine specimen. Since these requests are considered a threat to their masculinity and self-esteem, they will not comply. The women will undress, but the husband does not leave the room during an obstetric or urologic examination, since his role is to preserve her modesty. They usually look for a Catholic physician for prenatal care, and some will avoid care if one is not available.

They are very modest and may be especially embarrassed about venereal disease. They have more difficulty talking about it with dignity because of the language barrier.[36]

The family and their religion are very important. Few decisions are made without the husband, so problems result if the wife as a mother is asked to make a decision about practices such as birth control.[37] The cultural expectation is that girls should not obtain as high an educational level as boys. Adolescent girls receive less attention and few of the educational rewards. The conflicts they suffer may be seen in the form of obesity, anxiety, and sexual delinquency.[38]

The Chicano (Mexican-American) culture emphasizes that a male should never touch a strange woman's body, especially in the presence of another female; therefore, a male nurse should not care for the female patient. The body is "private," somewhat sacred, and should not be exposed.[39] The family comes first (the self second) and is usually a patriarchy. Few decisions are made without the husband so there may be problems if the wife is asked to make a decision about health care.[40]

Puerto Ricans. The Puerto Rican family is often matriarchal, large, and home related. When members move to the mainland, the wife may have to work in order for the family to survive, and the father leaves the family. Religion also plays a major role in their lives.[41]

American Indians. The American Indian values privacy, which is very important for some of their "illness" ceremonies. Religion and medicine are intimately mixed, religious beliefs being the most dominant factor influencing health care practice.[42] Lack of eye contact may be a sign of shame or guilt in some cultures, but the American Indian believes that when one looks into another's eyes one looks into the private soul and may take the soul away. Consequently, direct eye contact is avoided.[43]

The Navajo patient rarely makes a decision without consulting all family members. Modesty is very important, so permission to give a bath or even comb hair is obtained. Undressing before strangers is very discomforting.

The Navajo woman's role may include heavy work such as chopping wood and hauling water. When the patient's activity must be limited because of illness, instruction is given with the understanding that these activities are part of the life style and cannot be eliminated completely.[44]

Orientals. The oriental family is usually patriarchal, and the oriental husband may be the spokesman for his wife. They are extremely modest; the sexes are segregated in schools from childhood on.[45]

Blacks. The black family is not matriarchal as many may believe. The husband and wife work together. Children are valued, and usually there is a close relationship with parents.[46] A strong religious orientation is seen, and it has been important in the development, survival, and stability of the family.[47]

Appalachians. The Appalachians are identified as a subcultural group. The middle and upper classes share values and behavior similar to those of similar classes in the United States, but the poor and working classes may have different beliefs. The ethic of "neutrality" prevails among males and females. This ethic demands that one be nonassertive, nonaggressive, mind one's own business, and avoid direct eye contact, which is considered impolite. Consequently, nurses may feel the individual is shamed or guilty about something if they associate averted eyes with these responses.[48]

Although cultural factors are considered, nurses remember that each patient/client is an individual who may or may not conform to the culture's norms. Therefore, assessment, planning, and decisions for intervention are also made on an individual basis.

NURSING IMPLICATIONS

Decreased Sexual Self-concept (Self-esteem)

Assessment. Parameters of assessment to consider include the period in the life cycle, the marital status, and the presence and support of significant others. The occupation and interests are identified, since sexual identity and self-concept may rest heavily on ability to carry out usual tasks and roles. Any changes in role relationships, job situation, or ability to carry out activities of daily living are noted. The nature of the relationship with significant others—supportive, loving, hostile, punitive, minimal—has significance, since the nature of the support given by them can enhance or damage sexual self-concept.

The disease or surgical procedures are part of the data base. Pathology related to the skin, face, breast, genitalia, and internal sex organs are particularly assaultive on sexual integrity.

Conversational cues and behavior can provide significant data. Is the patient/client preoccupied with personal appearance, constantly looking in the mirror, questioning about attractiveness? Does the patient make statements indicating decreased self-worth, "I'm not good for anything, anymore," "Things have changed with me"? Comments about the sexual partner's disinterest or perceived disinterest may punctuate the conversation, "My husband sure can't be interested in an 'old hag' like me," was one patient's comment; "My boyfriend doesn't visit much, but I can understand," "After this surgery I'm all used up—no one will be interested in me," were another patient's comments.

Acting out or aggressive sexual behavior may be a sign of decreased sexual self-worth and the anxiety that accompanies it (see Chapter 14).

The nursing history is essential to provide necessary subjective data related to sexuality, expecially the patient's perception of how he/she may be affected sexually and of any changes in sexual function that have already taken place in the past. Are they already having potency or orgasmic problems or do they anticipate problems? If problems already exist additional data should be obtained (see Chapter 10).

Planning. The nurse's goal is to promote patients' sexual integrity, the feelings of worth as sexual beings, by increasing ability to carry out usual sexual role activities, and by helping them see themselves as valued sexual beings.

Intervention. Anticipatory intervention before certain surgery or therapies can at least decrease threat to sexual self-esteem based on misconceptions and myths. The effects of any therapy on sexual functioning is carefully explained. (See Unit V.) Of equal, if not greater, importance is allowing individuals to vent their feelings about what has happened to them and/or what they expect to happen in relation to their sexuality.

Nurses help the individuals maintain personal appearance. The female patient/client will experience fewer feelings of worthlessness if she is helped to apply cosmetics, if her hair is clean and done in her favorite style, and if she is encouraged to dress in clothes that make her feel attractive. The same meticulous personal care is needed by the male patient/client—a shave every day, pajamas instead of a hospital gown.

Nurses explain to the significant others the importance of attention, realistic compliments about appearance, and the expressions of affection that show the individual that he/she is still loved and wanted. Nurses, too, make positive comments about the patient's appearance and behavior, while accepting and intervening to decrease negative behavior such as tears, anger, and sexual acting out (see Chapter 14). Tender, loving care is never more vital.

As soon as appropriate, individuals should assume their usual role functions, whether they be decision making, household tasks, or the usual activities that are supportive of other family members. In their desire to protect the patient, the significant others may avoid talking about "little" problems. The patient is suddenly cut off from the satisfactions of counseling and giving attention to the loved ones.

Return to a job or the ability to pursue

accustomed hobbies and interests, especially for individuals who associate their masculinity or femininity with these activities, should be facilitated as soon as possible. If the illness makes this an impossibility, substitutes are found. The social worker or vocational counselor may help in these areas.

Individuals who suffer extreme negative self-concept may need definitive sex therapy (see Chapter 12). However, many individuals with reversible health limitations and with previous positive sexual self-concepts and relationships can maintain or regain sexual self-worth through the understanding and intervention of the nurses who care for them.

Privacy

Assessment. The nurse must be aware of the function of privacy for the individual. Is the patient from a large, extended family and used to noise and activity suddenly placed in a private room? Age is also considered. A 5-year-old child will more readily share information about himself than an adolescent who is struggling for sexual autonomy and who may have many conflicts and concerns.

What is the cultural background of the patient? Does the individual come from a background that considers some information personal and private? Is modesty an important concept? Religious beliefs may cause some individuals to feel that sexual topics are not appropriate for discussion.

Verbal and nonverbal clues indicate the patient/client wants to be left alone. Turning the face to the wall, glancing away frequently, drawing away, or frequent changes in subject may indicate the individual desires privacy in relation to a certain area. This behavior may occur during the interview or during a physical assessment.

Nurses clarify patients' statements that request privacy. A patient who says "I'll tell you but don't tell someone else," may be requesting privacy or may mean "How much do you share with others?" Is the setting conducive to privacy, or are there many people around, are doors and curtains open?

Interviewing to obtain information of a sexual nature requires tact and the ability to be an empathic listener. Probing and penetrating questions may require patients/clients to reveal more than they desire. Sensitivity of the nurses helps them respect the individual's privacy and at the same time interview therapeutically (see Chapter 10).

Planning. The sociocultural background of the individual, the nature of the illness, the amount of time needed with the patient, the environment, and the importance of the information needed should all be considered when privacy must be invaded. The nurse's goal is to minimize the experiences of threat, anxiety, and hostility that may accompany invasion of privacy.

Intervention. A private room may be necessary to preserve the privacy of patients and to preserve their worth and dignity. Patients with venereal disease may avoid invasions of privacy by isolating themselves. Going into a patient's/client's home unannounced may be considered an invasion of privacy, as is neglecting to knock on the hospitalized patient's door before entering.

If the patient needs the emotional release of sexual activity, the nurse provides privacy by closing the door, pulling the curtains, and insuring that there will be no interruptions by others.[49]

Self-evaluation, especially necessary when illness and altered body image affect perception of the sexual self, can be facilitated by allowing the patient uninterrupted time to think, yet nurses must be sensitive to times when the patients' needs to solve problems or ventilate requires their presence.[50]

At times, information given by the patient must be communicated to others responsible for the individual's care. When the patient attempts to extract a promise from the nurse not to tell, the nurse indicates that he/she cannot make that promise, especially if harm may come to the individual or others because information is not shared. The patient/client then has the option of sharing or not.

Shame

Assessment. The subjective experience of shame may be described by individuals as a sudden feeling of anxiety or painful self-consciousness. They may say they felt like hiding, or running away. Self-blame and self-derogation may be voiced along with statements such as "I was so embarrassed," "I was so ashamed," or "I was humiliated."

Body actions that are characteristic of anxiety may be observed. There may also be partial or complete withdrawal from visual contact by lowering the head, avoiding eye contact, or glancing up furtively. Blushing, flushing, or blanching of the skin may occur along with nervous gestures such as playing with hands or hair, twisting fingers, tremors, hesitating or subservient manner, tense muscles, and weak knees. There may be difficulty with speech, stuttering, a soft voice, high-pitched or low-pitched (or weakening) voice, dryness of the mouth, difficulty speaking, or incoherent speech.[51]

Adults may be able to shorten the response, while the individual who is chronically shamed may look bowed down and humble. Shame may be disguised by the opposite posture—head tilted back, chin out—while embarrassed laughter or anger may cover up the feeling. Playing with the mouth, covering the lower face to hide a quivering lip, cigarette smoking, or the cocktail glass may be used to handle shame reactions.[52]

Nurses also consider an individual's cultural background in identifying shaming experience, since the patient may be embarrassed by questions considered routine by the nurse. The nurse should be aware especially of nursing situations that may precipitate shame and assess the individual's response. Such events include what may be called "modesty" situations, such as bath, or the lack of privacy and the exposure of body, especially the genital areas during enemas, catheterization, or obstetric and gynecologic situations. Venereal disease and genitourinary conditions may also be shaming. Body changes, especially those of adolescence and those of the aging processes, may cause shame, especially when they threaten the individual's sexuality.

Planning. Nurses try to avoid causing shame. If shaming situations are inevitable the nurse considers the patient's sociocultural background and identifies ways to maintain sexual self-esteem. Prevention or minimizing shaming situations are her/his goals.

Intervention. The dignity and self-esteem of the individual is maintained when shaming experiences are avoided. Common courtesies, such as knocking on the door, providing a robe for the patient, minimizing exposure during the physical examination and nursing procedures, or calling the individual by name, may all prevent shame. Regaining control over body functions increases self-esteem and decreases shame, so the nurse gives expert physical care, encourages decision making and independence by the patient, and teaches self-help activities.

Nurses also teach parents the importance of avoiding shaming the child or adolescent by ridiculing his/her behavior, appearance, or lack of skill, especially in relation to others of their sex. "Other little boys can ride a bike, you can too," may cause shame and decreased feelings of sexual self-worth.

Talking about the shaming experience can defuse some of the anxiety. When nurses recognize that individuals are experiencing shame, they encourage them to acknowledge it, and then explore the reasons for the shame and the ways in which the patient feels inadequate or humiliated. In what ways did the patient fall short of his ego ideal and what is to be done about it? If a goal was involved, is it still desirable or reasonable? What steps can be taken to meet it? If the goal was inappropriate, the nurse helps the individual set other goals.[53]

Nurses apologize for shaming behavior that was caused by them or other staff members and try to make sure such behavior does not happen in the future. Team conferences may be necessary at times when staff become nonchalant about care and cause shaming experiences.

Evaluation. The patient's/client's decreased signs of anxiety and a more relaxed comfortable posture indicate that the nurse has minimized or corrected a shaming situation. Since prevention is the major goal, constant self-evaluation by the nurse and other staff members of their own conduct and behavior that may result in shame is necessary. It is easy to become nonchalant in the approach to patients/clients. Vigilance of nurses with regard to their behavior is essential.

Guilt

Assessment. As with shame, patients experiencing guilt may hang their head lower, avert their face, and take quick glances at other people. Eye-to-eye contact may be avoided. However, guilt may be distinguished from shame by two characteristics. The individual's face takes on a heavy look in intense guilt, while a blushed face (blushing) is more likely with shame. In addition, guilt affects the individual's demeanor longer than does shame.

Guilt-inducing events should be identified. These include pregnancy out of wedlock, venereal disease, abortion, masturbatory practices, disease or surgery of the genital organs, and homosexual or heterosexual experiences or practices. However, any experience that violates the individual's code of ethics may produce guilt. Consequently, nurses identify the individual's religious preferences and then determine if the individual puts high reliance on the religious beliefs and practices as a part of life, since much guilt results from transgressions of moral and religious codes of behavior.

The patient may express guilt openly to the nurse with whom there is a trust relationship, or she/he may express it covertly by expressing negative comments about events of the past life, "What did I do to deserve this?" "I should have been a better person!"

Conversation may be past instead of future oriented, a "Why did I do it?" focus.

The attitude and support of significant others should be assessed. Are they punitive and hostile, giving little understanding or positive support? Patients/clients may view their own behavior as causing this alienation of loved ones and may blame themselves.

Planning. The nurse analyzes the interrelationship of past events, religious beliefs, support of significant others, and the individual's feelings and knowledge about sexuality and sexual functioning. The nurse's goals are to increase the patient/client's spiritual and psychologic comfort by allowing discussion of guilt feelings, clarifying and correcting information about the causes of the illness, and by obtaining appropriate sources of spiritual or psychologic help for the individual.

Intervention. A frequent response of nurses to expression of guilt is "It wasn't your fault," "It couldn't be helped," "Everyone does it." The nurses act on their value judgment of the situation, identifying the "rightness or wrongness" on the basis of their beliefs. This inappropriate reassurance blocks communication and prevents the individual from ventilating feelings. Acting on the patient's perception, however, gives her/him the freedom to talk.

Some individuals may want to see a clergyman. If nothing is said, it is appropriate for the nurse to suggest that "I can get a priest (minister, rabbi) if you would like." Some individuals are hesitant to ask for a clergyman but are eager to discuss their feelings with one during a visit.

Teaching to correct myths and misconceptions about the cause of sexual and related problems may help allay some guilt feelings that are based on fallacious ideas about the cause of these disorders. However, if patients/clients believe that a sexual action of theirs was morally or ethically wrong, there is little teaching or reassurance that can be given by nurses that will eradicate the pangs of conscience. Other individuals, with scrupulous (overdeveloped) consciences or too low thresholds for guilt, will not respond to these approaches. Some may be helped by the intervention of their clergymen, while others with serious adjustment problems or psychopathology may need psychiatric help.

Evaluation. If goals are realistic, the patients will identify that they feel happier and can realistically describe their responsibilities in the etiology of life events while discussing the future in more optimistic terms. However, guilt is often not easily assuaged, so the nurse must constantly reevaluate interventions to identify not only if they are successful, but if outside help is needed.

Body Image

Assessment. Various objective behavior can be observed that indicates a body image disturbance. Absence of signs of anxiety, an unwillingness to acknowledge or discuss the loss, an unwillingness to accept help or care, and unwillingness to exhibit or look at the affected area may be signs of a body image disturbance. In more severe problems there may be depersonalization and intellectualization, the individual discussing the problem as apart from himself/herself.

The nature of the threat is assessed. Does the individual value beauty and wholeness and does adaptation to events depend on certain body organs? For example, if sexual organs are believed important for satisfactory life, their loss or disease provokes a greater threat than loss of other parts.

Age of the individual is considered because of differences in response at various age levels. The nurse also looks for signs that sexual roles are threatened or compromised.

The degree of support from significant others is assessed, since coping behaviors are enhanced by their concern and support. Of greatest importance is the nurse's assessment of the patient's perception of the situation. The "casual" patient is difficult to work with, since denial is usually operating.

Planning. The goals of intervention include decreasing threat and helping individuals feel accepted as worthy, loved, and wanted as sexual persons.

Intervention. Nurses help the individual acknowledge the loss and assist in the grief work. Grief and anger may need to be expressed. Encourage activities that support the individual's sexual self-esteem by providing meticulous personal care and the opportunity to make decisions.

The sexual partner must be helped to accept the change. Teaching to dispel misconceptions about the effect of the disease or therapy and encouraging expression of feelings will help individuals cope with the changes. Nurses can function to help the patient and significant others deal with concerns together by serving as intermediaries who facilitate expression of feelings and concerns.

By maintaining the modesty and privacy of patients, nurses show them that they are valued. Realistic compliments about appearance and behavior will focus attention on positive sexual characteristics. In addition, by providing opportunities for discussion of the changes, their meaning to the patient, and how he/she will compensate for the loss, the nurse facilitates adaptation to the altered body image.

Accepting the altered bodies or the changes in function by accepting the patients, the nurses serve as role models to them. For example, when nurses change a dressing on a breast incision carefully, without signs of aversion or distaste, the patient, seeing their acceptance, begins to accept herself.[54] Providing privacy so the patient can look at the altered body part or think about the internal changes gives the patient the opportunity to integrate the changes into an altered body image. By listening to what patients have to say, clarifying misconceptions about anatomy and physiology, and giving positive feedback nurses help patients gain positive perceptions of themselves as sexual beings.

Evaluation. Interventions have been effective if behavioral changes have occurred. Outcome criteria to be noted: (1) the patient expresses the intention to continue or begin sexual activity again, (2) the patient is relaxed and happy in interactions with the significant others, (3) the patient is able to look at the affected or altered part or is not unduly hesitant to talk about the changes that have occurred.

Sexual Dysfunction Related to Illness and Hospitalization

Assessment. The nurse collects information about marital status and significant others. Special note should be made of changes in body image or stressful life events and the presence of illness and therapy that have the potential for causing decreased potency in the male or orgasmic problems in the female or that pose threat to sexuality (see Unit V). The quality of interactions with significant others and changes in role relationships, job situation, etc. should be noted. Signs of anxiety, identified by Masters and Johnson as one of the major causes of sexual dysfunction, should be noted. Persistent questioning about the effects of illness may indicate problems. The nursing history, which contains questions about sexual function, may elicit the information that individuals have halted sexual activities or are impotent or nonorgasmic.

Persistent questioning about the effects of the illness, medication, or treatments may be a clue that the patient has problems, yet is too embarrassed to bring them out into the open. "What kinds of things does this medicine do to a fellow besides take down blood pressure?" was one patient's approach. Further discussion indicated he was experiencing potency problems as a side effect of the antihypertensive medication, and he felt he was "less of a man." "I hear you can't do all the things you used to do after a heart attack," may indicate the patient has concerns related to sexuality.

Concerns about changes in function and about role tasks may be more indirectly ver-

balized. The nurse follows up on subtle clues, since patients may hesitate to initiate the subject openly. If the nurse suspects a problem, a simple validating statement will often serve to open up the topic: "Have there been problems with your sex life (having satisfying sexual activity, getting sexual satisfaction, having sex, making love, or whatever words seem appropriate for the individual's age, sex, and sociocultural status)?"

If a trust relationship has not yet developed, the individual may say no, but later, remembering that the subject was not taboo to the nurse, will often bring up the concerns, fears, and problems. By asking the question, permission has been given to discuss these concerns.

Planning. The nurse's goal is to help the individual attain or maintain the level of sexual activity that is satisfying. If a change is necessary because of illness or other life events, the nurse helps the patient/client find alternate means of sexual expression or helps her/him accept the unchangeable. If other role activities are compromised, the nurse helps individuals make similar adjustment.

Intervention. The interventions appropriate for problems related to sexual self-worth also help alleviate problems of sexual function that are psychologic or sociocultural sequelae of illness. Since many individuals reduce coitus out of ignorance for fear that it may exacerbate symptoms, simple reassurance that sexual activity is permissible and that it should be resumed at the earliest possible moment consistent with health may be sufficient.[55]

In addition, the nurse teaches and counsels individuals about alternate means of obtaining sexual satisfaction after assessing any religious or other cultural beliefs and values that preclude any sexual activity different from what has been practiced. However, information such as different positions for intercourse, different times and places for sexual activity, or additional ways to stimulate the sexual response may be all that is needed to allay the problem (see Chapter 4). If no physiologic cause for dysfunction exists, simple reassurance that there is no physiologic abnormality plus a chance to discuss concerns may decrease anxiety, resulting in return of sexual response. The nurse with special training may engage in definitive counseling and sexual therapies (see Chapter 12). Other patients are referred for help.

If nurses anticipate the patient's concerns early in the onset of any illness or life event that has the potential for compromising sexuality the problems may be prevented.[56] (Interventions for specific illness and life events that may compromise sexuality are given in Units III, IV, and V.)

Evaluation. Behavioral signs that the nurse's goals were met include expressions of satisfaction with sexual activity by the patient/client, a resumption of role activities or substitute activities that the individual states are satisfying, and positive interactions with significant others.

NOTES

1. Littlefield V: The surgical patient's sexuality. AORN J 26:649–658, 1977
2. Alexander C: Nurses ignore the importance of sexuality in OR. AORN J 23:743–746, 1976
3. Tyler EA: Sex and medical illness. In Sadock BJ, Kaplan HI, Freedman AM (eds): The Sexual Experience. Baltimore, Williams and Wilkins, 1976, pp. 313–317
4. Ibid, p 314
5. Schuster E: Privacy, the patient and hospitalization. Soc Sci Med 10:245–248, 1978
6. Bloch D: Privacy. In Carlson CE (ed): Behavioral Concepts and Nursing Intervention. Philadelphia. Lippincott, 1970, pp 251–267
7. Schuster E: Privacy, the patient and hospitalization. Soc Sci Med 10:248, 1978
8. Ibid, p 253
9. Ibid, p 254
10. Hall ET: The Hidden Dimension. New York, Doubleday, 1966
11. Allekian CI: Intrusions of territory and personal space. Nurs Res 22:236–241, 1973
12. Meisenhelder JB: Boundaries of personal space. Image XIV:16–19, 1982
13. Webster's Third New International Dictionary, Springfield, Massachusetts, Merriam, 1965
14. Lange S: Shame. In Carlson CE (ed): Behavioral Concepts and Nursing Intervention. Philadelphia, Lippincott, 1970, pp. 67–91
15. Ibid, p 74
16. Ibid, p 75
17. Ibid, p 76
18. Ibid, pp 77–78
19. Ibid, p 83
20. Izard CE: Human Emotions. New York, Plenum, 1977, p. 411
21. Lange S: Shame. In Carlson CE (ed): Behavioral Concepts and Nursing Intervention. Philadelphia, Lippincott, 1970, p. 85
22. Izard CE: Human Emotions. New York, Plenum, 1977, p. 92
23. Ibid, p 424
24. Ibid, pp. 429–437
25. Ibid, p 451
26. Lederer HD: How the sick view their world. In Skipper JK Jr, Leonard RC (eds): Social Interaction and Patient Care. Philadelphia, Lippincott, 1965, pp 155–166
27. DiVasto PV, Pathak D, Fishburn WR: The interrelationship of sex guilt, sex behavior and age in an adult sample. Arch Sex Behav 10:119–141, 1981
28. Izard CE: Human Emotions. New York, Plenum, 1977, pp 445–450
29. Weinberg JS: Human sexuality and spinal cord injury. Nurs Clin North Am 17:407–419, 1982
30. Rubin R: Body image and self-esteem. Nurs Outlook 16(6):21–23, 1968
31. Kneisl CR: Body image, its meaning to self. J NY Nurses Assoc 2:29–35, 1971

32. Morris CM: The professional nurse and body image. In Carlson CE (ed): Behavioral Concepts and Nursing Intervention. Philadelphia, Lippincott, 1970, pp. 39–61

33. Tagliacozzo DL: The nurse from the patient's point of view. In Skipper JK, Leonard RC (eds): Social Interaction and Patient Care. Philadelphia, Lippincott, 1965, pp 219–227

34. Leininger M: Cultural diversities of health and nursing care. Nurs Clin North Am 21:5–18, 1977

35. Ibid, p 13

36. Lurie HJ, Lawrence GL: Communication problems between rural Mexican American patients and their physician. Am J Orthopsychiatry 42:777–783, 1972

37. White EH: Giving health care to minority patients. Nurs Clin North AM 12:27–39, 1977

38. Lurie HJ, Lawrence GL: Communication problems between rural Mexican American patients and their physician. Am J Orthopsychiatry 42:781, 1972

39. Leininger M: Cultural diversities of health and nursing care. Nurs Clin North Am 21:14, 1977

40. White EH: Giving health care to minority patients. Nurs Clin North Am 12:32, 1977

41. Ibid, p 34

42. Bullough VL, Bullough B: Health Care for the Other Americans. Norwalk, Appleton-Century-Crofts, 1982

43. Primeau M: Caring for the American Indian. Am J Nurs 77(1):91–94, 1977

44. Kniep-Hardy M, Burkhardt MA: Nursing and the Navajo. Am J Nurs 77(1):95–96, 1977

45. Chung HJ: Understanding the oriental maternity patient. Nurs Clin North Am 12:67–75, 1977

46. White EH: Giving health care to minority patients.. Nurs Clin North Am 12:29, 1977

47. Ibid, p 30

48. Tripp-Reimer T, Friedl MC: Appalachians: A neglected minority. Nurs Clin North Am 12:67–75, 1977

49. Bloch D: Privacy. In Carlson CE (ed): Behavioral Concepts and Nursing Intervention. Philadelphia, Lippincott, 1970, p 260

50. Ibid, p 262

51. Lange S: Shame. In Carlson CE (ed): Behavioral Concepts and Nursing Intervention. Philadelphia, Lippincott, 1970, p 73

52. Ibid, p 73

53. Ibid, p 84

54. McCloskey JC: How to make the most of body image theory. Nursing 76(6):68–72, 1976

55. American Medical Association Committee on Human Sexuality: Human Sexuality. Chicago, American Medical Association, 1972, p 127

56. Jacobson L: Illness and human sexuality. Nurs Outlook 21(1):50–53, 1974

Chapter 14

Sexual Behavior of Patients/Clients: Relationship to Nursing Care

Chapter 2 focused on the roles of nurses in relation to sexuality, emphasizing that nurses must be knowledgeable about and comfortable with the topic of sexuality and with their own sexuality. The culturally and professionally ascribed "laying on of hands" gives tacit permission to touch patients'/clients' bodies for therapeutic ends but with the implicit understanding that this is done in a "pure" and asexual sense. Nurses' white uniforms may be considered the explicit badge of their purity.

Sexual reactions from nursing contact are presumably not experienced by either party. Problems arise when the patients' behavior does not conform to nurses' expectations of sexual propriety or when nurses do not use their sexuality in a way that is therapeutic for their patients/clients. In either case, the quality of care suffers, while anxiety, guilt, and/or hostility may be experienced by all. Nurses may also hold some of the same misconceptions about sexuality and sexual expression that society has and usually acts upon. This may make it difficult for nurses to cope with sexual behavior and to intervene therapeutically.

The focus of this chapter is on the sexual behaviors of patients/clients and of nurses that are particularly problematic for nurses: aggressive or "acting out" sexual behavior by patients/clients, sexual attraction of the nurse to the patient, sexual activity with a partner and masturbation by patients in the care setting, homosexual patients/clients and their care, and other sexual problem areas such as "finishing the bath" and responding appropriately when the male patient has an erection.

Basic to nursing is the "laying on of hands"; touch may be used to help heal and to comfort. Because touch may cause discomfort for some nurses, the chapter begins with a discussion of this concept.

CONCEPT OF TOUCH

No matter what the explicit purpose of touch, implicitly it is a form of nonverbal communication. In primitive societies, it was precursor of speech, and it was associated with such benign activities as healing and magic. In later societies, touching became taboo, and society provided chaperones who maintained the distance between couples so that inappropriate touching would not occur.

Touch has an important reaching out function. Some types of touch are easily understood—a pat on the back, a handshake—while other types are poorly understood or may be misperceived.[1] Touch is essential for the development of individuals. The physical contact between mother and children fosters love, closeness, and security. Through it, the infant experiences pleasure, while the withdrawal of touch, the withholding of contact, is perceived as threat or a punishment. Prolonged withholding of touch early in life may result in loss of contact with reality and feelings of helplessness. Research in the behavior of monkeys demonstrated that when deprived of maternal care, the monkeys preferred mothers made of cloth and wire to no mother at all.

Children become aware of social taboos associated with touch through subtle social instruction. The social taboos against touching the genitals of self and others is often most forcefully communicated to them by parents and significant others. Touch, a means of communication at the most intimate and primitive level, is now restricted by the boundaries of social acceptability.[2]

Touch can communicate love and closeness and reduce physical and interpersonal distance, but it can be misperceived as a threat when none was intended unless the meaning is mutually understood. Individuals who have to assume the patient's role during illness accept without significant distress greater physical contact and more intrusion on their personal space than they would ordinarily tolerate. Given earlier prohibitions, however, nurses may experience considerable intrapersonal discomfort with touch, especially if touch involves care of the genitals of *either* sex. In addition, the nurse may fear that the patient ascribes sexual meanings to the interventions when none is intended.

Sociocultural backgrounds of the patients and nurses also affect attitudes toward physical contact. Some nurses and some patients/clients come from family backgrounds where embracing, touching, and holding are accepted as open and natural expressions of affection, while for others, these behaviors are reserved for the most intimate sexual contact.[3] Consequently, either nurses or patients may interpret a gesture as a sexual overture when none was intended, especially when there is lack of congruency in the meaning attached to these gestures by both parties.

Assessment

Assessment is made of how patients/clients use touch. Is reaching out in a physical sense part of their usual patterns of behavior, or are they individuals who are uncomfortable with physical contact? Nurses learn to identify patient signals not to touch them—a withdrawing, a stiffening, or excuses that care is not needed now, is not necessary or has been completed, when indeed the opposite is true.

Nurses assess their level of comfort with touch and their response to patients who reach out to them. Do they see these gestures as a normal response to threatening situations such as illness; a search for comfort, nurture, or protection; or do they see these overtures as a threat to their sexuality?

Intervention

Interventions that involve touch should be purposeful. Since the meanings vary and the gesture is so significant to nurses and to patients, touch should be used discriminately; it should be helpful, and its purpose should be understood by patients/clients.[4] If the meaning of touch is misinterpreted, these misperceptions are clarified by the nurse.

Touch involves risk taking, yet it surpasses words when verbal ability to communicate is interrupted. It is inherent in nurses' roles as nurturer and comforter, a potential source of support for the individual in distress.

PROBLEMATIC AREAS FOR NURSES IN RELATION TO SEXUALITY

Aggressive Sexual Behavior

Perhaps no area causes more anxiety and hostility on the part of nurses than patient behavior that has sexual overtones. This behavior may range from what has been called "personal advances"[5] to aggressive or "acting out" sexual behavior. Personal advances may include asking for the nurses' first name, address, or telephone number; inquiring whether they have boyfriends or girlfriends; or asking for a date. Often the nurse is of the opposite sex but in some cases the same sex, which produces even greater anxiety and hostility if the nurse is heterosexual.

Nurses may feel the questions are inappropriate but may fear that "putting the patient in his/her place" would hurt the patient, so the nurse involved avoids the room, warns other nurses about the behavior, or asks others to care for the patient.

The motivations for the personal remarks are diverse. Patients may fear the outcome of the illness and flirt with the nurses to alleviate some of the feelings of helplessness and to convince themselves that they have not lost complete control of their lives.[6] Other patients may fear they will not get attention unless they assure the nurses that they are attractive. The opposite may be true for patients who are frightened by the physical closeness involved in care. They hope that annoyance generated by their advances will cause the staff to maintain their distance.

Another group may be adults who fight dependence, especially if they had difficulty obtaining maternal love and affection as children, learning that it was not appropriate to ask for love. The adult with such a mother may feel the need to be "mothered" but fights it and converts the longing into "amorousness" which is "adult" behavior and therefore acceptable.[7]

Acting out or aggressive sexual behavior causes even greater discomfort, anxiety, and hostility on the part of the nursing staff. Manifestations of this behavior include frequent seductive comment and jokes with sexual connotation, often accompanied by overt attempts to hold, fondle, or kiss parts of the nurse's body. Some patients may deliberately expose their genitals while being bathed,

using the urinal, or when lying in bed. The patients' conversations focus on past sexual conquests, interests, and activities.[8]

There may be several causes of this behavior. Positions of dependency, loss of self-sufficiency, fear of or actual loss of physical strength and attractiveness resulting from illness, or the resultant change in life style may threaten the patient's feeling of sexual adequacy.[9] The perceived threat causes anxiety. The aggressive sexual behavior is an attempt to counteract this anxiety, which may be so great that the patient regresses. The sexual behavior is not an expression of adult sexuality, but rather a reflection of narcissism and pregenital behavior.

Sexually oriented behavior may also be a means of denying the severity of the illness. It says, in effect, "I'm not sick, I can pursue my sexual inclinations." To other patients, the realization that they are not strong and self-sufficient threatens their sexual identity. Sexual aggressiveness may be a reaction to the need to be passive and dependent. By acting aggressively, the patient denies his passive longing.[10]

Some patients are able to relate heterosexually only with a great expenditure of energy to suppress homosexual needs. The nursing care can stimulate these homosexual feelings, causing great discomfort. In order to compensate, males may behave in a hypermasculine or females in a hyperfeminine manner in order to feel less threatened.[11]

Nurses are frequently shocked by any behavior suggesting sexual interest by the aged individual, even though they can handle sexual advances of younger persons. Older persons make sexual advances for the same reasons younger ones do. In addition, some of their behavior may be in response to nurse behavior. One nurse admitted she would give the patient a quick hug goodbye, but when he tried to kiss her, she was shocked. He was from a middle-class cultural background, was not used to open display of affection, and misinterpreted the nurse's behavior. In other cases, the nurse may interpret a simple request for care ("Live with me and take care of me") as an implicit sexual advance instead of the need for nurturance and care. Not all patients' remarks are meant in a sexual sense.[12]

Humor is sometimes used by staff to deal with the anxiety caused by this behavior and to detoxify it. Consequently, the staff responds to the patient's sexual jokes with jokes of their own. However, by staff failing to understand the dynamics that underlie the behavior, the patient is not helped to verbalize concerns and may indeed view the nurse's behavior as rejection. Nurses may also feel they have lost control of the situation, so they may avoid the issue, ignore the comments, change the subject, or leave the bedside.

Assessment. Assessment includes identifying what the patient is seeking by the behavior. Is the patient terribly frightened by everything that is happening and afraid that death is possible? Are dependency conflicts involved, or is the behavior a simple ploy for attention?

Nurses assess their own feelings and behavior and how they may have contributed to the situation. By introspection, nurses get in touch with their feelings, responses, and the reasons for them. Getting feedback from coworkers and discussing their feelings are helpful. Self-monitoring or assessment of own behavior is important since some nurses send messages that are seductive by posture, clothing, or voice level.[13]

Intervention. If nurses go along with the overt behavior or if they reject the behavior and the patient by suitable negative comments, the anxiety or concerns that underlie the behavior still exist. By helping the patient identify the meaning behind the behavior, the underlying feelings, concerns, and fear can be verbalized.

Whatever the unconscious motivation, the nurse uses confrontation to address the subject promptly when overt sexual advances continue, explaining that he/she understands that anyone hospitalized for a period of time has sexual needs and frustrations. In addition, clearly and unambiguously, the nurse goes on to define the relationship between the patient and the professional. In response to requests of a sexual nature, the nurse might reply "I understand the needs and frustrations of being in the hospital, but I can't act on your suggestions." The approach must be firm but in no way hostile or delivered in a manner that puts the patient down.[14]

Patients whose behavior seems to be related to fears of dependency should not be forced to bring painful memories to the fore. If they start to dwell on subjects that indicate discomfort with dependency, listen to the complaints, identify areas where the patient is not dependent, and then explore areas where independence can be retained or regained.

If the flirtatious comments seem to be attempts to bolster the patient's ego or, in the case of the male patient, seem to be a culturally conditioned response to someone of the opposite sex, the nurse can acknowledge the behavior by simple acceptance.

This does not mean that nurses have to tolerate behavior that makes them uncomfortable or that is not acceptable by their standards. Some limit setting may have to be done before any helping interaction can take place. The nurse explains to the patient that the behavior makes him/her uncomfortable and that it makes caring for the patient difficult, or impossible.

In addition, nurses then should ask if there is something that he/she might have done to cause the behavior. This takes a considerable amount of ego strength on the part of the nurse, since the patient may feel comfortable enough to describe the nurse's behavior, which communicated more than professional interest in the relationship. However, by the willingness to acknowledge the possibility that the patient was responding to his/her behavior, the nurse removes some of the guilt, shame, and onus of blame that the patient experiences.[15]

The nurse may help patients sublimate behavior into socially accepted channels such as drawing, performing, speaking, and reading.[16] Others may substitute fetishism for interpersonal relationships, that is, stimulation by nonsexual objects such as panties, bras, or objects handled by the opposite sex, combs, perfumes, etc. It is easier for nurses to accept if gratification is through sublimation rather than fetishism, but a variety of patient behavior can be expected.[17]

Some patients will not accept limits to their behavior, especially if these are imposed by members of the opposite sex. They may have lack of respect for members of the opposite sex or may have the need to "cut the authority figure down to size." These patients may try to proposition the female nurse to take her out of her professional role to prove that women are no good. It is very difficult to maintain a therapeutic relationship with these patients, and outside help may be needed, since the nursing care can be disrupted by the continued patient behavior. Staff must have the opportunity to verbalize their resultant anxiety and hostility. The fact that the patient behavior continues indicates the depth of his/her distress and that outside counseling is necessary.

Nurses have difficulty intervening, partly because they are uncomfortable talking about sexual matters. It is difficult to take the initiative, and the patient will rarely do so. In addition, there may be difficulty in communicating the problem to other professionals. Role playing various interventions is very helpful, since this behavior rehearsal allows the nurse to say the words in an interaction with a simulated patient before the actual intervention.

Sexual Attraction of Nurse to Patient

Nursing textbooks devote considerable space to the development of and the significance of the nurse–patient relationship indicating that a professional rather than a personal relationship is important for therapeutic care. It is usually the young student who

voices the concern, "But what if I like the patient and feel attracted to him/her? What if I want to go out with him/her?" For whatever the reason, patients do seek to have further contact with the nurses after discharge from the hospital, and nurses are attracted to the patients on a human-to-human level.

When nurses become involved in a sociosexual relationship, they recognize that it is difficult to be therapeutic in an objective way. Friendship is in its own way helpful. However, it usually precludes empathetic intervention, and it definitely makes physical care embarrassing for both parties, who closely identify with each other. Rather than feel guilty about the abdication of the professional role, it is better for nurses to acknowledge their feelings and allow other staff members to care for their patient.

Because of their own needs, nurses may consciously or unconsciously behave seductively toward patients. These nurses may be distressed because they are such frequent targets of patients' aggressive sexual behavior. Pointing out their actions (often based on culturally defined social norms for their sex) that encouraged these responses may be enough to alleviate the problem. Nurses who continually need to prove masculinity or femininity by sexual conquests present a more serious problem and may need counseling to become more secure in their sexual identity.

Sexual Activity in the Inpatient Setting

Hospitalization imposes constraints on sexual activity but some patients are able to ignore these constraints as well as the written and unwritten proscriptions against sexual behavior. When it occurs, staff may respond, at the least, with humorous comments and snickering remarks, or at most, with overt censure and admonition that the activity be discontinued. Yet illness and/or institutionalization are times when some individuals especially need the closeness, comfort, and love, as well as the relief of sexual tension that sexual activity can provide. If sexual behavior is a part of our life and our being, then nurses will make opportunities for patients/clients to express their sexuality. Provision of a private place free from interruption is essential. The time and place must be appropriate both for the individuals involved as well as for other patients.

Roommates of patients who are expressing even mild expressions of affection may be acutely uncomfortable and distressed, so that some limits have to be set by the nurses. This can be done by straightforwardly explaining to the patient and the sexual partner that the open display of affection is upsetting the roommate and that the staff will provide them with privacy of an assured length of time. With ingenuity the time and the place can be arranged.

Masturbation

Masturbation has no pathophysiologic consequences, but nurses may consider it immoral and an unnatural activity that is wrong for themselves and for their patients.

Masturbation in the hospital may serve a variety of functions. Brooks[18] feels that these functions should be considered pathologic if they enable the individual to avoid recognizing unmet needs and inhibit use of more acceptable methods to meet these needs. Masturbation may serve to relieve sexual tension for adolescents and adults. For others, it may serve to reduce anxiety and produce pleasurable feelings. However, it may also serve to drive others away and help the patient avoid forming relationships with individuals of the same or other sex. Patients/clients who are discovered masturbating may be faced with censure equal to, if not greater than, individuals who engage in mutual sexual activity. Whatever their own feelings about masturbation, nurses can provide the privacy the individual needs.

When nurses enter the room of a patient who is masturbating, they can withdraw if they are unnoticed. When individuals see them, nurses can simply say "Sorry I walked in at just that moment, I should have knocked first."[19] The nurse may also offer to close the door.

If the patient's/client's health permits leaving the hospital, a pass to return home for a day or two can give individuals the time and privacy for the sexual activity that is desired and needed.

The Homosexual Patient

When the homosexual individual is hospitalized or seeks medical care, special problems present. Nurses may have difficulty accepting homosexuals' sexual orientation and seeing their sexual behavior as a variant rather than a deviant form of behavior.[20] They may not recognize the depth, variety, and the meaning of the life style to the homosexual patient. Whether the nurse sees these life styles as moral or immoral, deviant or variant, these patients, as all patients, are entitled to competent and loving care.

Hospitalization is an unpleasant and frightening experience to all patients, but homosexual patients may lose the support of the individual most important to their lives. Legally, partners' names cannot be inscribed on the records, so they are not called in emergencies. Any sign of affection or expression of concern may be viewed with curiosity, derision, or hostility by staff. Patients who are open about their life style may be avoided by staff, who have difficulty dealing with their anxiety about homosexuality.

The loved one may be unable to obtain information about the patient. Lawrence[21] describes the stress at having to hide love instead of providing it, dampening feelings at a time when they need to be expressed and censoring what is said since it might offend. Being described as "queer" provokes anger. Feelings of helplessness and hopelessness prevail; homosexuals are often at the mercy of a staff who believe the relationship is abnormal and immoral and who act out these beliefs.

When homosexuals seek mental health

care for feelings of depression, grief, "marital" difficulties, psychosis, or anxiety reaction, they are usually faced with the interpretation that their personal problems are evidence of the pathology of homosexuality. Lawrence[22] states that this is as logical as equating divorce with faulty heterosexuality. Treatment focuses on "curing" the homosexuality, rather than helping with the problems.

Caring For the Homosexual. Nurses who are caring for homosexual individuals can accept and respect the life style and the relationship as at least a potentially healthy alternative to heterosexuality. The patient's/client's sex mate and close friends should be regarded as significant others and be allowed to be a part of the therapy.

Nurses assess their attitudes and prejudices. If the homosexual patients are considered worthwhile, as they are, this itself is therapeutic and will be communicated. If staff is anxious about caring for homosexual patients, group meetings to express feelings and to give support for those with anxiety about giving care can help.[23]

Nurses who are comfortable about homosexuality may be able to help the individual who has problems by just listening. The gay who is still "in the closet" pretends to be straight but spends many evenings with gay friends. This almost inevitably results in anxiety about exposure, loss of job, and disgrace. Indecision and coming to terms with the real world may be the primary source of anxiety. The nurse may be able to help the homosexual person sort out feelings and decide whether to be open about the life style.[24]

Nurses also remember that it is considered an intrusion in the homosexual individual's privacy to discuss sexual orientation with the family unless permission has been given to do so or unless the family already knows.[25]

Parents may turn to the nurse for advice, however, when they learn their child is homosexual. If it is a young child who may often experiment with different sexual behaviors and if no other problems exist, reassurance of the parents is usually all that is necessary. If it is an older adolescent or young adult, parents' attitudes or exhortations will not change the sexual orientation. The individual needs acceptance and support, not anger, criticism, and rejection, and acceptance of the situation does not indicate approval.[26] The nurse also teaches about homosexuality after first allowing parents to ventilate their fears and concerns.

The lesbian may fear visiting a gynecologist or a nurse for routine care or when physical difficulties such as dysmenorrhea, abnormal bleeding, or venereal disease occur. Spoken or unspoken censure may be more than she can face, so needed care is avoided.[27]

Lesbians experience the gamut of female disorders that are experienced by heterosexual women. Vaginitis may be caused by fingers or a vibrator, anal or oral sex, or by the use of intravaginal devices rather than a penis. Partners are also treated, and to prevent reinfection, the individuals are taught to scrub fingers and fingernails and the vibrator, if used, before sexual activity. Physicians may prescribe providone–iodine soap or other antibacterial agents.[28]

In addition to infection, mechanical devices may cause periurethral and vaginal lacerations if the woman inserts the device before turning it on. Suturing may occasionally be required, but usually hot Sitz baths, warm douches, and application of antibacterial medications are sufficient treatment.[29]

Gay agencies sponsor "gay health nights" when problems are treated and preventive health care is given. Not all the staff members of these agencies are homosexual, but they accept the gay life style. Homosexual nurses can be advocates, and the Gay Nurses Alliance is attempting to deal with problems related to care of homosexual persons.

Other Problem Areas

The Bath. "Finishing the bath" may be a source of anxiety for nurses and for patients. Most texts devoted to beginning nursing care emphasize the importance of privacy when doing the perineal care but give little specific instruction. Indoctrinated with prohibitions against touching or manipulating their own genitals, much less those of others, nurses are faced with perineal care of the incapacitated patient or with telling others to do so. Embarrassing but amusing incidents can occur. A novice nurse set up soap and water, instructed the patient to "finish your bath," and hurried from the room. When she returned in what seemed an appropriate length of time, he was busily washing his hair. Finding the right words may be difficult.

In giving appropriate instruction for genital care, the nurse takes into consideration the patient's cultural, educational, and social background to choose language that the patient understands. One patient might understand "wash your privates," your "crotch," or "wash between your legs."

The nurse's assessment should indicate whether the individual is physically or mentally able to carry out the task. Nurses' embarrassment or values may blind them to the care needed, so they neglect genital care, rationalizing that the patients prefer to do it themselves and are able to do it.

Nurses may be just as uncomfortable doing the perineal care of patients of their sex as those of opposite sex, given the cultural prohibition against touching the genitals. Patients may be embarrassed, especially if nurses are embarrassed. In addition, patients are distressed if they perceive they have to be cared for like infants. Sexual self-esteem can be damaged.

A matter-of-fact approach, knowledge of the procedure, firm competent movements, along with the explanation to the patient why good perineal hygiene is so important (i.e., to prevent bladder, vaginal infections, and genital excoriation) serves to defuse the anxiety and focus the nurse's and patient's attention away from psychosexual implications of the procedure.

This author disagrees vehemently with the use of cotton balls to do perineal care of the incapacitated patient, as is outlined by an often-suggested reference. Cleansing the perineum is done with a washcloth, soap, and water. For the nurse to do otherwise is to suggest that there is something different about the genitals. Cotton balls do little to expedite the procedure. Use of gloves by the nurse is not indicated unless the patient has an infection in the perineal area or if the nurse has broken areas on her hands or fingers.

Gloves serve to suggest that the perineal area is dirty, should be untouched, and is untouchable. One nursing textbook states that the nurse uses a washcloth or towel to hold the male patient's genitals while she washes the folds of the body with another washcloth. Instead of expediting the procedure, one wonders if the nurses might not become tangled in washcloths and towels and these efforts to prevent sexual stimulation may accomplish just that.

Male Erection. The unspoken and unwritten fear, one suspects, involved in doing perineal care of male patients is that they will have erections. Any sexual response by the female patient is more subtle and so less anxiety-provoking for the care giver.

Erection occurs when arterial blood rushes into the body of the penis and venous outflow is cut off. It can be a rapid process, taking only 5 to 10 seconds. Erections are of two types—psychic and reflex. Psychic erections occur when thoughts and emotions from erotic fantasies, stimulating literature, or seeing a potential partner originate in the brain and send impulses via the spinal cord to the penis. Reflex erections are stimulated by tactile stimulation of the penis or genital area, by a full bladder, or irritation of the glans.

Consequently, the male patient may have an erection irrespective of the "asexual" behavior of the nurses caring for him, either because of his own sexual feelings or because of a reflexive response. Psychic erections are less likely to occur when the nurse is matter-of-fact and objective about care. Anxiety is communicated interpersonally, and the flustered care giver who is focusing on the sociosexual consequences of genital manipulation will communicate this discomfort to the patient.

Since reflex erection can occur with stimulation, "finishing the bath" in theory can evoke this response. In practice, the vast majority of patients unable to complete perineal care are either so physically ill, have such a low level of consciousness, or are victims of such incapacitating nervous system disease that erections rarely occur.

When they do occur, both the nurse and patient are embarrassed. One suggestion has been that the nurse excuse herself/himself when the erection occurs and leave the bedside, promising to return later. This may serve to shame the patient further, although it is probably the best response if the nurse is completely nonplussed. Another approach is to ask the patient if he would like the nurse to leave and to come back later. Finally, acknowledging that the patient has had an erection (and this may be happy news for neurologic patients or for those who have much anxiety about the effect of illness on potency) and finishing the care matter-of-factly can be the best approach.

Patients' with early morning erections may be exceedingly embarrassed if a nurse is present. If the nurse gives the patient time to use the urinal or go to the bathroom before starting care, the situation can be avoided.

Inherent in the male or female nurse's anxiety that the male may have an erection during care is the belief that in some way or other what happens has negative moral implications. Some male nurses may be just as anxious because they fear homosexual implications. The male erection is neither immoral nor indicative of homosexuality. When those connotations are erased, much of the anxiety suffered by the staff will decrease.

USING SEXUALITY THERAPEUTICALLY

A wise, warm, and loving nurse made a perceptive comment. She said, "I use my sexuality to help my patients. I'm not afraid to be mothering when a male patient needs mothering, and if I feel he needs his sexual self-esteem raised, I show him in subtle ways that he is still attractive and vital." She is comfortable with her own sexuality and can use it constructively to help patients having difficulty with their sexuality. Other nurses might be afraid that their behavior might be misconstrued as a sexual advance. That possibility exists, but one can only speculate that too often nurses become asexual because of rigidity, ignorance, and even prudery.

Whether male or female, nurses who are comfortable in their own sexuality, who do not restrict themselves to stereotyped role behavior, and who are risk takers when it comes to patient care can do much to help the people they serve maintain or regain sexual health.

NOTES

1. Hein EC: Communication in Nursing Practice. Boston, Little, Brown, 1973, pp 193–197
2. Ibid, p 195
3. Ibid, p 196
4. Ibid, p 197
5. Ujhely GB: Two types of problem patients and how to handle them. Nursing 76(16):64–67, 1976
6. Stockard S: Caring for the sexually aggressive patient—you don't have to blush and bear it. Nursing 81 11:114–116, 1981
7. Ujhely GB: Two types of problem pa-

tients and how to handle them. Nursing 76 (16):66, 1976

8. Scalzi C: Behavioral responses following acute M.I. Heart Lung 2:62–69, 1973

9. Coping with a seductive patient. Nursing 78 8:41–45, 1978

10. Robinson L: Psychological Aspects of the Care of Hospitalized Patients. Philadelphia, Davis, 1976, pp 30–31

11. Ibid, p 31

12. Pease, RA: Female professional students and sexuality in the aging male. Gerontologist 14:153–157, 1974

13. Assey JL, Herbert JM: Who is the seductive patient? Am J Nurs 83:530–532, 1983

14. Withersty D: Sexual attitudes of hospital personnel: A model for continuing education. Am J Psychiatry 133:573–575, 1976

15. Scalzi C: Behavioral responses following acute M.I. Heart Lung 2:67, 1973

16. Hampton P: Coping with the male patient's sexuality. Nurs Forum 18:304–310, 1979

17. Ibid, p 307

18. Brooks PA: Masturbation. Am J Nurs 67:820–823, 1967

19. Golub S: When your patient's problem involves sex. RN 38(3):27–31, 1975

20. Lanahan CC: Homosexuality—A different sexual orientation. Nurs Forum 15:314–319, 1976

21. Lawrence JC: Homosexuals, hospitalization and the nurse. Nurs Forum 14:305–317, 1975

22. Ibid, p 310

23. Ibid, p 315

24. When the patient is gay. Nurs Dig, March–April 1975, pp. 60–61 (condensed and reprinted from Nurs Update 5(2):12–15, 1974)

25. Ibid, p 61

26. Deisher RW: What is the best course for parents to take on learning their child may be homosexual. Med Aspects Hum Sexuality 11(2):20–30, 1977

27. Hornstein A, Cooke C: Counseling patients with sexual identity stresses. Interact 2(2) (Searle and Co., 1978) pp 1–12

28. Ibid, p 2

29. Ibid, p 6

Sexual Problems Throughout the Life Cycle

Chapter 15

Sexual Problems of Infancy and Childhood

Infants may be considered asexual by some, but in reality the foundations of sexuality are laid down at the moment of conception. Problems that have their origin in the formative years from the prenatal period onward may not only adversely affect the early stages of the life cycle but can be the genesis of problems in adulthood and later years.

It is in the family that the vast majority of individuals develop as sexual beings. Parents form the generation that leads and teaches. They are implicitly obligated to relate sexually to each other, and the offspring learn from the parents who are their gender models—for better or for worse. The tasks of parents, in addition to "teaching" sexuality, include overcoming such family evolutionary crises as the birth of other children, the oedipal phase, adolescence, and adversities such as illness or economic misfortunes.[1] With such major responsibilities, and usually with inadequate preparation for parenting, it is amazing that more developmental sexual problems do not occur.

Although the chapters in this unit are "problem" chapters, the word is used advisedly, since many sexual problems may be those identified by society and not by the individual involved or may be defined by the individual and not society. Problems may not be defined as such by all readers, depending on their own beliefs and orientation about sexuality. Contrary to the belief of some, problems of infancy and childhood are diverse in type, if not particularly frequent in occurrence.

Intersexuality is discussed as a problem whose origin is in the prenatal period. Psychosexual developmental problems of children, sexual activity, masturbation, sex play, sexual assaultiveness, and sexual precocity are also included in the content, along with their nursing implications.

Adult-initiated problems are presented. These include childhood guilt and negative feelings about sexuality because of adult proscriptions; adult nudity and sexual activity in front of the child; sexual victimization; incest, and rape; and childhood pregnancy, pornography, and prostitution.

Finally, the effects of childhood disability and the etiology and therapy of cross-gender behavior and identity are presented.

PROBLEMS ORIGINATING IN THE PRENATAL PERIOD, INFANCY, AND EARLY CHILDHOOD

Biologic Problems: Intersexuality
Each individual is a sexual being from the moment of conception. During the prenatal period, hormonal and genetic errors may oc-

cur that result in sexual problems in later life. Traditionally, individuals who have external genitalia of both sexes have been called hermaphrodites. However, true hermaphrodites have both testicular and ovarian tissue, a very rare occurrence.[2] True hermaphrodites should not be confused with cases in which an individual with only one kind of gonad possesses reproductive organs that have characteristics of the opposite sex. The terms *pseudohermaphroditism* or *intersexuality* may be used to describe these congenital abnormalities.

Intersexes are further divided, depending on the sex of the gonad, into male pseudohermaphrodites (when the gonads are testes) and female pseudohermaphrodites (when the gonads are ovaries). Intersexed infants may be born with such ambiguous genitals that clear visual determination of sex is impossible. In others, genital appearance is less ambiguous but is contrary to the chromosomal pattern, gonadal makeup, or other anatomic determination of sex.[3]

Genetic Anomalies

Turner's Syndrome. Turner's syndrome which occurs in 1 of 2000 female births is characterized by sexual infantilism and is a cause of sterility in the female. One sex chromosome is missing (an XO configuration), so only the female chromosome is present to influence the development. This results in the absence of or minimal development of the gonads. There is no significant production of male or female sex hormones; therefore, the tissues are considered to be in a female resting state. Since the second X chromosome necessary for full femaleness is missing, the girls have incomplete sexual anatomy, and since they lack adequate estrogens, secondary sex characteristics will not develop without treatment.[4]

The infants are born with normal-appearing female external genitalia, so they are assigned and raised as females, develop as feminine girls, and are heterosexually oriented. Later, medical management is neces-

sary to develop secondary sex characteristics.[5]

These females have abnormally short stature, and at least two of the following abnormalities: web neck, childlike chest with widely spaced nipples, cubitus valgus (an increase in the carrying angle of the arms), webbing of digits or of the axillae, senile facies, high-arched palate, and a high possibility of underlying abnormal development (coarctation) of the aorta or even the heart. Intelligence may be normal or slightly decreased.[6] Often the syndrome is not detected until puberty, when the female fails to develop secondary sex characteristics.

Klinefelter's Syndrome. Klinefelter's syndrome, which occurs in 1 of 500 male births, is a type of hypogonadism responsible for sterility in the male. These infants usually have an extra X chromosome (an XXY configuration). They usually have a penis and testes, but the testes are markedly decreased in size and serum testosterone levels are much lower than normal. In addition to testicular atrophy, there is azoospermia, a distinctive body habitus characterized by an elongated body, decreased facial and body hair, and gynecomastia.

In the more common type (XXY chromosomal configuration), intelligence is normal, but with additional X chromosomes (XXXY or XXXXY), mental retardation occurs and the persons have severe physical abnormalities, such as hypospadias, cryptorchidism, and more severe hypoplasia of the testes.[7] Sexual desire is weak. Clear sexual assignment at birth should lead to a clear sense of maleness, but these individuals often have a gender disturbance ranging from complete reversal (transsexualism) to homosexuality and cross-dressing.[8]

Hormonal Anomalies

Adrenogenital Syndrome. Adrenogenital syndrome occurs in females and is characterized by excesses of adrenal fetal androgens. This results in masculinization of the external genitals, ranging from slight clitoral enlargement to external genitals that look like a normal scrotal sack, testes, and penis. Hidden behind these structures are the vagina and uterus, and the person is otherwise a female.

The syndrome is caused by a congenital deficiency of one of the enzymes necessary for the synthesis of gluco- and mineral corticoids, resulting in increased synthesis of androgenic steroids and oversecretion of ACTH. This causes hyperplasia of the adrenal gland with an excessive production of androgenic steroids.[9]

If at birth the genitals appear to be male, the child is assigned the male sex and gets a sense of maleness and masculinity. If the child is diagnosed as female and reared as female, the child develops a sense of femaleness and femininity. If the parents are uncertain as to which sex the child belongs, hermaphroditic identity results.

Although these individuals demonstrate the power of rearing to determine gender identity, the resulting identity is masculine in direction because of the fetal androgens organizing the brain in masculine direction. The result is that those raised as girls have a tomboy quality more intense than usual but with a heterosexual orientation.[10]

Male Pseudohermaphroditism. Male pseudohermaphroditism may occur because of adrenogenital syndrome. The genitals appear more female than male but the individual is a biologic male. Since genital appearance determines sex assignment, core gender identity is male, female, or hermaphroditic, depending on the family's conviction of the child's sex.[11]

Androgen Insensitivity Syndrome. Androgen insensitivity syndrome results when fetal target tissues fail to respond to androgens. Therefore, the fetal tissue remains in the female resting state and the brain is not organized to masculinity. The infant appears to be female, although cryptoid testes are found. These produce testosterone, but the tissues do not respond. The child may have minimal or absent sex organs. The secondary sex organs, which develop at puberty, are female because of the small, but sufficient amount of estrogen typically produced by the testes. Individuals sense themselves as females and are feminine.[12]

Treatment of Intersexuality. The most significant criterion in deciding sex assignment of the infant is the sex indicated by the external genitalia. Money[13] states that it can be disastrous if a baby is assigned to a sex in which it will not be able to function erotically and coitally. This means that, pragmatically, an intersexual baby with female-appearing genitals should be assigned as female. There is no known method to construct a clitoris-type organ into a penis, and there is no hormonal treatment that will cause a hypoplastic penis to enlarge into normal or near normal size.

In contrast, a genetically female intersexed baby born with a hypertrophied clitoris may be assigned a female at birth, although the hypertrophied clitoris is morphologically a penis. These external genitalia can be feminized through surgery and the internal vagina externalized. This procedure must be performed soon after birth, or the child will have memories of being castrated. In addition, the parents will have difficulty treating their baby as a girl if she has a penis.[13]

There are two options considered when a genetic female is born with a penis. One is to treat the anomaly early and raise the child as a girl. The other is to remove the internal organs, implant prosthetic testes, and raise the child as a boy with hormonal treatment to ensure masculinization at puberty. Since genetic females who have been fetally masculinized invariably behave as tomboys even when raised as girls, there are strong arguments given for not surgically removing the penis neonatally, especially if it has a penile urethra, even if the child is a genetic female.

The guiding principle is that the child

should look like the sex to which he or she is assigned. Parents and significant others must see that the genitals do not lie. If there is congruity between genital appearance, the assigned sex, and rearing practices, then the gender identity develops in congruity with these factors.[14]

Psychosocial Aspects of Therapy. The etiology of intersexuality is rooted in biologic factors, but the response of individuals with these anatomic and physiologic alterations is predicated primarily on the psychosocial responses of significant others, especially the parents. The first conflict that occurs involves the decision whether the infant should be designated male or female and at what age the decision should be made. Many believe that the gender identity is due to sex assignment and rearing practices. Consequently, announcement of the newborn's sex if uncertain is delayed. It is imperative that the sex of the newborn intersexed infant not be dictated by the physician. The parents must have the diagnostic and prognostic facts. Only then will they be able to implement the decision with conviction and with certainty that they are correctly rearing their child. If they are beset by doubt as to sex, they will convey their anxiety and uncertainty.[15]

If the fact of intersexuality is not discovered until after the child's core gender identity is formed, certain principles apply. Attempts to change the gender orientation is done only after careful identification of the individual's present gender identity. The somatic state is not the criterion on which to base the decision to create a new personality. The judgment should be made on the basis of identity.[16] If there is an incompatibility, such as male chromosomes but an identity that is feminine with a sense of femaleness, then the identity should prevail. The decision about sex reassignment is based on the individual's sense of self, not anatomy.

In addition to the sex assignment and parental influence during raising as factors that contribute to the gender identity of the

intersexed infant, one biologic factor accrues. When an abnormal fetal hormonal central nervous system results in androgenization of the brain, the gender identity is toward masculinity. In the absence of androgenization, the child will tend toward femininity.

Other Biologic Problems
Anomalies of the External Genitalia.
Infants may be born with other anomalies. A genetic male baby may be born with no penis at all or with a severe hypoplasia of the penis (micropenis). The decision is usually to assign the infant as a girl, surgically remove the gonads, and institute hormonal therapy. These children are not technically considered intersexed (hermaphroditic), because a penile urethra exists, but the penis is too small to serve as an organ for coitus no matter what type of surgical or hormonal treatment is attempted.

The question of assigning a genetic male infant as a girl does not involve the ethical question that the surgical removal of the gonads will result in castration and sterility, since the gonads are already typically sterile. In addition, they are often undescended and have increased risk of becoming malignant. Even if left in, they may or may not function at puberty to masculinize the body, which may be resistant to the androgen. If this is true, administration of exogenous androgen will also be ineffectual.[17]

In borderline cases of micropenis, where the penis appears large enough to function, ointment containing testosterone is administered for 3 months. If androgen responsivity exists, the penis enlarges and public hair grows. However, the increase in penile size occurs only once and does not occur later during puberty.

In rare cases, the penis may be lost, sometimes as a result of circumcision accident, a condition identified as ablatio penis. In some cases the infant may be surgically and hormonally rehabilitated into a girl. Ethical considerations of castration exist along with ethical considerations of preserving fertility but allowing the child to live as a boy without a penis. The decision to assign female sex must be made by 18 or possibly 24 months of age, before gender identity is finally established. In the older child, the prescription of a prosthetic strap-on penis can be given to aid other lovemaking activity without a penis. It is possible to have an orgasm without a penis.[18]

The female infant may be born with genital tract obstruction, an imperforate vagina, double vagina, absence of a vagina or labial adhesions.[19] In counseling, parents are assured that the vaginal tract can be "opened," avoiding the word "created." Vaginoplasty is done and molds are inserted to maintain size and shape.[20]

Other developmental problems that cause concern are cryptorchidism, hypospadias, and epispadias, which are all discernible at birth. Cryptorchidism is the retention of one or both of the testes in the abdominal cavity. During fetal development, the testes first appear in the abdominal cavity, then start to descend to the scrotum. Sometimes the testes are halted in their descent in the abdomen, becoming undescended testes. Improperly developed testes may not produce the hormones that cause secondary sex characteristics. If they are fixed in the inguinal canal, they may produce secondary sex characteristics but no sperm, so the individual is sterile.[21]

The undescended testes may be treated surgically when the child is 5 to 7 years old. Often, however, the undescended testes can be brought down into the scrotum by medical therapy with gonadotropic hormone, which for physical and psychologic reasons is the preferred treatment.

Hypospadias and epispadias may occur in females and males. In the female it is significant only if urinary incontinence results. Hypospadias in the male is a developmental problem in which the urethra opens on the under side of the penis, or on the perineum. In the female, the urethra opens into the vagina. Epispadias in both sexes is a developmental abnormality in which there is absence of the upper wall of the urethra. In the male, the urethral opening is located anywhere on the dorsal side of the penis. Hypospadias is more common than epispadias and, since it is a genetic trait, occurs along family lines.

In addition to these problems of placement of the urethral orifice, there may be a scarred corpus spongiosum, which forms a chordee, or downward deflection of the penis. This may make erection difficult and intercourse impossible. Surgical cosmetic and functional correction is often possible.

These problems are discernible at birth and are discussed with the parents immediately. In addition, these infants are also examined for signs of intersexuality.[22]

Maternal Illness, Injury, Drugs. The effect of maternal illness and injury on prenatal development is equivocal. Ingestion of certain drugs may decrease fetal well-being. Excessive ingestion of alcohol and excessive smoking have been connected with small birth size. Infants born to mothers addicted to narcotics are born with a physical dependency on the drugs. Specific effects in sexuality of the infant, however, have not been verified.

Kester and associates[23] found that ingestion of pregnancy-maintaining hormones such as progesterone resulted in male children whose boyhood behavior was less "masculine" then the norm. Men whose mothers took diethylstilbestrol (DES) and natural progesterone reported high sex drive, but erectile failure, while those whose mothers took synthetic progesterone reported low sex drive.

Viruses, radiation, and cytotoxic drugs have also been incriminated.[24]

Psychosexual Problems

Even with the delivery of a normal child, some parents may be upset that the baby's sex is not that which was hoped and sometimes planned for. Parents may more or less reject the child or have ambivalent feelings, which result in parenting behavior that may be the cause of future sexual problems such as homosexuality and transsexuality, or bisexuality. (See Chapter 5.)

Other problems may have their roots in infancy. Both male and female infants are capable of sexual arousal but there is no way of knowing the nature of their subjective experience.[25] Male erection has been observed in utero[26] and it is not unusual for infants to explore or manipulate their genitals. Parents may become anxious about this activity, which they perceive as sexual, and as the children continue the behavior the parental anxiety may be communicated. In addition, children may be verbally reprimanded or physically chastised. Difficulty during adulthood accepting sexual activity as normal, good, and right may be rooted in these very early negative experiences.

Parenting practices begun in infancy also affect development of sexual roles. Daughters are handled gently by mothers, sons more roughly by fathers.[27] Social customs affect core gender identity and subsequent gender role behavior. Changing roles and relationships can be effected only if child-raising practices are changed.

During early childhood, problems may be caused by toilet-training practices which are punitive. When parents teach the 2-year-old that the contents are dirty, unclean, and need control and punish failure, future conflicts can result related to giving and receiving.[28]

From 3 to 5 years old, children may fondle their genitals, explore those of playmates or exhibit their own.

The quality of the communication between the parents and child concerning this sexual behavior is vital. If parents are too strict and shame the child or if they are too encouraging, that is, laughing at or showing how to engage in this behavior, the child may associate shame or guilt with something that gives pleasure and is associated with the genitals. If the parents threaten the child with statements such as "We'll cut off your hand if you don't stop playing with yourself," or worse "Your penis (or whatever euphe-

mistic term is used) will fall off if you play with it," the child may develop anxiety about losing something that is cherished (castration anxiety). Major neurotic problems related to sexuality may develop later in life. The female, however, does not develop this intense castration anxiety. (See Chapter 7.)

NURSING IMPLICATIONS

Assessment

Nurses working in hospital nurseries must be on the alert for any physical anomalies in the newborn, although the physician does the initial examination. However, nurse–midwives are the first health professional to see other newborns, so they must assess the infant for sexual anatomic anomalies and delay premature announcement of the infant's sex if it is equivocal.

If the diagnosis of intersexuality has been made and communicated to the parents, the nurse assesses their responses. Anxiety, depression, and guilt may occur. The ability of the parents to support each other should be ascertained. Depending on the relationship, one parent may blame the other, or both parents may be so devastated by the news that neither can provide support for the other.

The parents' attitude toward the normal infant should also be assessed. Is there inordinate disappointment that the infant is a girl instead of a boy, or vice versa, and are they able to accept the infant as the postdelivery period progresses?

Planning

The nurse's goal is to help all parents love their child. In the case of an intersexed infant, the nurse's goal is to help the parents cope with the anxiety, depression, and guilt that may accompany the birth and to help them accept and identify the child as a loved boy or girl, as the case may be.

Intervention

If it is not possible to identify the newborn intersexed infant's sex by inspection, the responsible individual's best approach is to advise the parents that the baby has unfinished or incompletely differentiated sex organs and that it may take a few hours or several days before the decision can be made. This allows the parents to delay the announcement of the baby's sex and then later having to retract it.[29] Avoid words such as intersex.[30] Explain to parents in words they can understand that the infant will undergo many tests: chromosome analysis, endocrine studies such as testosterone level, cortisol, 17-Ketosteroids and 17-hydroxyprogesterone assays, x-rays to assess skeletal maturation, and contrast pictures of any urogenital sinuses.[31]

The parents need support and the understanding that their new baby is not a freak. Stereotypes characterize the hermaphrodite as a half man, half woman and identify intersexuality as the cause of homosexuality.

Money[29] describes an effective destigmatization program in which the parents are shown and given charts and diagrams that show the formation of male and female sex organs. Next, the parents are shown color slides or photographs of what has been done in cases similar to their child's. These photos represent different age levels from infancy on, with details of the genitalia and adolescent physique, as well as ordinary portrait and group photographs of everyday activities.

What is the most surprising to most parents is that the gender identity is not preordained at birth but is developed under the influence of social factors. They are surprised that their child's gender behavior will reflect their own example, teaching, expectations, and reinforcements.

It is vital that the decision of the sex of the newborn not be dictated to the parents by the health professional. If the parents are not in full agreement, their uncertainty about how to rear the child will be conveyed to the child as contagiously as an infection. Later, parents may have to be counseled about the advisability of further pregnancies, the sex education of their child, and how to explain

to the child surgical procedures or frequent hospital visits and examinations. It is important that the parents not be overloaded with too much information in one sitting. Even if the nurse does not give the initial information, she can clarify and reinforce information given by the physician. Of even more importance, she can devote the time to listening to the parents' fears and concerns.

Counseling and teaching of parents is needed no matter what the sexual problem. Even if amenable to surgical or medical therapy, myths and misconceptions about sexuality may color and distort the parents' perception of the information given to them. Anxiety is inevitably present to further block their perception. The nurse considers these factors when planning and intervening. If surgery is performed, the parents are given a clear explanation of what has been done, and their questions are answered clearly and unambiguously. The parents should be allowed to be involved in the child's care and to work with the nurse whenever possible.[32]

As the child grows older and becomes concerned about sexual development, it is reassuring if he/she can meet with another person with similar problems to see that they can adapt.[33]

The parents who are disappointed by the sex of their normal child, wishing instead for a child of the opposite sex, need a ready ear to listen to their complaints without chastising them for their feelings. Verbalization of the disappointment may be enough to decrease the negative feelings. The statement "You have a beautiful, healthy baby; you should be glad he (she) doesn't have any defects," is not an appropriate intervention by the nurse, since it only serves to cut off communication and identify to the parents the nurse's insensitivity to their feelings.

As part of health teaching nurses give information about toilet-training practices that may be harmful to the child's psychosexual development, stressing that threats, verbal or physical punishment not only are harmful but are also self-defeating.

Evaluation

The nurse observes parents' interaction with the infant for signs of affection, willingness to participate in care, to look at the genitals, change diapers, etc., indicating acceptance of the infant. The parents' verbalization that the child is a boy (or a girl) and parenting practices that are congruent for the sex also indicate that the infant is accepted and seen as the designated sex.

SEXUAL PROBLEMS OF CHILDHOOD

The term *problem* is applied by adult society to childhood behavior and experiences that may not be considered problematic by the child. The label of *sexual deviation* should only be rarely used in childhood. In the child, problems are due more to immature emotional development. What is normal in one developmental period may be considered a deviation in a later period.

Biologic Problems

Biologic sexual precocity may occur in the male and female. In boys, sexual precocity is defined as the occurrence of signs of masculinization before the age of 10 years. Skeletal maturation is accelerated, and there is premature fusion of the epiphyses of the bones, leading to a short stature in adult life. Mental and dental development are not precocious. The condition may be due to organic lesions of the brain, adrenocortical and testicular tumors, and tumors that cause secretion of extra endocrine hormone.

True precocious puberty is manifested by maturation of the testes and spermatogenesis. When no organic cause is found, the condition is identified as idiopathic precocious puberty, which in some instances is transmitted as a sex-limited autosomal dominant trait.[34]

Incomplete sexual precocity or precocious pseudopuberty is a condition characterized by testes that remain more or less immature. The penis is enlarged, but true

puberty does not occur. The commonest cause is adrenocortical hyperfunction due to congenital virilizing adrenal hyperplasia or a virilizing adrenocortical tumor.

Sexual precocity is three times more prevalent in girls than in boys. It may be due to organic or idiopathic (constitutional) causes. Constitutional precocity is due to premature release of gonodotropin, which is sufficient to cause breast development, pubic and axillary hair, and menstruation in the 5- to 8-year age group. Menstruation may be the first symptom noted in some children. Because of premature closure of epiphyses the height is less than normal.[35]

Precocity may also be due to organic changes such as cerebral lesions or adrenal and ovarian hyperfunction. Precocious pseudopuberty in girls is commonly associated with estrogen-producing ovarian tumors. In pseudopuberty, ovulation does not occur.[36]

Although these children are treated medically and/or surgically, they present serious psychologic and social problems. They are obviously different from children their own age but also are not mature enough to cope with the sexual drive that parallels the physical changes. Some are capable of reproduction.

Psychosocial Problems

Freud's theories of psychosexual development are discussed in Chapter 7, but brief mention will be made here. Freud identified four stages of sexual development—oral, anal, phallic, and genital. He conceptualized problems as resulting from the needs of a given stage of development being either insufficiently or excessively gratified.

The task of resolving oedipal conflicts (Chapter 7) may go undone. If the child does not have a sustained relationship with both parents or adequate substitutes, she/he may not resolve the conflict. The boy will not resolve his strong sexual attachment to his mother (Oedipal complex) and the girl her attachment to the father (Electra complex). In addition, if one parent is openly seductive toward the child, or if the parents are hostile toward each other, the child's oedipal hopes are unrealistically increased and resolution of the conflict is more difficult. If the "rival" parent should become sick or should die, the child may blame self, ascribing the event to the hostile wishes.[37]

The boys who do not resolve their oedipal conflict become timid and sexually inhibited. If threatened by a punitive father, they may "give up" not only the mother, but all women, as erotic objects. The daughters of aggressive fathers may identify with them and develop masculine character traits. Those with punitive mothers may emulate them or may rebel.

Problems Related to Sexual Practices of Children

Masturbation. Masturbation is defined as genital self-stimulation resulting in sexual gratification. It usually begins by chance. The problem is usually more the parents' reaction, since there are no adverse biologic or psychologic consequences except those caused by guilt, anxiety, and fear.[38] These feelings may be evoked because of early prohibition and negative labeling of the activity. (See Chapter 4 for further discussion of masturbation.)

The responses of parents range from strict prohibitions with threats of or actual punishment, to moderate negative injunctions, benevolent neglect, or to positive reinforcement, which is qualified by describing the socially appropriate or inappropriate times and places for the activity.[39]

Some children and infants can achieve orgasm by masturbation. In societies that are sexually premissive in regard to prepubescent sexuality, most children masturbate by 6 to 8 years of age.

Excessive masturbation is difficult to define, since what is excessive rests with the evaluator. However, some persons speak of external pressure to masturbate and inability to stop. It is generally agreed that when masturbation becomes compulsive and is used to ward off anxiety or feelings of distress and not as a release of sexual tension, it can be considered as excessive and symptomatic of a deeper problem.

Children who fail to derive pleasure from social interchange and other kinds of interaction with the environment (the withdrawn or depressed child) may try to lift the mood and alleviate anxiety by masturbation.[40] The psychotic or retarded child may not understand the inappropriateness of the activity in the presence of others.[41] If the activity is a sign of a deeper problem, it is then treated as any kind of defensive behavior that is used to ward off feelings of distress. Compulsive masturbation is not usually associated with any real pleasure or satisfaction. Care is taken during therapy, however, to avoid the negative labeling of all genital self-stimulation or genital pleasuring per se.[42]

Small groups of boys sometimes use masturbation as acting out behavior. There may also be oral–genital activity and sexual deviations associated with it.[43]

Fantasies may accompany masturbation. The young child is usually only aware of the sensory experience. During the later part of the anal and during the phallic, latency, and adolescent periods, erotic and aggressive fantasies may accompany the activity. These may have a sadistic or masochistic character (see Chapter 4). The aggressive fantasies may be hostile, with the object one or the other parent. The child may suffer severe conflict about the fantasy and the possibility that actual acting out may occur, causing feelings of fear, guilt, and horror.

Heterosexual and Homosexual Activities. Heterosexual activities and homosexual activities involving children include childhood sex play (mutual childhood genital exploration) and genital exhibitionism. When children restrain all sexual impulses society is not concerned, but if the children develop "abnormal" sexual appetites, concern arises, although what is accepted as normal varies widely. The moral tone is set by the middle class, whose sexual codes are most organized.

Comparing of their genitals by children is not an unusual occurrence. A "you show me yours and I'll show you mine" attitude prevails. This behavior may occur with children of the opposite or same sex. Kinsey found that 40 percent of males[44] and 30 percent of females[45] had sex play with the opposite sex. Usually, the children were of approximately the same age. Genital exhibition was the most frequent behavior, but many children also engaged in manual manipulation of the other's genitals, while others engaged in oral–genital contacts and attempted intercourse.[46]

Preadolescents may use teasing and rough play as an excuse for physical and verbal contact among the sexes. Boys may gradually increase heterosexual childhood sex play until adolescence. Girls drop out of play as they near puberty. It is hypothesized that girls may be more aware of possible complications of sex play, or it may be that they are more carefully supervised.

The child rarely has a problem with this behavior, but the parents experience alarm and transmit their anxiety to the child. If there is intense disapproval expressed with the threat of punishment or even with mild scolding, the message may be imprinted that the genitals and sexual pleasuring are taboo. The child's sex play accompanied by fantasies and castration anxiety might then turn out to be a major complication of adult sexuality.[47]

The opposite effect may also occur. Instead of resulting in a halt to the sex play, the prohibitions impart to the behavior an aura of intrigue. This increases the appeal and the chance of probable recurrence. However, the behavior is more hidden and secretive.[48]

Homosexual activity may occur among children. Children play mostly with other children of their own sex until grade school age, so that sexual activity may occur with a child of the same sex. For the most part, childhood homosexual activities are confined to brief periods and are quickly forgotten as adolescence approaches. Sometimes, however, childhood homosexual activities are a source of guilt in later years.[49]

Seduction of an Adult. Children who may be starved for affection require and demand pleasurable, positive affective content to their lives. This may lead to seduction by the child and sexual activity. There is insufficient evidence of lasting consequences of the sexual behavior per se, but it may be harmful if it becomes public and the adult and child suffer the social consequences of the activity. The cause of the child's behavior must be identified so the problem in the child's social affectional experiences can be attended to.[50]

Sexually Assaultive Behavior. Sexually assaultive behavior toward other children may be exhibited by some children. The sexual aggressiveness may be toward same-aged or younger children of either sex. The behavior may be less sexual but more a search for control in the area of dominance, submission, and position within the peer group.

The victim needs supportive counseling in terms of the nature of the assaultive behavior, with the hope that the negative experience is not generalized to other sexual areas. The perpetrator is helped to learn alternate ways to gain social status and feelings of positive sexual self-esteem.[51]

Problems Initiated by Adult Behavior

Guilt. Guilt, as was mentioned earlier, arises from strict proscriptions against sexual activity voiced by adults and is often associated with religious beliefs. This results in a negative label being applied to sexuality and the natural curiosity of childhood. In the face of natural drives, the child gets a guilt response, which causes conflict and may lead to sexual difficulties. Children should develop a sexual value system that includes proscription against victimization of others, but without the development of a sense of wrongdoing regarding sexuality per se. (See Chapter 13 for a discussion of guilt.)

Household Nudity. Household nudity may be problematic. Some adult nudity is bound to occur in the family, although more frequently, parents hide their bodies from children. Children are naturally curious about the parents' appearance without clothes. In the early years, especially, children wonder about the distinguishing features of females and males. Discriminating cues such as hair length, clothing, and daily routine do exist, but they are less obvious during this period of "unisex," and do not help the children in their self-labeling as being male or female. Children need some cues for the development of appropriate sexual self-concept.[52]

Anxiety about nudity is primarily the parents'. In the early years, children are not embarrassed by their bodies and the bodies of others. The effect of the parents' embarrassment and anxiety about their bodies, the absence of cues for self-labeling as to sex, and the presence of negative connotations relative to the human body and particularly the genitalia may result in negative feelings about sexuality.

Excessive adult nudity may cause the problem of overstimulation, a term included in psychoanalytic and to a lesser degree general psychiatric dogma. This term is used to describe the consequences of household nudity. In this theoretic framework, the child and the parents experience overloading of erotic stimuli, and this damages the child's psychosexual development. The child develops harmful fantasies, and the parents' limited sexual control results in seductive influences in the child's direction. However, Green[53] states that most overstimulation is moderately experienced by parents, extensively experienced by psychoanalysts, and minimally experienced by the child.

Viewing Adult Sexual Activity. Childhood viewing of adult sexual activity may be problematic, even if nudity is not. There is an overlap between the physical activity that is typically involved in sexual conduct and that which is involved in aggressive conduct. Observation of adult sexuality by young children may be confusing and hazardous to them. The sex sounds, facial grimacing, and body movements may be misconstrued by the child as assaultive and painful, and children should be isolated from this experience. This does not mean that they should be kept ignorant about the process of sexual intercourse and its potential for reproduction.[54]

Viewing pictures of bizarre sexual behavior may also be problematic. Care should be exercised that children are not exposed to pictures depicting sadomasochistic behavior, rape, bestiality, or bizarre forms of sexual conduct. If sexual pictures are shown, they should be of body nudity and typical sexuality. The child will find pornography soon enough.

Sexual Victimization—Incest. Nationally, 800,000 sexual assaults against children are reported each year and 80 percent of these are committed by relatives, neighbors, or acquaintances, and this does not include unreported cases.[55]

Incest, sexual activity between persons of close blood relationship, or with surrogate family ties, occurs most commonly between father and daughter, but both parents are involved psychologically. Mother–son incest is rare.[56]

Incest has some typical characteristics. It occurs in girls under 17, usually the firstborn, by the father. It occurs over a long period of time, in unbroken homes with an intimidated, indifferent mother who may refuse sexual intercourse to her husband.[57]

The father usually initiates the activity, although in some cases the daughter is a willing partner. The incest is usually discovered when the daughter reports the relationship. Sibling incest between brother and sister in their early teens or younger is rarely reported.

Mothers who live alone with sons may in unconscious ways serve as a stimulus to the development of the child's sexuality. For example, the mother may sleep with the son, who may be aroused without conscious awareness. This may make the boy anxious and lead to his acting out and becoming sexually overactive as he goes into adolescence.

Incest is usually considered symptomatic of severe family disorganization. Family members may be so severely interdependent, so loosely organized, that the children never learn the importance of sexual restraint. In one study of convicted and institutionalized incestuous offenders, the fathers and brothers were usually unskilled workers with little education and below normal intelligence.[58] In contrast to these findings, Hunt[59] found that incest was more common among better educated and white collar people than among blue collar population or those who had not attended college.

Burgess and Holmstrom[60] describe children who are victims of sexual trauma as accessory sex victims. These children are pressured into sexual activity by someone in a power position over them because of age, authority, or some other way. The emotional reaction of the victims results from their being pressured into the activity or the tension of keeping the activity secret. These victims differ from victims of rape, in which the sexual assault is clearly against the victim's will as well as concomitant with a life-threatening situation (see Chapter 6).

The victim may not even be aware that sexual activity is part of the offer. Pressure for compliance may be applied by offering material goods (candy or money) or misrepresenting moral standards by statements such as "it's okay to do." Children under 6 and latency-age children may know the sexual situation is wrong, but the concept of sexuality is not part of their life style and they go along with the pressure.[61] The need of the victim for human contact may be another reason for agreeing to sexual activity.

After the sexual activity, the victim is pressured to secrecy, sometimes by threatening harm. The burden to keep the secret is psychologically experienced as fear of punishment, repercussion from telling, abandonment, or rejection. Barriers to communication because of the difficulty of describing the activity in words may also obviate disclosure, until direct confrontation occurs when the act is observed or the victim directly tells someone.[62]

Green[63] believes that most of this type of adult–child interaction is not violent and does not result in physical harm to the child. Some believe, however, that many adolescent prostitutes had incestuous relationships[64] that may also result in the child becoming a runaway, or subject of pornographic materials. Depression, self-mutilation, sexual dysfunctions such as promiscuity or frigidity may also follow.[65]

Finkelhor[66] believes that the fact that there is some empirical evidence that sex with adults causes harm is not the most compelling argument against such behavior. The stronger ethical argument is that such behavior ignores childrens' incapacity to give true consent. He believes American sexual ethics are increasingly confused and that this moral confusion about sex is partly responsible for the occurrence of sexual abuses as people interpret the sexual revolution to mean "all is permitted."

There has been little research in the psychologic consequences of the questioning and an ordeal of any civil action involving the child. Further research is needed to explore the effects of sexual trauma on the personality of the child and the right of children to their sexual development.

Sexual Exploitation of Children. Concern is being voiced about child sex exploitation in advertising. Television commercials and magazine ads show children in suggestive poses, apparently telling the world that children are ready for sex.

An image of a young temptress is projected. Yet encouraging children to be adults denies them childhood. Dolls now have breasts and boyfriends and infants wear makeup.[67]

Some argue that anything goes for children; that they should be allowed, perhaps encouraged, to lead a full sex life without interference from parents or the law. Some sexologists say that the latency period is a myth, children are sexual and may even develop problems if they do not have early sex. Others say incest can sometimes be beneficial. The Childhood Sensuality Circle, a pedophile sex group, advocates children beginning sex at birth. The results of these avant garde ideas about sexual behavior have not been assessed, but therapists see the traumatic results in children who have been involved in sexual situations. One concluded that childhood sexuality is like playing with a loaded gun.[68]

Prostitution. Childhood prostitution may be the result of parents pushing their children into early sexual experiences. Another factor is considerable sexual seduction of a girl by the father or another male resulting in a sex drive that may be increased, especially in adolescence.

When coldness and rejection exist in the family accompanied by an aura of depreciation, girls may seek the warmth and acceptance of physical contact even though it may be destructive. However, the children experiencing excessive sexual activity are almost always brought to it by being sexually exploited or stimulated by adults.[69]

Adults establish three types of child sex rings: sex initiation rings, youth prostitution rings, and syndicated prostitution and pornography rings. In the first, children are programmed by a familiar adult to provide sexual services in exchange for a variety of rewards. The second involves adolescents 14 to 16 years old who exchange sex with adults for money, attention, and/or material goods. The third type involves recruitment of children for pornography and for provision of sexual services to a network of customers.[70]

Pornography. Childhood pornography has increased. Children are used for commercial purposes to take part in sexual activity, both normal and bizarre. The newest "adult" mag-

azines are entitled "Lollitots," "Brat," and "Muppets," all featuring photographs of children, some as young as 6, simulating or actually engaging in sex acts and deviations.

In May 1978, legislation was enacted adding an amendment to the criminal code, setting fines of up to $10,000, a penalty of up to 10 years in prison, or both, for the first offense of child pornography. The law makes it a crime to induce anyone under 16 to engage in sex acts for the production of pornographic materials that are to be distributed through interstate commerce. It also makes it a crime to transport anyone under 18 across state lines to engage in prostitution or other sexually explicit conduct for commercial purposes.

Adults may also use children to provide them with vicarious sexual pleasure. Children are encouraged to indulge in sexual activity with animals and objects. In addition, they may be raped by adults (see Chapter 6).

Pregnancy. Childhood pregnancy is rare. If it occurs, it is typically in the female with precocious puberty. When it does occur, it presents severe problems, since the child is obviously not prepared for mothering.

Fetishism. Fetishism is the attachment to an object or body part that is charged with special erotic interest. A child separated from a parent may want to cling to an object such as a blanket or toy that for him/her represents the parent. This is normal developmental behavior. It becomes a deviation only if the object becomes the primary source of sexual satisfaction, a situation that usually happens later in life.

Sexual Ignorance. Sexual ignorance of children due to inadequate education may cause problems that may not surface until late in life. Children's questions about sexuality usually focus around how "babies are made" or "where did I come from." Too often, the children are either given obtuse or grossly misleading responses such as "The stork brought you," or some euphemism about "planting seed." The adult may avoid answering the questions with the reply, "We'll talk about it later." As a consequence children may engage in sexual behavior unaware of its consequences or they may be fearful of pregnancy as a result of behavior that does not have pregnancy as its consequence.

In addition, because parents and schools often give inadequate sex education, the children grow up with misconceptions about sexual anatomy and physiology. They hear peer group gossip, which is based on ignorance and exaggeration of individual sexual experiences, leading to feelings of incompetency and anxiety. (See Chapter 11.)

Childhood Disability. As with adults, society conveys a message to children that physical disability desexualizes them. The family may try to protect the child from rejection or exploitation and may avoid the topic of sex and interpersonal relationships so that the child is isolated from exposure to sexual situations. Disabled children worry about being normal, over- or undersexed, attractive or unattractive.[71] Unfortunately because of the social isolation, they may be thought of as being less than other children. The child may not know how to take responsibility for his or her social or sexual success.

The deaf child is particularly handicapped since there is a dearth of sex education material and it is difficult to learn about sex due to limited auditory and observational opportunities. Sex-related sign language is very regional and because the topic is so private and personal it is not often available to the child. Graphics are helpful and in schools for the deaf where sex education is provided the signing interpreter must be comfortable with the topic.[72]

Children with spina bifida have sexual response problems. The male will have difficulty getting an erection and only a minority ejaculate. The female can have intercourse and become pregnant but there is increased possibility of urinary tract infection and

those with lower motor neuron lesions do not have vaginal sensation or achieve orgasm.

Gender Disturbances of Childhood
Cross-Gender Behavior.
In Boys. The cross-gender behaviors of boys is characterized by an intense interest in clothes, activities, and toys of girls. Boys role-play girls and prefer girl playmates. Two-thirds are interested in cross-dressing (transvestism) by the age of 4, the other one-third by the age of 6. When they role-play house, they insist on being the mother. When shopping with the mother they may advise her what to wear at home. Transvestism usually occurs in a child involved in a pathologic relationship with a parent of the opposite sex. It can be prevented if it is recognized and treated early. Usually, parents make little effort to change the atypical behavior, "He'll outgrow it." Help is sought when the child reaches 7 or 8 and the behavior persists.[73]

Feminine boys have a greater than average possibility of maturing into adult transsexuals, transvestites, or homosexuals than nonfeminine boys (see Chapter 5).

In Girls. Cross-gender behavior in girls is not well studied. Tomboyishness is more common than feminine behavior in boys, and the saying "She'll outgrow it" is usually true. A neuroendocrine factor may be involved. Girls who are exposed to large amounts of androgenic hormones before birth—girls with androgenital syndrome or whose mothers received androgenic synthetic progesterone during pregnancy—may also exhibit cross-gender behavior. Cultural factors also operate. Diagnosis may not be made, since sexist pediatrics affords higher priority to boys. Mothers, too, do not consult a physician.

Differentiating normal from abnormal cross-gender behavior is difficult, since there is little clinical experience. Some girls insist on wearing boys' clothes, refuse to play with girls, and insist on sports, trucks, and guns.

Most girls change at adolescence. The

critical variable in diagnosis is differentiating the two components of sexuality, that of gender role behavior and of gender or sexual identity. The child may have the basic identity of being male or female but a preference for the opposite gender role behavior. Most tomboys know they are girls and do not wish to be male. They perceive correctly that the social system is giving more reward for boyish behavior. With the onset of adolescence and the attention and courtship by a male, the role behavior changes and there is no wish for sex reassignment. Those with a basic masculine identity, however, remain masculine. Tomboyism that lasts into adolescence, however, may be associated with homosexuality.[74]

With the advent of the Women's Liberation Movement and women's efforts to achieve equal rights, more children are taught to see the benefit of masculine behavior. In addition, women are eschewing the usual roles and relationships, preferring or combining a career with homemaking tasks. The effect of these changes has not yet been felt.

Cross-Sex Identity. This is the term used to describe a small number of children who are dissatisfied with their anatomic sex. They are anatomically normal but wish to belong to the other sex. It is difficult for these small children to understand why they cannot change sex, believing that modification of dress and hair length is enough. As they enter grade school, they may experience conflict with their peer group, since atypical gender role behavior usually accompanies cross-sex identity.[75] (See Chapter 5.)

Treatment of Gender Disorders. In the male, therapy is not directed toward the genital sex orientation but is directed toward teaching social skills to decrease stigmatization, promote more comfort with the anatomic sex, and permit the child to enjoy more boyish activites. Since gender role behavior and genital sexuality are related, therapy

may also affect the genital sexuality. The outcome of untreated behavior may be adult transsexuality, homosexuality, or transvestism (see Chapter 5). However, the long-term effects of treatment are unknown, and little is known about the percentage of children who will mature into heterosexual males without therapy. The goal is to make the child happier during childhood and permit a greater range of social and sexual options during adulthood.

Although much has been written about blurring of sex roles and about unisex and unigender child rearing practices, so far, the blurring of sex roles has had little effect on the pediatric population. The feminine boy still has the same social hardships, and therapy can help him be a happier boy.[76]

Some argue that the important aspect of adult sexuality is the adult's emotional feeling for others, not the individual's choice of genital partner, that everyone should be allowed to live and dress as he/she wishes. However, Green[76] believes that the child's immediate situation must be considered. In addition, as adults, the homosexual, transsexual, or transvestite individual suffers much distress because of society's negative attitude.

Two types of intervention may be used. In the first, the child is helped to develop one-to-one play relationships with other boys. At the same time, parents are counseled singly or jointly. The second type of intervention involves group meetings with several atypical boys and separate meetings of the parents. The male therapist serves as a role model. Effort is also made to decrease the boys' social distress by alerting them to behavior that causes teasing. Other boys who are not so rough and tumble may be recruited from the neighborhood in an effort to find boys with whom they are comfortable. Dolls are replaced with board games and handicrafts. The group experience may provide the first social experience with boys that is not threatening.

Parents who may have encouraged

atypical behavior in the past are sensitized to their role in the behavior. Alienation may exist between the child and his father, who views the son's behavior as personal rejection and evidence of his failure. The therapist points out the boy's need to have a sharing relationship with a male and attempts to get the boy and the father to take part in mutually enjoyable activities.

In the parents' group, there is an opportunity to share concerns and experiences. If the mother has been reinforcing feminine behavior of the boy, it is easier for her to see this in other group members. For the fathers, the group provides support. Usually, fathers feel that they are held responsible for the child's femininity. They become aware that they are not alone in this reasoning.[77]

Treatment of girls has not been systematically undertaken. Green[78] describes a pilot program in which the female therapist serves as a role model.

NURSING IMPLICATIONS

Assessment
Close observation should be made of the child's relationship with other children and with the parents. Play activities of the child and his/her acceptance by peers should be noted. The older child must develop trust in the nurse in order to feel free to share information and concerns.

In cases of possible adult victimization of a child, some clues may be evident and noted by the parents. These include walking home without clothes, staying out all night, or an accumulation of money or new clothes. Children may be able to describe activity that they cannot put into words by drawing pictures.[79] Some children may stay inside more, not want to go to school, or cry. They may bathe excessively or there may be sudden bedwetting. Change in sleep pattern may occur. Truancy, delinquent behavior, and running away may be withdrawal behavior symptomatic of incest.[80] Other somatic problems, such as stomach ache, urinary tract in-

fection, pneumonia, or infectious mononucleosis, may be less obvious reactions to victimization.[81]

Parents may identify and describe as problems such childhood activity as masturbation and hetero- and homosexual sex play. The nurse should assess the parents' beliefs about and attitude toward such activity before attempting intervention. Parents may have misconceptions about and/or may have strong religious beliefs that prohibit such practices (see Chapter 9). Information should be obtained about the frequency of sexual activity, whether it involves a few isolated activities or is constant repetitive behavior.

Planning
Whatever the problem identified, the nurse plans interventions that include both the child and the parent, since the behavior of the first and the response of the second are so intertwined that to intervene for one and not the other is to court failure. The nurse's goals are to correct myths and misconceptions about sexual behavior and to help the parents cope with the child's sexuality in a way that is supportive and nonpunitive.

Intervention
Parents need guidance in dealing with masturbation. Society does put restrictions on the activity, so parents need to find ways to help children see society's expectation without threats and misinformation. If they recognize the normality of the behavior during sexual development, they may be able to respond appropriately. Brooks[82] suggests paying special attention to children when they are *not* masturbating. Involving them in other activities is helpful, but if these activities are introduced after each episode of masturbation, they may only focus attention to the masturbation. What children need is love, attention, and creative stimulation along with limit setting as to the time and place where masturbatory activity is appropriate.

Intervention in cases of child victimization involves encouraging the child to talk about the experience. Parents may discourage the child from expressing feelings. Explaining that talking about the experience is normal and that it will stop when enough talking is done will enable the parent to accept the conversation. Some children are helped by allowing them to draw pictures of the activity and then talking about it. Burgess and Holstrom's[83] data indicate that the symptom reaction is a result of the pressure to keep the activity secret as well as the fear of disclosure.

It is essential to treat seriously reports by children of sexual experience.[84] If a gynecologic examination is necessary, presence of the mother may be a help or a hindrance depending on her reaction. The child fears pain since she may have been hurt before, and have difficulty lying still, so that efforts to gain rapport are essential.[85]

In cases of incest involving a parent and child, the nurse may be the health professional in whom the child confides.

Self-help groups of parents and children have been established. A team approach of physician, nurse, social worker, and attorney may be needed. There must be a family focus so the child is not placed in a vulnerable position.[86]

There is little other treatment. The child may be removed from the home, and behavior modification tried. Family therapy focuses on family dynamics rather than sexual activity.[87]

The nurse counsels parents of children with disabilities to let them take part in normal activities of childhood so that they can be comfortable with interaction with others of both sexes. After initial curiosity is satisfied most healthy children accept those with disabilities. It is the unknown that is frightening to them.

If assessment of the child's activities indicate atypical gender behavior that is distressing the parents and the child, referral for counseling may be necessary unless the nurse has been trained in counseling methods. The nurse may also be in a position to reinforce the counseling done by others. Encouragement of play activities appropriate to the sex is important. The male nurse and the female nurse may serve as appropriate role models for the children in learning social skills and behavior. Listening to the fears and concerns of the parents about the child's behavior also may serve to reduce their anxiety and guilt.

There is not full agreement among psychiatrists about the treatment of compulsive sexual activities. Understanding of what the behavior means to the child as a relief of tension is important. Most sex "deviations" in children are normal developmental processes that are exaggerated. The prognosis depends on how early the child receives treatment and how well the therapist can change unhealthy family patterns. A combination of psychologic and legal approaches may be needed. The younger child, treated along with the entire family, can be helped. The older child is less responsive, although behavior modification therapy has been successful in some cases.[88]

NOTES

1. Fleck S: The family. In Sadock BJ, Kaplan HI, Freedman AM (eds): The Sexual Experience. Baltimore, Williams and Wilkins, 1976, pp 155–180
2. Robbins SL, Angell M: Basic Pathology, 2nd ed. Philadelphia, Saunders, 1976, p 162
3. Stoller RJ: Gender identity. In Sadock BJ, Kaplan HI, Freedman AM (eds): The Sexual Experience. Baltimore, Williams and Wilkins, 1976, pp 182–195
4. Robbins SL, Angell M: Basic Pathology, 2nd ed. Philadelphia, Saunders, 1976, p 161
5. Money J, Ehrhardt AA: Man and Woman, Boy and Girl. New York, New American Library, 1972, pp 109–112
6. Robbins SL, Angell M: Basic Pathology, 2nd ed. Philadelphia, Saunders, 1976, p 161
7. Ibid, p 161

8. Stoller RJ: Gender identity. In Saddock BJ, Kaplan H , Freedman AM (eds): The Sexual Experience. Baltimore, Williams and Wilkins, 1976, p 194

9. Robbins SL, Angell M: Basic Pathology, 2nd ed. Philadelphia, Saunders, 1976, p 606

10. Money J: Sex assignment in anatomically intersexed infants. In Green R (ed): Human Sexuality: A Health Practitioner's Text. Baltimore, Williams and Wilkins, 1975, pp 109–123

11. Stoller RJ: Gender identity. In Sadock BJ, Kaplan HI, Freedman AM (eds): The Sexual Experience. Baltimore, Williams and Wilkins, 1976, p 194

12. Money J: Sex reassignment as related to hermaphroditism and transsexualism. In Green R, Money J (eds): Transsexualism and Sex Reassignment. Baltimore, Johns Hopkins University Press, 1969, p 91

13. Money J: Sex assignment in anatomically intersexed infants. In Green R (ed): Human Sexuality: A Health Practitioner's Text. Baltimore, Williams and Wilkins, 1975, p 111

14. Ibid, p 112

15. Ibid, p 114

16. Stoller RJ: Gender identity. In Sadock BJ, Kaplan HI, Freedman AM (eds): The Sexual Experience. Baltimore, Williams and Wilkins, 1976, p 194

17. Money J: Sex assignment in anatomically intersexed infants. In Green R (ed): Human Sexuality: A Health Practitioner's Text. Baltimore, Williams and Wilkins, 1975, p 112

18. Ibid, p 113

19. Dewhurst J: Genital tract obstruction. Pediat Clin N Am 28:331–344, 1981

20. Harkins JL, Gysler M, Cowell CA: Anatomical amennorhea. Pediat Clin N Am 28:345–354, 1981

21. Diamond M: Sexual anatomy and physiology: Clinical aspects. In Green R (ed): Human Sexuality: A Health Practitioner's Text. Baltimore, Williams and Wilkins, 1975, pp 21–34

22. Green R: Sexual problems of children. In Oaks WW, Melchiode GA, Ficher I (eds): Sex and the Life Cycle. New York, Grune and Stratton, 1976, pp 19–27

23. Kester P, Green R, Finch SV, Williams R: Prenatal "female hormone" administration and psychosexual development in human males. Psychoneuroendocrinology 5:269–285, 1980

24. Thi Tho P, McDonough PG: Gonadal dysgenesis and its variants. Pediat Clin N Am 28:309–329, 1981

25. Katchandourian HA, Lunde DT: Fundamentals of Human Sexuality, 2nd ed. New York, Holt, 1975, p 215

26. Money J: The development of sexuality and eroticism in humankind. Quart Rev Biol 56:388, 1981

27. Offer D, Simon W: Stages of sexual development. In Sadock BJ, Kaplan HI, Freedman AM (eds). The Sexual Experience. Baltimore, Williams and Wilkins, 1976, pp 128–143

28. Ibid, p 133

29. Money J: Sex assignment in anatomically intersexed infants. In Green R (ed): Human Sexuality: A Health Practitioner's Text. Baltimore, Williams and Wilkins, 1975, p 114

30. Pardridge WM, Gorski RA, Lippe BM, Green R: Androgens and sexual behavior. Ann Int Med 96:488–501, 1982

31. Bamford FN: Sexual development of children. Clin Obstet Gynecol 7:193–211, 1980

32. Lewis C: Nursing care of the neonate requiring surgery for congenital defects. Nurs Clin North Am 5:387–397, 1970

33. Thi Tho P, McDonough PG: Gonadal dysgenesis and its variants. Pediat Clin N Am 38:326, 1981

34. Beeson PB, McDermott W (eds): Cecil–Loeb Textbook of Medicine, 14th ed. Philadelphia, Saunders, 1975, pp 1756–1757

35. Ibid, p 1770

36. Ibid, p 1770

37. Katchadourian HA, Lunde DT: Funda-

mentals of Human Sexuality, 2nd ed. New York, Holt, 1975, pp 237–238

38. Godenne GD: Sexual development of children and adolescents. Nurs Clin N Am 14:475–482, 1979

39. Green R: Sexual problems of children. In Oaks WW, Melchiode GA, Ficher I (eds): Sex and the Life Cycle. New York, Grune and Stratton, 1976, p 21

40. Chess S, Hassibi M: Principles and Practices of Child Psychiatry. New York, Plenum, 1978, pp 230–235

41. Ibid, p 231

42. Green R: Sexual problems of children. In Oaks WW, Melchiode GA, Ficher I (eds): Sex and the Life Ccyle. New York, Grune and Stratton, 1976, p 24

43. Teicher JD: Sexual deviations in children. In Sadock BJ, Kaplan HI, Freedman AM (eds): The Sexual Experience. Baltimore, Williams and Wilkins, 1966, pp 391–397

44. Kinsey AC, Pomeroy WB, Martin CE: Sexual Behavior in the Human Male. Philadelphia, Saunders, 1948, p 173

45. Kinsey AC, Pomeroy, WB, Martin CE, Gebhard P: Sexual Behavior in the Human Female. New York, Pocket Books, 1965, p 110

46. Ibid, p 111

47. Belmont HS: Psychodynamic understanding of sexual development in childhood. In Oaks WW, Melchiode GA, Ficher I (eds): Sex and the Life Cycle. New York, Grune and Stratton, 1976, pp 29–39

48. Green R: Sexual problems of children. In Oaks WW, Melchiode GA, Ficher I (eds): Sex and the Life Cycle. New York, Grune and Stratton, 1976, p 21

49. DeLora JS, Warren CAB: Understanding Sexual Interaction. Boston. Houghton Mifflin, 1977, p 152

50. Green R: Sexual problems of children. In Oaks WW Melchiode GA, Ficher I (eds): Sex and the Life Cycle. New York, Grune and Stratton, 1976, p 24

51. Ibid, p 25

52. Ibid, p 20

53. Ibid, p 21

54. Belmont HS: Psychodynamic understanding of sexual development in childhood. In Oaks WW, Melchiode GA, Ficher I (eds). Sex and the Life Cycle. New York, Grune and Stratton, 1976, p 41

55. McIntosh R: Let the child speak. The Plain Dealer, March 2, 1983, Sec A, p 21

56. Fleck S: The family. In Sadock BJ, Kaplan HI, Freedman AM (eds): The Sexual Experience. Baltimore, Williams and Wilkins, 1976, p 177

57. VanderMey BL, Neff RL: Adult-child incest: A review of research and treatment. Adolescence XVII:717–736, 1982

58. Weinberg SK: Incest Behavior. New York, Citadel, 1955

59. Hunt MM: Sexual Behavior in the 1970's. Chicago, Playboy Press, 1974, p 347

60. Burgess AW., Holmstrom LL: Sexual trauma of children and adolescents. Nurs Clin North Am 10:551–563, 1975

61. Ibid, p 554

62. Ibid, pp 556–557

63. Green R: Sexual problems of children. In Oaks WW, Melchiode GA, Ficher I (eds): Sex and the Life Cycle. New York: Grune and Stratton, 1976, p 22

64. Kaplan SJ, Pelcovitz D: Child abuse and neglect and sexual abuse. Psychiat Clin N Am 5:321–332, 1982

65. James J, Myerding J: Early sexual experience and prostitution. Am J Psychiat 134:1381–1385, 1977

66. Finkelhor D: What's wrong with sex between adults and children. Am J of Orthopsych 49:692–697, 1979

67. Palumbo F: Growing up too fast. Pediatrics 69:123–124, 1982

68. Leo J: Cradle to grave intimacy. Time, September 7, 1981, p 69

69. Teicher JD: Sexual deviations in children. In Sadock BJ, Kaplan HI, Freedman AM (eds): The Sexual Experience. Baltimore, Williams and Wilkins, 1966, p 396

70. Burgess AW, Birnbaum HJ: Youth prostitution. Am J Nurs 82:832–834, 1982

71. Cole TM, Cole SS: Rehabilitation of problems of sexuality in physical disability. In Koltke FJ, Stillwell GK, Lehmann JF (eds). Krusen's Handbook of Physical Medicine and Rehabilitation. Philadelphia, Saunders, 1982, pp 889–905

72. Ibid, p 897

73. Green R: Atypical sex role behavior during childhood. In Sadock BJ, Kaplan HI, Freedman AM (eds): The Sexual Experience. Baltimore, Williams and Wilkins, 1976, pp 196–205

74. Ibid, p 200

75. Green R: Sexual problems of children. In Oaks WW, Melchiode GA, Ficher I (eds): Sex and the Life Cycle. New York, Grune and Stratton, 1976, pp 22–23

76. Green R: Atypical sex role behavior during childhood. In Sadock BJ, Kaplan HI, Freedman AM (eds): The Sexual Experience. Baltimore, Williams and Wilkins, 1976, p 204

77. Ibid

78. Ibid, p 205

79. Burgess AW, Holmstrom LL: Sexual trauma of children and adolescents. Nurs Clin North Am 10:562, 1975

80. Luther SL, Price JH: Child sexual abuse: A review. J School Health 50:161–165, 1980

81. Teicher, JD: Sexual deviations in children. In Sadock BJ, Kaplan HI, Freedman AM (eds): The Sexual Experience. Baltimore, Williams and Wilkins, 1966, p 397

82. Brooks PA: Masturbation. Am J Nurs 67:820–823, 1967

83. Burgess AW, Holmstrom LL: Sexual trauma of children and adolescents. Nurs Clin North Am 10:562, 1975

84. Weaver BM, McCarthy P: Sexual misuse of children: An emergency department nursing perspective. J Emerg Nurs 7:59–62, 1981

85. Cowell CA: The gynecologic examination of infants, children and young adolescents. Pediat Clin North Am 28:247–266, 1981

86. Brant RS, Tisza V: The sexually abused child. Am J Orthopsych 47:80–90, 1977

87. Rist K: Incest: Theoretical and clinical views. Am J Orthopsych 49:681–691, 1979

88. Teicher JD: Sexual deviations in children. In Sadock BJ, Kaplan HI, Freedman AM (eds): The Sexual Experience. Baltimore, Williams and Wilkins, 1966, p 397

Chapter 16

Sexual Problems of Adolescence

Puberty brings profound changes in biologic, psychologic, and sociologic aspects of sexuality. Adolescents are faced with new tasks to master and new crises to face. Society, too, is confronted with children's increased demands for autonomy, often coupled with a rebellion against authority. It is a period when sexuality looms large and adolescents must learn to cope with their changing sexual roles and relationships and to live with their sexual urges and concerns. It is a time of conflicts and, for some, problems.

The term *deviation* is rarely used to describe adolescent problems. Fixed disorders in adolescence may warrant this diagnostic term, but it should only be used if it is regarded as a major personality disorder that is chronic and so pervasive that it may cause problems in the adult orientation toward social life.[1]

This chapter focuses on the biologic changes facing the young person with the advent of puberty, especially those that cause anxiety and concern—in girls, the onset of menstruation, and in both sexes, changing body shape and size, masturbation, heterosexual and homosexual activity, and pregnancy and its consequences. The sexually uninterested adolescent and atypical sexual behavior are also briefly discussed. Finally, the problems associated with adolescents' development of autonomy are presented—parent–adolescent conflict over appropriate sexual behavior, sexual acting out, ignorance about sexuality, and inadequate health care.

BIOLOGIC PROBLEMS

Adolescents worry about the "normality" of change in their bodies. Breast size may be a source of self-consciousness in girls. Those who have changes in breast size before their peers may be embarrassed, while girls who are slow in development feel inadequate. Others worry if their breasts are too large or are too small or are unequal in size. In rare cases there may be inflammation, supernumerary breasts and nipples.[2]

Girls may also feel self-conscious if they are too tall, especially in relation to boys. A young girl who is unprepared for menstruation may worry that she has injured herself internally (through masturbation) or she may fear she has some disease.

The mother does much to shape her daughter's attitude toward menstruation. Some girls become moody, withdrawn, quarrelsome, or despondent. A mother who focuses on "sickness" in connection with menses, takes to her bed when menstruating, or acts like an invalid may set up negative reactions in the daughter.

Dysmenorrhea, a spasmodic cramping of the uterus, occurs only in ovulatory periods and is usually absent until age 15. Its peak occurrence is at about 18, and it usually diminishes by mid-20s. Primary dysmenorrhea is believed caused by release of prostaglandins from the endometrium.[3] Secondary dysmenorrhea is pain caused by organic pelvic conditions such as endometriosis, pelvic stenosis, pelvic inflammatory disease, etc. The role of emotional factors is not well identified, but some girls seem to follow the behavior pattern exhibited by their mothers.

Delayed menarche may be a cause of concern. For some, menses may not occur until past 16 years because of constitutional factors and familial traits. If menarche is delayed past 18, primary amenorrhea is said to exist. It is at this time that some of the hormonal and genetic errors present since birth may be first identified and treated (see Chapter 26).

Secondary amenorrhea is the cessation of previously normal menstrual cycles. It may occur abruptly, or it may follow menses of decreased frequency. In the absence of pregnancy, amenorrhea may be due to hormonal imbalances, inadequate dietary intake (especially "crash" diets), ovarian lesions, and certain systemic diseases such as diabetes, anemia, and hepatic and renal disease. In any case, the amenorrhea may be a cause of anxiety for adolescent girls.

Boys carry their own burden of worries about biologic changes. Delayed adolescence, a failure to undergo sexual maturation, is usually due to normal variation in pubertal development. Although puberty usually occurs by 16 years, occasionally it may be later. Even if no pathology exists, it is a cause of anxiety to boys and their parents. In addition to "idiopathic" delay in puberty, the problem may be caused by gonadal or pituitary disease, inadequate dietary intake, or chronic illness. Boys also worry about their anatomy and physiology. Height, weight, the presence of acne, and penis size may be cause of concern.

Gross and Duke[4] found that there is an advantage to boys and girls who physically mature earlier. Those that do were found to be more attractive and popular with more positive body image than later developers who seemed to be educationally disadvantaged, and had feelings of inadequacy and rejection.

Spontaneous erections and nocturnal emissions "wet dreams" first occur when the boy is between 12½ and 14 years old and continue at a frequency of every 10 to 35 nights provided that boys have little, if any, voluntary sex activity. During adolescence, however, emissions may occur on two or more successive nights, usually during REM sleep and without penile manipulation. Erection occurs during an erotic dream and orgasm is reached while the boy is asleep. Some individuals will awake just before orgasm and in half sleep may produce climax by some masturbation. More awaken for a brief period after orgasm. In the morning, there may be no recollection of the orgasm, and the stained clothes and sheets may be a surprise.[5]

Boys should be prepared by their fathers, who stress that all boys have emissions at this age, that they are natural and harmless, and since they are not under their will, are not an immoral or unchaste act. Some boys are frightened that they may injure themselves internally or afraid parents will discover the evidence in the morning and will not understand or will criticize the mess they have made.[6]

With the rapid change in appearance and function, plus the fear of being "different" from the peer group, integrating the changing appearance into body image is another formidable task for many adolescents. (See Chapters 7 and 13 for discussion of body image.)

Venereal disease is increasing among adolescents. It is becoming a young single person's disease. Lack of information about its cause, its effects, and its prevention contribute to its epidemic status. The greatest number of cases occur in the 15 to 29 age group. It is estimated that 50 percent of American young people contract syphilis or gonorrhea by age 25, about 200,000 each year. (See Chapter 22.)

ILLNESS-RELATED SEXUAL PROBLEMS

Whether the genitals are involved or not, illness or surgery that results in change in body appearance is especially devastating for adolescent sexuality. Disfigurement presents the greatest threat to body image during adolescence,[7] when there is need for conformity in appearance, dress, and behavior. Young persons rate themselves against their peers in these areas. Inability to measure up is threatening especially when expertise in heterosexual relationships is being developed. Self-esteem may be tenuous at best. Changes in appearances interfere with their perceptions of self as male or female resulting in depression, anxiety, and withdrawal from sociosexual interactions. (See Chapter 13 for discussion of body image and illness.)

PSYCHOSEXUAL PROBLEMS

For some adolescents, sexual activity may initiate psychologic distress. In others, sexual activity may be the response to psychologic distress. Anxiety, guilt, and shame related to sexual practices and experiences may be pervasive.

Masturbation

Masturbation may be a particular cause of concern. Viewed developmentally, many believe it serves to help the adolescent. However, because of myths and misconceptions and parental condemnation, adolescents may experience guilt and shame about the activity. Along with these factors, Teicher[8] also believes that unconscious repressed fantasies from the oedipal period tend to become conscious again during masturbation, causing concern. The adolescent is unconsciously afraid the fantasies will return and come true. (See Chapter 7 for discussion of oedipal conflict.) Moore[9] sees the masturbatory fantasies as a developmental necessity, since they are necessary for final sexual identity and the establishment of adult relationships.

The adolescent struggles to control sexual impulses and fantasy. At the same time, paradoxically, the adolescent boy, in particular, is an avid reader of pornographic literature and may brag about embellished sexual experiences in order to maintain sexual self-esteem.

Heterosexual Activity

Sexual activity among girls in cities is increasing from 30 percent in 1971 to 43 percent in 1976 and 50 percent in 1979,[10] yet this activity may cause anxiety. The adolescent is often caught between the advocates of free sexual license and the rules and regulations set down by parents or the larger society. The girl who wants to remain a virgin may be pressured by both male and female friends to engage in sexual activity.[11] Lieberman[12] believes that virginity is devalued today and that many in society act as if no girl beyond 12 should be a virgin. Girls may be charged with being repressed; some may wonder if something is wrong with them and feel that to be a virgin is to be an outcast.

The young female may be torn in three directions: to bow to the pressures of peers, to be good and obey the parents, or to obey her inner feelings and wait to develop social intellectual strengths so that she is able to engage in sexual activity with security and pleasure.

Others may refrain from sexual activity because of religious convictions or because aspects of sex may be so frightening or threatening that they do not let feelings surface.[13] Girls who are pressured into sexual activity by peer groups do not usually enjoy sex but do it to get acceptance of the group. Others engage in sex to establish friendship or even marry in hope of finding themselves in each other.[14]

Although little information is available in the literature, one might speculate that many adolescent males also lose their virginity because of peer pressure to engage in sexual activity, and to prove masculinity and power.

The initial coital experience is almost universally disappointing, if not actually painful, unless orgasm occurs. If it is in the context of an affectional relationship with mutual consent, the girl usually has more satisfaction and less guilt, shame, anxiety or disgust.[15]

In a Gallup survey, premarital sex appeared to be accepted with equanimity by a

majority (62 percent) of teenagers. Paradoxically, however, although accepting premarital sex in principle, 51 percent felt that
virginity is very or fairly important in a marriage partner.[16]

Some adolescents are sexually active by
the age of 12 or 13. The focus of most adult
concern is the young female. Adults seem to
have little concern about the psychologically
harmful effects on the young male, a sign of
society's double standard.[17]

In adolescence, acting out behavior may
be characterized by rebelliousness, delinquency, and involvement with drugs and sexual activity. Sex may be used in an effort to
cope with authority—parents, school. Acting
out may reflect the sexual problems of parents and adolescents and the conflict that
may occur between them. Daughters may be
encouraged to date and develop heterosexual
interests, but limits placed on their activities
cause rebellion. In other situations, no limits
are placed on the adolescent's activities so
that the adolescent impulses are unchecked
and unrestricted.

Early heterosexual activity may be an
attempt to deny the fact that adult responsibilities and adult sexual function are interdependent if one is to function appropriately.
Some cases of irresponsible premature heterosexuality may represent conflicting unconscious attitudes. On the other hand, it
may be a demand for adult status for which
the ego is not prepared or a prolongation of
childhood by treating sex as a form of play
without real consequences, one reason adolescents ignore the possibility of pregnancy
so frequently.[18]

Pregnancy. Pregnancy does not occur
often in the young adolescent girl, since the
menstrual cycle may be anovulatory, but by
midadolescence, heterosexual activity may
be followed by unplanned and unwanted
pregnancy; an estimated 1,000,000 occurring
each year.

The pill has been credited for the increased evidence of sexual activity, but few
adolescents use contraceptives, suggesting
that the pill may not be a factor in promoting
sexual activity. Only 20 percent of sexually
active teenagers use contraceptives regularly, the rest relying instead on such ineffective practices as Coke douches, laxatives,
avoidance of orgasm, withdrawal (coitus interruptus), standing up, and prayer.[19]
Thornbury[20] found that one-third of a group
of adolescents had distorted or highly distorted information about contraception.
Many boys used "luck" as a birth control
method.[21]

Many reasons for avoiding contraceptives are presented, some based on the myths
and misconceptions about the entire process
of reproduction. These beliefs may be summarized as follows[22]:

1. Some adolescents believe that they will
   not become pregnant if they have infrequent intercourse; others do not believe
   they can get pregnant very easily.
2. Some think that they are having intercourse during the safe period (often believing erroneously that the safe period is
   midway through the menstrual cycle).
3. Even when adolescents desire to use a
   contraceptive, they have difficulty getting
   oral contraceptives and intrauterine devices (IUD), which require a doctor's prescription and legally, in some states, need
   the parent's permission. Few teenagers
   feel comfortable talking about any aspect
   of sex with their parents, much less admit
   they are sexually active.
4. Because of general disapproval of premarital sex, adolescents do not want to
   admit to themselves or their parents that
   they are sexually active.
5. Parents resist the request for permission
   to use contraceptives, equating the use
   with promiscuity and believing that the
   adolescent girls will not be sexually active
   if not using contraceptives.
6. Finally, adolescent girls refuse to use contraceptives and especially oral contraceptives because they want to be "carried
   away," and to "plan ahead" takes away
   the romance.

One-half of illegitimate births in the United States are to teenage mothers. From 1940 to 1970, there was a threefold increase in illegitimacy in the United States. Moreover, contraception alone cannot solve the teenage pregnancy problem. Unmarried teenage girls, even with available contraceptives, become pregnant. Some teenagers have little motivation to avoid pregnancy. For other unmarried teenagers, the pregnancy may be a symptom of an emotional disturbance, or the pregnancy itself may cause a disturbance. (See Chapter 19.)

Research is needed on premarital coitus, the use and nonuse of contraception. Strahle[23] has formulated a two-stage causal model that can be used to estimate the impact of variables, such as parental and adolescent religiosity; degree of independence from parents; age; sexual socialization; sex role norms; educational and occupational aspirations; knowledge of contraception, and situational perception (aggression, control, embarrassment).

Although the pregnancy may appear to be an accident, most adolescents get pregnant because they want to. The general motivation is unconscious, but some reasons given by girls who admit to wanting pregnancy include: to prove she is woman, to have a baby to love, to please the man, to get back at parents who hassled her over sexual behavior, to get away from a rejecting home, "boring" school or "awful" town, to satisfy parents' covert wish for her to have a baby, to get a man to marry her, and to relieve loneliness and depression. Tragically, the pregnancy does not often accomplish these ends. Some adolescents select abortion, a few allow adoption of the baby, and 55 percent keep the baby and raise it as single parents. Marriage resulting from unwed, unwanted pregnancy has a high probability of ending in divorce (over 50 percent),[24] and 80 percent of pregnant teenagers drop out of school.[25]

Boys may desire to impregnate a girl and may deliberately choose the girl but drop her when she gets pregnant. Others act responsibly and assist the girlfriend through the stressful period of pregnancy or abortion but have no desire to get married. The response of adolescent boys ranges from support to denial of responsibility: from the belief of one that he is a partner in the sex act and is responsible for the consequences, to views of others who felt that if a girl got pregnant they would blame her. "If she didn't want to get pregnant, she shouldn't have done it." Another boy admitted that there should be communication between the boy and girl but that the girl should be more involved with contraception than the boy— "After all, she has the pill to take.[26]

Programs are being established to help teenage fathers and to head off a second pregnancy that often happens to the same girl. Leaders feel that prevention of pregnancy must involve the boys who often have tremendous influence and who often get girls pregnant to improve poor self-image and feelings of powerlessness. The poorer and less educated the community, the more need to exploit.[27]

Ramsey[28] believes that the answer is not more sex education and contraception but that there must be a change from our normless society in which anything is permitted. Others agree that the difficulty with most solutions are that they are based on the mistaken assumption that teenagers must (or will) be sexually active[29] and that no moral guidance is needed.

In 1983 the federal government established the Adolescent Family Life Program, a $13.5 million plan to discourage teen sex. One of its goals is to "promote self-discipline and other prudent approaches to the problem of adolescent premarital sexual relations." The program has been criticized by the American Civil Liberties Union because it allows grants to religious groups and by the Alan Guttmacher Institute because it discourages teenagers from having sex, and "then forgets about them until they get pregnant."[30]

Abortion. Abortion is one solution to teenage pregnancy. In 1974, the United States

Department of Health, Education and Welfare reported 900,000 abortions. One-third of these were to teenagers. Anxiety and guilt may overwhelm the young girl unless she has the support of significant others and effective counseling so that the decision is freely arrived at without coercion (see Chapter 20).

Homosexual Experiences

Homosexual experiences are more common in boys than in girls. These experiences are not the result of deep emotional attachment but are often called a homosexual "crush"—mostly a friendship or an intense nonsexual companionship that primarily satisfies dependency needs. A crush or incident of actual homosexual genital activity rarely leads to later overt homosexuality. The activity usually involves mutual genital masturbation or manipulation. Fellatio may be used occasionally. Girls' experiences are usually limited to touching, caressing, or kissing.

Although the experiences may be erotic, the heterosexually-oriented adolescent does not usually seek them out. Young males who have homosexual activity in late adolescence may have guilt feelings about the experience and may develop an acute anxiety reaction.[31]

SEXUALLY UNINTERESTED ADOLESCENTS

Some girls and boys may be threatened by sexual urges they are unable to handle. Others keep them under control by avoiding socialization with those of the opposite sex.[32] A delay in the development of normal sexual interests may also be related to a wish to deny or avoid oncoming authority and responsibility, an unconscious effort to remain a dependent child.[33]

These adolescents become "sexless" and involve themselves in nonsexual activities such as hobbies, sports, music, and arts. They avoid their peers except on a superficial level. These activities are an important and

necessary part of development but become problematic when they result in inadequate development of interpersonal relationships. For some young persons, they may become a pattern of behavior, for others, they just become part of a temporary adjustment followed by sexual maturity in late adolescence or in the 20s.[34]

ATYPICAL SEXUAL BEHAVIOR IN ADOLESCENCE

This behavior includes homosexuality and transvestism. (See Chapter 5 for discussion of alternative forms of sexual expression.) Erickson[35] describes the bisexual confusion of adolescence. Young individuals may not feel themselves as clearly members of one sex or another, so they are easy victims of pressure from homosexual cliques. The bisexual confusion in adolescents joins their identity consciousness, or self-consciousness. The result is excessive preoccupation with the question of what kind of men or women they might become. An adolescent may feel that to be a little less of one sex means to be much more, if not all, of the other.

In contrast to the isolated or occasional homosexual experience of the heterosexual adolescent, some young men may establish homosexual identity. To most adolescents (and adults), *homosexuality* implies a male who is slight of build, not interested in girls, with nonmasculine interests. The adolescent who feels he meets these criteria begins to believe he may be homosexual. The chronic anxiety that results may lead to the avoidance of girls, followed in turn by the belief that he is incapable of being interested in the opposite sex. The self-label of *homosexual* also carries with it the expectation of failure in heterosexual relationships. Self-fulfilling prophecy may operate.

As an outcome of these fears, the troubled adolescent may inspect the genitals of little girls, may try to become interested in girls, but only "looks."[36] The adolescent who repeatedly and eagerly seeks out homosexual experiences is more likely to establish homosexual identity in later life, the majority of homosexuals "coming out" between ages 15 to 25.[37] There is a paucity of information about homosexuality and adolescent girls.

SOCIOCULTURAL PROBLEMS

The critical task of the adolescent is to obtain awareness of him/herself as independent from parents and to arrive at a sense of ego identity.[38] In order to arrive at this identity, some rebellion is necessary. Adolescence is a period of conflict between the child and society. The first conflict occurs in the home. It results from the parents' feeling that the child's sexuality must be controlled by them. However, adolescents have the autonomy to do what they wish sexually, so conflict ensues. Conflict may also arise between the parents' cultural background and values and those of adolescents' school and peer society. The debate about hetero–homosexuality is also part of the adolescent culture and confusion.[39]

Parents' confusion and ambivalence results in girls having to struggle through double talk and the double standard. The Women's Liberation Movement may give intellectually oriented parents the chance to abdicate the parents' role. This, along with advice that emphasizes adolescent freedom and fewer restraints, results in parents who have difficulty setting limits. The sexual acting out of teenage girls may also be due to pathologic encouragement by mothers who have their own unresolved sexual fantasies. Today, many of these activities may be encouraged under the guise of the Women's Liberation Movement.[40]

Peers are of vital importance to adolescents. What friends and classmates think of the adolescent takes precedence over anything else. Peers are important factors in terms of sexual behavior, since they may discourage or pressure the adolescent to engage in sexual activity. Adolescents who have not reached the psychologic maturity to cope with this pressure may become unhappy and troubled.

Society, and especially the parents and the schools, must also bear the blame for the problems arising from inadequate sex education. Teachers are as uncomfortable discussing the topic as are parents. (See Chapter 11.)

Adolescents obtain most of their information from peers—information that is distorted and inaccurate. Adolescents want to talk about: moral issues, homosexuality, contraceptives,[41] and sexual variations such as voyeurism, masturbation, venereal disease, and pregnancy.[42]

Obtaining health care for sexual problems is difficult for adolescents. They lack information about sources of care and are usually afraid to tell their parents about problems. In many states, adolescents cannot get treatment for venereal disease, counseling and care during pregnancy, or information about contraceptives without parental consent.

NURSING IMPLICATIONS

Assessment

Adolescents and their parents are reluctant to seek help, usually feeling uncomfortable about bringing sexual concerns to health professionals. Sexual problems often become known during legal, medical, or psychologic treatment for other problems. Consequently, nurses who have contact with adolescents and their parents must be alert to subtle signs that difficulties exist.

Problem identification should be a mutual task of the nurse and the adolescent. As with any age group, it is important that nurses not impose their definition of a problem on the adolescent. If they do, there is little chance that the interventions will be effective. Data collection should include the adolescent's chronologic age, level of psychosexual development, exposure to sexual activity, environmental pressures and support systems, and general physical development and health.

The adolescent is very self-conscious and can be intensely modest.[43] Physical examination is done in privacy without the parents' presence. This time can also be used to teach examination of the breasts by girls and examination of the testes by boys.[44]

Intervention

Adolescents need a chance to discuss their views of self and their feelings about the opposite and the same sex. They want to develop their values and are very responsive to empathetic adults. The ability to build trust is vital. Being open about sex with an authority figure (and the nurse may be viewed as such) is difficult. Patience to listen and not indicate shock or embarrassment is also vital.

Moralizing is a way to block communication. Adolescents like hearing about adult morals and values, but they do not want the values preached to them. Jensen[45] believes that the ability to reassure and give information about where to go or what to do for help is of greatest help. However, others believe that health professionals have the responsibility to give some moral guidance, that it should be emphasized to adolescents that intercourse should take place only when there is a deep and lasting relationship between two people—something different from infatuation. It should be pointed out that intercourse without deep respect for the other person is exploitative and immoral.[46]

Adolescents can gain clearer understanding of their beliefs through values clarification and use of a decision-making model, a process of developing a plan with a proposed course of action toward some goal.[47] When counseling, nurses learn first what the adolescent believes and values and then incorporates principles of decision making.[48] A buddy system in which each adolescent brings a best friend to a group helps provide the adolescent with a feeling of comfortableness and security.[49]

Assurance of confidentiality is essential since much information, particularly about sexual behavior, will be withheld if the teenager fears betrayal to parents. Parents may be concerned that confidentiality is an attempt to interfere with their rights and responsibility as parents. This rarely happens and most teenagers are willing to have summaries of sessions shared with parents.[50]

If parents arrive with the adolescent, the teenager is usually seen first, although some argue for initially interviewing families together.[51]

Specialized adolescent programs or clinics whose staff is knowledgeable, informative, personable, and interested in adolescent feelings are excellent resources.[52] It is estimated that in 1979, 417,000 unintended pregnancies were prevented by special programs in these clinics.[53]

Communication with adolescents can be difficult and frustrating, but with patience they will share concerns. Avoid rapid fire questions or waiting in silence. Keep appointments short and allow the adolescent some choice of date and time. Confronting silence with statements such as "I bet there are a hundred places you'd rather be right now" serves to relax the teenager. If the teenager is angry, address the anger directly. Limit setting may be necessary for inappropriate behavior or language.[54] There are pitfalls that the nurse avoids. Overidentification with the adolescent or the parent may cause the nurses to impose their own value system. Stereotyping, anger, and frustration of the nurse when progress does not seem to be being made may limit therapeutic effectiveness.

No matter what the approach, adolescents must be accepted and valued as they are without pressuring them to meet certain standards, since they are already frustrated by the expectations of parents and society and their inability to meet these expectations. They can grow through communication that is essentially an exchange of meaningful thoughts and feelings.

Masturbation. Many health professionals consider masturbation a normal part of adolescent development and necessary for control and integration of sexual urges. Adolescents should be told that it is not an unusual sexual practice, that it does not cause mental deterioration or physical decay, and that it has some advantages. Kinsey found that girls who masturbated to orgasm were more likely to enjoy intercourse when they reached sexual maturity.[55] Masturbation to orgasm can also relieve premenstrual tension and dysmenorrhea.

Pregnancy. If the adolescent girl becomes pregnant, she and her sexual partner need help and understanding to make decisions about the future direction of their lives.

The nurse can help the boy see that he has some obligations to the girl and the child. He must also be prepared for the girl's emotional commitment and dependence on him, since what may have been only a casual encounter to him may have been considered a love relationship by her. The nurse also helps him work through his feelings about the pregnancy.[56]

When a nonmarital pregnancy occurs, the nurse may be in a position to help the adolescent arrive at a decision about abortion, adoption, marriage, or keeping the baby. The nurse determines first who the girl has told about the pregnancy, then her sources of support, her relationship with her family and the father, and her feelings about the pregnancy and its meaning to her. If the girl has not told her parents, the nurse may be the one to help her break the news and to try to draw their anger and bitterness from their daughter before they make statements that they may regret in the future.

Rather than suggesting solutions to the pregnancy, an important question the nurse puts to the girl is, "Do you understand what the alternatives are?" The girl then has the opportunity to share her feelings about the pregnancy and what she wants to do about it.[57] The nurse helps her discuss alternatives

and arrive at her own solution. Since her feelings are usually ambivalent, this may not be possible immediately.

Each solution produces its own problems: possible guilt and depression after abortion or adoption; unstable and unsuccessful marriage if neither the boy nor the girl is mature enough for its responsibilities; economic, social, and child-rearing problems if the girl decides to keep the infant and raise it herself. The nurse's responsibility to help in the decision process may be great.

Adolescents who have had a pregnancy followed by abortion, birth, and/or adoption of the child need counseling to relieve the anguish and guilt. If the decision has been for abortion or adoption, girls particularly need help to work through their loss and grief. They may need support to help them keep up with school work and maintain peer relationships so they can go back to school.

Some adolescents describe absence of sexual interest after abortion. They may be helped by talking about their conflicts and their relationships with boyfriends and family, usually responding to reassurance that sexual interest will return in time. If there is evidence of depression or other emotional problems, they may need referral for psychiatric help. (See Chapter 20.)

Help is especially needed to avoid another pregnancy, since many continue to use ineffective contraceptive practices. Others enter into unsatisfactory marriages, get divorced, or have repeated unwanted pregnancies.[58] School nurses particularly can be in the forefront of casefinding and counseling.

Teaching

Adolescents need information about anatomy and physiology of sexuality. This information must be clearly, succinctly, and openly communicated. They need reassurance that isolated homosexual experiences do not mean that one is homosexual. Those with neurotic guilt may need the benefit of counseling or psychiatric therapy.

If contraceptive information is sought,

the nurse can be a valuable source of help. In most states, minors can get contraceptives without parental permission if they are emancipated, living away from home, and primarily self-sufficient. Most planned parenthood clinics are sources of help, and many physicians will prescribe the oral contraceptives without the parents' permission. Jensen[59] feels that the pill is not necessarily best for adolescents with infrequent intercourse, suggesting a combination of condom and foam, which he feels is almost 100 percent effective. Use of the condom and foam is inexpensive, does not have undesirable side effects, and prevents the spread of venereal disease (see Chapter 22).

The prevalent attitude that favors sexual intercourse makes it difficult for those who believe intercourse is reserved for marriage to feel comfortable with their sexuality. Virgin men may expecially feel that their masculinity is threatened. Women may be apologetic about themselves or may feel less than adequate. They need sources of support for their beliefs that sexual intimacy is reserved for marriage. Nurses working in schools or health clinics can be that source of support. In addition, nurses can suggest peer groups with similar values. Church groups are most effective.

The school nurse, who initiates teaching programs not only for students but for parents, can help all members of the family. In addition to content about sexuality, adolescents should be given a chance to discuss such questions as: "Should I have sex with my boyfriend?" "Is virginity valuable or not?" "What do others do?"

Concerns and guilt about sexual activity need to be ventilated by some. Others need to talk of their fears of being involved in sex at all, even after marriage. Group discussion is particularly helpful. (See Chapter 11.)

Evaluation
If adolescents can make their own thoughtful decisions about sexual behavior based on carefully identified and developed values as a result of nursing intervention, intervention will certainly have been successful. That is a major accomplishment not possible in some short-term care settings. However, the adolescent's ability to identify the consequences of certain sexual behavior and willingness to accept help and guidance from the nurse is evidence that the nurse has begun to increase sexual health.

NOTES

1. Teicher JD: Sexual deviations in children. In Sadock BJ, Kaplan HI, Freedman AM (eds): The Sexual Experience. Baltimore, Williams and Wilkins, 1976, pp 591–597
2. Dewhurst J: Breast disorders in children and adolescents. Pediat Clin North Am 28:287–338, 1981
3. Brown MA: Primary dysmenorrhea. Nurs Clin North Am 17:145—153, 1982
4. Gross RT, Duke PM: The effects of early versus late physical maturation on adolescent behavior. Pediatr Clin North Am 27:71–77, 1980
5. Oliven JF: Clinical Sexuality, 3rd ed. Philadelphia, Lippincott, 1974, p. 129
6. Ibid, p 130
7. Wilbur J: Sexual development and body image in the teenager with cancer. Front Radiat Ther Oncol 14:108–114, 1980
8. Teicher JD: Sexual deviations in children. In Sadock BJ, Kaplan HI, Freedman AM (eds): The Sexual Experience. Baltimore, Williams and Wilkins, 1976, p 393
9. Moore WT: Genital masturbation and adolescent development. In Oaks WW, Melchiode GA, Ficher I (eds): Sex and the Life Cycle. New York, Grune and Stratton, 1976, pp 53–66
10. Zelnick M, Kantner J: Sexual activity, contraceptive use and pregnancy among metropolitan-area teenagers: 1971–1979. Family Plan Persp 12:320–337, 1980
11. Ramsey P: Adolescent morality—a the-

ologian's viewpoint. Postgraduate Medicine 72:233–236, 1982

12. Lieberman F: Sex and the adolescent girl: Liberation or exploitation. In Gottesfeld ML (ed): Modern Sexuality. New York, Behavioral Publications, 1973, pp 224–243

13. Katchadourian H: Adolescent sexuality. Pediatr Clin North Am 27:17–28, 1980

14. Ibid, p 23

15. Rosenbaum MB: Female sexuality, or why can't a woman be more like a woman. In Oaks WW, Melchiode GA, Ficher J (eds). Sex and the Life Cycle. New York, Grune and Stratton, 1976, p 91

16. Gallup G: Sexual attitudes reveal conflict. The Plain Dealer, December 20, 1981, Sec c, p 7

17. Jensen GD: Adolescent sexuality. In Sadock BJ, Kaplan HI, Freedman AM (eds): The Sexual Experience. Baltimore, Williams and Wilkins, 1976, pp 142–154

18. Gadpaille WD: Adolescent sexuality and the struggle over authority. J School Health, 40, November 1970, pp 479–483

19. Jensen GD: Adolescent sexuality. In Sadock BJ, Kaplan HI, Freedman AM (eds): The Sexual Experience. Baltimore, Williams and Wilkins, 1976, p 147

20. Thornbury HD: Adolescent sources of information on sex. J School Health 51:274–277, 1981

21. Teen boys use luck as birth control. The Cleveland Press, March 12, 1982, Sec A, p 6

22. Reiss IL: Adolescent sexuality. In Oaks WW, Melchiode GA, Ficher I (eds): Sex and the Life Cycle. New York, Grune and Stratton, 1976, pp 45–52

23. Strahle WM: A model of premarital coitus and contraceptive behavior among female adolescents. Arch Sex Behav 12:67–89, 1983

24. Jensen GD: Adolescent sexuality. In Sadock BJ, Kaplan HI, Freedman AM (eds): The Sexual Experience. Baltimore, Williams and Wilkins, 1976, p 148

25. McCormack P: Most pregnant girls drop out of school. The Cleveland Press, June 18, 1981, Sec B, p 4

26. The Plain Dealer, April 27, 1978, p 12-D

27. Jensen C: The reluctant fathers. The Plain Dealer, Sunday Magazine, June 4, 1982

28. Ramsey P: Adolescent morality—a theologian's viewpoint. Postgraduate Medicine 72:236, 1982

29. Hinkelman D: Teenage sexuality: Making the responsible choice. Liguorian 69:20–33, 1981

30. Isikoff M: Critics howl, but move to stem teen sex moves ahead. The Plain Dealer, April 26, 1983, Sec C, p 1

31. Jensen GD: Adolescent sexuality. In Sadock BJ, Kaplan HI, Freedman AM (eds): The Sexual Experience. Baltimore, Williams and Wilkins, 1976, p 149

32. Ibid, p 146

33. Gadpaille WD: Adolescent sexuality and the struggle over authority. J School Health, 40, November 1970, p 482

34. Jensen GD: Adolescent sexuality. In Sadock BJ, Kaplan HI, Freedman AM (eds): The Sexual Experience. Baltimore, Williams and Wilkins, 1976, p 146

35. Erickson EH: Identity: Youth and Crisis. New York, Norton, 1968, p 27

36. Teicher JD: Sexual deviations in children. In Sadock BJ, Kaplan HI, Freedman AM (eds): The Sexual Experience. Baltimore, Williams and Wilkins, 1976, p 395

37. Jensen GD: Adolescent sexuality. In Sadock BJ, Kaplan HI, Freedman AM (eds): The Sexual Experience. Baltimore, Williams and Wilkins, 1976, p 149

38. Erickson EH: Childhood and Society. New York, Norton, 1963, pp 261–263

39. Lieberman F: Sex and the adolescent girl: Liberation or exploitation. In Gottesfeld ML (ed): Modern Sexuality. New York, Behavioral Publications, 1973, p 241

40. Ibid, p 242

41. Jensen GD: Adolescent sexuality. In Sadock BJ, Kaplan HI, Freedman AM

(eds): The Sexual Experience. Baltimore, Williams and Wilkins, 1976, p 153

42. Gordon S: What adolescents want to know. Am J Nurs 71:534–535, 1971

43. Cowell CA: The gynecologic examination of infants, children and young adolescents. Pediatr Clin North Am 28:247–266, 1981

44. Marks A: Aspects of biosocial screening and health maintenance in adolescence. Pediatr Clin North Am 27:153–161, 1980

45. Jensen GD: Adolescent sexuality. In Sadock BJ, Kaplan HI, Freedman AM (eds): The Sexual Experience. Baltimore, Williams and Wilkins, 1976, p 154

46. Gordon S: What adolescents want to know. Am J Nurs 71:535, 1971

47. Smith D, Hamrick M, Anspaugh S: Decision story strategy: A practical approach for teaching decision making. J School Health 51:637–639, 1981

48. Tauer KM: Promoting effective decision-making in sexually active adolescents. Nurs Clin North Am 18:275–292, 1983

49. Ibid, p 281

50. Adams BN: Adolescent health care: Needs, priorities and services. Nurs Clin North Am 18:237–248, 1983

51. Ibid, p 241

52. Resnick M, Blum RW, Heden D: The appropriativeness of health services for adolescents. J Adol Health Care 1:137, 1980

53. Forrest JD, Hermalin AI, Henshaw SK: The impact of family planning clinic program on adolescent pregnancy. Family Plan Persp 13:109–115, 1981

54. Adams BN: Adolescent health care: Needs, priorities and services. Nurs Clin North Am 18:245, 1983

55. Kinsey AC, Pomeroy WB, Martin CE, Gebhard PH: Sexual Behavior in the Human Female. New York, Pocket Books, 1965, p 172

56. American Medical Association: Human Sexuality. Chicago, AMA, 1972, pp 51–56.

57. Ibid, p 56

58. Osofsky HJ: Pregnant Teen-Ager. Springfield, Illinois, Thomas, 1968

59. Jensen GD: Adolescent sexuality. In Sadock BJ, Kaplan HI, Freedman AM (eds): The Sexual Experience. Baltimore, Williams and Wilkins, 1976, p 148

Chapter 17

Sexual Problems of Adulthood and Middlescence

If the sexual problems and concerns of adolescence are resolved, one might hope that adulthood would be free of problematic areas. However, the task defined by Erik Erikson of developing intimacy rather than living in isolation can be a formidable one both for those who chose marriage or for those who by choice or by circumstances are involved in other sexual life styles. Problems identified in this chapter include those defined by the individual and those identified by society. Sexual problems, like beauty, may be in the eye of the beholder, so there may be a lack of congruence between the individual's and society's concerns in relation to sexuality.

Since the vast majority of individuals chose marriage at some time in their life as a means of forming a permanent sexual relationship, much of this chapter will focus on the problems related to the marital relationship, as well as to the stable sexual relationship that may not include marriage. Sexual dysfunction, differences in sex drive, ignorance of arousal technique, anxiety about failure, and destructive interpersonal relationships may initiate problems. Changing roles and relationships and conflicts over family responsibilities are discussed along with the possible sequelae of these events, infidelity, and divorce. The problems of the single individual who is seeking a permanent relationship are more briefly mentioned.

Middlescence brings its own concerns—menopause, the male climacteric, and fears aroused by aging and changing relationships and family constellations.

MARRIAGE

Traditionally, marriage has been a stabilizing factor in society. Reed[1] identifies four apparent advantages of marriage for the achievement of sexual stability in a culture. First, with the formalized and permanent contact (at least in theory), a clear definition of the sexual domain and responsibilities occurs. The woman and man have clearly identified each other as sexual partners. Indiscriminate sexual activity may lead to social chaos, so there is value in the identification of a sexual choice. In addition, marriage helps insure the orderly distribution of property and insures the rights of the spouse and family when one of the partners dies, thus providing stability not only to the economic system but also to the family for the continued development of sexual roles and relationships. Marriage, in addition, combines the responsibilities of the sexual relationship with that of reproduction and socialization. Traditionally, the couple is expected to become parents and then to transmit the values, sexual and otherwise, of the culture so that the children learn the way of life of their society. Finally, marriage has some religious significance to much of society. This significance is rooted in the mystical view of sex and procreation, which many feel should take place within the marriage relationship.

Traditional views of the value and necessity of marriage have been under attack, however. Sexual relationships before marriage or outside of marriage are defended and/or advocated.

PROBLEMS OF ADULTHOOD

Biologic Aspects

Adulthood is not usually plagued with the health problems that may begin to surface in the middle and older years. It is a period of physical well-being and maturity. Significantly, there is a lack of parallelism in the development of the female and male's sexual responsiveness. Males peak at 17 or 18 years of age, after which there is steady decline in responsiveness. Females peak in their late 30s or early 40s and then decline at a slower rate than males. Since the usual practice in American society is for women to marry men older than themselves, problems may arise if the male is unable or uninterested in satisfying his sexual partner's desires. From the standpoint of sexual satisfaction, it might be wise for women to choose younger sexual partners.

Male impotence may become a problem, although the etiologic factors may be psychologic, rather than physiologic. With the emphasis on performance in a stable relationship, anxiety and a fear of failure may have a negative effect on potency.[2] Even when erections occur, premature ejaculation may contribute to the male's inability to satisfy his sexual partner (see Chapter 3).

The female may be troubled with orgasmic dysfunction. This, too, is usually related to anxiety over sexual satisfaction and orgasmic potential, excessive attention to

whether the orgasm is clitoral or vaginal, or whether her sexual appetite parallels that of the male.[3] Fear of intercourse may cause vaginismus and dyspareunia (see Chapter 3). Orgasmic dysfunction may also have a simpler etiology—inadequate personal hygiene by the marital or sexual partner. Vigorous use of a toothbrush and dental floss, a shower or bath, followed by use of a deodorant and a change of clothes may be the solution to some sexual problems.

The woman should also be aware of the importance of personal hygiene. Regular bathing, changing of perineal pads or tampons and use of deodorant will all increase sexual attractiveness.

There may be a conflict in beliefs about the suitability and/or morality of the use of alternate methods of sexual expression, either as foreplay or as a substitute for penile–vaginal intercourse. Oral–genital and manual–genital stimulation may be desired by one of the sexual partners and not the other, leading to discord in the relationship.

Differences in sexual drive may also contribute to problems. (See Chapter 4 for discussion of sexual drive.) Fatigue in either of the partners may decrease interest in sexual activity. If household tasks and care of children are still the major responsibility of the woman in addition to employment outside the home, she may have difficulty developing sexual tension. The male may also be fatigued by the physical and/or mental responsibilities of his job so that he is unresponsive to his partner's sexual advances.

Finally, one of the sexual partners may control the relationship by refusing sex because of minor physical problems—a headache removes the responsibility for engaging in sex, since the illness takes it out of the individual's control.

Despite having various sexual dysfunctions, however, 80 percent of 100 married, well-educated couples reported their marital sexual relations happy and 90 percent stated they would marry the same person again.[4] Frank and Anderson report from a study of 100 couples that it is possible to have a successful marriage without a highly active sex life and that emotional atmosphere is much more important than a feeling of satisfaction.[5] In an age that has emphasized sexual performance, there may be a new emphasis on intimacy and caring[6] and these may sustain the relationships.

Psychologic Aspects

Anxiety and fear of failure in sexual performance during adulthood may have their roots in adolescence. Adolescents may be subjected to social pressures to engage in premarital sexual activity. In an atmosphere usually characterized by secrecy, urgency, and perhaps discomfort, they may be disappointed with intercourse, discovering that the world did not revolve around sex and the experience did not meet its fantasized expectations. The male may have experienced some potency problems and the female orgasmic dysfunction. This initial failure coupled with fear and embarrassment leads to a vicious cycle of fear and failure, which may continue into adult relationships.

Paradoxically, with marriage, the socially ascribed freedom to involve oneself in erotic pleasure without fear of detection or censure may bring its own anxiety. Failure to achieve sexual satisfaction cannot be ascribed to adverse environmental factors as before. Concern about one's own pleasure as well as the partner's response may also decrease sexual response. This, combined with unrealistic expectations and sexual ignorance, easily leads to failure.

Poor self-esteem may contribute to feelings of insecurity in the male or female. Intrapsychic as well as interpersonal conflicts arise. Destructive interactions, coupled with poor communication regarding wants and needs of the sexual partner, leads to additional concerns.[7] Sexuality, an important part of the self-concept and self-identity, also serves as a form of communication. Through it, affection, love, hate, or anger can be expressed. Withholding of coitus may be used by one of the sexual partners to intimidate, antagonize, and punish the other.

Sociologic Aspects

The family has been called the critical unit of social change and some question if it is going out of existence.[8] Women may feel they have to choose between love and children and work and accomplishment. In the marriage relationship, the decision may be mutually made to delay the start of the family or not to have children at all.[9] However, if one partner feels pressured into the decision, conflict will inevitably occur—if not at the time of decision, later.

The birth of a child may also cause difficulties in the sexual relationship if the woman directs her attention and energy toward the child and the man feels that his needs—sexual and otherwise—are being neglected (see Chapter 21).

Changing roles and relationships may be threatening to the sexuality of the female or male. Traditionally, in the white middle class, the male has the role of the leader in the family. His education and activities determine the family's position in the community.[10] The female's responsibility was the affective life of the family. With the Women's Liberation Movement, women are frequently combining a career and the care of the family. Problems in the sexual relationship may occur if the woman feels guilty about her dual role, if she feels she is neglecting either the family or the career, and if the man is not supportive, either verbally or by accepting some of the responsibility for care of the children or the home.

Role conflict may occur between husband and wife over the division of responsibilities. The man may be threatened by the need to do tasks that he feels traditionally belong in the woman's domain. The man with a wavering self-esteem may also be severely threatened if his career achievements fail to match those of his spouse. Moreover, traditional beliefs and practices change slowly. A total of 23,000 *Psychology Today* readers returned questionnaires in response to the question "How do you like your job?" which in addition to disclosing feelings about jobs, also disclosed feelings about dual-career families. A random sample of the questionnaires returned showed that despite the influence of the women's movement, men's careers came first in two-career families. In addition, women were still left with most of the housework, most of the grocery shopping, cleaning, cooking, and child care. The younger the woman, the more likely that the household tasks were shared equally. Men and women also showed traditional attitudes on the issue of whose career comes first when both partners work. About 65 percent of the men said their career came first in decisions affecting both partners, while only 9 percent of the woman said theirs came first. The higher the man's income, the more resistant he was to moving. His mate's income had nothing to do with his decision.[11] If the marital partners share the same beliefs, conflict will probably be avoided. If there is lack of congruence in beliefs regarding employment priority, problems in the relationship may occur.

The years from 35 to 45 may be marked by an authenticity crisis. The roles that have been chosen earlier now seem too narrow and the life structure seems too confining. Any husband, wife, mother, father, or child to whom the individual has given faith in the past can be felt to be hemming one in. This may lead to depression, promiscuity, hypochondriasis, and such self-destructive conditions as alcoholism, drug-taking, suicide, and violent mood swings.[12]

With the advent of the Women's Liberation Movement, women are becoming more sexually aggressive, and some husbands or sexual partners may have difficulty handling the changing role behavior. The change in the woman's role during sexual intercourse may threaten some men's sexuality. Sex, historically, was something men did to women. The male may sense her demand for sexual satisfaction and not feel able to handle the pressure. Guilt and shame may follow inability to bring her to orgasm. This is especially true in the middle and upper class groups.

Ninety-eight percent of men questioned in a recent survey believed it was important for woman to have an orgasm, and the majority blamed themselves if the woman did not.[13] The survey's findings indicated that the man's enjoyment of sex may be greatly diminished by his partner's incomplete response; that he prefers an eager, active sexual partner; and that he tries to delay his own orgasm until the woman is satisfied.

Contrary to these findings, women respondents to a survey by Hite[14] complained that men were interested in their own satisfaction, were not interested in pleasing their female partners, and did not want to be taught how to do so. Abernathy[15] compared self-reported sexual satisfaction of a small sample of 24 feminists with 26 more traditionally oriented women. The findings gave no support to the supposition that woman's sexual response is enhanced by being dominated. Instead, a sense of power and aggressiveness were positively associated with sexual arousal in both sexes.

In the lower class groups, the male usually focuses on his performances and the female may put up with this without question, since as a group, the members are not psychologically oriented toward sexual relationships.[16]

The contradictory findings of these studies are significant in that they indicate not only that problems exist in some male–female relationships, but also that there are different views as to the nature of the problems that do exist. Perhaps of most importance is that sexual partners can mutually achieve sexual satisfaction with each other. Their inability or discomfort in communicating their sexual needs, feelings, fears, and what is pleasurable, what is not is the most pervasive problem.

Specific Problems Affecting the Sexual Relationship

Sexual Infidelity. Although actual figures indicated that 27 to 37 percent of men reported infidelity, in 1948, Kinsey suggested that it was safe to suggest that 50 percent of all men "cheat" on their wives and girlfriends.[17] Pietropinto and Simenauer's[18] findings from a survey of 4000 men confirm this figure. The response to the question "Have you ever cheated on your wife or steady girlfriend?" was 49.5 percent no, 28.5 percent yes with one or two others, 13 percent yes with many different women, 5.5 percent yes with partner's knowledge and consent, 2.8 percent never had a wife or steady girlfriend, and 1.0 percent no answer.

However, there is a considerable difference between those over 55 and those under. Excluding those who never had a wife or steady girlfriend, only 36 percent of those men 55 years and older were unfaithful, despite having lived longer. In contrast, half of the men between 30 and 54 and 52 percent of the men below age 30 were unfaithful. Although half of the men admitted being unfaithful, a higher percentage admitted thinking about it. Some stated they would cheat only if the affair was brief and casual or if the relationship with the regular partner was bad. Others (13 percent) stated they would cheat only if they were away from the partner for a long period, 12 percent would to have a different sexual partner, and 7 percent only if they fell in love.[19]

Reasons given for infidelity were usually poor sex or fighting with the partner—"poor communication at home," "Puritan hang-ups," or "arguments, especially nagging, or indifference." Some men admitted that the infidelity was prompted by an attractive brief opportunity. Extramarital activity in the adult years may also be due to a kind of age 30 crisis when individuals make an assessment of their life goals and styles. Often some precipitating event such as the death of a friend causes the reevaluation and desire for a different life style; as a consequence, extramarital sex and general marital dissatisfaction may occur.

Some seek help when extramarital sex is involved, some spouses tolerate it, and the involved partner may be confused as to how to manage the situation.

Pietropinto and Simenauer have concluded that there has been a definite increase in cheating, and this cheating has a deleterious effect on marital stability, pointing out that divorced men have a higher incidence of cheating than men currently married.[20]

Kinsey reported that 25 percent of women admitted that they had at least one extramarital affair.[21] On the basis of a survey of readers of *Redbook* in October 1974. Levin[22] has concluded that 40 percent of married women now engage in extramarital sex. However, his figures are open to question, since the study suffers from sampling errors that accompany surveys in popular journals. (See Chapter 8.)

Reasons given by women for sexual infidelity include search for excitement and romance, a variety of partners and sexual techniques, dissatisfaction with the present sexual partner, and/or a need for reaffirmation of sexual attractiveness.[23]

Moral considerations aside, it has generally been believed that sexual infidelity within or out of marriage indicates a weakness in the relationship. Currently there are some counterclaims that extramarital relations can strengthen a marriage. However, there is no evidence of major change in attitude regarding extramarital behavior. Eighty to 90 percent of couples in a Playboy Foundation survey felt that the prospect of infidelity by a spouse was unacceptable, and this applied to younger as well as older couples.[24]

Divorce. Infidelity is the chief reason for one of three divorces in the United States,[25] but conflict that leads to divorce may have many causes: partner disenchantment, often due to a secret desire to change the other, life processes such as personal growth and changes, comparison of the marriage with others and finding it wanting, inability to maintain the emotional "cost" of a relationship, and physical and emotional attraction to another. Destructive verbal fighting at a personal level that destroys trust and love and money problems may also be involved.[26]

In the period before the initiation of the divorce, there may be a period of emotional separation marked by hostility and alienation accompanied by an agonizing appraisal of the situation. The sexual pattern is not predictable. The emotionally separated male may commit adultery to drive his spouse away and to provoke desire for revenge. Other couples do not allow interpersonal antagonism to affect the sexual relationship, in fact describing it as adding new excitement to their sex life. However, after separation and withdrawal from the sexual relationship, the average woman may have lowered sexual responsiveness and the male may experience secondary impotence.[27]

The sexual response that takes place after divorce depends on personal attitudes and the meaning of the divorce in one's life. Some spouses eschew sex for several months or longer, others are promiscuous, seeking casual relationships. The most typical response is depression and with it a loss of libido. Anxiety over the future may also be present. Men may develop drinking problems and lowered work efficiency. Women may be left with the old circle of friends but may be considered a threat by their married peers.[28]

Some individuals desiring remarriage may suffer severe conflict about the decision if their religious beliefs prohibit remarriage after divorce. Financial considerations may also present obstacles to remarriage. Divorces that are followed by remarriages may result in families with children who are "hers, his, and theirs." Friction between the children and hostility of the children toward the new parent may interfere with sexual relationship of the woman and man.

Problems of the Single Life and Single Parenthood.

The number of individuals who have never married has increased. In the past, the derogatory terms "old maid" and "spinster" were applied to the unmarried female, and she was characterized as frigid, lonely, unhappy, and emotionally starved. Now she may be sterotyped as a carefree, promiscuous woman, seeking only sexual pleasure. Neither of these stereotypes is valid, but like all stereotypes they may operate to decrease the woman's opportunity to develop a sexual relationship.[29]

The image of the bachelor is more likely to be one of carefree, swinging male with many opportunities for sexual liaisons. He is less likely than the female to be characterized as emotionally starved. He may suffer additional pressures because of belief that he needs to perform sexually: always ready, willing, and able to have intercourse. Men like women, however, are not always "in the mood."

In their study of 3000 single men and women, Simenauer and Carroll[30] found that the singles were not swingers, only 20 percent of men and 6 percent of women approved casual sex and over 90 percent of the group agreed that platonic relationships are rewarding.

In reality the attitudes of singles, male and female, vary from individual to individual. Some are looking for any kind of relationship, casual or committed, to enrich their lives. Others vehemently deny any desire for marriage or sexual intimacy. Finding companionship and/or a permanent relationship is especially difficult for the single woman, especially if she is of low income and lives in a smaller town or rural area. Furthermore, the likelihood of marriage decreases with age.[31] Other single individuals freely choose their life style and enjoy the freedom to grow.

Single parents have additional problems especially if following divorce or death of a partner. Women may not be prepared to head a household since they are used to negotiating through men.[32] Other unmarried men and women choose single parenthood by adoption as a means of sharing their love with a child. Single parenthood, however, may cause logistic problems in establishing social and sexual relationships with others. Patton and Wallace[33] found that single parents stress the need for a close relationship and that 92 percent of the men and 81 percent of the women had engaged in intercourse after becoming single.

More research is needed on the effects on the sexual behavior of children raised by one parent.

NURSING IMPLICATIONS

Assessment

A careful gathering of data is necessary, since problems are diverse and varied in scope. Age, sex, marital status, and marital history should be ascertained. A listing of significant others, family members, and the occupations of the individuals should be obtained. The presence of and number of children and/or the beliefs of the partners about having children should also be part of the data base. Information about the sexual relationship should be obtained:

1. Who is the initiator of sexual activity?
2. Is there compatibility of beliefs about various forms of sexual activity and the frequency of intercourse?
3. Are there similar attitudes in both sexual partners toward sexual activity in general?
4. What have been the early experiences with intercourse, negative or positive?
5. Is there conflict or congruency of beliefs about the morality of sexual practices?
6. Has there been a change in relationship since children have arrived?

If the woman remains at home, information about her satisfaction with this life style should be obtained. If both partners work outside the home additional information should include (1) the degree of the partners' satisfaction with their own and their spouse's job, (2) the presence of division of home responsibilities that is satisfactory to both partners.

The nurse should question about the degree of sexual role satisfaction of each partner and the history of extramarital sexual relationships and generally ascertain if there are any life practices of either sexual partner that offends the other. Finally, the nurse assesses the level of self-esteem and the ability of the sexual partners to communicate with each other. (See the Appendix for specific information to be obtained in the history at various stages of the life cycle.)

If the patient/client is not married, data relating to the sexual life style and the individual's degree of satisfaction with that life style should be obtained. Concerns about sexual functioning and sexual role should also be ascertained to identify areas of teaching and counseling that may be needed.

Planning

The nurse's initial and primary goal is to facilitate communication between the sexual partners so that concerns can be shared and problems mutually resolved. The nurse also plans to teach about sexuality to clarify misconceptions and provide information about sexual behavior and response.

Intervention

Many sexual problems can be alleviated by health teaching to correct myths and misconceptions about sexual activity. Giving of information about intercourse, the importance of foreplay, the male and female response cycle, the importance of good hygiene practices, and suggestion of different times for intercourse to decrease fatigue and enhance pleasure may be all that is needed to increase sexual well-being.

If there is conflict in role relationships, the nurse may serve as a catalyst to increase communication and problem solving of the sexual partners. However, if the problems are severe, referral to a sexual counselor may be necessary.

If the individual is faced with divorce, the nurse can provide the empathetic ear to help the persons verbalize concerns, identify solutions, and to generally reduce tension. Nurses particularly can help increase the communication between sexual partners by providing a climate of care and concern in which each partner feels free to verbalize concerns and feelings, and sexual issues related to divorce.

It may be necessary to work with the woman to help her develop independent self-identity, positive self-esteem, and the ability to assume financial responsibility for herself and the family[34]

Single individuals may need or desire teaching about alternate forms of sexual expression. They may have concerns if they use masturbation as a way of reducing sexual tension yet fear adverse physiologic and psychologic effects. Teaching to correct myths and misconceptions may be all that is necessary. However, if the individuals have strong religious beliefs prohibiting masturbation, nurses should not urge it as an acceptable form of sexual activity, since patients/clients may experience severe guilt responses if they do masturbate. In addition, the patient's/client's trust in the nurse as a reliable source of health information in the future may be destroyed.

Nurses who are knowledgeable about the community's social activities may also serve as a resource person to suggest activities and organizations where the individual may find opportunities to meet others. Church groups, philanthropic organizations, and groups organized around special interests such as nature clubs, biking clubs, travel clubs may all provide opportunity for social interaction with both sexes and the possibility of the formation of a deeper sexual relationship.

Groups such as Parents Without Partners have been organized to help single parents meet others, share problems, and provide support for each other. Churches have also organized groups to offer support to those who are trying to rebuild their lives after separation, divorce or remarriage. Reassurance and encouragement to initiate these social activities may be all that is needed as an impetus to widen sociosexual relationships.

THE MIDDLE YEARS

The middle years include the period from 47 to 65 years of age. Many of the problems that

may occur in young adulthood and adulthood for some persons surface in the middle years for others. However, there are certain problems which more especially occur in this period of the life cycle.

Biologic Aspects

During the middle years, hair may begin to thin and gray, wrinkling of the skin occurs, and both sexes may struggle to avoid the sagging abdomen and thickening waistline that herald middle age. These changes become problematic when individuals are unable to accept or cope with them. Midlife and menopause are often used interchangeably but this puts undue emphasis on one event in a passage to another developmental phase. Middle age may also need to be redefined as couples start their families in the late 30s.[35]

In the female, menopause signals the end of monthly menstruation. The average age of onset is around 50, although the "change of life" includes the years from 46 to 60. Menstruation commonly stops between the ages of 46 and 50. The changes in menopause are related to decreased production of estrogen by the ovaries. Atrophy of the reproductive organs follows. In the years after menopause, the fat in the breast decreases and the soft glandular tissue is replaced by fibrous cords. The vagina shrinks in size and loses some of its elasticity. The vulva becomes thinner and loses the engorgement response to sexual stimulation. There is a decrease in vaginal secretions necessary for lubrication during intercourse. The lining of the vagina becomes less acid, increasing its susceptibility to infection.[36-37] Hormone therapy may decrease these physical changes; natural vaginal secretions may be replaced by estrogen-containing creams or suppositories (see Chapter 18). Additional symptoms resulting from endocrine imbalance may include insomnia, "hot flashes," headaches, heart palpitations, and depression. Supplemental hormones may decrease these symptoms.

Reaction to sexual stimulation changes, usually decreasing. Breast engorgement and nipple erection, engorgement of the clitoris and labia, and vaginal secretions decrease. Contractions of the pelvic platform that occur during orgasm are less vigorous and less frequent.[38] (See Chapter 3 for details of the sexual response cycle.)

The physiologic changes in the male and female are biologic givens; how individuals respond to them and to other life changes is dependent on psychologic and sociocultural factors. Anxiety and depression may accompany the physiologic changes. Fears of loss of sexual attractiveness and loss of the partner to a young individual may affect sexual responsiveness in one or both partners. Men fear age, women fear that menopause will reduce their sexual capacity.

Uphold and Susman[39] found that women low on marital adjustment had significantly more frequent and severe symptoms during climacteric than women high on marital adjustment. Some women have thought of menopause as a disease[40] but a study of 152 middle-class white females 18 to 55 indicated that women are reversing this trend. These women did not attribute pathopsychologic characteristics to women in menopause.[41]

Changes in sexual activity and interest may occur. Not all are negative. Many women report an increase in subjective feelings of pleasure and satisfaction after menopause, and others report no change. Increased satisfaction in intercourse may result from the freedom from fear of pregnancy. Others may use menopause as an excuse to halt sexual activity, causing severe conflict in the relationship if it is not a mutually agreed upon decision.

Males also experience sexual changes with increasing age. Androgen levels decrease slowly until the age of 60. Sperm production does not cease, and although fertility may be decreased, viable sperm can be produced in elderly men.[42] The decrease in hormones is slower and milder than in women, and males may have a reproductive decline without clinical symptoms comparable to those of menopause. Physical changes include a decreased amount of ejaculate and

less forceful ejaculation. The testes become smaller and less firm, and erections may be less frequent and less rigid. By the age of 50, the refractory period increases and the male may require 8 to 24 hours after orgasm before another erection can be achieved. Resolution proceeds more quickly.[43] One advantage to men and their sexual partners is that the male needs a longer period of stimulation to achieve erection and to reach orgasm.[44] Thus, the male is able to prolong intercourse and lengthen the period of pleasure for his partner and himself.

Middle aged men may experience irritability, fatigue, restlessness and insomnia, urinary irregularities, fluid retention, and hot flashes that interfere with sexual activity.[45] They may complain of decreased libido. Midlife impotence may occur, but in 90 percent of the cases, results from a combination of ignorance about the normal changes in response to sexual stimulation and to male sexual anxiety. Masters and Johnson state flatly that the male is tremendously susceptible to the power of suggestion with regard to his sexual prowess to an almost unbelievable degree. The slightest suggestion that sexual capability is decreasing may cause free-floating anxiety and subsequent secondary impotence.[46]

Although sexual activity may decrease, George and Weiler[47] found in their longitudinal study of 278 women and men 46 to 71 years of age, that sexual activity remained more stable over time than has been suggested. Women reported significantly lower interest in sexual activity than did the men, although both sexes attributed responsibility for cessation of sexual activity to the male partner. The findings may indicate the importance of the male role as the *initiator* of activity.

Other health deviations may affect sexual response. The chronic diseases of the middle years—diabetes, cardiovascular disease, and cancer—may cause cessation of sexual activity (see Unit V). Excessive indulgence in alcohol and in food may cause problems. Chronic alcoholism may be marked by decrease in potency and orgasmic function (see Chapter 30).

Psychologic Aspects

The biologic changes may be accompanied by anxiety and depression. Much attention has been given to the menopause as a stressful period for the woman. The male climacteric may also be a period of stress. It is a time when the male should have reached his peak of socioeconomic achievement. Self-evaluation may find the male concluding that he has not reached his expected potential. Fear of what he can accomplish in the future and dissatisfaction with what has been accomplished in the past may lead to depression and decreased self-esteem. He may suddenly resent the family responsibilities that he had accepted eagerly in adulthood. His solution may involve extramarital sexual activity, since sex may symbolize status and bolster his wavering self-esteem.

Extramarital activity by both partners may be due to monotony and a mechanistic approach to sexual activity. The man may choose a more youthful partner whose inexperience he can control and who poses less of a threat to his decreasing sexual capacity. The wife, frightened because the husband avoids sex and shows less interest, may have an extramarital affair to test if she is still desirable.[48,49]

Communication problems that have been hidden during the child-raising and career-focusing years of adulthood may surface during the middle years as the partners in the marital relationship once more focus on each other and their relationship instead of child-raising concerns.

Sociologic Aspects

As children grow and leave the home, the woman is suddenly faced with an "empty nest." For some it may be a period of stress, since much of their energy and talent has been directed toward child-raising and housekeeping, the mother role. Suddenly the children are gone and the house is too large.

To another woman the empty nest represents freedom to extend her concern to others, into political reform or national movements. She may become aggressive in the service of her convictions rather than directing her energies to her children's and family's needs. Society is the beneficiary. As the male may struggle to defeat his stagnation and continue his generativity, the comparable task for women is to transcend dependency through self-declaration.[50]

This may cause additional stress on roles and relationships that have developed over the years. If the woman aggressively seeks to resume or to increase her commitment to a career, the man, suffering through his own crisis, may feel threatened and anxious. If open communication about concerns is not present, the relationship may be fractured.

NURSING IMPLICATIONS

Assessment

Many of the problems that can occur in adulthood may surface in the middle years. It is important that nurses note whether an identified problem is of long-standing duration or whether it is of recent occurrence. The parameters of assessment identified for adulthood apply to the middle years, with some additions.

Information about menopause should be obtained—whether it is completed or whether the individual is still experiencing any physiologic and psychologic consequences. In the male, objective and subjective data indicating the male climacteric should be gathered. Presence of other health deviations in both sexes should be identified. The meaning of these changes to both sexes should be ascertained, since many individuals accept these events with equanimity, requiring little assistance, while others need counseling and much emotional support. (See the Appendix for specific information to be obtained in the history at various stages of the life cycle.)

Careful assessment should be made to determine the presence of depression, anxiety, and/or hostility that may be affecting the sexual relationship or that may be caused by changes in sexual relationships. It is especially important to assess the degree of satisfaction with the sexual role responsibilities, changes in role due to changes in the family constellation, and finally, job satisfaction, since these may all affect the sexual relationships.

Planning

The nurse's goals are essentially the same as those applicable to problems of adulthood.

Intervention

LaRocco and Polit[51] found that women are deficient in their own knowledge about menopause. Teaching to dispel myths and misconceptions about the "change of life" is essential. Referral to a physician for estrogens may be needed but therapy is as brief and low as possible while still alleviating symptoms.[52] A willing and compassionate listener may be all that is needed by other patients/clients to help them solve problems.

Myths and misconceptions that sexual activity is not suitable for those past menopause and the climacteric can be dispelled by the nurse. If the woman is experiencing vaginal atrophy and decreased lubrication during intercourse, the nurse can recommend the use of water-soluble jellies (such as K-Y jelly), saliva, or insertion of the finger in the vagina to bring out secretions deeper in the vaginal barrel. The physician may order vaginal medication containing estrogen to inhibit the atrophic process.

Hot flashes may be relieved by removing clothing, seeking cooler surroundings, bathing, or changing activities. Women can be reassured that they are temporary and not dangerous.[53]

Educational programs stress body changes, the role of hormones, the role of and need for exercise of the pubococcygeus muscle, and permission and reassurance to be sexual. Postmenopausal zest (PMZ) depends on a healthy life style, proper nutrition, proper weight, maintenance of friends and activities.[54]

The etiology of changes in sexual drive and interest by one or both of the sexual partners must be determined before intervention can take place. If due to illness, treatment of the underlying problem must be initiated. If due to monotony in the sexual relationship, teaching about alternate lovemaking techniques may be all that is needed to meet the partners' changing needs for stimulation and gratification.

Giving accurate information about the normal changes the male experiences in his response cycle during the middle years and allowing him to verbalize fears and concerns may prevent the occurrence of secondary impotence. The nurse points out that his greater ejaculatory control and ability to maintain an erection may improve the quality of his sex life. Prolonged lovemaking is possible, and his ability to satisfy his sexual partner may increase. There is no rigid standard of performance. Masters and Johnson[55] indicate that the man of 60 can experience sexual satisfaction if he reserves his ejaculation altogether. In this way, sexual tension will increase to a climax that meets his expectation.

For both the female and the male, the best defense against the problems related to aging is regular intercourse, once or twice a week over a period of years. Consistency of sexual relations maintains sexual vigor.[56] If mutually agreed upon, the decision to decrease the frequency of intercourse may not cause sexual conflicts. Problems may ensue, however, if it is a decision by one of the partners. Counseling may be necessary if no resolution of the problem can be reached.

Interpersonal conflicts that take place over change in sexual roles may also require in-depth counseling, although the nurse's ability to promote communication between the couples may help them share concerns and decide on a mutually satisfactory solution, especially if the relationship has been a positive one in the past.

Evaluation

Accurate identification of the problems and setting of realistic goals is essential. Changes in behavior that indicate teaching and counseling has been successful include lifting of depression, expressions of satisfaction with the life situation, and increased

communications between the sexual partners.

NOTES

1. Reed DM: Traditional marriage. In Sadock BJ, Kaplan HI, Freedman AM (eds): The Sexual Experience. Baltimore, Williams and Wilkins, 1976, pp. 217–230

2. Masters WH, Johnson VE: Human Sexual Inadequacy. Boston, Little, Brown, 1970, pp 157–192

3. Reed DM: Traditional marriage. In Sadock BJ, Kaplan HI, Freedman AM (eds): The Sexual Experience. Baltimore, Williams and Wilkins, 1976, p 222

4. Crown S, D'Ardenne P: Symposium on sexual dysfunction: Controversies, methods, results. Brit J Psychiat 140:70–77, 1982

5. Heckmann N: Sex doesn't determine a happy marriage. The Cleveland Press, November 9, 1981, Sec B p 10

6. Phillips D: Sexual Confidence: Discovering the Joy of Intimacy. New York, Houghton Mifflin, 1983

7. Ficher I: Sex and the marriage relationship. In Oaks WW, Melchiode GA, Ficher I (eds): Sex and the Life Cycle. New York, Grune and Stratton, 1976, pp 81–86

8. Johnson M: The Health of Families in a Culture of Crisis. Kansas City, American Nurses Foundation, 1981

9. Morrow L: Wondering if children are necessary. Time, March 5, 1979, pp 42–47

10. Fleck S: The family. In Sadock BJ, Kaplan HI, Freedman AM (eds): The Sexual Experience. Baltimore, Williams and Wilkins, 1976, pp 155–181

11. Renwick PA, Lawler EE: What you really want from your job. Psychol Today 11(12):53–65, 1978

12. Sheehy G: Passages. New York, Dutton, 1976

13. Pietropinto, A, Simenauer J: Beyond the Male Myth. New York, New York Times Books, 1978, pp 153–158

14. Hite S: The Hite Report. New York, Macmillan, 1977

15. Abernathy V: Feminists heterosexual relationships. Arch Gen Psychiatry 35:435–438, 1978

16. Ficher I: Sex and the marriage relationship. In Oaks WW, Melchiode GA, Ficher I (eds): Sex and the Life Cycle. New York, Grune and Stratton, 1976, p. 84

17. Kinsey AC, Pomeroy WB, Martin CE: Sexual Behavior in the Human Male. Philadelphia, Saunders, 1948, p 585

18. Pietropinto A, Simenauer J: Beyond the Male Myth. New York, New York Times Books, 1978, p 278

19. Ibid, pp 279–282

20. Ibid, p 290

21. Kinsey AC, Pomeroy WB, Martin CE, Gebhard PH: Sexual Behavior in the Human Female. New York, Pocket Books, 1965, p 417

22. Levin RJ: The Redbook report: Study of female sexuality, premarital and extramarital sex. Redbook 145 (6):38–44, 190, 1975

23. Pauly IB: Premarital and extramarital intercourse. In Sadock BJ, Kaplan HI, Freedman AM (eds): The Sexual Experience. Baltimore, Williams and Wilkins, 1976, pp 256–267

24. Hunt MM: Sexual Behavior in the 1970's. Chicago, Playboy Press, 1974, pp 255–257

25. Bartusis MA: Infidelity, separation and divorce. Curr Psychiat Ther 20:95–101, 1981

26. Turner NW: Sexual issues in separation and divorce. Top Clin Nurs 1:39–44, 1980

27. Reed DM: Sexual behavior in the separated, divorced and widowed. In Sadock BJ, Kaplan HI, Freedman AM (eds): The Sexual Experience. Baltimore, Williams and Wilkins, 1976, pp 249–255

28. Ibid, pp 252–253

29. Proulx C: Sex as athletics in the singles

complex. Saturday Review, May 1973, pp 23–29

30. Simenauer J, Carroll D: Singles: The New Americans. New York, Simon and Schuster, 1982

31. DeLora JS, Warren CAB: Understanding Sexual Interaction. Boston, Houghton Mifflin, 1977, pp 27–29

32. Duffy M: When a woman heads the household. Nurs Outlook 30:468–473, 1982

33. Patton RD, Wallace BC: Sexual attitudes and behaviors of single parents. J Sex Educ Ther 19:39–41, 1979

34. Berman WH, Turk DC: Adaptation to divorce, problems and coping strategies. J Marriage and the Family 43:179–189, 1981

35. Carroll JS: Middle age does not mean menopause. Top Clin Nurs 4:38–44, 1983

36. Rubin I: Sexual Life After Sixty. New York, Basic Books, 1965, pp 122–135

37. Stanford D: All about sex . . . after middle age. Am J Nurs 77:608–611, 1977

38. Master WW, Johnson VE: Human Sexual Response. Boston, Little Brown, 1966, pp 223–247

39. Uphold CR, Susman EJ: Self-reported climacteric symptoms as a function of the relationships between marital adjustment and childbearing stage. Nurs Research 30:84–88, 1981

40. MacPherson K: Menopause as disease. The social construction of a metaphor. Adv Nurs Science 3:95–113, 1981

41. Muhlenkamp AF, Walker MM, Bourne AE: Attitudes toward women in menopause: A vignette approach. Nurs Research 32:20–23, 1983

42. Rubin I: Sex Life After Sixty. New York, Basic Books, 1965, pp 112–121

43. Masters WH, Johnson VE: Human Sexual Response. Boston, Little Brown, 1966, pp 248–270

44. Ibid, p 251

45. Ruebsaat HJ: The Male Climacteric. New York, Hawthorn Books, 1975

46. Belliveau F, Richter L: Understanding Human Sexual Inadequacy. New York, Bantam, 1970, pp 134–135

47. George LK, Weiler SJ: Sexuality in middle and later life. Arch Gen Psychiat 38:919–923, 1981

48. Ficher I: Sex and the marriage relationship. In Oaks WW, Melchiode GA, Ficher I (eds): Sex and the Life Cycle. New York, Grune and Stratton, 1976, p 85

49. Hotcher B: Menopause and sexuality: Gearing up or down. Top Clin Nurs 1:45–52, 1980

50. Sheehy G: Passages. New York, Dutton, 1976, p 294

51. LaRocco S, Polit D: Women's knowledge about menopause. Nurs Research 29:10–13, 1980

52. Pearson L: Climacteric. Am J Nurs 82:1098–1100, 1982

53. Shaver J: Women's physiologic adaptations to reproduction. In Smith ED (ed): Women's Health Care: A Guide for Patient Education. New York, Appleton-Century-Crofts, 1981, pp 9–22

54. Caldwell LR: Questions and answers about menopause. Am J Nurs 82:1100–1101, 1982

55. Masters WH, Johnson VE: Human Sexual Response. Boston, Little, Brown, 1966, pp 251–256

56. Ibid, p 270

Chapter 18

Sexual Problems of Aging

The author has chosen 65 as the onset of older age, not because it necessarily represents the advent of sexual old age but because symbolically for some, at least, 65 may represent the passage into the realm of the aged. It must be emphasized that chronologic age is not what defines sexual senescence. Some individuals are "old" at 50, others are vigorous and sexually active into their 90s.

Although generalizations are made, the aged are not a homogeneous population and life styles differ according to social class, health status, and education. The needs and desires of a funloving "swinger" in a retirement community may differ from the aged poor in a large city or an aging farmer. Individuals in a lower socioeconomic class are more likely to "give in" to aging and accept dysfunction and disability.[1]

Some of the sexual "problems" associated with the older years are those defined or created by society and not necessarily by the individuals. Sociocultural factors may contribute to bio-psychologic problems of age. For this reason, this chapter will begin with a discussion of sociocultural factors and sexuality in the older population.

SOCIOCULTURAL ASPECTS

Masters and Johnson[2] have stated that reasonable good health and an interesting and interested partner should ensure an active sexual life even into the 80s. Ignorance is one of the greatest deterrents to successful sexual function in all ages, but it is the most crippling in the aging. Myths and misconceptions have continued because information was lacking. Many couples, when faced with the male's slower erection and quicker detumescence in the middle years may have severely curtailed sexual activity, believing "It will all be over soon."[3] Kuhn[4] identified five such myths. The first is that sex does not matter and is not important in the later years, which are supposed to be (and usually are, in society's eyes) sexless: a belief possibly linked to the religious tradition that considers sex as virtuous only if related to reproduction of the species.

The second misconception is that an interest in sexual activity is abnormal for older people. Giving compliments to members of the opposite sex and a certain amount of conversational sexual innuendo is often quite acceptable in much of society when done by a 30-year-old male. If the same behavior is evidenced by a 70-year-old male, he may be considered "a dirty old man." The woman who continues a high level of interest in her personal appearance in her 70s may be described as a silly and vain woman. Children reject the idea that their older parent remains sexually active and may view an aged parent's interest in sex as unhealthy, unnatural, or a sign of second childhood. Young people have negative fantasies when they think of two older people making love. By and large, elderly people want to do the conventional thing. If society says sexuality is wrong, they conform. Guilt feelings about sexuality develop if their feelings are not acceptable to the people with whom they associate.[5]

The third myth is that remarriage should be discouraged after the loss of a spouse. Often children are especially vehement in their disapproval, and the surviving parent, fearful of alienating the family, changes plans.[6]

The fourth myth is that it is acceptable for the older man to seek younger women as sexual partners but ridiculous for the older woman to become involved with younger men. The problem is particularly acute if children are negative about the relationships. The older man offers experience in sexual relationships and knowledge of the world to the younger woman. It is equally true that younger men may find the older woman desirable and attractive, notwithstanding society's attitude.[7]

The final myth is that older people should be separated by sex in institutions and privacy between the sexes should be prohibited. This is usually done primarily to avoid problems for the staff and to avoid criticism by families and the community. Consequently, the patients are denied the opportunity to form satisfying sexual relationships, relationships that may or may not involve physical sex. Sexuality is more than sexual intercourse. Isolating patients denies them the opportunity for a deep psychologic and spiritual relationship with someone of the opposite sex.[8]

Many health professionals hold some of the same misconceptions as the larger society. In three studies of nursing homes and their staffs, findings indicated severe negative attitudes toward sexuality in the aged by staff and the aged themselves who internalize society's negative attitudes.[9–11]

Perhaps attitudes are changing, however. In a random sample of female nursing students, Damrosch[12] found that the subjects saw the sexually active 68-year-old as more alert, cheerful, well adjusted, and physically attractive. Although the subjects favored the sexually active patient, they felt that nursing home staffs would like them less.

Society, however, should not bear the brunt of censure for absence of sexual activity in older individuals. Some, by choice, have discontinued sexual activity and are satisfied and fulfilled. Negative comments about what was viewed as promotion of sex for the elderly were expressed by the author of a "golden years column"[13] who feels older people are being bombarded with information about sexual activity. It may provide some recreation, perhaps, and some feeling of well-being, but he questions its social value.[14]

He goes on to say that what an older man and woman do in their bedroom is nobody else's business: that ultimately the decision about what is normal or abnormal rests with the individuals.

BIOLOGIC ASPECTS

Myths accrue to the biologic aspects of sexuality, also. One is that the elderly could not make love if they wanted to. Another is that they are too fragile and may hurt themselves with sexual relations. Another is that the emission of semen is debilitating,[15] and finally, that the elderly are physically unattractive and therefore sexually undesirable.[16] Older individuals may adopt these ideas, and the myth of sexless older years becomes a self-fulfilling prophecy.

Many older individuals have great curiosity and want to learn about sexuality. They have had considerable experience but lack information.[17]

The biologic changes women experience after menopause may also cause problems. Sex steroid starvation may result in uncomfortable or even painful penetration, vaginal burning, pelvic aching, or irritation on urination due to continued thinning of the vaginal mucosa and decreased elasticity of the vaginal barrel. Some women may experience spastic uterine contraction during or shortly after orgasm and pain in the abdomen and/or the labia majora. These symptoms are more likely to occur with infrequent intercourse of only one time a month or less. Regular and more frequent sexual activity results in a higher capacity for sexual performance.[18]

The decreased hormone levels of the male may continue to cause changes that began in the middle years (Chapter 17). As long as these biologic changes are not misinterpreted and do not result in anxiety, men may be sexually competent into their 70s and 80s with regular sexual activity and reasonable good health. It is a sexual myth that the aging process per se will cause erectile incompetence in the older male[19] (see Table 18-1).

When sexual dysfunction occurs, health professionals may not be interested in the problems of the aged. In a study of 35 older men with sexual dysfunction, Kofoed and Bloom[20] found that physicians were often uninterested in initiating therapy.

General poor health may result in one or both of the sexual partners deciding to stop sexual intercourse. However, a survey indicated that four of five males in good health still had sexual interest, although actual sexual intercourse decreased with advancing age.[21]

In order to determine why some older men are more or less sexually active, Martin[22] conducted a study of 188 60- to 70-year-old married men. He found that none stopped coitus because they thought the aged should be sexless. In spite of good health, however, 35.6 percent of the respondents reported no more than 6 sexual events each year, while those in the "most active" groups reported having coitus 93.5 times within the year. Findings suggested that a low level of sexual activity was due to decreased motivation and that subjects generally maintained high or low patterns over their life span.

Sources of sexual stimulation seem to change also. Money,[23] on the basis of anecdotal data, indicates that the older individuals have decreased dependence on imagery and fantasy and increased dependency on touch for stimulation.

In a population of 800 aged 60 to 91, Starr and Weiner[24] found that older people express their sexuality in more diffuse and varied ways with more emphasis on pleasuring, touching, cuddling, and less goal orientation, but they maintained continued interest in sex and remained sexually active.

There is no complete explanation why some postmenopausal women remain sexually active or become more so while others lose interest.

Christenson and Gagnon[25] found that sexual behavior continues into later life, though its frequency decreases with age. At age 50, seven-eighths of the women were still having coitus with their husbands well over once a week. By age 60, however, participation in sexual activity dropped to 70 percent of the group, and by age 65 to 50 percent.[26] The male was the strongest factor in setting the frequency of intercourse. After marriage ends, the woman's previous capacity to reach orgasm appears to be a strong factor in her desire to continue coitus and to seek out sexual activity.[27]

Masters and Johnson[28] question why every episode of sexual interaction should end in orgasm, that a warm sensual experience of holding and being held should not be viewed as a failed sexual experience because one or both partners did not attain orgasm. They also question our society's "orgasmic mania."

PSYCHOLOGIC ASPECTS

Sexual dysfunction in the older couple in the absence of physical illness may be due to lack of information about changing physiology, resulting in anxiety. It may also be due to a dysfunctional marital relationship, either short-term because of life stresses or long-term because of long-standing problems.[29]

The stresses and crises of aging are related to the growing number of losses experienced by the elderly; losses due to relocation to different communities after retirement, withdrawal, and death of the people around

TABLE 18–1. VAGINAL AND PENILE CHANGES IN SEXUAL RESPONSE WITH AGING

	Female	Male
Excitement	1. Rate and amount of vaginal lubrication decreases 2. Decrease in degree and rapidity of expansion of inner two-thirds of vaginal barrel	1. Speed of penile erection doubled or trebled or longer 2. Erection maintained for extended periods without ejaculation 3. When erection is attained and then lost without ejaculation, there is more difficulty returning to full erection with further stimulation, i.e., a refractory period occurs in the excitement phase
Plateau	1. Expansion of vaginal barrel continues 2. Vasocongestion in outer third of vagina reduced (orgasmic platform) 3. Once platform developed, lumen of vagina constricted to degree proportional to that of younger woman	1. Full erection not attained until just before ejaculatory phase 2. Involuntary increase in glans circumference and increased length and diameter of entire penile shaft prior to ejaculation
Orgasmic	1. Contraction of orgasmic platform develops as in younger women, but phase decreased in duration 2. Orgasmic platform contractions recur three to five times (five to ten times in younger women)	1. Decrease in amount and ejaculatory force (semen expelled 6 to 12 inches rather than 12 to 24 inches of younger man) 2. If extended penile erection, ejaculation may be one of fluid seepage, rather than under pressure 3. Fewer expulsive contractions (one to two) and increased interval between contractions
Resolution	1. Rapid collapse of inner two-thirds of vagina and entire vaginal barrel	1. Extended refractory period, especially after age 60 2. Rapid penile detumescence after ejaculation

Masters, William W. and Johnson, Virginia E.: Human Sexual Response. *Boston, Little, Brown, 1966, pp. 233–236, 251–254.*

them (friends, relatives, spouses). Many more older women, especially, are left, since the tendency has been to marry older men.

Loss of role and that status associated with employment and the concomitant loss of income may cause depression and anxiety. Loss of the parental role may cause feelings of uselessness, loneliness, and boredom. Decrease in cognitive functioning, although less likely to occur with good nutrition and intellectual stimulation, may be noted by the aging individual and also cause depression and anxiety.

Sexual activity may cease in older individuals who disengage from other activities. Much of their emotional energy may be tied up in fears about death, disability, and dependence on significant others. Life may seem meaningless, with little that is positive to look forward to. Self-concept may be poor. By Western norms, a beautiful body and physique is equated with sexual desire. The aging body may be seen as unattractive, obscene, or repulsive.

Some may resort to cosmetic surgery. It may prove helpful for some but it is no guarantee in restoring libido, increasing potency or sexual bonds in a couple.[30]

DEATH OF THE PARTNER

Although death may take away a sexual partner at any stage of the life cycle, it is a problem that most often confronts older individuals. Both men and women describe the loss of a love object and a source of support. Both suffer a marked change in their social interaction system, especially if most friends and acquaintances are still married and social activities are couple oriented. Loneliness may be described as a frequent response the first year or two. The death rate of surviving partners tends to increase, and there are an increasing number of suicides.[31]

Women respond with a grief reaction, depression and guilt[32] and decreased interest in all activities. If grief work is completed satisfactorily, previous levels of function returns. Some major problems described by a group of widows included jealousy of old friends who were happily married, missing someone who cared, a feeling of being socially arid, anger and resentment at the husband for dying and leaving, and finally, lack of money. The sexual adjustment is liable to go in any direction based on attitudes, sexual drive, and opportunity. For some women, death of the sexual partner is an escape or rescue from undesired sexual activity. A study by Pfeiffer and Davis[33] found that 90 percent of women stopped having intercourse after their husbands became ill, disinterested, or died. For other women, finding sexual outlets is difficult. Society censures sexual activity outside of marriage, and marriage between older individuals is often viewed as a joke.

The older women, particularly, have difficulty finding sexual companionship, since there are a relatively smaller number of older men available. In addition, women's inhibitions about assertive seeking out of male friends may additionally limit their opportunities. Polygamy has been suggested as an alternate solution.[34] Older widowed men experience less social prohibition to seeking out female companionship. In addition, numberwise, there is more opportunity for developing a relationship. No matter which sex, older persons usually have no one with whom to share their sexual concerns and problems.

Some may masturbate to relieve sexual tension although others who turn to self-pleasuring may be overcome with anxiety, guilt, and shame. Homosexuality and bisexuality have not generally been chosen as acceptable outlets.[35]

Socioeconomic factors may present additional conflict-laden situations for older persons. "Sin versus marriage" has become a question facing older couples who wish to remarry. Because of some pension laws and limitations set forth in some wills, individuals may suffer a considerable decrease in income with remarriage.[36] Some older individuals are willing to go against their consciences and live together without marriage, but guilt may ensue. Others forego marriage.

One suggestion is that couples seek out an understanding clergyman who would perform a religious ceremony, which would unite them in the eyes of God. Without a license, the marriage would not have the legality to change pension and other benefits. Another solution suggested is that if the sin label bothers the couple, they can move to a town where nobody knows them, cohabit, and get on with their lives.[37] This solution, however, does not resolve any guilt feelings that the couple might experience after their decision.

RESEARCH ON SEX AND AGING

Research is needed in many areas. In institutions focus should be on patient behavior not only staff attitudes. Research is needed on the effect of "petting rooms" or areas where patients may have sexual activity and the effects of segregated or integrated age groups. Different measures of sexuality may be needed for the aged individuals including a measurement of sexual attractiveness and self-esteem.[38]

Ludeman[39] reviewed research on sex and aging and pointed out that all studies were based on biased samples, all provided information primarily on genital sex and ignored the relationship and sensual aspects of the sexual experience.

NURSING IMPLICATIONS

Assessment
Interviewing the elderly requires more time and more patience. Memory impairment and need to remember may slow down the data collection process.[40]

A sexual history must be taken to distinguish between physical illness, sexual ignorance, genuine sexual disinterest, and short-term problems in sexual relationships as a cause of sexual dysfunction. Those with long-term problems in their sexual relationship do not usually respond to sexual

therapy. Individuals should have a history of pleasure with sex and a desire to continue or resume sexual activity. Some couples may not have had sexual intercourse or enjoyed each other's company for many years. Since sex in the later years depends on good sexual function during the middle years, the sexual history should include this information.[41] (See the Appendix for specific information to be obtained in the history at various stages of the life cycle.)

The other general information that is obtained from adult or middle-aged patients/clients should be obtained from aging persons (see Chapter 17). Special effort should be made to assess the quality of the interpersonal relationship between the sexual partners—whether supportive and positive or accusatory and negative.

The general health status of persons should also be assessed to obtain information about previous illnesses, surgeries, and medications taken by both sexual partners, since any of these factors may be causes of sexual dysfunctions. (See Unit V relating to specific disease processes and to drugs that effect sexuality.)

It is important that the nurse consider the client's religious beliefs. Research findings indicate that about one-half retain earlier religious beliefs and about one-half become more religious.[42]

It is crucial to question the persons about sex and not be surprised at their answers. Health professionals' own biases and misinformation about the older person and sex make them hesitant to ask questions. When problems are identified, mutual goal-setting of nurse and client is essential.

Intervention
Counselors should approach sexuality, disability, and aging concerns as though they are related since the systems interact.[43]

Any health problem that may interfere with sexual activity should be corrected if possible. Teaching to dispel myths and misconceptions about sexuality and the older individuals may be all that is necessary for some older couples to attain a satisfying sex life. Information about the physiologic changes that take place and adaptations that the couple should make in length and type of foreplay is important. Erection takes longer to achieve, and more direct stimulation may be needed. Since vaginal lubrication is slower in the older woman, the longer foreplay works to the advantage of both sexual partners. Vaginal lubrication can be supplemented with a water-soluble lubricant or estrogen creams. Spastic uterine contractions may decrease with the use of oral estrogen–progesterone.

Less physically strenuous positions for sexual intercourse can be suggested. Side-by-side position or the female superior position may be less fatiguing. Change in time of day for sexual activity is helpful. The early morning after a night's rest rather than late evening may result in increase in physiologic and psychologic response to sexual stimulation.

Providing a willing ear and supportive words of encouragement may be the only counseling needed by some couples to resolve their concerns about sexuality. Reassurance that the aging couple's interest in sex is normal may do much to dispel fear and shame. The nurse remembers, however, that some sexual partners may be satisfied with just lying together, holding, touching, and sharing expressions of love. Intercourse itself is not necessarily the "be all and end all."

In conducting formal courses on sexuality, nurses consider that the aged have their own biases. One group was threatened by mixed-sex groups,[44] another group reacted negatively to being tested and to explicit content. A slower pace, time for teacher acceptance by the group to develop, and sensitivity to feeling as individuals with less liberal views are needed.[45] Classes should be on a volunteer basis only for those who wish information. Professionals must be cautious that they do not press their own attitudes about sexual activity on those who are satisfied with abstinence.[46]

Touch may be an important means of communicating between nurse and patient. Costello states that rapport can be established with an elderly patient if the nurse touches the individual at appropriate times, since this indicates that the nurse is human and understanding.[47] The older person who reaches out to touch a young nurse is not a "dirty old man" (or woman); sexual acting out in older individuals may be more a way of offering oneself.[48]

Staff in nursing homes assess their attitudes and values, knowledge of sexuality, and practice communication about the topic. Starr and Weiner[49] were shocked by the general attitude of rejection and repression of health professionals who were shocked with the idea of even helping with research.

If they have difficulty dealing with sexual behavior of the aged, they may promote behaviors they wish to prevent. Scolding about or punishing masturbation or sexual activity may provide reinforcement in the form of attention. Don'ts must be accompanied by dos. Positive alternatives such as private masturbation and sexual activity are suggested.[50]

Nurses can be instrumental in changing the isolation of patients by sex in nursing and retirement homes. The pleasure of interacting with individuals of the opposite sex can do much to increase interest in appearance and activities and provide intellectual and affectional satisfactions for older persons.

Encouraging older individuals to become active in "golden age groups" may give them the impetus to seek interaction with others of both sexes. When no sexual partner is available, there may be times when teaching a patient to masturbate effectively is indicated, and a wider range of sexual expression may need to be explored for the elderly.[51]

Nurses can also serve as mediators if children object to a parent's interest in remarriage.

Evaluation

If the goals of intervention are mutually chosen by patients/clients and nurses, evaluation is not difficult, since aging individuals are then able to identify whether intervention has been appropriate and adequate to meet these goals. The danger is that unrealistic goals have been set by the nurse and that these goals have not been mutually decided upon. Careful reassessment is done to determine problems and change the plan. Verbal expression of satisfaction by the aging individuals will indicate that nursing intervention has been helpful.

NOTES

1. Berman EM, Lief HI: Sex and the aging process. In Oaks WW, Melchiode GA, Ficher I (eds): Sex and the Life Cycle. New York, Grune and Stratton, 1976, pp 125–134
2. Masters WH, Johnson VE: Human Sexual Response. Boston, Little, Brown, 1966, pp 223–260
3. Rubin I: Sex Life after Sixty, New York, Basic Books, 1965
4. Kuhn ME: Sexual myths surrounding aging. In Oaks WW, Melchiode GA, Ficher I (eds): Sex and the Life Cycle. New York, Grune and Stratton, 1976, pp 117–124
5. Ibid, p 120
6. Ibid, p 121
7. Ibid, p 122
8. Ibid, p 123
9. Cameron P: The generation gap: Beliefs about sexuality and self-reported sexuality. Devel Psychol 3:272, 1970
10. Falk G, Falk UA: Sexuality and aged. Nurs Outlook 28:51–65, 1980
11. LaTorre RP, Kear K: Attitudes toward sex in the aged. Arch Sex Behav 6:203–213, 1977
12. Damrosh SP: Nursing students' attitudes toward sexually active older persons. Nurs Research 31:352–355, 1982
13. Collins T: Nature should dictate in the bedroom. Cleveland Plain Dealer, November 2, 1975, Sec 4, p 22
14. Ibid, p 22
15. Stenchever MA, Stickley WT: Human Sexual Behavior. Cleveland, Press of Case Western University, 1970
16. Stanford D: All about sex . . . after middle age. Am J Nurs 77:608–611, 1977
17. Boyer G, Boyer J: Sexuality and aging. Nurs Clin North Am 17:421–427, 1982
18. Masters WH, Johnson VE: Human Sexual Response. Boston, Little, Brown, 1966, p 241
19. Ibid, p 263
20. Kofoed L, Bloom JD: Geriatric sexual dysfunction: A case survey. J Am Geriat Soc 30:437–440, 1982
21. Berman EM, Lief HI: Sex and the aging process. In Oaks WW, Melchiode GA, Ficher I (eds): Sex and the Life Cycle. New York, Grune and Stratton, 1976, p 127
22. Martin CE: Factors affecting sexual functioning in 60–79 year old married males. Arch Sex Behav 10:399–420, 1981
23. Money J: The development of sexuality and eroticism in humankind. Quart Rev Biol 56:379–403, 1981
24. Starr B, Weiner MB: On Sex and Sexuality in the Mature Years. New York, Stein and Day, 1981
25. Christenson CV, Gagnon JH: Sexual behavior in a group of older women. J Geriatr Psychiat 6:351–356, 1973
26. Ibid, p 352
27. Ibid, p 356
28. Masters WH, Johnson VE: Sex and the aging process. J Am Geriat Soc XXIX: 385–390, 1981
29. Berman EM, Lief HI: Sex and the aging process. In Oaks WW, Melchiode GA, Ficher I (eds): Sex and the Life Cycle. New York, Grune and Stratton, 1976, p 127
30. Filstein I: Sexual function in the elderly. Clin Obstet Gynecol 7:401–420, 1980
31. Reed DM: Sexual behavior in the separated, divorced and widowed. In Sadock BJ, Kaplan HI, Freedman AM (eds): The Sexual Experience. Baltimore, Williams and Wilkins, 1976, pp 249–254

32. Toth SB, Toth A: Empathetic intervention with the widow. Am J Nurs 80:1652–1654, 1980

33. Pfeiffer E, Davis GC: Determinants of sexual behavior in middle and old age. J Am Geriatr Soc 20(4):151–158, 1972

34. Ross CH: Geriatrics and the elderly woman. J Am Geriatr Soc 22(5):230–239, 1974

35. Ludeman K: The sexuality of the older person: Review of the literature. Gerontologist 21:203–208, 1981

36. Collins T: When God's laws run afoul of man's laws. Cleveland Plain Dealer, May 14, 1978, Sec 4, p 30

37. Ibid, p 30

38. Gurland BJ, Gurland RV: Methods of research in sex and aging. In Green R, Weiner J (eds). Methodology of Sex Research. Alcohol, Drug Abuse and Mental Health Association, Rockville, Maryland. U.S. Department of Health and Human Services, Public Health Service, National Institute of Mental Health, 1980, pp 67–92

39. Ludeman K: The sexuality of the older person: Review of the literature. Geronolotogist 21:203, 1981

40. Bacley PA: Physical assessment of the elderly. Top Clin Nurs 3:15, 1981

41. Pfeiffer E, Davis GC: Determinants of sexual behavior in middle and old age. J Am Geriatr Soc 20(4):157, 1972

42. Devine BA: Attitudes of the elderly toward religion. J Gerontol Nurs 6:679–687, 1980

43. Woodard WS, Rollin SA: Sexuality and the elderly: Obstacles and options. J Rehabilitation 47:64–68, 1981

44. Guarino SC, Krowlton CN: Planning and implementing a group health program for the elderly. J Gerontol Nurs 6:600–603, 1980

45. Brower HT, Tanner LA: A study of older adults attending a program in human sexuality. Nurs Research 28:36–39, 1979

46. McCarthy P: Geriatric sexuality: Capacity, interest, opportunity. J Gerontol Nurs 5:20–24, 1979

47. Costello MK: Sex intimacy and aging. Am J Nurs 75:1330–1332, 1975

48. Ibid, p 1331

49. Starr B, Weiner M: Sex and Sexuality in the Mature Years. Briarcliff Manor, New York. Stein and Day, 1981

50. Aletky PJ: Sexuality of the nursing home resident. Top Clin Nurs 1:53–60, 1980

51. Yeaworth RC, Friedeman JS: Sexuality in later life. Nurs Clin North Am 10:565–574, 1975

Sexuality and the Reproductive Cycle

Chapter 19

Conception Control

Children who are wanted, loved, and carefully nurtured are more likely to grow up into loving and nurturing adults. Conception control to insure only planned pregnancy is one suggested, albeit limited, means to achieve this end.

Conception control is imperfect, to say the least. Contraceptive efficacy is related not only to the method used, but to variables such as age, parity, availability of the method, motivation, economic factors, cultural factors, religious factors, needs, and side effects.[1] Lack of knowledge is less a cause of contraceptive failure than the individual's norms and culture, fads and fancies, values placed on children, personalities, and pressures of the subcultures.[2] Changes in practices depend on changes in values, attitudes, norms, roles, and relationships. These do not change rapidly, and their change depends on social, economic, educational, and legal factors.

This chapter will present a discussion of specific methods and the psychologic and sociocultural factors that influence their use, misuse, and nonuse.

HISTORICAL OVERVIEW

Contraception has been used throughout history. Early medical treatises written on papyrus 4000 years ago in Egypt detail contraceptive and abortifacient information for women of the court.[3] Modern contracep-

tion began in 1876 when the first vulcanized rubber condom was offered for sale at the Philadelphia Centennial.[4] Early vaginal spermicides included vinegar or lemon juice in water, 20 percent salt solution.[5] In the 1960s, the pill and intrauterine device were developed and, in the 70s, the use of sterilization procedures, vasectomy, and fallopian tubal ligation have become increasingly popular.

There were no laws in the United States before 1873 concerning contraception, although in some areas it was forbidden under existing obscenity laws. In 1873, however, the United States Congress passed the federal antibirth control law.[6]

Although there were voices raised against this law, the first full-time proponent and crusader for liberalization of birth control was Margaret Sanger, a nurse. Her experiences in nursing in the slums of lower Manhattan led her to focus on birth control.[7] Her motivation in espousing birth control was prevention of unwanted conception among the married poor. Sanger opened the first birth control clinic in Brooklyn in 1916. She was immediately arrested, the first of eight times. Despite legal restrictions, under her leadership, federal and state antibirth control statutes were gradually eroded.[8]

In 1936, the prescription of contraceptives for health reasons was legalized, and in 1965, the United States Supreme Court's decision declaring the prohibitory law of Connecticut unconstitutional ended legal statutes against conception control. Beginning in 1966, federal funds have been increasingly used for both domestic and foreign voluntary programs. At the present time, the United States is working with voluntary agencies and especially Planned Parenthood Federations of America to expand knowledge and availability of birth control techniques.[9]

The Planned Parenthood–World Population (PPWP) is a national organization with headquarters in New York and affiliates in 190 American cities. It provides contraceptive services, male sterilization, genetic counseling, and in some offices, abortion services. Its aim is to have each child wanted joyfully by responsible parents.[10]

RESPONSIBILITY FOR CONCEPTION CONTROL

Women's burden for responsibility for birth control is a relatively recent one. For centuries before the invention of the diaphragm, women depended on men to prevent pregnancy by use of the condom and withdrawal (coitus interruptus). The diaphragm was a breakthrough that gave women control of their bodies, yet women have at times found total responsibility a burden, since they must obtain the supplies, see the physician, suffer the side effects, and say no when intercourse is suggested but conception control is unavailable.[11] Increasingly, members of the Women's Liberation Movement and others are urging that the man be responsible for conception control. The condom is becoming more widely advertised and more easily accessible. Major magazines such as *Playboy, Penthouse,* and *Redbook* now carry advertising for its use.

Interestingly, 20 to 30 percent of condom purchasers are women, and the sales approach is to women who are worried about the birth control pill or IUDs.

With the passage or liberalized abortion laws, abortion has now become more easily available as a method of birth prevention, but again, the burden of decision and its sequelae are primarily the woman's.

CONCEPTION CONTROL VERSUS ABORTION

The issue as to which is the better method of birth control, abortion or contraception, has been debated since antiquity. Soranus, a famous gynecologist, wrote in about 130 A.D., "It is better to prevent conception than eliminate it." There are very few who disagree. Guttmacher stated that, on physical and psychic grounds, contraception is preferred and that abortion should not be viewed as a first line of defense in family planning, but as a second-line measure. He expressed the hope that as contraceptive methods improved and as family-life education became part of education in schools, the need for abortion as a family planning measure would decrease.[12] (See Chapter 20 for discussion of abortion.)

David and Friedman[13] studied the relationship between abortion and contraceptive practices transnationally. They found that women with repeated abortions ranked lowest in the use of contraceptives and that in countries where there is a high level of contraceptive use, the abortion rate has dropped. However, women who use contraceptives are more likely to resort to abortion with failure than those who do not. Contraception has not solved the problem of unwanted pregnancies.

In spite of increased contraceptive services, the number of adolescents who bear children in or out of wedlock has increased in the United States.[14] There has been a 50 percent improvement in contraception success since the 1950s, but there is still a 34 percent failure rate among American women.[15] Abortion may be the chosen solution to the undesired pregnancy. Until the development of universally acceptable means of contraception along with change in social attitudes and responsibility, it appears that abortion services will still be relied on by a significant number of the population when contraception fails.[16]

CONCEPT OF FAMILY PLANNING

The concept of family planning has superseded the narrower "birth control" concept. The goals of family planning are to insure that people of childbearing age have the knowledge and ability to plan the number and spacing of their children. On the governmental level, federal support of family planning programs has three objectives: (1) to improve the health of the American people, (2) to assist families to avoid poverty, and (3) to provide freedom of choice in determining the number and spacing of their children.[17]

Fischman[18] points out that the "freedom of choice" phrase implies that couples have the right to choose the size of their families but that programs serving the poor and disadvantaged do not stress freedom of choice but on getting people to make a particular choice—to have fewer children. Although many couples want fewer babies, programs often do not allow for individual differences and desires.

Those arguing for fertility reduction stress that this will help decrease economic, social, and educational deprivations and hardships. However, research has not established a definite association between contraception use and these benefits to low-income families, and infant mortality rates have not declined rapidly.[19]

Ewer and Gibbs[20] studied contraceptive use of black adolescent mothers, and their findings suggest a lack of fit between most service programs and the life styles of many patients. The service operated on the assumption that the patient had a continuous need for contraception, but the girls had not defined themselves as having this need, or any need at all. Much instruction was given that the clients saw as irrelevant.

Fischman[21] states that too many family planning workers do not consider these facts, but rather perform their duties zealously, transmitting the message that tells the client not to become pregnant again. She raises some provocative questions in relation to family planning and the workers' attitudes. Do they contribute to feelings of guilt or failure in women when pregnancies occur? Have some women learned that an "unplanned" pregnancy "caused" by method side effects results in more acceptance and support by health workers than a planned pregnancy? As women use contraception, will their problems change from dealing with anxieties of unwanted pregnancies to coping with anxieties and ambivalence toward contraceptive methods and conflicted and disrupted relationships with sexual partners? How does a woman who has adjusted to being a mother and childbearer adjust to her freedom from pregnancy? What new programs can family planning programs offer?

Coercion and harrassment by health professionals should not be a part of any family program. The goals of the women served must be considered—the number of children they desire, their hopes for fulfillment and enrichment. This involves much more effort and involvement for the nurse and others helping in family planning than in prescribing and teaching about a contraceptive method.

Patient/Client Role

The patient/client chooses the contraceptive method, at least in theory. Health care workers should not impose their values and beliefs in the efficacy of a specific contraceptive measure. However, family planning personnel appear to place methods they actively dispense in a favorable light and may be biased against traditional contraceptives, such as foam and the condom. Difficulty does exist in objectively giving efficacy rates to clients because of a variety of reporting methods, yet the woman has the right to know the contraceptive's effectiveness based on objective data so she can make an informed choice.[22] In considering patients' rights, one must also consider their right to refuse to use any contraceptive. In the age of "population explosion," "zero population growth," and "planned parenthood," the nurse or other health care provider may have difficulty in accepting the decision of the partners to eschew contraception, even after teaching and counseling. However, if nurses support the rights of the individual to make his/her own informed decision, then care must be given within the framework of this decision.

Permanent Infertility

Some women and men may choose permanent infertility through use of contraceptives or sterilization procedures. Women may have wide personal experiences and do not wish the 20-year responsibility of child rearing. Others are aware of ecology and population pressures or wish to preserve their dyadic relationship with their spouse. Katreider and Margolis[23] studied one group of women and found that they were high-achievement oriented, had strong psychologic motivation to avoid pregnancy, or feared being bad mothers or being emotionally destroyed by children. They were strikingly nontraditional and negative toward the concept of husband, home, and children. Baum[24] found similar attitudes in a group of 38 childless couples, most of whom made their decision after much debate and soul searching. When there is agreement that both want their freedom and want to find happiness together without children, the decision can be a mutually satisfactory one.

CHOOSING A CONTRACEPTIVE METHOD

Choosing a method of conception control is the responsibility of the client, but the nurse can supply information and aid in decision making. Bio-psychosocial factors are considered, and the known effectiveness of various contraceptives can be a starting point for sharing information.

Contraceptive Effectiveness

Contraceptive effectiveness can be evaluated in several ways. One method is in terms of the number of pregnancies per 100 women years (HWY) of method use; (of 100 women using the method, the number who would get pregnant each year). By this rating system, in order of decreasing effectiveness for couples who wish to delay pregnancy are the pill, IUD, condom, diaphragm, foam, rhythm, and douche.

In couples who intend to prevent further pregnancies in order of decreasing effectiveness are the pill, IUD, condom, diaphragm, rhythm, foam, and douche. Withdrawal (coitus interruptus) has effectiveness somewhere between that of the diaphragm and rhythm.[25] Sterilization procedures are chosen by those who wish to permanently limit the family and do not wish the bother of contraception.

Guttmacher[26] stresses that there is a tremendous psychic component in sexual satisfaction, and a couple should not choose a contraceptive in which they lack confidence or fear because of its side effects or that is unesthetic or objectionable to either partner. Contraceptive effectiveness is a combination of three factors of equal importance: the efficacy of the method, the consistency of use, and the correct use by the couple. Different methods differ in their biologic effectiveness, but psychosocial factors affect the consistency of use of the contraception chosen, or indeed, if it is used at all.

Information relating to biologic action of various conception control methods is widely available, so this aspect will be only briefly discussed.

Natural Methods of Conception Control

Rhythm Method. Basically, the rhythm method is the avoidance of coitus during the fertile phase of the menstrual cycle. Ovulation occurs, theoretically, 14 days prior to menstruation. However, there is considerable variation in the growth of the ovarian follicle in each individual. Consequently, the time from the previous menstrual period to ovulation cannot be always predicted.

Recording of basal body temperature can improve determination of the safe period. Using a basal thermometer that is calibrated in tenths of a Fahrenheit degree, the woman records her temperature on arising before beginning her daily routine. The temperature rises following ovulation as a result of progesterone and some of its metabolites, which act on the hypothalamic thermoregulatory center, possibly with norepinephrine or the catecholamines serving as mediators. The length of the preovulatory safe period is always uncertain, but the woman can assume that conception will not take place after the third day following the rise in basal body temperature.[27] (Table 19-1).

Ovulation Method (Billings Method).
This method is another form of conception control that utilizes the body's "rhythms" of ovulation and involves identification of physiologic differences during ovulation by the woman herself. Cervical mucus accompanies ovulation and is necessary for the viability and mobility of the sperm. This mucus is produced in cyclic fashion and varies in character during the menstrual cycle. The woman is taught to concentrate on sensations of wetness and dryness from the vagina. Observation of wet or dry days is made in the evening after impression made throughout the day.[28]

During the preovulatory period, the cervical mucus is yellowish, thick, or cloudy.[29] The closer to ovulation, the clearer and more watery is the mucus. It changes to a colorless liquid, more watery, but with a "stringy" consistency. The mucus can be stretched into a fine thread without breaking. Its stretchability is such that the length can be measured.[30]

An applicator can be inserted into the vagina to the cervix and the mucus can then be stretched out with cover glass or wooden spatula to more than 6 cm and up to 15 cm. This is referred to as *Spinnbarkheit* and indicates peak of ovulation. These changes favor

sperm survival and mobility by providing a more alkaline environment.[31]

Sex contact is avoided on all wet days and especially 3 days after the peak. As with the basal temperature method, women keep charts or graphs of mucus observations daily. They may take their temperature with a basal thermometer. The temperature will rise and remain at a consistently high level when the mucus becomes watery.[32] (See Table 19-1.)

Special thermometers, observation charts, a workbook,[33] and textbook[34] are available for use by women interested in natural family planning.

Coitus Interruptus.
The technique involves the withdrawal of the penis prior to ejaculation. It is probably the oldest method of contraception known. Theoretically, it should be very effective. It is probably the first method used by most adolescents, who should be warned about the presence of sperm in the preejaculatory fluid and who should also be warned that ejaculation of semen on the woman's external sex organs has resulted in pregnancy, probably related to extension of the cervical mucus, which is copious in midcycle. (See Table 19-1.)

Douche.
Douching after coitus has been used by some women, but its risk of failure is very high. Spermatozoa have been found in the fallopian tubes 5 minutes after exposure to cervical mucus. Aside from its ineffectiveness, it puts a time limit on coitus, since the woman has to quickly douche after ejaculation takes place. (See Table 19-1.)

Mechanical Methods of Conception Control
Condom. The "rubber," "prophylactic," or "safe" is a rubber sheath, which is sometimes lubricated and which comes in various shapes and forms. It is the chief contraceptive in Japan, Sweden, and Britain, and the third most popular in the United States. The condom is moderately effective if used by it-

self. If used with spermicidal foam, cream, or jelly, effectiveness approaches that of the pill and IUDs. Newer condoms are coated with a spermicidal jelly which reduces the ability of the sperm to move by 50 percent within 30 seconds. This provides added protection if the condom breaks or the contents spill.[35]

In instructing men in the use of the condom, the nurse suggests that the condom be applied by the sexual partner as part of the lovemaking, so that mutuality is involved. She/he also stresses that at least 1 cm should be left at the end for collection of the semen and that the individual should remove the condom immediately after intercourse, holding on to the base tightly to prevent leakage of semen, while withdrawing the penis. Lubrication of the condom with water-soluble jelly or spermicidal creams increases sensation and decreases irritation and breakage[36] (Table 19-2).

Diaphragm and Polyurethane Sponge.

The diaphragm consists of a rubber dome supported by a rubber-encased metal spring that fits over the cervix. It should always be used with a spermicidal preparation to increase effectiveness, which is high when it is used with a spermicide. The diaphragm interrupts the movement of sperm up the cervical canal, and the spermicidal jelly or cream kills any that reach the rim of the diaphragm.

In instructing women in the use of the diaphragm and spermicidal creams, the nurse stresses that the diaphragm can be inserted as part of sexual foreplay, the man and woman inserting it together. This sharing is best in a long-term relationship. Many women prefer to insert the diaphragm in advance. This should be done within 2 hours before intercourse, the closer to the time of intercourse, the better. If the diaphragm is properly inserted, it should not be felt. It should be left in at least 6 hours after intercourse, since it takes the spermicide that long to be effective. If intercourse takes place within 6 hours, more creams or jellies must be added.[37,38] (See Table 19-2.)

The newest barrier contraceptive is a soft polyurethane sponge 5.5 cm wide and 2.0 cm thick permeated with a spermicide, nonoxynol-9. In tests it has been as effective as the diaphragm, is easy to use and to buy without prescriptions. It can be inserted up to 16 hours before intercourse and stays effective for 24 hours regardless how many times intercourse takes place. A small polyester loop makes removal easy.[39]

IUD. Intrauterine devices come in many shapes, sizes, and materials, but their mode of action is unknown. It is known that with the device in place, the endometrium is infiltrated by leukocytes producing an endometrial exudate, which may be spermicidal, prevent fertilization, be blastotoxic, or inhibit implantation. There is no effect on ovulation, ovarian steroids or tubal transport.[40]

Some IUDs contain copper on a plastic base. The copper IUD has the advantage of causing less pain on insertion, a decreased expulsion rate, decreased incidence of abnormal bleeding and heavy menses, and of possible protection against gonorrheal salpingitis.[41] (See Table 19-2.)

When pregnancy takes place, there is also increased risk of uterine infection if the IUD is left in place. Consequently, it is usually removed. With the IUD in place, abortion rate is approximately 50 percent; removed, it is 30 percent. The chance of a live birth being premature is four times greater when the IUD is left in place.[42]

The IUD is contraindicated with pregnancy, pelvic inflammatory disease, undiagnosed vaginal bleeding, severe anemia, congenital uterine anomalies, a uterine cavity distorted by fibroids, and severe uterine flexion with fixation of the fundus.[43]

Some physicians recommend that patients who have just received an IUD use an overlap method of contraception such as foam for the first few months, since most expulsions occur then.[44] Others recommend use of foam during the most fertile days of the menstrual cycle as backup protection. It can be inserted in early postpartum or

TABLE 19–1. NATURAL METHODS

Billings Method (Rhythm)	Coitus Interruptus (Withdrawal)	Douche
Advantages: acceptable to religious groups; involves no chemical or mechanical interference with coitus, no medical risk, need for prescriptions or complicated manipulation; involves both sexual partners reinforcing sexual equality	*Advantages:* no medical risk; can be used with unexpected coitus; no chemical or mechanical interference	*Advantages:* none
Disadvantages: higher method failure if ovulation time is irregular; need high motivation and intelligence; prolonged period of abstinence. Vaginitis, cervical infection produce leukorrhea; may make Billings observation difficult	*Disadvantages:* need for male self-control, alertness, timing and motivation; coitus terminated with male orgasm; female may not be satisfied; pre-ejaculatory fluid may contain sperm	*Disadvantages:* puts time limit on coitus; considered a nonmethod; little or no protection from pregnancy
Chance of pregnancy: method failure 5–10 per HWY; use failure 9–28 per HWY	*Chance of pregnancy:* method failure 20–25 per HWY	

postabortion, although there is an increased expulsion rate for postabortion insertions.[45]

The male cannot feel the strings during coitus, but strings may become entangled with pubic hair fragments or a tampon, thus causing irritation to both sexual partners. Long strings can be cut. The patient is taught how to check the IUD periodically, particularly following a menstrual period, by inserting her fingers in the vagina to feel the strings. She should also check each sanitary napkin or tampon before discarding it to make sure the device has not been expelled. If the woman cannot feel the strings, she should use an alternate method of contraception and return to the clinic or physician for a checkup.[46]

Chemical Conception Control

Antispermicidal Preparations. These preparations include foams, creams, jellies, and suppositories containing a spermicidal chemical in an inert base. This is inserted into the vagina with an applicator and is spread by coital movements. These are moderately effective when used by themselves. When used as an adjunct to the condom or diaphragm, their efficiency increases greatly. Some are effective against gonorrhea and other sexually transmitted diseases.[47] (Table 19-3).

Oral Contraceptives. The birth control pill is the most commonly used contraceptive in the United States. Depending on brand, it contains varying amounts of estrogen and progestin.

The pill prevents fertility in several ways: (1) inhibition of the hypothalamus and pituitary gland, resulting in inhibition of ovulation; (2) change in fallopian tube motility and secretion; (3) endometrial changes; and (4) antagonistic action of cervical mucus to spermatozoa.[48]

Oral contraceptives have a protective, preventive effect against menorrhagia, be-

TABLE 19–2. MECHANICAL METHODS

Condom	Diaphragm	Intrauterine Device (IUD)
Advantages: no prescription needed; some protection against VD; male assumes responsibility; inexpensive, easy to use, no medical risks	*Advantages:* no side effects, medical risks; may be used during menstruation to contain menstrual blood	*Advantages:* nothing to do at time of coitus; little motivation or intelligence needed
Disadvantages: incorrect use; self-control by male to apply; some report decreased sensation	*Disadvantages:* need medical prescription; may become dislodged if uterine displacement or relaxed vagina; privacy needed for insertion; may interfere with pre-coital lovemaking; woman must be comfortable touching genitals; some report less cervical stimulation	*Disadvantages:* infection; uterine perforation (usually at insertion); expulsion; bleeding; dysmenorrhea; pelvic pain; pelvic inflammatory diseases (PID); some report dyspareunia with deep penetration; penile laceration from string
Chance of pregnancy: method failure 2–4 per HWY; user failure 6–13 per HWY	*Chance of pregnancy:* method failure 2–4 per HWY; user failure 10–15 per HWY	*Chance of pregnancy:* method failure 2 per HWY; user failure none

nign breast neoplasm, dysmenorrhea, anemia, acne, and various cysts. Garcia[49] states that they may help relieve premenstrual tension. Morris and Udry[50] found, however, that most women do not feel any day-by-day differences when taking the hormones, a few feeling better, a few worse. Age is particularly significant, and the Federal Food and Drug Administration cautions against the use of the pill by women over 40.[51] The relationship of oral contraceptives and heart disease is still being investigated. In 1978, researchers at Ohio State University announced that women who take oral contraceptives may not be as susceptible to heart attacks as previously believed.[52]

The National Centers for Disease Control (CDC) announced that the risk of endometrial cancer is less and the risk of ovarian cancer is 40 percent less for those who take the pill than for those who do not. Women on the pill run no increased risk of breast cancer.[53]

There has been concern that oral contraceptives are associated with the development of cervical cancer. The results of various studies are contradictory but it appears that the risk of cervical cancer is highest in women who are most sexually active and who have used oral contraceptives for 4 to 6 years.[54] (See Table 19-3.)

The pill may result in increased libido and enjoyment in sexual activity, since fear of pregnancy is limited. However, Masters and Johnson[55] have reported that some women after 18 months to 3 years on the pill lose interest in sexual activity. They postulate that it may have a long-range depressant effect on the libido. Those on progestin-dominant, low dosage estrogen pills, particularly, complain of lack of sex drive, lack of vaginal lubrication, decreased sensitivity of vulval tissues, and decreased ability to reach orgasm.[56]

In considering the risks involved in taking the pill against the risks of using other methods or none at all, Garcia[57] concludes that although the pill is not innocuous, the relative risk is very low, the pill is safer than pregnancy, and the pill is safer in the younger patient, below the age of 35.

Minipills. These contain microdose quantities of 19-nortestosterone or progesterone

TABLE 19–3. CHEMICAL METHODS

Antispermicides	Oral Contraceptives (Pill)	Sterilization
Advantages: quick and easy; no medical risk; no prescription needed; decrease VD	*Advantages:* most effective temporary method; convenient to use; separates contraception from sexual activity	*Female—Advantages:* low failure rate; if "belly button" type, done under local anesthesia as outpatient, no scar
Disadvantages: motivation needed; "messiness"; leaking out; may interrupt prolonged sex since must be reapplied after each coitus; allergic reactions; vaginal, penile irritation	*Disadvantages:* minor: depression; breakthrough bleeding; hyperpigmentation of skin; nausea; vomiting; weight gain; edema. Major: urinary tract infection; gallbladder disease; leg vein thrombosis; cerebrovascular disease; myocardial infarct especially with increased age (over 40); hypertension; smoking hypercholesterolemia	*Disadvantages:* general anesthesia for some procedures; abdominal incision; hospitalization; irreversible; "belly button" type complications—intestinal perforation, hemorrhage, infection, occasional recanalization, vaginal ligation, occasional dyspareunia
Chance of pregnancy: method failure 2–4 per HWY; user failure 13–16 per HWY	*Chance of pregnancy:* method failure less than 1 per HWY, user failure 2–3 per HWY	*Male vasectomy—Advantages:* effective, safe, easy to perform
		Disadvantages: permanent

derivatives. With the elimination of the estrogen component, there may be few hazards with its use. Its disadvantages include menstrual spotting and a wide variation in cycle length.[58]

Depo-Provera. This progesterone derivative given by intramuscular injection every 3 to 6 months has proven highly effective as a contraceptive. It requires minimal effort by the patient, is simple to administer, and is particularly effective for individuals incapable of using other methods. It has been widely used in developing countries. In March 1978, however, the Federal Food and Drug Administration decided not to approve its use for contraception in this country because of safety questions raised in studies with dogs.

Controversy continues about its safety, proponents arguing it is as safe or safer than oral contraceptives or IUDs.[59] The World Health Organization, International Planned Parenthood, and the American College of Obstetrics and Gynecology favor its approval but coalitions of consumer and feminist groups support the ban.

Monthly Pill. Quinestrol is a synthetic estrogen that is stored in adipose tissue and slowly released into general circulation. Its effectiveness is lower than the combined pill. It has the same disadvantages as other oral pills plus more frequent undesired bleeding episodes.

Postcoital Chemical Contraceptives. The "morning-after" pill or postovulatory contraceptive is given to the woman shortly after intercourse and results in either inhibition of fertilization, inhibition of egg development, or lack of implantation.[60] The morning-after pill utilizes high doses of estrogen given over several days. It can be given up to 72 hours following unprotected coitus, but it will not interrupt an implanted pregnancy. It is moderately reliable, but should only be used as an emergency method, e.g., in cases of rape.

It has the same medical risk as oral contraceptives, plus it may be harmful to the developing fetus. If pregnancy occurs in spite of its use, abortion is suggested.[61,62]

Male Contraception

Research is being conducted to develop anti-spermatogenic compounds. The difficulty is that these drugs cause chemical castration, decrease in the size of the testes. The psychologic factors resulting from the loss of testes size and consequent threat to masculinity preclude use of some methods. The ideal agent will interfere with the fertilizing capacity of spermatozoa stored in the epididymis or influence the metabolism and transport and fertilizing capacity of spermatozoa. Promising drugs are cyproterone acetate and the α-chlorohydrins, which render epididymal sperm immotile and infertile.[63] Other methods being studied include hypothalamic–pituitary suppression, immunologic techniques, and prevention of sperm maturation.[64]

Surgical Conception Control: Sterilization

Approximately one couple in five choose sterilization for permanent conception control, and the incidence is increasing in the United States. In the structure of contemporary society, many physicians believe it can be done for social and economic reasons as well as therapeutic.[65]

Female Sterlization. A variety of techniques may be used for sterlization of women. Abdominal tubal ligation can be done immediately postpartum under local anesthesia or during cesarean section. The procedure is not considered reversible, although spontaneous recanalization has sometimes occurred. Surgical reanastomosis has also been effective occasionally.

Laparoscopy tubal ligation, known as the "belly-button" or "bandaid" surgery, involves cutting or cauterizing the tubes under direct visualization with the fiber optic laparoscope.

Hysterectomy may be performed in the presence of pelvic pathology. Hysteroscopy involves obstructing the opening of the fallopian tubes into the uterus by use of a cautery, sclerosing chemicals or even silicone plugs via a transcervical intrauterine approach. (See Table 19-3.)

The majority of patients are satisfied with sterilization procedures. However, psychologic problems may occur if the patient is not carefully counseled before surgery. Coital enjoyment and responsiveness may be adversely affected if there are strong religious beliefs, marital instability, fear of loss of a spouse and the ability to reproduce, and especially if there is misunderstanding about the reversibility of the procedure.[66] Individuals must be counseled that the procedure should be considered irreversible.

Male Sterilization. Vasectomy is becoming increasingly popular, and it is effective, safe, and simple to perform. Interest in vasectomy has been stimulated by a number of social changes—interest in family planning by the man, better understanding of the separation of sex and reproduction, knowledge that the man's sexuality is unaffected by the procedure, the failures and unacceptability of other methods of birth control, and the emancipation of women.[67]

Men are told the operation is irreversible. Even if reanastomosis of the vas deferens is successful, most of the time fertility is not immediate and there is a time interval before there are enough sperm for impregnation. There is no explanation for the problem in getting an adequate number and motile sperm, but it may be due to the body producing antibodies against the sperm.[68]

Negative psychologic reactions sometimes occur, so presurgical counseling of both sexual partners is important. In a longitudinal study of 75 men postvasectomy, Williams[69] and associates found that the response to vasectomy involves a compensatory process in which men who view the surgery as demasculinizing develop increased desire for sex. The most stereotypically masculine males are most threatened by the vasectomy.

Individuals who have had difficulty with sexual function before vasectomy are more likely to have increased difficulty postoperatively. A smaller number have relief of sexual dysfunction when it was partly due to fear of pregnancy. Depression akin to that of menopausal women occurs in some men with the realization that male childbearing years are ended. Problems may also arise when a change in life situation—the death of a child, divorce and remarriage—causes a change in desire for reproduction.[70]

Future Research on Contraception

Research focuses on the ideal and more universally acceptable contraceptive—one that is effective, easily used independent of coitus, reversible in effects, nontoxic, inexpensive, and able to meet individual needs predicated by religious beliefs, cultural mores, socioeconomic background, emotional needs, and intellectual motivation.[71]

Study of male contraception continues. However, strict, costly government restrictions, problems associated with animal testing, and lack of knowledge about reproductive physiology all cause difficulty in research.[72]

Gossypol, derived from cotton-seed oil, has been tried in more than 4000 men in China but safety has not been established. High doses of the hormone LHRH (luteinizing hormone releasing hormone), produced by the hypothalamus, suppress sperm development, but undermine sexual performance.

The newest chemical contraceptive is RU-486, a pill taken two to three times a month, that induces menstruation and terminates pregnancy if it has occurred.[73]

Research continues on the use of prostaglandins (see Chapter 26), new IUD designs, once-a-month pills, and subdermal implants of contraceptive capsules which provide 6-month contraception.

Effects of contraceptive methods on sex of infants is being investigated. In a study of a cohort of 33,205 newborns, Shiono and associates[74] found that births after failure of oral contraceptives, IUD, mechanical or chemical methods, showed no shift in sex ratios but there was an excess of male births after failure of the rhythm method.

FACTORS INVOLVED IN MISUSE OR NONUSE OF CONTRACEPTION

Psychologic Factors

Omitting nonuse of conception control because a couple desires pregnancy or misuse because the couple is ignorant of the correct method, Sandberg[75] has identified numerous factors that contribute to contraceptive failure.

Denial. Unwillingness to acknowledge reality may operate during the first coital experience, and especially in high school and college students. They deny that coitus may occur or that pregnancy could result. One college student stated after discovering she was pregnant, "All the others get away with it. Wouldn't you know that I'd be the one to get caught. We were trying to be careful!" Some deny that contraception works, rationalizing that their friends "got pregnant anyway." Others deny a personal responsibility for contraceptive use as a response to hostility and interpersonal gamesmanship.[76]

Guilt. For some individuals, aside from religious etiology, guilt occurs because to be sexually accessible at all times is tantamount to prostitution and promiscuity. For some women, contraceptive use is an open invitation to be used (or raped) rather than to be romantically seduced and loved. Those who believe that sex was designed by God only for babies may view contraception as used for sinful and lustful pleasure. Some cannot emotionally accept this thought and may take risks, since the potential for pregnancy must exist to obviate this guilt.[77]

Guilt seems to limit use of effective contraceptive methods. Gerrard[78] found that in 109 college women in 1973 and a comparable group in 1978, there was an increase in sexual activity in 1978 but a decreased use of effective contraception. He felt that guilt, as measured by the Mosher Sex-Guilt Inventory, was effective in inhibiting sexual activity in 1973 but not in 1978. Those using ineffective contraceptive methods, however, had a higher guilt score than those using effective methods.

Hostility. Resentment and hostility is seen in the woman, who by rejecting contraception, rejects the sexual partner, using fear of pregnancy as a weapon. A man may desire to evoke fear or he may revengefully force pregnancy on a wife or mistress for a number of reasons. In others, misuse or abuse of contraception may be a means of using pregnancy to cause pain to a parent, rebel against society, or punish a mate who is unfaithful with guilt and additional responsibility.

Hostility may also exist if one partner feels he or she has the major contraceptive responsibility or if it has shifted from one to the other. In other cases, rejection of contraception is not directed toward pregnancy, but is simply an expression of some anger or discontent that exists.[79]

Shame. Some sexually active individuals may be ashamed or embarrassed to admit their ignorance of contraceptive practices to the partner, a physician, or the peer group and consequently do not seek information. Others are fearful of discovery by parents, relatives, or friends that contraception is being sought or used. This is especially true of adolescents and those who are acting contrary to their social or religious norms. Shame or embarrassment will limit use, es-

pecially if the community is small, peer group support is minimal, or if the physician, nurse, or clinic personnel are considered too inquisitive, distant, judgmental, or disapproving.[80] (See Chapter 13 for discussion of shame.)

Sexual Identity Conflicts. Self-esteem is closely connected with sexual identity and adequacy. In men, it may be based on virility demonstrated by impregnating a woman. In women, femininity may be based on fecundity. The necessity for demonstration of sexual identity is inversely proportional to the number of other life accomplishments and to the degree of ego strength in the entire area of sexuality. If the person's rewards of life and self-esteem are poor, bringing forth a baby may be a compensatory mechanism.

The man with weak ego strength may be afraid that contraceptive use by his partner may decrease her desire and responsiveness. Conversely, he may fear that use of a contraceptive will eliminate her fear of pregnancy and increase her sexual demands to a degree that he is unable to satisfy. This would further injure his pride and self-esteem, leading to impotence and other sexual dysfunctions.[81]

In some cases, contraceptives are not used, since pregnancy is an objective proof of worth. Some childless women in their 30s fear aging and may demonstrate their femininity with motherhood, either in or out of wedlock.[82]

Fear and Anxiety. Some individuals eschew contraception because of fear of manipulating, altering, or harming their body via cancer, infection, blood clots, or unknown diseases. These fears contribute to the choice of method, but they may also serve as rationalization for avoiding contraceptive use.

Some women may feel loss of sexual control if fear of pregnancy is removed, while others fear that contraceptive side effects may result in frigidity and loss of libido. Anxiety may also occur because of the responsibility of controlling reproductive activities and the need to accept personal blame for failures. It may be easier to "accept fate" and "suffer" at its hands.

Opportunism. At times, coitus is available and the individuals are unwilling to put it off until contraception can be obtained. Coitus may also be viewed as an opportunity to initiate, cement, or continue a relationship; gain status; obtain affection; or be accepted or for other reasons that offer some reward for immediate intercourse. The reward may be just to please the sexual partner.[83]

Entrapment. Individuals may avoid contraceptive use to achieve pregnancy as a means of forcing another into marriage, into a closer commitment to self or the family, to prevent separation and divorce, or to force the partner into greater emotional or financial support. Hostility and masochism may be underlying dynamics. If the ploy fails and the partner leaves or does not respond appropriately, expressions of long-standing resentment are justified.

Coital Gamesmanship. In the struggle for personal control in a relationship, partners may use coitus and contraception as a manipulative ploy. Partners may struggle over who controls the frequency of coitus and who will be forced to accept the role of contraceptor and responsibility if pregnancy ensues. The balance of power in a relationship may be the deciding factor in the type and use of contraception.[84]

Nihilism. Feelings of apathy or hopelessness may exist, especially in cultures marked by poverty. Not enough effort can be mobilized to prevent pregnancy, although it is not actively sought. An attitude of fatalism prevails, and contraception is low on the priority of needs until more urgent needs are met.[85]

Affectional Poverty. Poverty may occur in more than the physical or social forms. Some individuals have chronic or acute deprivations of love, companionship, and the feelings of being needed, sometimes accompanied by concerns about sexual identity. Coitus may be a way to fulfill this need for some. Others, with an extremely strong unfulfilled need, may meet it by pregnancy and the acquisition of a dependent and loving infant, in or out of marriage. The middle-aged woman with children leaving the nest and a husband with other interests is another who may seek pregnancy, the new child stopping the affectional poverty.[86]

Masochism. Hostility directed inward may be evidenced by self-deprecation and self-punishment. The individual may allow herself to be used sexually and may eschew contraception, which adds the threat of pregnancy for punishment. Self-abortion may add life-threatening injury. Pregnancy may be also sought as demeaning, degrading, imprisoning, figure-destroying subjugation, the price to be paid for sins or for simply existing.

Eroticism. Sexual risk taking through nonuse of contraception may be a source of sensual and erotic pleasure. Although probably infrequent, Sandberg[87] feels that this element may exist to some extent in all instances of unprotected coitus. Risk is anxiety provoking, but to "win" is thrilling, and the thrill is directly proportional to the initial degree of anxiety. In the game of risking pregnancy, people win most of the time, so repetitive risks continue as long as anxiety is not too great.

Love. Risk taking may take another form. It may be seen as self-sacrifice and a romantic and realistic sign of love. It may exist on the part of both partners, but more often it is unilateral, an offering of one to another. This may be very satisfying and fulfilling to the giver and equally so for the receiver. Risk taking may not be enough; the gift of pregnancy may be chosen with or without the knowledge of the partner.

Contraception rejection may also occur out of naive and idealistic adoration and what are believed to be the requirements of love: "I must surrender myself to him entirely," "To use contraception would be to deny the love I feel." In addition, contraceptive use destroys the illusion that coitus is the spontaneous, uncontrollable, and overwhelming result of love. It is the objective demonstration of one's search for sensual pleasure.[88]

Abortion Availability. Abortion provides a rational basis for contraceptive nonuse or for use of less effective contraception, especially with couples with infrequent coitus and low fertility. Abortion may be especially desired by the individual who has to demonstrate femininity by pregnancy but has no desire for the infant. It offers the "best" of two worlds, the achievement of pregnancy without the sequelae of prolonged responsibility.[89]

Iatrogenesis. The health professional may cause nonuse of contraceptives. Instead of focusing on the individual's needs and desires and on those of the sexual partner (who may be rarely consulted), the professional prescribes the contraceptive of his/her choice, rather than taking the time to help the patients/clients arrive at a personal choice. Unless individuals are given the opportunity to express their fears and concerns and identify their needs, their use of the contraceptive imposed upon them is doomed to failure.

Sociocultural and Demographic Factors

Age—Adolescent Conception Control.

The sexually active adolescent girl who desires contraception presents a challenge to health professionals. Use of contraception is a complex multidimensional behavior and variables such as self-concept, cognitive skills, motivation, vulnerability, locus of control, and availability of method must be considered when working with adolescents.[90] The adolescents' preference must be considered or they will stop using the method, especially if they feel ambivalent or guilty.

Lane[91] stresses matching the girl to the method. The diaphragm may be effective for a girl who is suspicious of chemicals or who fears something foreign in her uterus. The girl must be comfortable about her body and reasonably in control of her emotions. She may have some problems with the device, such as a palpable rim or cramps when it is in place, so may discontinue its use, or if coitus is frequent, she may consider it too much of a hassle.

The girl who fears the possibility of forgetting to use contraception or who does not want to have to do something about it repeatedly often chooses the IUD. The ideal IUD for the nulliparous teenager is one that is easily and painlessly inserted, not readily expelled, delicate and flexible enough for comfort, yet covers sufficient area for effectiveness. However, she must be alerted to the dangers associated with the intrauterine device.

The pill is usually chosen by the girl who wishes no risk of pregnancy and is not afraid of side effects or of ingesting "chemicals." She is confident that she will remember to take the medication and likes the convenience of routine. Some feel the pill should not be given to the young adolescent, because it may cause long bone epiphyses closure prematurely or it may suppress the pituitary gland, adversely affecting stimulation of ovulation and ovarian hormone production when the pill is discontinued. Lane[92] argues otherwise, that pregnancy is an even greater risk. The hormonal effects of pregnancy may have these same effects on long bones. In addition, grand multiparas are subject to much higher estrogen levels than in the pill, without subsequent loss of ovulatory function.

The condom has the added advantage over other contraceptive methods of preventing venereal disease. In addition, it is low in cost, easy to use, and provides a high degree of protection if used correctly. Unfortunately, the adolescent male may feel that the responsibility for conception control rests with the girl, not himself (see Chapter 16).

A higher proportion of younger patients/clients will experience contraceptive failure than older ones. They may express interest in contraceptive use but not follow through with use or not return for followup visits.[93]

It also appears that the adolescents with above average educational background are at greater risk either because they are not served by existing agencies or because they have more sporadic sexual activity.[94] Free conception control care is available at federally funded clinics, but arguments in court still exist about requiring these family planning clinics to notify parents within 10 working days of the time their children (17 and under) receive prescription contraception. In February 1983, the so-called "squeal rule" was blocked by federal district judges who asserted that the rule blocked the will of Congress to combat the problems of teenage pregnancy. Opponents of the rule maintain that parental notification would cause teenagers to boycott family planning services but not stop sexual activity. Those for the rule felt it would have had the opposite effect: reduce sexual activity, pregnancies, and abortion. From a legal viewpoint, the regulations appeared to violate the rights of minors and cause gender discrimination because they would affect only teenage girls.

Contraceptive failure was frequent in a group of young black adolescent girls studied by Gispert.[95] Among those who had been given contraceptives, the numbers who always used contraceptives were rare. Those who had been given the pill took it irregularly or had independently discontinued its use. Reasons given by the adolescents for contraceptive failure were an IUD that slipped or a "busted" condom. Shelton[96] found that among young adolescents, contraceptive clinics and teaching did not result in decrease in fertility. It was only when abortion became increasingly available that the escalating numbers of illegitimate births to girls under 14 stopped.

Duncan,[97] feels that education is not the answer for the failure to use contraception, since many sexually active adolescents have adequate knowledge and availability of contraception. Moreover, nonuse cannot be explained by the fact that the initial sexual experience is rarely planned. The adolescent more likely prefers the risk involved to the alternative—carrying an image of herself/himself as continually prepared for intercourse. In a rather pessimistic view, Duncan states that health professionals can offer the information or advice, but should not hold any illogical expectations of its effectiveness. (See Chapter 16 for discussion of the reasons for adolescent pregnancy other than contraceptive misuse or disuse.)

Social Class. In studying contraceptive use of lower-socioeconomic-class black women, Gebhard et al.[98] found that little was known about contraception, that it was considered a nuisance at best and at most dangerous and unnatural. Many saw pregnancy as an inevitable part of life. Whether it was in or out of wedlock was a secondary issue. However, black women of middle and upper socioeconomic classes have attitudes similar to those of white women, seeking and accepting conception control as a part of their sexual experience.[99]

Rainwater[100] identified some of the underlying values and assumptions about family planning that working class Americans hold based on interviews with 46 men and 50 women. Working class families were defined as those in which the breadwinner work is manual, blue collar occupations or lower-level service jobs. Their housing was modest, and high school was their highest level of education. Some couples practiced sporadic and careless contraception, with responsibility strictly up to the wife. At times, doing nothing was the easiest way out when there was conflict about family planning. There was difficulty in communicating and poor interpersonal relationships.

Many of the women had and expected to have larger families than women of higher class.[101] Even when conception control was desired, some of the women had to struggle against the wishes of their spouses, who had a greater interest in having many children than upper class men. This may have much to do with the males' need for repeated proof of potency. Since they tended to feel weak and ineffective in relation to their world, fathering children represented a demonstration that they were real men.[102]

Sexual Roles. Changing sex roles and relationships are considered in choosing a contraceptive method. Scanzoni[103] investigated sex role modernity in relation to contraceptive practice. He found that women oriented toward individuality and achievement were more likely to choose a more efficient technique, with less risk of failure. In his sample, he found that blacks and non-Catholics, especially, were more likely to choose more efficient methods such as the pill and IUD. He suggests that sex role definition is more basic for family planning than whether a woman works or whether contraceptives are available and distributed.[104]

Rainwater[105] found that working class women have difficulty thinking of themselves in any roles other than wives and mothers. Being a good wife fosters a sense of being a worthwhile person and of being a real woman. Moreover, they are unsure of their ability to hold their husbands and may be afraid to assert themselves. "Holding their husbands" means giving in to their wishes. Lower-class husbands may like to think of themselves as masters of the house.[106] Given the woman's difficulty in being assertive and the man's view of himself as master, it may be difficult for the working class woman to either suggest contraception or dictate type of contraception. She will also use less effective methods.

Scanzoni notes that in the third world, there is increased fertility control along with greater sex role equality. However, he also points out that couples will not forego what they see as the benefits of having children unless there are some visible compensatory alternatives, such as individual gratification

and socioeconomic benefit.[107] Unfortunately, many women have difficulty talking about conception control, fearing that the man may react negatively.

Religious Beliefs. Religion and religious convictions must be considered in the use or lack of use of conception control. With concerns increasing about global overpopulation, the use of contraception is increasingly accepted as a matter of religious teaching. The methods used, however, are a matter of individual beliefs.[108]

The Catholic Church, in particular, teaches that contraception and sterilization are illicit, recognizing, however, that there may be reasons for limiting family size.[109] It is licit to take into account the "natural rhythms" of the "generative function" to regulate birth, a method that does not impede natural processes.[110]

The rhythm method and the Billings ovulation method of conception control are accepted as licit methods, others are not. Katchadourian and Lunde[111] report, however, a change in contraceptive behavior among married American Catholics. The proportion of Catholic women using a method other than rhythm increased from 30 percent in 1955, to 51 percent in 1965, and between 1965 and 1970 to 68 percent.

Charles Westoff of the Office of Population Research of Princeton University reported that by 1975, 90 percent of Catholic women who were married less than 5 years were using contraceptive methods not approved by the Roman Catholic Church and that the acceptance of artificial birth control was shared by practicing as well as nominal Catholics.[112]

Scanzoni[113] agrees that the trend indicates increased use of contraceptives by Catholics. However, he found that Catholics still tend to want and have more children than non-Cathlics. The Catholic woman who is more egalitarian in her beliefs about the sexes will have children early in marriage and then follow individual gratification later in life, while non-Catholic women defer the costs and rewards of children until later in the marriage.

Catholic women who seek contraceptive counseling from Catholic clergymen may obtain conflicting information. Official teaching may prohibit contraception other than by approved methods, but individual priests may feel differently (see Chapter 9). Catholics are not the only religious group that may experience conflict over contraception. Mormons, liberal and conservative Protestants, and Jews also hold divergent views within and between groups.

Race. Some black leaders see a relationship between population control and political power. Some cry genocide when conception control is advocated and taught in black neighborhoods and in the third world countries. During the Watts riot in Los Angeles, the first structures burned were family planning trailers situated in the neighborhood.

Cultural Beliefs. Cultural norms influence acceptance and use of conception control methods. In the Puerto Rican culture, it is important that the daughter marry and enter into marriage as a virgin, the father being held responsible for the daughter's virginity. To give the girl information about the pill and suggest she be free to go out may be tantamount to asking the father to allow the daughter to do something immoral. Today, many "enlightened" people are so concerned with sexual expression that they voice opposition to any repressive behavior and confuse having sexual relations with freedom from repression.[114] One may argue that it is better to give the girl information. However, she will be living within her cultural milieu and must face the consequences of breaking its rules and regulations. A more difficult but satisfactory approach would be to counsel and teach the girl and the family to find a solution that is acceptable to all.

Some ethnic groups value large families

and do not want to limit pregnancy. The American Indians want children to help with tasks, to help them become complete and adequate parents, and to be with them in old age. They also believe that one should have at least six children, a sacred number.[115]

Cognitive Factors. Educational level and intellectual ability must be considered in conception control. The rhythm method or the ovulatory method requires a certain degree of intelligence, as does the use of the pill. In either method, conception failure may result from improper procedure being followed because the woman is not able to understand or follow written or verbal directions.

Economic Factors. The cost and availability of the contraceptive and the opportunity for medical followup must be considered when helping the woman choose a contraceptive method. Large urban areas may have planned parenthood clinics or hospital-based programs within short distances of the woman's home. In rural areas, facilities may be farther away and transportation a problem when followup visits are needed or when side effects occur and the woman needs medical attention. Return visits for a supply of pills may also be difficult, because babysitters and carfare are not available for many women.[116] In these situations, instruction in the use of the condom for the male partner, insertion of an intrauterine device, or the diaphragm may be the most efficient methods. Costwise, use of the diaphragm, condom, or IUD is much less expensive than use of oral contraceptives, unless public funding is available for their purchase.

In 1969, Guttmacher[117] stated that there would be no difference between family size among the poor or the affluent if both had the same opportunity to control conception and that the poor actually want slightly smaller families than the affluent. The poor have had a higher fertility rate in this country, but he felt that this was due to differences in knowledge and sophistication, in their willingness and ability to use contraceptive methods, and in the availability of family planning services. He felt that if all hospitals and clinics supplied information, fertility rates would equalize.

NURSING IMPLICATIONS

A survey of health professionals and pre-professionals in 47 schools of nursing, 11 schools of medicine, and 15 schools of social work indicated that the great majority of faculty and students (over 90 percent) approve of birth control and believe that family planning should be a part of health counseling (95 percent). However, more than three-fourths of the faculty and over half the students indicated that the average health professional is not knowledgeable in the area of human sexuality and family planning.[118]

Attitudes of senior nursing students toward providing contraception services to all who want them were assessed by Elder.[119] In general, the students had permissive attitudes toward dispensing contraceptives to all but very young teenagers. They were also reluctant to endorse educating young people about contraception prior to puberty. Elder[120] felt the reluctance to teach contraception to adolescents under 15 is understandable but disturbing. Although there are few studies of young people under 15 years of age, those done indicate a sizable number are sexually active. Based on what teenagers say, at least, the major reasons they do not use effective contraceptives are lack of knowledge and problems in obtaining contraceptives.[121] Both of these factors are amenable to nursing intervention.

The nurse who is involved in family planning needs to have achieved personal growth and knowledge, not only about herself, but about family planning. Sister Mary Helen[122] gives nine objectives that must have been realized by the family planning nurse:

1. A realistic, satisfying personal attitude about sexuality and his/her sexual role.
2. Ability to apply the problem-solving process to patient situations as well as his/her own.
3. Skill in the use of interview techniques.
4. Understanding that family planning is a problem affecting not only the individual family but society as well.
5. Recognition that the goal of family planning is the strengthening of the family.
6. Recognition of and respect for the rights of individuals to choose the size of their family and support for their decision as to the method to employ.
7. Knowledge of the various methods of birth control and ability to explain their use.
8. Understanding of the nurse's role in family planning and actively searching for ways to legitimately participate in such programs.
9. Awareness of his/her limitations, seeking counsel when necessary and referring patients to appropriate sources.

Increasingly, family planning nurse practitioners are being utilized to care for normal patients, with medical backup for special pathologic or managerial problems. Beginning with a comprehensive history and physical examination, the nurse collects information to help the patient choose the appropriate contraceptive method. Unfortunately, as with other new programs, physician acceptance has been poor in some areas, and salaries are not yet at an acceptable level.[123]

Assessment

Biologic Data. The nurse collects data about the woman's medical problems, the extent of sexual activity, her knowledge of biologic and physiologic components of human sexuality, and the present understanding of contraceptive technique. Feelings about touching the genital area, having preparations leak out of the vagina, or taking chemicals into the body are explored. Other data include how often intercourse takes place, whether the individual is forgetful, the degree of self-control, and whether there are facilities to store contraceptive supplies.

Psychosocial Data. The individual's religious and ethical beliefs and sociocultural and economic status, as well as those of the sexual partner are assessed. It is essential to consider a couple as a bio-psycho-social unit.

The motivation for family planning must be considered. Are the woman and partner interested in spacing the pregnancies or do they want to limit the family size permanently? The rate of failure is high if the intention is to delay rather than to prevent pregnancy. If acceptable for other reasons, the pill or IUD are more effective for limiting pregnancy.

The woman is allowed to express her feeling about contraception, the method, if any, that she feels would be acceptable to her and to her sexual partner. If there is lack of agreement as to methods or if conception should even be prevented, the conflict that exists almost insures failure.

While listening, the nurse assesses the woman's intellectual ability and tries to determine to some extent the woman's degree of motivation for contraceptive use.

Planning

The nurse considers the bio-psycho-social–economic factors that may significantly affect conception control and the woman's and her partner's willingness to use contraception. In some instances, the man may be willing to take responsibility for conception control by use of the condom or by vasectomy. It is important that the nurse follow the same assessment parameters and obtain comparable data from him. The goal is to help the individual make an informed, responsible decision that best meets his/her needs and the needs of the sexual partner.

Intervention

The nurse's attitude toward the patient/client is of prime importance. Warmth, interest, ob-

jectivity encourage the patient/client to share information and to accept information. Women may be embarrassed about the gynecologic examination and about the questions asked. If the nurse works in a family planning clinic, it is important to avoid a "speed up," "production belt" environment, which may result in total failure to help the patient/client.[124] The nurse's primary concern is the individual.

Contraceptive Method. The nurse helps the sexual partners, or the individual, choose a method by providing information about the effectiveness and the advantages and disadvantages of each method. Individuals select one method based on their life styles and their feelings about their bodies, after weighing whether effectiveness, safety, or convenience is the most important. In addition, it is important that individuals choose the method that they feel most comfortable with and will use consistently.[125]

In the enthusiasm to suggest and urge the use of a certain contraceptive, the nurse may neglect to assess carefully the patient's acceptance or response to its use. There is no ideal method of conception control for all, and the nurse needs to develop tolerance and understanding in dealing with the infrequent or nonuse of contraception.

If there is lack of agreement between the sexual partners, not only in relation to the type of method that is acceptable, but also whether pregnancy is to be delayed or prevented permanently, counseling is needed to help the couple come to a mutually agreeable decision. The condom may seem to be the ideal solution for some women, but if the man has reservations about its use, the chance of effective conception control is minimal. Mutual cooperation is also needed when rhythm or ovulatory methods are used, since there are considerable periods of time when coitus is not advised.

Teaching. Use of pamphlets, charts, and other audiovisual materials that are written on a level that will be understood by the individual helps clarify information. Individual teaching is beneficial, but group teaching is more economical of the nurse's time and allows women to share their experiences and concerns.[126] (See Chapter 11.)

Programmed instruction regarding oral contraceptives has been found effective in teaching nursing students. It replaces "lecture" presentation and is followed by group discussion.[127] This approach might be effective in teaching patients/clients about conception control if modules are constructed at the appropriate intellectual levels. The nurse then can focus on answering questions and counseling.

Teaching and counseling on an individual basis are valuable to help the patient absorb instructions about her specific contraceptive method and to allow the nurse to better evaluate if the patient/client has learned the essential information.

When working with adolescents, the nurse may have to function not only as a teacher and counselor, but also as a friend. She may have to assume responsibility in planning their health care. At times, the nurse is a mother surrogate who listens to the adolescent girl air her views about sex, but who does not judge her harshly for them. The nurse listens, does not impose her values, but permits the girl to clarify her own views.[128]

Some patients/clients may appear to welcome information about use of the pill, IUD, etc., but many persons suffer various degrees of guilt with contraceptive use. This may be a carryover from conflict between deep-rooted childhood-grounded religious restrictions and the person's modern, intellectualized disagreement with these restrictions. This guilt is magnified when both partners are faced with such conflicts, although to different degree and extent for each.[129] The nurse is sensitive to these responses and conflicts and helps the individuals come to an acceptable decision. (See Chapter 13 for information about guilt.)

It may appear overwhelming to consider all the variables involved in helping individuals choose a method of conception con- trol. Time may be limited and the pressures to "get the job done" great. However, to be effective, with effectiveness measured by not only spacing and limitation of children, but also in greater happiness and satisfaction for the sexual partners, more than pills, condoms, and diaphragms must be given. When the patients'/clients' bio-psycho-social problems are overwhelming, prescribing contraception may be the least effective intervention. It is then that the members of the health team are needed—the psychologist, social worker and professional counselor.

Evaluation

If clients return with an unplanned pregnancy or with expression of dissatisfaction with regard to the method being used, reevaluation and reassessment are indicated. Failure may be due to psychologic processes, sociocultural influences, or biologic difficulties with the specific method. To prescribe another method of contraception without this reassessment is to court further failure.

Contraception is just one aspect of a person's existence and its impact and meaning change with all other aspects of personality and emotional life. Nurses also realize that what is acceptable at one point in time may not be acceptable at another.

The following outcome criteria are observed. The individual:

1. Chooses a method of conception control.
2. States satisfaction with that method.
3. Is able to space or prevent pregnancy according to her own goals by use of that method.

NOTES

1. Garcia C-R: Human Fertility: The Regulation of Reproduction. Philadelphia, Davis, 1977, p 60
2. Fischman SH: Change strategies and their application to family planning programs. Am J Nurs 70:1773, 1973
3. Bennett JP: Chemical Contraception.

New York, Columbia University Press, 1974, pp 7–20

4. Bennett JP: Chemical Contraception. New York, Columbia University Press, 1974, p 41

5. Ibid, p 7

6. Guttmacher A: Pregnancy, Birth and Family Planning. New York, Viking, 1973, p 268

7. Ibid

8. Ibid, p 269

9. Ibid

10. Ibid, p 270

11. Boston Women's Health Book Collective: Our Bodies, Ourselves, 2nd ed. New York, Simon and Schuster, 1976, pp 181–215

12. Guttmacher A: Pregnancy, Birth and Family Planning. New York, Viking, 1973, p 271

13. David H, Friedman HL: Psychosocial research in abortion: A transnational perspective. In Osofsky H, Osofsky JD: (eds): The Abortion Experience. Hagerstown, Maryland, Harper & Row, 1973, pp 310–333

14. Menken J: The health and social consequences of teenage childbearing. Fam Plann Perspect 4:45–53, July 1972

15. Garcia C-R: Human Fertility: The Regulation of Reproduction. Philadelphia, Davis, 1977, p 65

16. Editorial: Am J Public Health 67:604–605, 1977

17. U.S. Office of Economic Opportunity, Family Planning Program: Need for Subsidized Family Planning Services: United States, Each State and Country, 1969. Washington, D.C., Office of Economic Opportunity, 1972, p 3

18. Fischman SH: Change strategies and their application to family planning programs. Am J Nurs 70:1771–1774, 1973

19. Ibid, p 1771

20. Ewer P, Gibbs JO: Relationship with putative father and use of contraception in a population of black ghetto adoles-

cent mothers. Public Health Rep 90:417–423, 1975

21. Fischman SH: Change strategies and their application to family planning programs. Am J Nurs 70:1774, 1973

22. Trussel TJ, Faden R, Hatcher RA: Efficacy information in contraceptive counseling: Those little white lies. Am J Public Heath 66:761–767, 1976

23. Katrieder N, Margolis AC: Childlessness by choice: A clinical study. Am J Psychiatry 134:179–182, 1977

24. Baum FE: Orientation toward voluntary childlessness. J Biosoc Sci 15:153–164, 1983

25. Garcia C-R: Human Fertility: The Regulation of Reproduction. Philadelphia, Davis, 1977, p 65

26. Guttmacher A: Pregnancy, Birth and Family Planning. New York, Viking, 1973, p 274

27. Garcia C-R: Human Fertlity: The Regulation of Reproduction. Philadelphia, Davis, 1977, p 69

28. Temby BK: Ovulation method of birth control. Am J Nurs 76:928–929, 1976

29. Ibid, p 928

30. Ibid, p 929

31. Dickason E, Schult MO: Maternal and Infant Care. New York, McGraw-Hill, 1975, pp 13–15

32. Ibid, p 15

33. Natural Family Planning: The Couple to Couple League. P.O. Box 11084, Cincinnati, Ohio, 45211

34. Kippley J, Kippley S: The Art of Natural Family Planning. Cincinnati, The Couple to Couple League International, Inc., 1977

35. Graedon J: New contraceptives on the horizon. The Plain Dealer, March 6, 1983, Sec. C, p 14

36. Garcia C-R: Human Fertility: The Regulation of Reproduction. Philadelphia, Davis, 1977, p 74

37. Boston Women's Health Book Collective: Our Bodies, Ourselves, 2nd ed. New York, Simon and Schuster, 1976, p 202

38. Garcia C-R: Human Fertility: The Regulation of Reproduction. Philadelphia, Davis, 1977, p 75
39. One from Egypt. Time, March 28, 1983, pp 48–49
40. Garcia C-R: Human Fertility: The Regulation of Reproduction. Philadelphia, Davis, 1977, p 102
41. Ibid, p 105
42. Tatum HJ, Schmidt F, Jain AK: Management and outcomes of pregnancies associated with copper T intrauterine contraceptive device. Am J Obstet Gynecol 126:869–879, 1976
43. Garcia C-R: Human Fertility: The Regulation of Reproduction. Philadelphia, Davis, 1977, p 105
44. Manisoff MT: Intrauterine devices. Am J Nurs 73:1118–1192, 1973
45. Ibid, p 1192
46. Ibid, p 1190
47. Jick H, Hannan MT, Stergachis A, et al: Vaginal spermicides and gonorrhea. J Am Med Ass 248:1619–1623, 1982
48. Garcia C-R: Human Fertility: The Regulation of Reproduction. Philadelphia, Davis, 1977, p 80
49. Ibid, p 81
50. Morris N, Udry JR: Contraceptive pills and day by day feelings of well-being. Am J Obstet Gynecol 113:763–765, 1972
51. FDA Drug Bull 8(1):9, 1978
52. Research lessens pill's link to heart ills. Cleveland Plain Dealer, August 2, 1978, p B-12
53. Byrd R: Confirmed: Pill cuts cancer risk. The Plain Dealer, March 5, 1983, Sec. B, p 3
54. Swan SH, Brown WL: Oral contraceptive use, sexual activity and cervical carcinoma. Am J Obstet Gynecol 139:52–57, 1981
55. Masters WH, Johnson VE: Conference on human sexuality for nurses, St. Louis, Missouri, October 1975
56. Boston Women's Health Book Collective: Our Bodies, Ourselves, 2nd ed. New York, Simon and Schuster, 1976, p 191
57. Garcia C-R: Human Fertility: The Regulation of Reproduction. Philadelphia, Davis, 1977, p 87
58. Ibid, p 98
59. Effective, but how safe? Time, January 24, 1983, p 67
60. Bennett JP: Chemical Contraception. New York, Columbia University Press, 1974, p 68
61. Ibid, p 99
62. Garcia C-R: Human Fertility: The Regulation of Reproduction. Philadelphia, Davis, 1977, p 102
63. Bennett JP: Chemical Contraception. New York, Columbia University Press, 1974, p 134
64. Bremner WJ, deKretser DM: The prospects for new reversible male contraceptive. N Engl J Med 295:1111–1115, 1976
65. Siegler AM: Tubal sterilization. Am J Nurs 72:1625–1629, 1972
66. Garcia C-R: Human Fertility: The Regulation of Reproduction. Philadelphia, Davis, 1977, p 114
67. Davis JE: Vasectomy. Am J Nurs 75:509–513, 1972
68. Schmidt SS: Reanastomosis of the vas deferens: Techniques and results. Clin Obstet Gynecol 25:533–539, 1982
69. Williams D, Swicegood G, Clark MP, Bean FD: Masculinity-femininity and the desire for sexual intercourse after vasectomy: A longitudinal study. Soc Psych Quart 43:347–352, 1980
70. Zinsser HH: Sex and surgical procedures in the male. In Sadock BJ, Kaplan HI, Freedman AM (eds): The Sexual Experience. Baltimore, Williams and Wilkins, 1976, pp 303–307
71. Garcia C-R: Human Fertility: The Regulation of Reproduction. Philadelphia, Davis, 1977, pp 59–119
72. Bennett JP: Chemical Contraception. New York, Columbia University Press, 1974, p 175
73. Clark M, Lord M, Nater T, Witherspoon D: The Depo-Provera debate. Newsweek, January 24, 1983, p 70

74. Shiono P, Harlap S, Ramcharan S: Sex of offspring of women using oral contraceptives, rhythm and other methods of birth control around the time of conception. Fert, Steril 37:367–372, 1982

75. Sandberg EC: Psychological aspects of contraception. In Sadock BJ, Kaplan HI, Freedman AM (eds): The Sexual Experience, Baltimore, Williams and Wilkins, 1976, p 342

76. Ibid

77. Ibid, p 344

78. Gerrard M: Sex, sex guilt and contraceptive rise. J Pers and Soc Psych 42:153–158, 1982

79. Sandberg EC: Psychological Aspects of Contraception. In Sadock BJ, Kaplan HI, Freedman AM (eds): The Sexual Experience. Baltimore, Williams and Wilkens, 1976, p 345

80. Ibid, p 344

81. Ibid, p 343

82. Ibid

83. Ibid, p 342

84. Ibid, p 345

85. Ibid, p 346

86. Ibid, p 345

87. Ibid

88. Ibid, p 344

89. Ibid, p 347

90. Urberg KA: A theoretical framework for studying adolescent contraceptive use. Adolescence 17:527–540, 1982

91. Lane ME: Contraception for adolescents. Fam Plann Perspect 5:19–20, 1973

92. Ibid, p 20

93. Smith E: Family planning coordinator in a city hospital. Am J Nurs 70:2363–2365, 1970

94. Kreutner AK: Adolescent contraception. Pediat Clin North Am 28:455–473, 1981

95. Gispert M: Sexual experimenting and pregnancy in young black adolescents. Am J Obstet Gynecol 126:416–417, 1976

96. Shelton JD: Very young adolescents in Georgia: Has abortion or contraception lowered their fertility. Am J Public Health 67:616–620, 1977

97. Duncan JW: An essay on adolescent girls. Med Clin North Am 58:847–855, 1974

98. Gebhard PH, Pomeroy WB, Martin CE, Christenson CV: Pregnancy, birth and abortion. In Weinberg MS (ed): Sex Research. New York, Oxford, 1976, pp 100–113

99. Ibid, p 107

100. Rainwater L: And the Poor Get Children. Chicago, Quadrangle, 1967, p 4

101. Ibid, p 28

102. Ibid, p 85

103. Scanzoni JH: Sex Roles, Life Styles and Childbearing. New York, Free Press, 1975

104. Ibid, p 187

105. Rainwater L: And the Poor Get Children. Chicago, Quadrangle, 1967, p 72

106. Ibid, p 78

107. Scanzoni JH: Sex Roles, Life Styles and Childbearing. New York, Free Press, 1975, p 187

108. Sandberg EC: Psychological aspects of contraception. In Sadock BJ, Kaplan HI, Freedman AM (eds): The Sexual Experience. Baltimore, Williams and Wilkins, 1976, p 339

109. Pope Paul VI: Of Human Life. Boston, Daughters of St. Paul, 1968, p 9

110. Ibid, p 13

111. Katchadourian HA, Lunde DT: Fundamentals of Human Sexuality. New York, Holt, 1975, pp 145–171

112. Contraception curbs Catholic birth rate. Cleveland Press, 1978

113. Scanzoni JH: Sex Roles, Life Styles and Childbearing. New York, Free Press, 1975, p 176

114. Lieberman F: Sex and the adolescent girl. In Gottesfeld ML (ed): Modern Sexuality, New York, Behavioral Publications, 1973, p 235

115. Leininger M: Cultural diversities of health and nursing care. Nurs Clin North Am 12(1):5–26, 1977

116. Fischman SH: Choosing an appropriate contraceptive. Nurs Outlook 15:28–31, 1967

117. Guttmacher AF: Family Planning: The needs and the methods. Am J Nurs 69:1229–1234, 1969

118. Shea FP, Werley HH, Hudson Rosen RA, Ager JW: Survey of health professionals regarding family planning. Nurs Res 22(1):17–35, 1973

119. Elder RG: Orientation of senior nursing students toward access to contraceptives. Nurs Res 25:338–345, 1976

120. Ibid, p 344

121. Shah F, et al: Unprotected intercourse among unwed teenagers. Fam Plann Perspect 7:39–44, 1975

122. Sister Mary Helen: Family planning within the curriculum. Nurs Outlook 15(5):42–45, 1967

123. Manisoff M, Davis LW, Kaminetsky HA, Payne P: The family planning nurse practitioner: Concepts and results of training. Am J Public Health 60(1):62–64, 1976

124. Arnold E: Individualizing care in family planning. Nurs Outlook 15(12):26–27, 1967

125. Boston Women's Health Book Collective: Our Bodies, Ourselves, 2nd ed. New York, Simon and Schuster, 1976, 187

126. Fischman SH: Choosing an appropriate contraceptive. Nurs Outlook 15:30, 1967

127. Guimei MK: Effectiveness of a programmed instruction model on oral contraceptives. Nurs Res 26:452–455, 1977

128. Cassidy JT: Teenagers in a family planning clinic. Nurs Outlook 18:31, 1970

129. Sandberg EC: Psychological aspects of contraception. In Sadock BJ, Kaplan HI, Freedman AM (eds): The Sexual Experience. Baltimore, Williams and Wilkins, 1976, p 339

Chapter 20

Abortion

Abortion, the termination of a pregnancy before the fetus is viable, may be spontaneous or artifically induced. The focus of this chapter will be on abortion as a voluntary interruption of pregnancy. Types of abortion procedures and the psychosocial and philosophic factors that influence abortion-seeking and the individual's response to abortion will be discussed. Whether nurses work in an agency that includes abortion as an intervention or not, they must be knowledgeable about this still debated procedure, since individuals present concerns and questions not only in relation to their unwanted pregnancy but to those of others. Whatever the nurse's beliefs and feelings about the procedure, individuals make their own decisions about using abortion as a solution to their problems. The nurse's role is to help them make informed choices, based on their own beliefs and needs.

HISTORICAL OVERVIEW

Although the laws governing abortion and attitudes toward abortion have varied, it has been practiced since the beginning of society. The primary purpose of the first laws enacted were social—to preserve the structure of the existing society. Consequently, the fetus was considered to be without rights and could be aborted for sufficient reason. Primitive societies sanctioned abortion for fear of child-

birth or pregnancy resulting from rape or improper paternity.[1]

Rome sanctioned abortion, but Judaism and Christianity condemned the practice. Early Christian arguments about abortion were related to the question of when the fetus became a human and when life started. The earliest views were that the fetus was a part of the mother until birth. Later, life was said to begin in the fetus at the time of its physical formation (40 days after conception). Some fathers of the Church held that the human soul was infused at this time, while others argued that the soul was infused at the moment of conception and that abortion was killing of a human being.[2]

Eventually, the social reasons for which abortion was sanctioned gave way to medical indications; abortion was permitted if the fetus was harming the mother's health or was aggravating an existing illness.[3] With advances of medical technology, those indications for abortion were less viable, so that by 1950, psychiatric indications accounted for more than 50 percent of all abortions. By the late 1960s, psychiatrists were becoming aware that they were being asked to solve a social problem and felt that they were being exploited to meet society's need for easier abortions.[4]

By 1970, four states had liberalized abortion laws. In January 1973, the United States Supreme Court overruled all state laws that prohibited or restricted women's rights to obtain an abortion during the first 3 months of pregnancy, emphasizing that during the first trimester the right to have an abortion was between the woman and her physician and that the state's interest in her welfare did not warrant interference. The court also ruled that for the next 6 months of pregnancy, the state does have the right to regulate the procedure in matters related to maternal health such as licensing and regulating abortion facilities. During the last 10 weeks of pregnancy, when the fetus is judged to be capable of surviving if born, any state may prohibit abortion if it wishes, except where it may be necessary to preserve the life or health of the mother.

Medicaid payments for abortion began in 1971 but in 1976, Congress passed the Hyde Amendment which restricted use of these funds except when the woman's life was in danger. In 1979 permission was given for use of funds for abortion after rape and incest. In 1980 the Supreme Court ruled on the constitutionality of the fund restriction, stating that the federal government and the states may deny use of Medicaid funds for elective abortions. The result is that the poor have limited access to legal abortion.[5]

The Helms–Hyde bill (Human Life Statute) was introduced in Congress in 1981. It states that life begins at conception. In 1983 it was defeated on the floor by Congress. Legislative efforts continue to pass an amendment to the Constitution giving the states and Congress the right to decide whether abortion is legal.

State and local governments have tried to circumvent the Supreme Court decisions by enacting laws that are designed to discourage abortion. One of these is the informed consent requirements which tell physicians what specific information must be given to the patient as a precondition of her informed consent. Some of these provisions have been declared unconstitutional because in essence they would force the woman to hear unpleasant details not pertinent to her condition, subjecting her to unwarranted punishment.[6]

In 1981 the Supreme Court ruled that states have the right to require parental notification of unmarried minors' abortions. A survey of 141 white teenagers in an abortion clinic found that most (71 percent) told their girlfriends, but not the parents of their plan, because they were concerned about parents' feelings and feared physical retaliation. The findings raise the question: Might fear of parental notification cause some adolescents to carry the pregnancy to term?[7]

Pro-Life Versus Pro-Choice

Induced abortion is a topic that is often argued with fanaticism by those either for or against the procedure. It is an issue that has been approached from political, social, religious, medical, legal, moral, and ethical viewpoints—an issue that is difficult to discuss without bias. Proponents and opponents of abortion argue genocide, murder, the right for life versus the right of freedom and privacy and control of one's body. The three major points that are debated are: (1) the question of when life begins, (2) the individual's right over her own body, and (3) psychologic consequences of abortion, if any. Differences of opinion exist over the impact of abortion on the emotional health of the woman versus the effects of an unwanted pregnancy and possible subsequent rejection on the child's physical and mental welfare.

The antiabortion groups oppose abortion but prefer to be known as "pro-life," because they are concerned with more issues than just abortion. They believe that from the moment of conception the embryo has a genetic identity separate from the mother and should be entitled to due process under the law;[8] that from the moment of conception it is human.[9] They argue that abortion is the first in a series of steps toward a society in which individuals will be judged by their social usefulness, eventually leading to euthanasia for the aged, the incurably ill, the handicapped, or the severely retarded. They also argue that abortion is not so medically and psychologically safe as its advocates claim.

The antiabortion campaign was originally led by the Catholic Church but today the largest antiabortion group is the American National Right to Life Committee which has an estimated 13 million members, its leadership including Protestant, Jews, and Catholics, liberals and conservatives. It has also come under the influence of the New Right, the Moral Majority and other conservative pro-life groups.[10]

Groups such as the American Life Lobby argue that a constitutional amendment giving states the right to regulate abortions would be inadequate. What is needed is an amendment that prohibits abortion because the lives of persons (the fetuses) are involved.[11]

Others believe that women have the right to their own bodies and to decisions about their bodies. Pro-choice advocates are led by groups such as the National Organization for Women (NOW), and the National Abortion Rights League (NARL). Organizations like The Abortion Fund have been established to provide indigent women with money for wanted abortions.

While recognizing the sincere disagreement of others, these groups do not agree that the unborn fetus's right to life is greater than the rights of the woman who is carrying it. In addition, they point out that the quality of life of the child, including the woman's emotional and situational readiness for a child, is as important as life itself.[12]

POSITIVE EFFECTS OF LEGALIZED ABORTION

In addition to arguing women's rights to choice, advantages of legalized abortion have been noted. When abortion is utilized, data indicate an easing of population growth, decline in maternal mortality due to illegal abortions, decrease in the number of septic and incomplete abortions (most due to illegal abortions), decrease in infant mortality (probably related to reduction in the number of illegitimate births), decrease in child

abandonment, and decrease in out-of-wedlock births.[13]

Voluntary interruption of pregnancy in clean, adequate facilities was available to women with money and information on how and where to obtain an abortion. In addition, the number of complications of abortion have decreased, especially since women are having earlier abortions, more than half before 8 weeks' gestation.[14]

With change in the law relating to Medicaid payment for abortion. Petitti[15] predicts mortality rates will probably rise from the present 4 per 100,000 for legal abortions to 40 per 100,000 for nonlegal and unsafe abortions. There may also be increased mortality from legal abortions, since women will delay the procedure in order to seek funds, resulting in more midtrimester procedures and greater risk.

Other positive effects of abortion have been noted. Women receive medical screening at the time of abortion, which identifies conditions that might have escaped unnoticed (gonorrhea, abnormal Pap smears). There is no agreement on the effects of abortion on contraceptive use. Improved contraceptive utilization by women who received an abortion has been identified by some studies.[16,17]

NEGATIVE EFFECTS OF LEGALIZED ABORTION

In addition to arguments that abortion is immoral, that a human being is "murdered," concern has been voiced that there will be an ever increasing number of abortions. This appears to have happened. Statistics indicate that there has been an annual increase in the number of abortions since legalization. In 1983, however, the Center for Disease Control reported that the rate of increase appears to have leveled off. Nearly 1.3 million legal abortions were performed in 1980, but there was only a 3.6 percent increase from 1979 to 1980.[18] However, there is no way to compare these figures with the number of illegal abortions done anually before liberalization of laws.[19]

Some argue that many abortions may be used as a safe method of fertility regulation and that repeat abortions will be common. Results of studies conducted are equivocal. Schneider's[20] investigation indicated that women with one abortion were more likely to seek several and that an increased number and rate of repeat abortions were occurring among some women. Those who cure an unwanted pregnancy by abortion seem more likely to have another unwanted pregnancy. Reasons given for second abortions are failure of contraception and an impractical method, but an underlying desire to become pregnant,[21] guilt, and game playing may be involved. (See Chapter 19.)

Other studies have shown that where contraceptive information and availability are poor, repeat abortion is common; where information is utilized, incidence of repeat abortion is low (among New York City residents in 1976, 16 percent were repeaters).[22]

There have been studies indicating that abortion negatively affects the patient's health and future reproductive capability. The possibility of tubal occlusion, infection, and uterine perforations does exist. Conflicting data exist concerning the increased possibility of premature births and a higher rate of second trimester abortions with planned pregnancy after a woman has had a therapeutic abortion.[23,24]

Mortality and morbidity statistics indicate that the timing of abortion is important, since earlier abortions are much safer than those performed in the second trimester and are much safer than pregnancy. In a study by Rovinsky[25] mean obstetric mortality rate was 23 per 100,000 deliveries, while first trimester abortion mortality rate was 1.2 per 100,000 abortions, and second trimester mortality was 17.7 per 100,000 abortions. Delay is generally found in women who are of younger age, low or very high parity, lower socioeconomic group, unmarried, nonutilizers of contraceptives, and who have not completed high school.[26]

Mortality and morbidity rates are also related to type of procedure, D & E (suction curettage) having the lowest and saline and hysterotomy, the highest. Infection, emboli, hemorrhage, and anesthesia problems are the most common complications.[27]

Cates[28] found that there may be a increased risk of breast cancer in women if abortion occurs before 3 months' gestation, and if the woman is nulliparous. More research is needed, however, to establish a relationship.

BIOLOGIC ASPECTS: TECHNIQUES OF ABORTION

Because of differences in mortality and morbidity associated with legal abortion in the first or in the second trimesters, laws, medical practices, and educational programs should enable and encourage women to have it in the first 3 months of pregnancy.

First Trimester Abortion

Four first trimester procedures are most commonly used in the United States. Menstrual regulation often called menstrual extraction, endometrial aspiration, or mini-abortion, is performed with a flexible plastic cannula used with negative pressure supplied by a suction apparatus or by use of 20- or 50-ml syringe (Table 20-1).

Dilation and curettage (D&C) involves dilating the cervical canal and scraping the walls of the uterus. (See Table 20-1.)

Dilation and evacuation under suction (D&E suction) is the most widely used abortion technique at the present time. The cervix is exposed with a speculum, grasped, dilated, and evacuated under suction pressures from 30 to 70 mm Hg. Curettage may be performed to ensure complete evacuation and oxytocin or ergotrate administered for hemostasis. (See Table 20-1.)

Laminaria tents are made from the stems of the brown algae *Laminaria digitata*. They are sterilized and are available in different diameters and lengths. By hygroscopic swelling they slowly and steadily mechanically dilate the cervix. They are usually inserted into the cervical canal just beyond the internal os the day before the abortion. A tampon is then inserted and left in place. The laminaria is removed several hours later or the next day. A medium-sized laminaria in place more than 16 hours will dilate the cervix to 13 mm. (See Table 20-1). They are usually used in conjunction with other methods.

Midtrimester Abortion

There are two methods primarily used for midtrimester abortions.

Intrauterine saline instillation, the most commonly used midtrimester procedure involves the instillation of 50 to 250 ml of a 20 percent sodium chloride solution into the amniotic sac following amniocentesis. After injection, there is immediate damage by the hypertonic saline to decidual cells and chorionic villi, congestion, and thrombosis in blood vessels, causing placental and fetal death. Uterine contractions, probably resulting from release of prostaglandins from the decidua, begin 12 to 24 hours after instillation, unless an oxytocic drug is given.

The popularity of this procedure is decreasing because of the development of better and safer techniques.

It is difficult procedure prior to 14 weeks, where there is less than 100 ml of amniotic fluid. The time interval from injection to abortion is long, ranging from 22 to 40 hours (a mean of 35 hours), and in 10 to 15 percent of patients over 72 hours. Complications are also high. (See Table 20-1.)

Prostaglandins are a group of 20-carbon unsaturated hydroxy fatty acids. Fourteen are found in most human tissues and are readily synthesized from essential fatty acids. Synthetic derivatives are being developed. They function intracellularly as possible regulators of metabolic processes through a modification of cyclic AMP production. They cause abortion by their ability to cause uterine contractions. Prostaglandins F_{2a} and E_2 are generally used, although another form, 15(S)-15-methylprostaglandin E_2 methyl es-

ter, a synthetic derivative, has been found effective without the necessity of the frequent administration needed for the naturally occurring forms.[29]

Administration of prostaglandins is not superior to suction curettage for early abortion, but they have much value for midtrimester abortion.[30] Routes of administration that are used are intraamniotic, intrauterine extraamniotic, intravaginal, and intramuscular (Table 20-2).

Whitehead suggests that the time may come when drug companies will be allowed to market prostaglandins in intravaginal suppositories. The question that arises is whether individuals should be able to terminate their own pregnancies without the counseling of a physician or health worker, an important aspect of abortion practice.[31]

Early claims for prostaglandins hailed them as abortifacient and contraceptive agents and claimed that they might supply once-a-month birth control. However, research is still needed.[32]

Midtrimester abortions are subject to increased complications due to the difficulty in preventing untoward systemic effects. However, Kerenyi[33] reports that it is not so much the effects of specific abortifacients that make midtrimester abortion difficult, but the complex and poorly understood regulatory mechanism of pregnancy.

Other Procedures During Midtrimester.

Hysterotomy may be used if the patient has had previous cesarean sections, the pregnancy is advanced, the cervix is firm, and hypertonic saline or prostaglandins have failed.[34]

Hysterectomy is indicated only when other techniques cannot be used. It has a high mortality and morbidity rate and is limited to use when the patient requests sterilization and there is pelvic pathology to justify its use.[35]

Rivanol is a disinfectant used in Japan. It is injected through a catheter, and oxytocin is given concomitantly.[36]

Bougie, also a Japanese technique, is an

TABLE 20–1. FIRST TRIMESTER PROCEDURES

Procedure and Time	Advantages	Disadvantages and Complications
Menstrual regulation (extraction, endometrial aspiration, miniabortion) Up to 6th week	Done in office or clinic, little or no analgesia, no cervical dilation, rapid, easy, inexpensive, activities resumed same day	Perforation, cervical trauma, cramping, nausea, syncope, heavy bleeding, 5% failure to terminate pregnancy, may be done unnecessarily when woman is not pregnant
Dilation and curettage D&C Up to 10th week	Done as outpatient, requires no sophisticated equipment, local anesthesia with parenteral analgesia	Uterine perforation, hemorrhage, infection, trauma to cervix, bowel, bladder, pelvic infection
Suction curettage Up to 13th week	Rapid, done as outpatient, minimal risk, reasonable cost, fewer complications than D&C	Uterine perforation, laceration of cervix by dilator, hemorrhage, scarring of endometrium with repeated abortion
Laminaria tent (used with suction curettage)	Slow safe dilation of cervix, decreases incidence of cervical lacerations, uterine perforation, decreases amount of operating time, analgesia needed	Requires visit to clinic day before abortion, premature expulsion of tent, difficulty of removal, possible increased infection

Adapted from Quilligan EJ, Zuspan FP: Douglas-Stromme Operative Obstetrics. New York, Appleton-Century-Crofts, 1982; Smith ED: Abortion: Health Care Perspectives. Norwalk, Connecticut, Appleton-Century-Crofts, 1982.

elastic gum inserted in the uterus until contractions begin. Failure rate is high and fetuses are born alive, making this procedure usually unacceptable.[37]

Metreurynter is also a technique used in Japan. A rubber tube with a balloon on the end is inserted in the uterus and filled with 100 to 300 ml of saline. The tube is suspended over the front of the bed with weights of 300 to 800 grams. This procedure is also generally unacceptable. The failure is 15 percent and the fetus is born alive.[38]

PSYCHOLOGIC FACTORS

Motivation for Abortion

Pregnancy itself causes emotional and physiologic stress. No matter how planned or desired the pregnancy, the first trimester is characterized by ambivalence. Changes in physiologic processes, new feelings, and new concerns all require adaptation on the part of the woman. With quickening in the twelfth to fourteenth week of gestation, the fetus becomes a reality, and the woman usually accepts the need to mother. If the fetus is not accepted as a reality, conflict continues, usually with psychosomatic symptoms, denial of pregnancy, and efforts at abortion.[39]

There are many psychologic motivations for abortion. Early in the pregnancy, the woman may wish to remove a disrupting factor in her life. Social and moral factors such as out-of-wedlock pregnancy may contribute to feelings of shame and disgrace. Concern over the responsibility of raising a child and the economic factors involved also cause stress.[40] Abortions are also sought after rape, incest, sexual acting out, and "accidents." Physical and mental diseases are infrequent indications for abortion.

TABLE 20–2. MIDTRIMESTER PROCEDURES

Procedure and Time	Advantages	Disadvantages and Complications
Intrauterine saline instillation (hypertonic saline—amniotic fluid exchange) After 16th week of pregnancy, usually 16–18 weeks	Can be used later in pregnancy	Higher failure to abort, need to carry pregnancy past 3 months, requires inpatient 2–3 day stay. Complications: retained placenta, hemorrhage, hypernatremia from saline in maternal circulation, water intoxication, myometrial necrosis, abdominal wall endometriosis,[27] infection, convulsions, coagulation defects
Prostaglandins E_2 and F_{2a}		
1. Intraamniotic installation	Shorter abortion time than saline	Need for repeated administration, cervical laceration, higher failure rate than saline, nausea, vomiting, diarrhea, headache, pyrexia, chills
2. Intrauterine extraamniotic	Fewer side effects, lower doses needed	Difficulty placing intrauterine catheter, infection
3. Intravaginal suppository or pessary	Ease of administration, may be used after missed menses	Vomiting, diarrhea, increased failure rate and incomplete abortion
4. Intramuscular (serial injections)	High success rate, easy, safe to administer, can be used after membranes rupture	GI symptoms, pyrexia, headache, flushing, depression, repeated injections uncomfortable

Refusal, however, does not necessarily have adverse physical effects. Binkin[41] and associates found that in 316 women who were refused abortion and continued the pregnancy, neither the rate of serious maternal complications nor neonatal death increased when compared with the rest of the hospital population.

Pregnancy under the best conditions brings its share of fears and conflicts. Abortion is second assault, stopping a process already set in motion.

Psychologic Responses to Abortion

One of the disadvantages attributed to abortion by its critics is the psychologic damage that may be initiated by the procedure. However, analysis of responses is difficult, since one is unable to compare the impact of the procedure with the trauma of undesired motherhood and the negative effects on the children.

The abortion itself may be a crisis situation. During abortion, some women describe anxiety and fear of dying, mental and physical injury, disgrace, and punishment. They also fear disruption of interpersonal relationships, withdrawal of love from significant others, isolation, and separation. They may express fear of destroying living tissue.[42] After saline abortion, some women are shocked that the labor was painful, that the baby was so big, and despite thorough orientation, many do not know what was involved and how the fetus would be removed.[43]

In their longitudinal study of the psychologic impact of abortion in 742 patients, Howard and Joy Osofsky[44] noted that women who had abortion prior to its legalization had only rare instances of negative emotional sequelae. Emotionally healthy women had less negative response than did those with severe psychiatric disorders. Relief and happiness have been the predominant moods.

After legalization of abortion, similar responses were found. Negative reactions were guilt, depressive reactions, and fear of men, but the difficulties were transient.

Older, married, and better educated individuals experienced less emotional difficulty with the procedure, while Catholics had somewhat more emotional difficulty. Race did not relate significantly to psychologic variables. In followup interviews, patient satisfaction with the decision was high, only 5 percent expressing dissatisfaction, most women feeling a sense of release from emotional symptoms.[45]

Niswander and associates[46] administered the Minnesota Multiphasic Personality Inventory preoperatively and 6 months postoperatively to 65 patients. Preoperatively, the patient was less "normal" in overall adjustment, anxiety, depression, and impulsivity than a control group of maternity patients. The abortion patients showed im-

provement in their psychologic state 6 months after abortion, except in impulsivity, so that there was little difference from the control group, suggesting that abortion decreases psychologic stress for the patients and betters their overall adjustment.

Smith[47] found some sexual dysfunction, a mild and self-limiting guilt, and depression in some women, but in most cases, the abortion was therapeutic if the woman desired the procedure. Most of the women in the study resumed sexual activity and only 6 percent sought psychiatric treatment. Most of the women, however, did not see abortion as a preferable means of birth control.

A study at Temple University Health Science Center indicated significant differences in psychologic responses of first and second trimester patients. Two percent of the first and 10 percent of the second trimester patients noted some degree of guilt after the procedure. Two percent of the first and 12 percent of the second trimester women reported feelings of depression. However, only 4 percent of either group had any uncertainty that their decision had been a right one.[48] Rosenthal and Young[49] also report that second trimester abortions, especially after quickening, seem to produce more depression, sadness, and a period of mourning. A woman denies the existence of the fetus during early pregnancy, but once she admits the pregnancy, she begins a process of unconscious attachment to it. The longer the pregnancy endures, the more it becomes a part of her. Therefore, the sense of loss in a recently aborted woman is not surprising—part of her is gone.[50]

In a study involving 62 women, Moseley[51] and associates found that the degree of support of significant persons rather than any demographic variables was most predictive of a positive reaction to abortion. A statistically higher level of anxiety, depression, and hostility were present in women who had made the abortion decisions while coping with opposition of significant others. Women who made their own decision scored higher on hostility pre- and postabortion, however. The investigators speculated that hostility may be a major defense response to guilt.

White[52] found that 50 randomly sampled women having midtrimester D&E abortions did not have the expected level of anxiety during the preoperative period and fell within the normal range in six mood characteristics after delivery.

Frank psychiatric problems are not a usual sequela to abortion. Twenty-one consulting psychiatrists did a progressive study of postabortion psychosis. During a 15-month period, only one case was reported in a woman who had had a past history of postpartum psychosis after previous deliveries.[53]

Adolescents who have abortions may be at risk for suicide on the anniversary of what would have been the aborted fetus' first birthday, although they too usually have a history of psychiatric disturbances.[54]

Induced abortions performed in a medical setting in psychiatrically healthy individuals seem to have few sequelae. However, long-term effects in shaping and changing the life pattern of the woman are still not determined,[55] and longitudinal studies are needed.

If abortion is refused, the impact on the unwanted child must also be considered. Rejection is the one single factor that can be responsible for psychopathology. In a study in Sweden, Forssman and Thuwe[56] investigated the mental health, social adjustment, and educational level of 120 children born after therapeutic abortion was refused. In comparison with a control group, these children received more psychiatric care, exhibited more antisocial and criminal behavior, received more public assistance, and less often continued their education beyond that which was obligatory.

The woman who comes in later pregnancy may have more ambivalence about abortion and more difficulty in making the decision. It is important that patients who contemplate abortion or who have terminated pregnancy have an opportunity to talk to a health professional, since sequelae may be minimized if adequate counseling is given. The woman needs to talk in an atmosphere that is nonjudgmental, both before and after the procedure. Unfortunately, it may be difficult for some health care personnel to provide this opportunity.

Psychologic Reactions of Health Care Personnel

Both physicians and nurses have their own feelings, attitudes, and beliefs about the emotionally charged subject of abortion. Most individuals enter the health professionals to heal and preserve life. Those working in maternity areas particularly may feel distressed about caring for the abortion patient,[57] when their usual role is to bring life into the world. Nurses and physicians may have difficulty relating to the patient or deciding whether to offer congratulations or to be sad.

Strongest reactions have been by staff working with patients who had saline injection with delivery of fetuses that have almost formed human features. Some become angry at the physician, who is blamed for performing the abortion but leaving the "dirty work" to them. Intrastaff hostility and jealousy may develop, especially in hospitals that respect the religious restrictions of some staff and do not assign these nurses to abortion service. Other staff become resentful and may displace their negative feelings on patients.[58]

Dream analysis of nursing students who have had a 1-day clinical experience in abortion units indicated that the abortion experience was more stressful for them than other experiences.[59] Other students respond differently. Estok[60] found that 80 nursing students became more positive toward abortion after a clinical experience with abortion.

Many physicians are reluctant to do abortions, and many hospitals also make restrictive rules related to patient age, length of time into pregnancy, and availability of beds and personnel. Some physicians refuse to perform abortions. Data from a survey of all private obstetricians in one state indicate, however, that private physicians may perform abortions even if they are personally opposed to the procedure if the practice community provides normative and structural support. Low level community support for abortion is a significant obstacle to expansion of services.[61]

There is little question that women need some sources of support, but women may not turn to the physician for advice about abortion. In a sample of 1746 women, only 17 percent turned to their physicians. Forty-one percent spoke to no one, while the male sexual partner was the main source of support, 31 percent consulting with him. Rosen believes that women do not turn to the physician for counseling because of many physicians' negative attitudes and the woman's desire to avoid negative sanctions.[62]

Reactions of the Sexual Partner

Abortion, like sexual intercourse, is an interpersonal event, but it is too often treated as if only one person were involved. Men have their own fears and conflicts about the abortion, and being able to talk to someone may relieve their psychologic stress. Rothstein[63] investigated the reactions of 60 men who accompanied their wives and girlfriends when they came for abortion. Most felt responsible along with their partner for preventing the unwanted pregnancy. The men had a striking lack of knowledge about contraception and abortion, indicating that this was a neglected area of health education.

The role of the sexual partner in the initiation of request for abortion cannot be ignored. Some men may pressure the woman into having an abortion, causing anger in the woman, who feels that she is being coerced into doing something that is against her wishes.[64]

ABORTION CLINICS

Free-standing abortion clinics have been established.[65] Most of these legal clinics are well run and provide counseling as well as abortion service. However, some have been found to be assembly-line operations, concerned primarily with making money. Women may not be counseled to consider their decision, and high-pressure tactics and false information may be used to urge the operation. Abortions may be performed under unsanitary and unsafe conditions, resulting in subsequent infections and internal injury.[66]

In contrast, women's clinics, many started by feminists, have been set up after the Supreme Court decision. They stress self-help and self-education, not just abortion. Individual counseling and followup after the abortion and contraceptive information are provided.[67]

SOCIOCULTURAL FACTORS

Data to Be Considered

Data about women seeking abortion are relatively easy to collect and report, but there is the ever present danger of oversimplification and misunderstanding. Steinhoff[68] has found that these data reveal both attitudinal and situational factors involved in the abortion decision. Attitudinal factors are influenced by a combination of social and cultural experiences, including religious training, ethnic or cultural background, education, and social class.

Race and Ethnicity. From 1972 to 1974, the legal abortion rate was 2.2 times higher and the abortion ratio was 1.5 times higher among nonwhite women than among white women.[69] This is a change from earlier studies that showed that white women obtained most abortions, although nonwhite women had abortion ratios one-third greater.

Steinhoff[70] states that it is difficult to attribute black–white differences to cultural factors. However, these factors may account for other ethnic differences in abortion use. There is a consistently lower rate of abortion among Puerto Ricans in New York City. Lower rates in Hawaii for Filipino, Hawaiian, Puerto Rican, and part-Hawaiian women suggest religion may be a critical factor. However, a study by Gebhard and others[71] indicated that in black women, the educational level correlates with reproductive behavior in the same way as in white women. Negro wives of less than college education as a group were rather opposed to induced abortion as were white women of the same educational status.

Religion. Although the Catholic Church teaches that abortion is immoral, attitudes of Catholic women about the procedure vary. The National Fertility Study of 1965 indicated that Catholic and Morman women were least approving of abortion and white Catholic women with college educations were least approving of all.[72] Some studies indicate that the attitudinal effect of Catholicism depends on how religious the person is.[73] Data reported on Catholic patients in several studies show that the proportion of abortion patients who are Catholic is larger than the Catholic representation in the geographic areas, suggesting that some Catholic women may oppose abortion in the abstract but will resort to abortion with an unwanted pregnancy.[74]

However, Catholic women may be still using abortion less frequently than non-Catholics. In Hawaii, a study of maternity and abortion rates shows a higher pregnancy rate and a smaller rate of abortion in Catholic than non-Catholic women.[75]

Most Catholic clergymen support the Church's teaching on abortion. However, a study by Traina[76] indicates that some difference exists in the extent of agreement by age and job category; younger priests and those working in deprived neighborhoods having a more liberal attitude.

Officially, the Jewish religion is as strongly opposed to abortion as an elective procedure for limiting size of families as is Catholicism. Abortion is sanctioned to save the mother's life or when the child will be born diseased or defective. However, Jewish women and those who report no religion have been found to be the most accepting of abortion. Paradoxically, however, Jewish women utilize abortion the least.[77]

Most Protestant denominations have more liberal rules about abortion. However, statistics at birth control and abortion clinics show little relation to population percentages of the various denominations.[78] The Planned Parenthood Poll found that differences in attitudes about abortion were not so great between Catholics and Protestants as between frequent churchgoers of either faith and those who attend only occasionally.[79]

Gebhard[80] found that religious devotedness correlated positively with live births and negatively with induced abortion and relatively few religious women had induced abortion. Religiosity rather than specific religious denominations per se seems to be the major factor in attitudes toward utilization of abortion.

Social Class and Education. Studies have demonstrated that abortion is more widely used in middle and upper classes. In the Hawaii study, 22.8 percent of white collar or middle class pregnancies ended in abortion, while only 14.9 percent of blue collar or working class pregnancies ended similarly.[81]

Liberal attitudes toward abortion are positively correlated with educational attainment and modern conceptualization of the feminine role. In the National Fertility Study, a series of probability sample surveys of married women taken at 5-year intervals, people who completed college scored 4.4 (where 6 means the subject accepts all six major reasons for abortion and 0 means the subject rejected all six) compared to 2.5 for those who completed only elementary school,[82] but they may still seek abortion.

In the Hawaii study, a quarter of all pregnancies of women with higher education, as opposed to only a fifth of pregnancies of women with high school education or less, were terminated by abortion. A direct motive given for abortion was a desire for further education. Contrasting figures from those of Hawaii were reported from Maryland, where 40 percent of abortion patients had a high school education or less, while 13 percent had some higher education. Gebhard and associates[83] found that in terms of absolute numbers, women with grade school education had the most induced abortions, those with postgraduate education the least.

Women who seek first trimester abortion tend to be the better educated, and non-teenagers than women seeking midtrimester abortions.[84]

Demographic Factors—Age, Marital Status, Parity. Between 1972 and 1978, the abortion rates and ratios (abortions per 1000 live births) have increased for all American adolescents, but those for teenagers of black and other races have increased faster than those of whites.[85] Factors of age, marital status, and parity are interrelated and heavily influence a woman's decision to chance abortion. Two types of patients are seen. One type is the young, unmarried woman who has not begun a family but plans to do so at a later date. The other type is the older, previously or presently married woman who has already completed her family. Women who do not want children at all or who want to space their children make up only a fraction of patients.[86,87] Abortion is also more common among women who are separated, divorced, or widowed.

Situational factors seem more important than attitudinal. Steinhoff[88] suggests that attitudinal variables are more likely to predict how Americans vote for change in abortion laws than to predict if women will utilize abortion.

NURSING IMPLICATIONS

Nurses must recognize their feelings and deal with them honestly if they are to pro-

vide adequate care. Those who work in settings where abortion services are not segregated from other patient care must subscribe to the philosophy of care, or their punitive attitudes will be communicated to the patient and negatively affect care. Harper and associates[89] found that women having abortions perceived nursing care as less supportive in a hospital where nursing staff held negative views toward abortion than did women having abortions in another hospital where nurses viewed abortions more favorably.

In 1972, the Nurses Association of the American College of Obstetricians and Gynecologists published a statement in which they urged concern and compassion for the woman having an abortion. They also stressed that nurses have the right to refuse to assist with abortions or sterilizations in keeping with their ethical, moral, or religious beliefs, except when the patient's life is clearly in danger. When nurses decline to participate in abortion, failure to assist should in no way jeopardize the nurse's employment.[90] In Doe vs. Bolton, the Supreme Court upheld the section of the abortion statute that provided for conscience protection. The Federal Civil Rights Act states that the employer bears the burden of proving undue hardship to accommodate the religious needs of an employee.[91] However, nurses who oppose abortion should not impose their personal views on peers or on clients.

Assessment

Initial assessment begins with the nurse who analyzes her/his attitudes and ethics relating to abortion, sex, and the quality of life.[92] If the nurse holds negative attitudes toward the woman who elects abortion, it is usually wiser for someone else to give care. The patient may be anxious and conflicted, and she needs someone who is sensitive to her feelings and compassionate in approach to care. Lack of understanding can be devastating.[93]

During the initial conference, relevant medical, obstetric, and social history is obtained. Abortion may be considered a crisis situation, so that the nurse is alert for subtle signs of stress. Since there is some evidence that Catholic women may have more ambivalent feelings about abortion, the nurse particularly gives them the opportunity to verbalize their feelings and concerns so she can assess their willingness and desire for the procedure.

The patient will usually bring up the reasons the pregnancy is unwanted, but a helpful introduction is, "We feel it is important that you have a chance to talk to someone who is not a friend or relative and to talk about how you feel about this pregnancy, and what it is you want to do. It is a good idea if you go over some of your choices and express some of your feelings about them."[94] It is important that the decision be made by the woman herself and that she not be coerced by others, since there is probably nothing more harmful than an abortion that a woman feels has been performed against her will.[95]

Data are obtained concerning options available to the woman and what plans there might be for a baby. Other questions to have answered include: What does the pregnancy mean to the woman and what are the reasons for the pregnancy? Was it planned or accidental? Other information obtained relates to her attitudes toward abortion, the relationships involved in this pregnancy, past contraceptive use, and the general past sexual history.[96]

It is important that the nurse determine how people important in the patient's life consider the procedure and whether the woman feels it will affect her relationship with her family. The attitude and degree of support of the sexual partner is assessed. Is he supportive and understanding? Is he against the procedure, or has he not been involved in the decision for abortion?

The patient's coping mechanisms should be assessed. Is she able to make her own decisions, or is she more likely to let others make the decisions for her? Is she managing satisfactorily at her job or at school? Is there a history of emotional disturbance in the past.[97] Finally, the nurse determines the patient's/client's knowledge about the procedure.

It is helpful if the initial assessment interview can be done a day or two before the procedure, rather than the same day, so the woman can think over what has been discussed and talk with the sexual partner if he has not been at the initial interview.[98]

The assessment procedure provides the opportunity to identify women who might benefit by either brief or intensive psychiatric care. In interviewing to provide referral, the nurse looks for severe ambivalence, a decision made under coercion, psychiatric illness, abortion for medical reasons in a patient who really desires to continue the pregnancy, and repeat abortions, especially ones late in pregnancy.[99]

If the patient's decision is for abortion, she must be given the chance to ventilate her feelings in order to lessen the anxiety, guilt, and conflict before the procedure.

Planning

The goal of the initial interview is not only to gather preliminary information before an abortion, but to help the woman make the decision that is right for her. The nurse also analyzes the information to plan for teaching and provision of needed support if the patient chooses to have the abortion or chooses not to have the procedure. The nurse also plans care to help the patient and her family utilize their coping mechanisms.[100]

Intervention

Before the Procedure. Patients may show signs of distress such as crying, shaking. A calm approach, a gentle touch, and statements such as "I understand that you feel sad" may help deal with feelings. Other patients deny feelings, appear stoic, overconfident, and avoid eye contact.[101] They may appear hostile to staff. These behaviors are accepted and the patient given an opportunity to talk.

Preoperative teaching is directed to explaining what is involved in the abortion procedure. Patients are often misinformed about the procedure, some believing that it causes physical damage, sterility, or death. They do not know what the procedure involves, especially that in the case of midtrimester abortions, uterine contractions take place to expel the baby. Some think the saline "dissolves" the baby.[102] Even though anxious, patients need careful explanation of the steps of the abortion procedure.

During the Procedure. In some areas, for midtrimester abortions, nurses give total care to saline abortion patients, except for the saline instillation. The nurse remains with the patient during the injection. If the nurse has given careful explanation, the patient will more likely trust her, and this trust may help augment the patient's psychologic strength.[103]

The nurse listens to the patient. Often the patient may again talk about reasons for the abortion and her fears about the labor. She begins to resolve the consequences of the procedure. Some patients may express regret about the decision. Nurses need skill and comfort with their own feelings to supply needed tender, loving care.

During labor, some patients may have severe pain while others have little. Psychologic response may accentuate pain, and there is no joy during an abortion to make pain tolerable such as with childbirth. Basic comfort measures, in addition to giving medication, include perineal cleansing and linen changes. Solid food is discouraged during the labor stage, since nausea and vomiting may occur near the time of abortion. Careful record is kept of urinary output in order to detect oliguria due to water intoxication from the antidiuretic action of oxytocin drugs. The patient has bathroom privileges until her cervix is partially dilated or until she complains of rectal pressure. She is then kept at bedrest.[104]

Then the nurse instructs the patient to exert pushing force until abortion occurs. If the placenta is not expelled immediately, the cord is clamped and cut and the fetus removed. The patient is not allowed to have anything to eat or drink until the placenta is expelled, since surgical removal may be required. Precautions against infection are important through all stages of abortion, but especially when expulsion of the placenta is delayed.[105]

First trimester abortions are shorter in duration but require as careful explanation of the procedure, which is usually easier to perform than midtrimester procedures. Since these can be done in free-standing clinics, the women will have shorter contact with health professionals than in midtrimester procedures.

After the Procedure. Contraceptive teaching is an important aspect of the care of the abortion patient. In addition, the nurse has the opportunity to teach about other aspects of sexual functioning, clarifying myths and misconceptions about sexuality.

Women also need time to verbalize their feelings about the procedure. Some women may have negative feelings about sexual activity or their sexual partner, guilt feelings, and a sense of loss, especially if the abortion took place in the second trimester. They may feel angry and express their hostility by criticism of the staff and the procedure. Listening and accepting the anger is important. Other women express a sense of relief, but they, too, should be given an opportunity to talk about the procedure.

Doing health teaching before the woman has recovered from analgesic medication is futile, and little information will be retained or understood. One-to-one teaching and counseling is preferred to group intervention. Written information about complications and health measures to follow after returning home are essential to fill in the gaps in the woman's memory. After first trimester procedures, patients are instructed to use sanitary pads only, since tampons may introduce infection. Showers are preferable for the following 2 weeks, but tub baths may be taken if showers are not available. Douching is prohibited for 4 weeks. Intercourse should be avoided until the bleeding has completely stopped for 48 hours. Mild or moderate cramping and a moderate amount of bleeding may occur for 24 to 48 hours after the procedure, and spotting may occur for up to 3 weeks.[106]

After saline abortion, women are given instructions to avoid intercourse, douching, tub baths, and use of tampons until heavy bleeding stops.

In many instances, the patient seeking abortion has had no prior use of contraception. Hearing about conception control measures and provision of some contraceptive method is part of the abortion experience. Since the woman may be emotionally and physically fatigued, written information is essential.

Intervention: The Woman Who Chooses Not to Have an Abortion

A woman, after discussing alternatives, may decide not to have the abortion but elects to continue the pregnancy and keep the baby or give it up for adoption. The nurse can direct her to agencies that can be of help. Various adoption and foster home agencies are available. Planned Parenthood and United Fund Agencies have lists of agencies that provide help as well as homes in which the woman can live during the pregnancy if she cannot remain at home.

Groups such as Heartbeat, Lifeline, and Birthright vary in operating policy, but agree to provide confidential service without charge, offering emotional support, and medical, legal, or material assistance for women during their pregnancy. Birthright chapters, in addition, offer help in arranging adoption through licensed agencies, provide financial assistance and shelter if necessary, and supply maternity clothes, baby clothes, and baby furniture without charge. The services are free and confidential. Psychologists and so-cial workers volunteer their services; doctors and lawyers arrange their fees on a sliding scale.[107] Pro-life persons are realizing that tangible steps must be taken to help the woman with a problem pregnancy—urging her to avoid terminating her pregnancy is not enough intervention.

Evaluation

Intervention is successful when the woman has made her own informed choice based on adequate knowledge about abortion and other options open to her. The following outcome should be noted. The woman

1. Discusses her feelings about abortion.
2. States the options open to her and where she can get help if she decides not to terminate the pregnancy.
3. Describes in simple terms the procedure that will be performed if abortion is chosen.
4. Identifies her health care after discharge with written instructions to guide her.
5. Has information about conception control methods and where she can obtain further information.
6. Has an opportunity to discuss her feelings and concerns after the procedure.

NOTES

1. Babikian HM: Abortion. In Sadock BJ, Kaplan HI, Freedman AM (eds): The Sexual Experience. Baltimore, Williams and Wilkins, 1976, pp 349–357
2. Connery JR: Abortion: A philosophical and historical analysis. Hosp Prog 58(4)49–50, 1977
3. Babikian HM: Abortion. In Sadock BJ, Kaplan HI, Freedman AM (eds): The Sexual Experience. Baltimore, Williams and Wilkins, 1976, p 350
4. Ibid
5. Smith, ED: Abortion: Health Care Perspectives. Norwalk, Appleton-Century-Crofts, 1982

6. Kapp MB: Abortion and informed consent requirements. Am J Obstet Gynecol 144:1–4, 1982

7. Clary F: Minor women obtaining abortion. A study of parental notification in a metropolitan area. Am J Pub Health 72:283–285, 1982

8. Balides C, Danzger B, Spitz D: The abortion issue: Major groups, organizations and funding sources. In Osofsky HJ, Osofsky JD: (eds): The Abortion Experience. Hagerstown, Maryland, Harper & Row, 1973, pp 496–529

9. Connery JR: Abortion: A philosophical and historical analysis. Hosp Prog 58(4):50, 1977

10. Isaacson W: The battle over abortion. Time, April 6, 1981, pp 20–28

11. Rice CE: An analysis of Eagleton reveals awful outcome. About Issues American Life Lobby, May, 1983, pp 4–8

12. Boston Women's Health Book Collective: Our Bodies, Ourselves, 2nd ed. New York, Simon and Schuster, 1976, pp 216–238

13. Garcia C-R: Human Fertility: The Regulation of Reproduction. Philadelphia, Davis, 1977, pp 129–132

14. Cates W: Legal abortion: The public health record. Science 215:1586–1590, 1982

15. Petitti D, Cates W: Restricting medical funds for abortion: Projection of excess mortality for women of childbearing age. Am J Public Health, 67:860, 1977

16. Garcia C-R: Human Fertility: The Regulation of Reproduction. Philadelphia, Davis, 1977, p 131

17. Steinhoff PG, Smith RG, Palmore JA, et al: Women who obtain repeated abortions: A study based on record linkage. Family Plan Pers 11:30–38, 1979

18. Steinhoff PG, Smith RG, Palmore JA, et al: Abortion increase seen leveling off. The Plain Dealer, February 17, 1983, Sec. C, p 9

19. Garcia C-R: Human Fertility: The Regulation of Reproduction. Philadelphia, Davis, 1977, p 133

20. Schneider SM, Thompson DS: Repeat aborters. Am J Obstet Gynecol 126:319, 1976

21. Steinhoff PG, Smith RG, Palmore JA, et al: Women who obtain repeat abortions: A study based on record linkage. Family Plan Pers, 11:37, 1979

22. Garcia C-R: Human Fertility: The Regulation of Reproduction. Philadelphia, Davis, 1977, p 134.

23. Levin AA, Schoenbaum SC, Monson RR: Association of induced abortion with subsequent pregnancy loss. JAMA 243:2495–2499, 1980

24. Chung CS, Smith RG, Steinhoff PG, Ming-Pi M: Induced abortion and spontaneous fetal loss in subsequent pregnancies. Am J Publ Health 72:548–554, 1982

25. Rovinsky JJ: Impact of a permissive abortion statute on community health care. Obstet Gynecol 41:781–787, 1973

26. Garcia C-R: Human Fertility: The Regulation of Reproduction. Philadelphia, Davis, 1977, p 139

27. Smith, ED: Abortion: Health Care Perspective. Norwalk, Appleton-Century-Crofts, 1982, p 86

28. Cates W: Legal abortion: The public health record. Science 215:589, 1982

29. Lauerson NH, Secher NJ, Wilson KN: Midtrimester abortion induced by serial intramuscular injections of 15(S)-15-methyl prostaglandin E_2 methyl ester. Am J Obstet Gynecol 123:665–670, 1975

30. Speroff L: Prostaglandins and abortion. In Osofsky HJ, Osofsky JD (eds): The Abortion Experience. Hagerstown, Maryland, Harper & Row, 1973, pp. 415–433

31. Whitehead S: Abortion practice: Could drugs replace doctors. Nurs Times April 15, 1976, pp 564–565

32. Speroff L: Prostaglandins and abortion. In Osofsky HJ, Osofsky JD (eds): The Abor-

tion Experience. Hagerstown, Maryland, Harper & Row, 1973, p 415

33. Kerenyi TD: Midtrimester abortion. In Osofsky HJ, Osofsky JD (eds): The Abortion Experience. Hagerstown, Maryland, Harper & Row, 1973, pp 383–399

34. Quilligan EJ, Zuspan FP: Douglas-Stromme Operative Obstetrics. New York, Appleton-Century-Crofts, 1982

35. Garcia C-R: Human Fertility: The Regulation of Reproduction. Philadelphia, Davis, 1977, p 150

36. Ibid

37. Ibid

38. Ibid

39. Babikian HM: Abortion. In Sadock BJ, Kaplan HI, Freedman AM (eds): The Sexual Experience. Baltimore, Williams and Wilkins, 1976, p 353

40. Ibid

41. Binkin N, Mhango C, Cates W, et al: Women refused second trimester abortion: Correlates of pregnancy outcome. Am J Obstet Gynecol 145:279–284, 1983

42. Lanahan CMC: Anxieties and fears of patients seeking abortion. In McNall LK, Galeener JT (eds): Current Practices in Obstetric and Gynecologic Nursing. St. Louis, Mosby, 1976, pp 201–204

43. Goldmann A: Learning abortion care. Nurs Outlook 19:350–352, 1971

44. Osofsky JD, Osofsky HJ, Rajan R: Psychological effects of abortion with emphasis upon immediate reactions and followup. In Osofsky HJ, Osofsky JD (eds): The Abortion Experience. Hagerstown, Maryland, Harper & Row, 1973, pp 188–205

45. Ibid, p 203

46. Niswander KR, Singer J, Singer M: Psychological reaction to therapeutic abortion. Am J Obstet Gynecol 114:29–33, 1972

47. Smith EM: A follow-up study of women who request abortion. Am J Orthopsychiatry 43:574–585

48. Ibid, p 202

49. Rosenthal MB, Young F: The psychological effects of abortion. In Unwanted Pregnancy: A National Health Issue. Cleveland, Case Western Reserve University, 1976, p 52–57

50. Lanahan CMC: Anxieties and fears of patients seeking abortion. In McNall LK, Galeener JT (eds): Current Practices in Obstetric and Gynecologic Nursing. St. Louis, Mosby, 1976, p 204

51. Moseley DT, Follingstad DR, Harley H: Psychological factors that predict reaction to abortion. J Clin Psychol 37:276–279, 1981

52. White LD, White PF: Midtrimester abortion patients. AORN J 34:756–768, 1981

53. Brewer C: Incidence of post-abortion psychoses. Br Med J 1:476–477, 1977

54. Tischler CL: Adolescent suicide attempts following elective abortion: A special case for anniversary reaction. Pediatrics 68:670–671, 1982

55. Babikian HM: Abortion. In Sadock BJ, Kaplan HI, Freedman AM (eds): The Sexual Experience. Baltimore, Williams and Wilkins, 1976, p 355

56. Forssman H, Thuwe I: One hundred and twenty children born after application for therapeutic abortion refused. Acta Psychiatr Scand 42:71–88, 1966

57. Fonseca JD: Induced abortion: Nursing attitudes and action. Am J Nurs 68:1022–1027, 1968

58. Babikian HM: Abortion. In Sadock BJ, Kaplan HI, Freedman AM (eds): The Sexual Experience. Baltimore, Williams and Wilkins, 1976, p 354

59. Hurwitz A, Eadie RF: Psychological impact on nursing students of participation in abortion. Nurs Res 26:112–119. 1977

60. Estok PJ: Abortion attitude of nurses: A cognitive dissonance perspective. Image 10(3):70–74, 1978

61. Nathanson CA, Becker MH: Professional norms, personal attitudes and medical practice: The case of abortion. J Health Soc Behav 22:198–211, 1982

62. Rosen RH: The patient's view of the primary care physician in abortion. Am J Public Health 67:863, 1977

63. Rothstein AA: Men's reaction to their partner's elective abortion. Am J Obstet Gynecol 128:831–837, 1977

64. Boston Women's Health Book Collective: Our Bodies, Ourselves, 2nd ed. New York, Simon and Schuster, 1976, p 222

65. Hall RE: Abortion: Physician and hospital attitudes. Am J Public Health 61:517–519, 1971

66. Risky abortions: Chicago clinics exposed. Time, November 27, 1978, p 52

67. Gray MJ, Tyson J: Evolution of a women's clinic: An alternate system of medical care. Am J Obstet Gynecol 126:760–765, 1976

68. Steinhoff PG: Background characteristics of abortion patients. In Osofsky HJ, Osofsky JD (eds): The Abortion Experience. Hagerstown, Maryland, Harper & Row, 1973, pp 206–231

69. Tietze C: Legal abortions in the United States: Rates and ratios by race and age. Family Plan Perspect 9:12–15, 1977

70. Steinhoff PG: Background characteristics of abortion patients. In Osofsky HJ, Osofsky JD (eds): The Abortion Experience. Hagerstown, Maryland, Harper & Row, 1973, p 211

71. Gebhard PH, Pomeroy WB, Martin CE, Christenson, CV: Pregnancy, birth and abortion. In Weinberg MS (ed): Sex Research. New York, Oxford, 1976, pp 100–113

72. Shain RN: Abortion practices and attitudes in cross-cultural perspective. Am J Obstet Gynecol 142:245–251, 1982

73. Steinhoff PG: Background characteristics of abortion patients. In Osofsky HJ, Osofsky JD (eds): The Abortion Experience. Hagerstown, Maryland. Harper & Row, 1973, p 211

74. Ibid, p 212

75. Ibid

76. Traina FJ: Catholic clergy on abortion: Preliminary findings of a New York State survey. Fam Plann Perspect 6(3):151–156, 1974

77. Fineman RM, Gordis DM: Occasional essay: Jewish perspective on prenatal diagnosis and selective abortion of affected fetuses, including some comparisons with prevailing Catholic beliefs. Am J Med Genetics 12:355–360, 1982

78. Franzblau A: Religion and sexuality. In Sadock BJ, Kaplan HI, Freedman AM (eds): The Sexual Experience. Baltimore, Williams and Wilkins, 1976, pp 611–625

79. RL Associates (Princeton, New Jersey): Public attitudes toward birth control, sex education and abortion. Commissioned by Planned Parenthood Federation of America, Inc., New York, 1979

80. Gebhard PH, Pomeroy WB, Martin CE, Christenson CV: Pregnancy, birth and abortion. In Weinberg MS (ed): Sex Research. New York, Oxford, 1976, p 113

81. Steinhoff PG: Background characteristics of abortion patients. In Osofsky HJ, Osofsky JD (eds): The Abortion Experience. Hagerstown, Maryland, Harper & Row, 1973, p 214

82. Shain RN: Abortion practices and attitudes in cross-cultural perspective. Am J Obstet Gynecol 142:249, 1982

83. Gebhard PH, Pomeroy WB, Martin CE, Christenson CV: Pregnancy, birth and abortion. In Weinberg MS (ed): Sex Research. New York, Oxford, 1976, p 103

84. Fielding W, Sachtlebein M, Friedman L, Friedman E: Comparison of women seeking early and late abortion. Am J Obstet Gynecol 131:304–311, 1978

85. Ezzard NV, Cates W, Kramer DG, Tietze C: Race-specific patterns of abortion use by American teenagers. Am J of Publ Health 72:809–814, 1982

86. Steinhoff PG: Background characteristics of abortion patients. In Osofsky

HJ, Osofsky JD (eds): The Abortion Experience. Hagerstown, Maryland, Harper & Row, 1973, p 224

87. Gebhard, PH, Pomeroy WB, Martin CE, Christenson CV: Pregnancy, birth and abortion. In Weinberg MS (ed): Sex Research, New York, Oxford, 1976, pp 101–103

88. Steinhoff PG: Background characteristics of abortion patients. In Osofsky HJ, Osofsky JD (eds): The Abortion Experience. Hagerstown, Maryland, Harper & Row, 1973, p 214

89. Harper MW, Marcom BR, Wall VD: Do attitudes of nursing personnel affect the patient's perception of care. Nurs Res 21:327–330, 1972

90. Tyrer L: The new morality, ethics and nursing. J Obstet Gynecol Nurs 2:54–55, September–October 1973

91. Creighton H: Refusing to participate in abortion. Nurs Management 13:27–28, 1982

92. Keller C, Copeland P: Counseling the abortion patient is more than talk. Am J Nurs 72:102–106, 1972

93. One day you will understand. Nurs Mirror 155:40–41, 1982

94. Rosenthal MB, Young FR: Voluntary interruption of pregnancy. In Lytle NA (ed): Nursing of Women in the Age of Liberation. Dubuque, Iowa, Brown, 1977, p 157

95. Bolognese RJ, Carson SL: Interruption of Pregnancy: A Total Patient Approach. Baltimore, Williams and Wilkins, 1975, p 17

96. Branch BM: Extramural abortions: Why bother. In Osofsky HJ, Osofsky JD (eds): The Abortion Experience. Hagerstown, Maryland, Harper & Row, 1973, pp 122–134

97. Rosenthal MB, Young FR: Voluntary interruption of pregnancy. In Lytle NA (ed): Nursing of Women in the Age of Liberation. Dubuque, Iowa, Brown, 1977, p 158

98. Ibid, p 157

99. Rosenthal MB, Young, FR: Voluntary interruption of pregnancy. In Lytle NA (ed): Nursing of Women in the Age of Liberation. Dubuque, Iowa, Brown, 1977, p 158

100. Cronenwett LR, Choyce JM: Saline abortion. Am J Nurs 71:1754–1757, 1971

101. White LD, White PF: Midtrimester abortion patients. AORN J 34:58, 1981

102. Goldman A: Learning abortion care. Nurs Outlook 19:351, 1971

103. Cronenwett LR, Choyce JM: Saline abortion. Am J Nurs 71:1756, 1971

104. Ibid

105. Ibid, p 1755

106. Bolognese RJ, Carson SL: Interruption of Pregnancy: A Total Patient Approach. Baltimore, Williams and Wilkins, 1975, p 97

107. Balides C, Danzger B, Spitz D: The abortion issue: Major groups, organizations, and funding sources. In Osofsky HJ, Osofsky JD (eds): The Abortion Experience. Hagerstown, Maryland, Harper & Row, 1973, p 511

Chapter 21

Pregnancy, Birth, and Postpartum

Pregnancy, especially the first, can be viewed as one of the most important developmental crises in a woman's life. For many it is a time of stress. For all it is a period of profound biologic and psychosocial changes. Unfortunately, there is a paucity of objective data about how persons deal with and meet their sexual needs and maintain their sexual relationship during this time.

Butler and Wagner[1] believe part of the problem lies in society's attitude toward sexuality, indicting the medical world particularly as having difficulty accepting sexuality and pregnancy simultaneously in the same person. Society's attitude may be summed up in the statement, "Whoever saw a sexy pregnant lady?"[2] It is speculated that the impending motherhood in women raises unconscious resistance in physicians, who are usually male, "by mixing the unmixables, lover and mother."[3] Consequently, the nurse, who is usually female, has the opportunity to play a needed and essential role in helping couples meet their sexuality needs during pregnancy, childbirth, and postpartum, and the woman may sometimes turn to the nurse rather than the doctor.[4]

Increasingly, nurses are expanding their roles in maternity clinics and inpatient services to include not only education, supportive guidance, and assessment, but also comprehensive health supervision to women who are experiencing normal pregnancies.[5,6] Nurse–midwives assist in delivery and direct postpartum care.

This chapter includes discussion of the biologic changes that occur in the sexual response cycle during pregnancy and the postpartum, as well as changes in the subjective experiences of pregnant women during coitus. Changes in the pattern and frequency of sexual activity of both the woman and the man and the biologic and psychosocial factors that cause or influence these changes are presented. Sexual responses during the intrapartal and postpartal periods and their influencing factors are also discussed to help nurses identify when problems exist and intervene therapeutically.

PREGNANCY

Biologic Changes in the Sexual Response Cycle

Masters and Johnson[7] were able to compare physiologic sexual responses of six women during pregnancy with nonpregnant sexual response. After conception, the breasts enlarged and became tender due to increased amount of vascular and glandular structures. During the first trimester, when the multiparous woman responded to sexual stimulation, the venous congestion of the breast became more noticeable than in the nonpregnant state (see Chapter 3). This was accompanied by tenderness localized to the nipple and areolar area. As the pregnancy continued, there was decreased tenderness, although the breast increased in size by one-third. In nonpregnant women, sexual tension causes an increase in breast size, nipple erection, and areolar tumescence, but this was not true of the pregnant woman.[8]

Increased vascularity of pelvic viscera takes place. All six subjects experienced increased sexual tension levels toward the end of the first and during the early stages of the second trimester. Sexual tension reached a high level during the second and continued into the third trimester. The women also had increased uterine irritability after effective sexual stimulation.[9] Masters and Johnson also reported changes in relation to the four phases of the sexual response cycle. (Table 21-1).

Subjective Reports of Changes in Sexual Activity and Response

Women's sexual response to pregnancy has been studied with both contradictory findings and agreement (Table 21-2). In general, studies indicate a general decline in sex interest, libido, frequency, and satisfaction with sexual activity and coitus, but in all studies there was considerable number of women for whom this was not true. There are methodologic problems with all the studies so general trends can be reported but each couple must be evaluated separately.

For example, the direction of changes in sexuality reported by Falicov corroborates the findings of Masters and Johnson: very reduced sexual function in the first trimester, relatively increased by the second trimester and the first part of the third trimester, followed by sharp decline in the last month of pregnancy. In Masters and Johnson's subjects, however, second trimester sexual interest moved beyond the prepregnancy norms of sexual performance, while Falicov's subjects did not escalate that high.

Pregnancy can be a time of increased libido for many women. Some report that in-

---

TABLE 21–1. CHANGES IN SEXUAL RESPONSE CYCLE

Excitement phase: Dramatic vasocongestive response more than myotonic; labia majora in nullipara—no change, multipara—engorged and edematous; labia minora—engorged and enlarged in both; vaginal lubrication, increased from end of first trimester throughout pregnancy; vaginal expansion and distension same as nonpregnant state; tenting or ballooning of proximal ⅓ of vagina absent.[10]

Plateau phase: Skin color change of labia minor same as nonpregnant state; orgasmic platform, even more pronounced due to extensive vasocongestion.[11]

Orgasmic phase: Altered, uterus may go into tonic spasms instead of rhythmic contractions; contractions of distal ⅓ of vagina and of uterus occur throughout pregnancy,[12] orgasm does not reduce sexual tension for long period.

Resolution: Pelvic vasocongestion—not relieved completely by orgasm and becomes increasingly less as pregnancy progresses—may explain subjective experience of higher sexual tension levels.[13]

TABLE 21-2. STUDIES OF CHANGES IN SEXUAL ACTIVITY AND RESPONSE

Study	Year	No. of Subjects	Findings
Masters and Johnson[14] (retrospective interview)	1966	111 women, 79 husbands participated	Eroticism and response; 1st trimester: nulliparas decreased in multiparas same; 2nd trimester: increased eroticism and response in both groups beyond nonpregnant state, increased sexual fantasies and dreams and demand for sexual performance by male; 3rd trimester: decreased interest in sexual activity as delivery date neared.
Solberg, Butler, and Wagner[15] (retrospective interviews)	1973	260	Coital activity, orgasmic response, sexual interest and noncoital sexual behavior decreased in linear fashion; activity tending to decrease more with greater age and longer marriage; coital frequency independent of age, religion, education, negative feelings about pregnancy, planned or unplanned pregnancy; those with decreased sexual interest tended to have lower rates of coitus before pregnancy than those whose level stayed the same or increased; decrease in intensity of orgasm in some, increase in others; rate of orgasm significantly related to sexual interest level; decrease in number who masturbated, or use of hand stimulation by sexual partner; no difference in use of oral–genital stimulation; coital positions, decrease in male superior and increase in others, especially side by side, rear entry.
Falicov[16]	1973	19 primigravidas	First trimester: 8 had moderate or marked decrease in desire, coital frequency, eroticism, 1 had increased satisfaction; second trimester: coital frequency, sexual satisfaction slightly increased from first trimester but below prepregnancy level, sexual relationship improved over first; third trimester: 7–8 months, 7 women had fluctuation in desire, at times disinterest, other times above prepregnancy level; half felt coitus more relaxed and enjoyable; by 8th month 15 of 18 couples stopped intercourse, 2 stopped at 3 weeks before due date, one not at all.
Holtzman[17] (retrospective)	1976	25	Coitus and orgasm decreased as pregnancy advanced; orgasm from masturbation and oral–genital sex more difficult to achieve.
Robson, Brant, and Kumar[18] (longitudinal)	1981	119	Coitus, libido and enjoyment decreased especially in third trimester.

(continued)

TABLE 21–2. *(cont.)*

Study	Year	No. of Subjects	Findings
Perkins[19] (retrospective survey)	1982	155	Coital frequency, interest and positive attitude toward coitus progressively decreased; masturbation persisted or increased in inverse relation to coitus; poor conjugal relationship before pregnancy resulted in more rapid deterioration after than did a good relationship; majority felt pregnancy improved feelings about marriage, partners, and babies.
Reamy, White, Daniell, and LeVine[20] (prospective study)	1982	52	Coital frequency, enjoyment and orgasm decreased linearly through pregnancy; mid-trimester increase in sex desire followed by progressive decline; sexual satisfaction correlated with feeling (1) happy about pregnancy, (2) more attractive in late pregnancy than before pregnancy, (3) experiencing orgasm; male superior position, primary position throughout, female superior next, side by side, rear entry used by more subjects as pregnancy progressed; no difference between parous and nulliparous in desire, coital frequency and orgasm; nulliparous had more sexual enjoyment than parous in early pregnancy.

terlocking physiologic processes between the mother and the fetus make the woman's body "abound with libidinous feelings," that metabolic and emotional processes replenish the libido reservoir of the pregnant woman. Rosenbaum[21] states that activity usually considered reproductive may be associated with a considerable level of genital excitement. The movement of the fetus has been described as stimulating by some women.

Etiology of Change in Sexual Activity

During the first trimester, there is general agreement that gastric distress, nausea and vomiting, and general physical discomfort, fatigue, sleepiness, and breast and vaginal discomfort were major causes for decreased sexual interest. The severity of symptoms was associated with a concomitant decrease in sexual activity. Ptyalism, increased sali-

vation, may also limit sexual activity for physical and esthetic reasons.[22]

Other somatic complaints voiced by six women in the Falicov[23] study included changes in the sexual organs, such as the vagina feeling smaller making penetration painful, or a feeling of vaginal numbness interfering with the experience of orgasm. Fear of harming the fetus or provoking a miscarriage was voiced by women in all studies. In some women, this fear was a greater inhibitor of sexual enjoyment than physical symptoms. Feelings of loss of attractiveness and loss of interest were expressed by women in all studies. As the delivery date approached, fear of infection, anxiety, fatigue, and sleeplessness were additional factors.[24,25] Some women reported their husbands lost interest in them.

Recommendation from others than the physician were also reasons for cessation of sexual intercourse.[26] Medical indications such as separation of the symphysis pubis due to relaxation of support ligaments of the bony pelvis may cause severe pain on pelvic motion, making sexual activity very uncomfortable. Bleeding may occur at any point in the pregnancy, but most likely in the first and third trimester, and is also a reason for cessation of coitus.[27]

Women who have had several spontaneous abortions are usually instructed to avoid intercourse during the first trimester. In rare cases, intrauterine fetal death is not followed immediately by labor. Some physicians prefer to wait for spontaneous labor, and as a result the woman and her husband have to spend a difficult waiting period. Along with a feeling of loss, the woman feels she must rid herself of this dead thing. Both partners may feel that sexual activity is undesirable.[28]

Physician Instruction

There was considerable lack of uniformity in the teaching and counseling regarding sexual activity during pregnancy that was given to women. Of Masters and Johnson's subjects, 77 of 111 women were warned by physicians, sometimes during the last trimester, not to engage in sexual intercourse until the baby was born. Some doctors forbade intercourse the last 3 months, others for specified periods as short as 1 month.

Twenty-nine percent of the 260 women in Solberg's[29] study were told to abstain from coitus, beginning at times ranging from 2 to 8 weeks before the estimated date of confinement. Only 10 percent received recommendations about positions for coitus that might be more comfortable during pregnancy; side by side or rear entry was recomended to 5 percent. Only 2 percent were instructed about sexual activities that could be substituted for coitus.

Five of 19 women in Falicov's study were told to stop coital activity 6 to 7 weeks prior to the delivery date. Holtzman[30] reported that 60 percent of the women in her study received no medical recommendations about sexual activity, others received false or minimal information.

Effect of Coitus and Orgasm on the Fetus

There are differences of opinion and conflicting reports regarding the effect of sexual activity on the continuation of the pregnancy, on the rate of infection, and on the fetus. It has been postulated that prostaglandins that stimulate uterine contraction may play a part in initiation of premature labor after coitus, since some of these compounds are present in the male ejaculate.[31] A summary of findings of various studies is found in Table 21-3. In general, coitus and orgasm were not found to have deleterious effects.

TABLE 21-3. EFFECT OF COITUS ON FETUS

Study	Year	No. of Subjects	Findings
Pugh and Fernandez[32]	1953	500	No significant relationship between time of last coitus, infection or premature rupture of membranes.
Masters and Johnson[33]	1966	111	Postorgasmic uterine contractions; decrease in fetal heart rate but no fetal distress or early labor.
Goodlin, Keller, and Raffin[34]	1971	200	Incidence of orgasm significantly higher in women who subsequently delivered prematurely than those at term (even those at term described painful uterine contractions or lower abdominal discomfort with orgasm).

TABLE 21–3. *(cont.)*

Study	Year	No. of Subjects	Findings
Goodlin, Schmidt, and Creevy[35]	1972	10	Fetal heart rate decreases with contractions, whether due to coitus, manipulation of breasts, genitalia or other erotic areas.
Solberg, Butler, and Wagner[36]	1973	260	No association found between birth weight, gestational age, APGAR scores at 1 minute and frequency of coitus or rate of orgasm in 7th, 8th or 9th month.
Perkins[37]	1979	25	No association between premature birth and coitus, orgasm and other sexual experiences; orgasmic women had lower percentage of early delivery; coitus apparently a stronger stimulus to contractions than orgasm.
Grudzinskas, Watson, and Chard[38]	1979	70	No association between sexual activity and any indicator of maternal or neonatal condition but a higher incidence of meconium staining of amniotic fluid and low APGAR scores at 1 minute of a few infants whose mothers were sexually active the last 4 weeks of pregnancy.
Naeye[39]	1979	26, 886 pregnancies	Increased amniotic fluid infection rate from 117/1000 to 156/1000; increased respiratory distress; jaundice also two times as common with mothers who were sexually active, the last month.
Rayburn and Wilson[40]	1980	111	No association between frequency of coitus and onset of premature labor in those who delivered prematurely and a matched control group.

Coitus During Pregnancy

Guttmacher[41] suggests that, in the absence of vaginal bleeding or a history of miscarriages, it is safe to have coitus up until 3 or 4 weeks before the expected delivery date, the frequency and positions for intercourse being modified as the pregnancy progresses. Goodlin[42] concurs that, although it is difficult to get data supporting a cause–effect relationship between orgasm, labor, and prematurity, orgasmic abstinence during coitus and other sexual activities is indicated in women with prior difficulty carrying pregnancies to term.

Masters and Johnson state that for the majority of women there is no reason to refrain from intercourse during the first trimester. However, women who are habitual aborters may be cautioned to refrain from intercourse and from orgasm by other means during these months. During the second trimester, there is no reason to refrain from coitus for the overwhelming majority of women. Late in the third trimester, they feel that the problem of coition should be individualized for each woman and her sexual partner. They do not consider that potential infection is an indication for abstention. However, toward the end of pregnancy, when the fetus's head is engaged and the cervix descends into the main axis of the vagina, vigorous coital thrusting may cause the penis to strike the cervix, causing spotting and bleeding. In this case, intercourse should be halted. In other women, the baby's head does not engage, and there is little reason to prohibit intercourse.[43]

Negative feelings may be engendered by

coital prohibitions. These can be avoided or minimized if counseling is individualized, and when necessary, the reasons for abstinence are carefully explained.[44]

Psychologic Factors Affecting Sexuality

Mann[45] sees pregnancy as ideally suited to meet woman's and man's need for creative self-realization, although at times it may be overidealized to meet emotional needs. However, the joy of the accomplishment of pregnancy may become muted by the physiologic and concomitant psychologic changes that accompany the pregnancy experience, adversely affecting the sexual relationship.

Women's Reaction. Childbirth may be considered a part of the maturation process for the woman, reactions throughout the maternity cycle affecting relationships with the sexual partner, other children, and the larger family. Invariably, an increased amount of tension exists. The ability to cope with these tensions is directly related to a close relationship with the mother, a happy home life, social and sexual compatibility with the husband, and economic security.[46] In many situations, however, these beneficent conditions do not exist.

Pregnancy can mean many things, and the woman's reactions can range from happy hope to utter disgust, anger, bitterness, and depression. The motives for having a child differ; because she loves the sexual partner, wants to make new life, likes children, or because she wants to hold a mate, raise faltering self-worth, or to get love from someone even if she has to create him/her. Depending on the factors that operate in each woman, her sexual response to the pregnancy will be affected.[47] Rubin states that women differ in what they perceive, how they interpret the situation, and how they respond to interpersonal relationships during pregnancy. She describes pregnancy as having a cognitive style of its own, a style characterized by inconsistency, questioning, and

uncertainty. Few women who become pregnant are sure they are ready "now."[48]

Responses vary depending on the point in the pregnancy. During early pregnancy, the presence of the child is intangible and the woman may be very introverted, searching for validation of her pregnancy. During the second trimester, usually a happy time, the woman focuses on the condition of the child. As the third trimester commences, she becomes increasingly protective of the child. She feels vulnerable to loss or rejection, danger, or insult. She may seek isolation, feeling a sense of vulnerability, and may become impatient and irritable with her husband. The seventh month is the hardest for the woman to cope with, since she frequently feels that no one cares. During the eighth month, the woman drives herself hard, and her coping resources improve with this activity. By the ninth month, she is "ready."

Jessner and others[49] also associate psychologic fears with the pregnancy experience. Some women see pregnancy as proof of really being a woman and reassurance from the fear of being unable to conceive. Consequently, the first trimester is a period of satisfaction. During the second trimester, the woman loses her enthusiasm and capacity to become involved, partly because of concern about harm to the baby, partly because a concept of sex as sinful and impure is irreconcilable with the idea of a mother. Paradoxically, however, some women have increased sexual needs induced by these anxieties.

Body image changes are a factor affecting her attitude toward pregnancy and in turn toward her sexuality. As her body grows, the changes make her proud, but also distressed because of perceived loss of beauty and growth. Throughout pregnancy, she must cope with altered patterns of sleeping and eating, nausea and vomiting, minor discomforts, pigmentary changes in her skin, enlarging breasts, and an expanding waistline. She may complain of feeling "cow-like" and may wonder if she will ever be the same again. Her thoughts eventually include the child. "Am I big enough and can I stretch to deliver the baby?" "What if I can't?" "Will the baby be all right?"[50] Along with these concerns come those about waning sexual attractiveness and fear of disinterest and loss of her husband's love. At the same time, her introversion and her tendency to focus within herself create a distance between them. Redefinition of femininity is common; a shift from being a girl to being a woman. However, for the woman to whom a career is a form of self-actualization, motherhood may be a dilemma,[51] since she must decide what career changes, if any, will be necessitated by the birth of the child.

Falicov[52] reports the psychologic reactions of 19 women to change in sexual activity during pregnancy. A variety of attitudes were present, ranging from intense frustration to a bland, almost indifferent acceptance. During the early months, half the couples in her study took the changes in stride, but over one-third had difficulty adjusting. By the second trimester, sexual interaction was regarded by 10 of 19 women as a means of affective communication rather than for its erotic value.

During the third trimester, seven women expressed frustration and resentment at having to abstain from sexual relations at a time when they had just become more enjoyable. As delivery approached, nine women stated they had gotten used to decreased sexual activities but felt intensely guilty about their husbands' forced abstinence.[53]

Falicov[54] determined a sexuality index based on frequency of sexual intercourse before pregnancy, affective investment, the importance attributed to intercourse and orgasm, and attitude toward anticipated pre- and postchildbirth sexual abstinence. Women with high ratings on sexuality were less ambivalent or conflicted about sexual relations during pregnancy and experienced fewer and milder changes and more sexual enjoyment than women with low ratings. Falicov concluded that although physical and possible hormonal and psychologic factors were affecting the majority of women when they had decreased sexual adjustment,

those women with a low investment in sexuality may have used the discomfort and fears of pregnancy as a further means of avoiding a tense situation.

Psychologic etiologies may be responsible for biologic problems of pregnancy, especially nausea and vomiting and abortion. Grimm[55] found that some women with hyperemesis gravidarum had a history of gastric disturbances in response to disorders of sex life, usually frigidity. However, in the majority of women, nausea and vomiting are more likely due to biochemical changes and not psychologic maladjustment. In general, Grimm states that sterility, habitual abortion, and premature labor seem to be associated with immaturity and resentment of the feminine role, and in some cases, dependency on or hostility toward the mother.

Semmens[56] investigated the relationship of women's view of their sexual role and the incidence of nausea and vomiting. Contrary to Grimm's observations, he found that patients with nausea and vomiting were far less threatened by their female role, their pregnancy, or by their ability to respond sexually than had been believed. However, the data suggest that the nausea and vomiting represented a reaction to forces that interfered with the women's projection of self-image. Their anxieties were caused more by life situations, family, friends, and society, which threaten that image, rather than problems with sexual role.

Men's Reaction. Benedek[57] describes the instinctual drive of fatherhood, rooted in the instinctual drive for survival. Rainwater[58] found that working class fathers viewed pregnancy as confirmation of their masculinity. Fatherhood is as essential to being as motherhood. However, pregnancy may be a time of conflict for the man as well as the woman. Tenderness, gentleness, and a capacity to empathize with others, to respond emotionally, and to value a love object are all parts of fatherliness as well as motherliness, but for the adult male to express these feelings is too often considered evidence of repressed femininity.[59] Consequently, the man may be faced with the dilemma of responding in an appropriate and socially acceptable way to fatherhood, yet feeling the need to assert masculinity.

In the working class families, Rainwater[60] found that it was during pregnancy that husbands were the most considerate of, close to, and interested in their wives. And in fact, most men are considerate of their wives' vicissitudes of pregnancy, but sooner or later they may resent her "pathologic" state, since they are often deprived of coitus, the gratification of virility.[61] In a study of 15 white men 22 to 34 years of age, McNall[62] found that sexual abstinence resulted in frustration or feelings of rejection or both. One father felt so rejected by his wife that he regretted the pregnancy. Another, whose wife could not tolerate intercourse after the sixth month of pregnancy, felt like a "sexual pervert." In general, many fathers expressed uncertainty as to whether it was all right to have intercourse during pregnancy. Many felt a decrease in love and attention from their wives and were left feeling a little resentful. Most of the men were accepting of or took pleasure in the change in their wives' figures, although several expressed negative feelings. Some expressed feelings of jealousy and fear of losing their wives' attention and love after the baby was born.

Masters and Johnson[63] found that of 79 men participating in the interview project, 71 were married to women whose doctors had forbidden intercourse for periods of from 2 to 6 months. Only 21 of these men understood, agreed with, and honored the prohibition. Eighteen of the husbands engaged in extramarital sex activities during this period, and several insisted this had been the first time they had been unfaithful.

Shereshefsky and Yarrow[64] studied the reactions of 60 young middle class urban families to pregnancy. Especially with the advent of fetal movement, half of the husbands were disinclined to engage in coitus because of fear of harming the baby. Some men evidenced envy of the pregnancy and

the woman's body to the extent of taking pictures of her developing body. Others felt uneasy about the pregnant figure and did not want to be seen about the woman, seeing the changing figures as public evidence of what he "had been doing." Some husbands experienced some of the same physical discomfort as the woman. One man was made so unwell that he could not approach the wife for intercourse and she could not convince him he would not harm the baby.

For some men, passive femininity may be activated. Latent homosexuality may surface, and the husband may resist sharing the wife's interest in pictures and diagrams of the changing figure. The woman's genital area is frightening, and the larger breasts give rise to anxiety about sexual adequacy. The most burdensome and pervasive stress is marital disharmony at a time when support from the spouse is needed by both partners.[65] By the third trimester, particularly, the couple need ingenuity as well as mutual understanding, tenderness, and a sense of humor to work out sexual adjustment.[66] Both the woman and man need to respond sensitively to each other's needs. There is much that is exciting and gratifying about pregnancy along with the uncertainty and anxieties. New depth to the sexual relationship may be the additional outcome.

Sociocultural Factors Affecting Sexuality

Sexual Role. As was mentioned earlier, pregnancy is an unmistakable sign of femininity. Many women accept and take pride in their sexual identity and role, but those who are dissatisfied with their sexual role reject femininity. They claim pregnancy is an unfair burden thrust upon the female sex and feel resentful and humiliated by being pregnant.[67] Especially if the pregnancy is unplanned, they may tend to blame the partner and withhold sexual activity.[68] Others become pregnant to satisfy their need to compete with men. Becoming pregnant is something men cannot do. Unconsciously, the woman who feels deprived of a penis and who envies the male's physical characteristics may try to compensate for being female by imagining the fetus as a male organ.[69]

Jessner and associates[70] report the difference in roles fathers assume during pregnancy. Fathers who were romantically oriented were awed by the responsibility of parenthood, and fathering became a maturational experience. Those who were career oriented regarded parenting as a burden and wished to postpone it. Husbands who were family oriented saw pregnancy as a gift and felt their relationship with their wives became closer. The effect of these responses on sexual relationship may be inferred. Those who saw fatherhood as a burden might view their wives' increasing size and discomforts as evidence of the burden that was being imposed on them. Those who accepted impending fatherhood received joy and satisfaction. In either case, the sexual relationship may be adversely or positively affected.

Cultural Patterns of Sexual Behavior.
In many cultures, males have experienced couvade, the mimicry of labor pains and postpartum fatigue and weakness, which supposedly promoted closeness between father and child. The trend of encouraging the father to be actively involved in the pregnancy by attending prenatal class and permitting him to support the wife during labor and delivery may relate to these early practices.

A sense of responsibility for the unborn child is evident in many cultures. Parents' behavior is linked with the health and welfare of the fetus. Fear that coitus may harm the fetus is common in many women and in many men.

In many cultures, pregnancy is a sign of sexual adequacy. In Bolivia, the Aymara tribe arrange the wedding after the woman is pregnant. Trial marriages are accepted and the permanent union is not formalized before children are certain.[71]

In Jordan, pregnancy is used to solidify marriage and is a sign that the women still receives attention from her husband. This same motivation sometimes functions in the

United States.[72] In some cultures, such as the Punjab in India, however, pregnancy is a time of shame and reticence, related to feelings of embarrassment about the coitus that precedes it. Bulgarian villages view people who are pregnant as rather "immoral," while the Nahave of North Canada do not discuss the pregnancy or comment about it, but ignore the condition.[73]

Sexual intercourse during pregnancy is encouraged by some societies, discouraged by others. Chaggu men are taught restraint after the fifth month and practice coitus interruptus. In most of six primitive cultures studied by Mean and Newton,[74] restrictions are imposed gradually, so that fewer than 30 percent approved of intercourse in the ninth month.

Mexican-American[75] and Pueblo Indian[76] women are shy, modest, and reticent. Female nurses, midwives, and physicians should perform the physical examinations and provide prenatal care.

Economic Factors.   No matter how much pregnancy is wanted, many couples will experience anxiety about finances and feelings of inadequacy about being able to cope.[77] If both have been working, the question of managing on one salary or of the wife working may be a source of conflict affecting their sexual relationship. If the pregnancy is unplanned and financial resources are marginal, the partners tend to blame each other rather than themselves, and problems with the sexual relationship may follow.[78]

Unwed Pregnant Adolescents

Pregnancy for the unwed adolescent is a crisis situation, not just for the girl but for her family. The mother, particularly, may feel that the pregnancy is a sign of her inadequacy as a parent, a reflection on her past life and practices, a failure of her daughter to conform to expected behavior, and a threat to her daughter's achievement of potential goals.[79] The mother feels ashamed and may blame herself, experiencing a sense of guilt, because of her own sexual behavior as an adolescent.

The entire family is placed in a state of unbalance. The mother may be faced with talking with the expectant father and his family, negotiating marriage for the daughter, or deciding if a marriage should take place and arranging for pre- and postnatal care for her daughter.[80] Financial problems may also surface.

The nurse recognizes that this is a crisis situation, both for the girl and the family, and focuses on strengthening their communication and their relationship. The nurse must also help the family work through role relationships. Finally, it is essential that the nurse deal with the issue of sex with the girl and her mother and that he/she help them set realistic goals for future behavior.[81]

NURSING IMPLICATIONS

Assessment
The nursing history focuses on obtaining information about bio-psycho-social variables that affect sexuality. The nurse assesses the attitudes of both partners toward the pregnancy, their desire for the pregnancy, their feelings about the pregnancy, and their knowledge of pregnancy and its effect on sexuality. Jensen and associates[82] suggest questions to assess sexual knowledge: "What has your family (partner, friends) told you about sex during pregnancy?" "What are your feelings about sex during pregnancy?" "Is it all right for married people to masturbate?" "How do your ideas about sex differ from your partner's?" "What changes have already taken place in your sexual relationships?"

Sexual self-concept and body image changes are also assessed, using questions such as: "How do you feel about changes in your appearance?" "How does your partner feel about your body now?" "Do you think maternity clothes make the pregnant woman attractive?"

Information about the marital relationship and expected changes in life style is also elicited. "What will it be like having a baby in your home?" "How is your life going to change?" "Your partner's life?" "What plans were interrupted by having a baby now—later?" "What concerns do you have about the pregnancy and afterward?"

The nurse collects information about the woman's physical status. "Tell me about your general health: before pregnancy, after pregnancy." "When do you feel the best, most alive?"[83]

Finally, the nurse obtains information about sexual activity, both before pregnancy and since pregnancy has progressed; the usual frequency of coitus and noncoital sexual activity; the usual frequency of orgasm; general level of comfort of both partners in the area of sexuality; interest and concern for the partner; the overt and covert need of both partners for sexual activity.

This information plus the past obstetric history, closeness to the estimated date of confinement, and the usual repertoire of sexual positions for coitus are especially important for the nurse to be able to answer the woman's question, "Is it all right to make love during pregnancy?"

Planning
The nurse plans care with the following goals: helping the woman and her partner grow in their sexual experience and relationship; attending to the concerns of the partner; providing information about sexual function before, during, and after pregnancy; giving emotional support; and mobilizing sources of love and affection.

The nurse plans for anticipatory guidance; telling the partners beforehand what to expect, the differences in responses, and the normalcy of responses helps decrease anxiety and promotes sexual adjustment.[84] Problems of dyspareunia, differing sexual drives of both partners during stages of pregnancy, and concerns of harm to the mother can be prevented or alleviated by appropriate intervention.

Intervention

Teaching and counseling is most beneficial if it involves both sexual partners. The counselor focuses on psychologic preparation for the stresses of pregnancy, delivery, and postpartum.

Sexual Activity. Individualized response is needed to those who ask about sexual activity during pregnancy. If the woman has a history of abortion, the couple is usually counseled to avoid orgasm for several weeks at the end of the first trimester, when placental support is being firmly established. Providing that the pregnancy is uneventful, without bleeding or pain, there does not appear to be a need to restrict orgasm, whether by manipulation or coitus. The problem of infection resulting from coitus is easily treated, but if membranes have ruptured, coitus should be avoided.[85]

The nurse suggests alternative positions for coitus as the pregnancy progresses. The female superior position allows the woman to control the depth of penile thrusting, and she can lift off if it becomes painful or uncomfortable. Side by side may be comfortable in early pregnancy and a "spoon" position, with partners lying on the same side, with the man penetrating the vagina from the rear, can be comfortable during late pregnancy, since the bed supports the woman's abdomen and she does not feel the man's weight on her. Rear entry or "dog fashion" is also recommended. If coitus becomes too uncomfortable, couples can achieve sexual pleasure and orgasm by manual manipulation or oral–genital activity, if desired, but blowing air in the woman's vagina must be avoided, since cases of air embolism have been described. The nurse encourages the couple to identify what is most satisfying and acceptable to them.

The nurse can counter myths and misconceptions, explaining that the fetus is not harmed by coitus and that it cannot hear or see in utero. Some persons see the baby's role as a third person in lovemaking, causing disruption in sexual activity.[86] The nurse can also combat the myth that the birth process brings about a change in the woman's genitals.

Relieving Discomfort. If breast tenderness is severe in the first trimester, the nurse suggests positions for intercourse that do not cause pressure on the breast and avoidance of breast fondling. During the first and third trimester, the woman may have lower abdominal cramping and backache. Particularly during the third trimester, when tonic contractions replace rhythmic ones during orgasm, the sexual partner can give a backrub to relieve discomfort and provide a pleasant experience.[87]

If prohibition of intercourse is necessary, it is crucial that the woman be informed that the prohibition concerns orgasm and not coitus per se. Consequently, it must be emphasized that masturbating to orgasm may have more potential for fetal harm than intercourse, since the orgasm response tends to be more intense than that of intercourse.

By being an empathic listener, the nurse can enable the couple to discuss their concerns about change in sexual drive and activity, body image, fears associated with the pregnancy, and concerns about changing roles within the family. By acting as a facilitator of communication between the couple, she can help them share problems and identify solutions.

McNall[88] stresses that the more the father knows about the ups and downs of pregnancy, especially in relation to his feelings and concerns, the easier the period of pregnancy and its adjustments will be. Sexual exploration with different techniques of foreplay and coital positions during pregnancy can be a change for growth in patterns of sexual expression that can be used after pregnancy.

Nurses also need to help prospective parents begin to think and talk about their new roles, what they will entail and who will assume the new activities that accompany parenthood.[89]

Evaluation

See outcome criteria given at the end of this chapter.

INTRAPARTUM: BIO-PSYCHO-SOCIAL FACTORS AND SEXUALITY

Labor and Delivery

Delivery of the infant without anesthesia has been described as an intensely orgastic experience. Newton describes several similarities. During early sexual excitement and during early labor, breathing becomes deeper. The woman may hold her breath and make gasping noises as orgasm approaches as well as during the second stage of labor. She tends to have a tortured expression as orgasm nears and a strained look as birth approaches. Rhythmic uterine contractions accompany both processes, and contraction of abdominal muscles during orgasm is much like the bearing down activity. Muscle strength and flexibility are enhanced during coitus and childbirth, and finally, the decreased sensory perception of orgasm and delivery are usually followed by feeling of well-being of joy.[90] One patient described her second delivery without anesthesia as the biggest orgasm she had ever experienced.[91] Another spoke of "exploding."[92]

Shereschefsky[93] questions whether watching childbirth has a sexualized meaning for some women. Some women with voyeuristic tendencies may find some sexual need gratification in watching the birth process. Seeing the use of forceps, however, may be frightening to others. Body image change occurs throughout pregnancy, and it is possible that in the process of labor and delivery, the woman may again be faced with an experience that is threatening and damaging.

If local anesthesia is used, what may be the effect on body image to have part of the body numb, a part the woman can see but not feel, as if watching someone else? The possibility exists that fragmentation of body image and depersonalization may occur.[94] Others, when watching, may perceive delivery as an anatomic assault, and fear of bodily changes precipitated at early months of pregnancy may be intensified. They may become concerned about the body's intactness, with further change in body image and sexual self-esteem.[95]

Increasingly, husbands are being allowed to accompany and assist their wives during labor and delivery. This activity helps to prepare them for the father role and to make them feel an important person in the childbearing process. Cronenwett and Newmark[96] found that attending the childbirth process increased male role satisfaction, self-worth, and sense of growth and positively influenced the couple's relationship. It seems fitting and proper that a process that started with the union of two individuals should be concluded with the presence of both. If feelings of self-worth and sense of growth are associated with childbirth, Cronewett felt it will positively affect other aspects of the father role.[97]

Cultural factors must be considered when inviting the father to be present during the labor and delivery. Some husbands may seem to be apathetic about supplying support and encouragement to the wife during this period. In some cultures, Mexican-American,[98] Pueblo Indian,[99] Arab-American,[100] and oriental[101] men do not usually participate in the labor and delivery process although this custom is beginning to change. Birth is considered a female affair and many of the women do not want their husband's involvement in work they feel is their own. These deeply held beliefs must be recognized and respected, or the experience, rather than facilitating growth in the parent's relationship, may promote dissension.

POSTPARTUM

Biologic Factors Affecting Sexuality

Mann[102] describes postpartum as a time when the parents forget the problems and tensions of the antepartal period in the pride of reproduction. However, the postpartum period has its own set of tensions and problems.

The physiologic reactions to sexual stimulation for the first three postnatal months are marked by decrease in both the rapidity and intensity of response. The vasocongestion of the labia major and minora is delayed until well into the plateau phase. The walls of the vagina are thin and pink, a condition similar to senile vaginitis, due to the hormonal starvation of the involutional period. Finally, the size of the orgasmic platform and the strength of the orgasmic contractions are reduced.[103] However, at the end of the third postpartum month, responses resemble those before pregnancy.

Sexual Activity. In general, there is decreased sexual tension during this period because of fatigue, weakness, and vaginal discharge or spotting. Physical discomfort may limit interest in sexual intercourse and make achieving orgasm more difficult than before pregnancy. Pain in the perineal area, vaginal muscles that seem tighter making intercourse painful or that seem stretched (which women fear might detract from husband's sexual enjoyment),[104] aching from muscular exertion during labor, and breast discomfort whether the woman is nursing or not[105] all serve to decrease sexual response.

Women in Masters and Johnson's[106] sample reported that perineal pain or vaginal barrel irritation were deterrents to full resumption of coital activity. Vaginal barrel lubrication may be decreased during the first 6 weeks to 6 months postpartum because the steroid depletion inhibits the vasocongestion response to sexual stimulation. Interestingly, 11 women reported increased sexual pleasure from tenderness of the episiotomy site or tightness of the postpartum vaginal barrel.

Just as there is lack of uniformity in instructions about sexual intercourse before delivery, there is difference in beliefs about the proper interval for resumption of sexual activity after delivery. "After the 6-week checkup" has been the traditional instruction, but more liberal attitudes are being evidenced. Guttmacher[107] states that coitus can be resumed immediately if no abnormality is present, and in fact, many couples, in the absence of bleeding, discharge or perineal pain, resume intercourse before the date suggested by the physician. Others recommend resuming intercourse 3 to 4 weeks after delivery if the bleeding has stopped.[108]

The presence of an episiotomy and fear of injury to the area before healing has taken place is a frequent cause of coital prohibition. Contrary to popular belief, Richardson and associates[109] report that in a sample of 800 women with vaginal deliveries and median episiotomies, the majority could resume intercourse 14 to 21 days after delivery without adversely affecting the healing of the perineum.

Masters and Johnson[110] found that strong sexual interest returned within 2 to 3 weeks in some women, while others were still sexually uninterested during the third postpartum month. Women who were breast feeding their babies at the time of the third-month checkup as a group reported a quicker return to sexuality and interest in resuming sexual intercourse with their husbands. They also reported higher levels of sexual tension than others, although they have a longer delay in return to ovarian sex steroid production.

In Falicov's[111] study of 19 women, postpartum sexual activity was considerably less frequent than before pregnancy in ten couples, primarily due to fatigue and psychologic tension. However, sexual desire and eroticism had returned to normal or heightened levels. Nine women reported their capacity for orgasm to be increased beyond prepregnancy levels. The timing and level of resumption of postpartum sexual activity were related to the woman's physical condition and her husband's attitude toward abstinence, rather than to their characteristic investment in sexual interaction before pregnancy. In general, the prepregnancy degree of sexual adjustment was related to sexual adjustment during the late postpartum period, but not during the early postpartum period.

After delivery, one-third of 119 primiparas in Robson and associates'[112] study resumed intercourse by 6 weeks and nearly all did by 6 months, but 77 and 57 percent were having intercourse less often at 3 and 12 months respectively, in comparison with the month before they became pregnant. Libido was still down for 57 percent of the subjects at 3 months postpartum, 33 percent had no change, and 10 percent stated it had increased. Pregnancy and childbirth seemed to reduce sexual activity at least for some in the first year although by 12 months postpartum 80 percent had returned to prepregnancy levels and 25 percent were enjoying sex more than before conception.

Breast Feeding. Breast feeding had erotic potential for some women, who reported sexual stimulation to plateau or orgasmic level when nursing their babies. Some felt guilty about their response. Others reported that they decided not to nurse their babies because they found themselves sexually aroused when nursing a previous baby.[113] Moreover, the woman's spouting nipples and tender breasts may serve to compromise sexual ardor of both parents.[114]

Infants may also respond sexually to breast feeding. Kaufman[115] reports that pleasure in breast feeding is present in older babies, as their total body response shows signs of eagerness and rhythmic motion of the hands and feet while nursing. Along with the rhythm of sucking, penile erection is common in male babies, and after feeding, there is relaxation characteristic of the conclusion of satisfactory sexual response.

Psychologic Factors Affecting Sexuality

Postpartal "blues" or depression in the woman is a common phenomenon. Pervasive fatigue, feelings of unworthiness and inadequacy, and fear of pregnancy may operate to cause a depressive reaction with a concomitant aversion to sexual activity and/or a decreased capacity for orgasm.[116] Body image changes of stretch marks, loss of breast tone, and still bulging abdomen also serve to cause feelings of depression.

Fifty-eight of 111 women in the Masters and Johnson[117] study expressed concern

about forced abstinence from sexual intercourse and how it might affect their husband's attitude toward them. They especially complained that they should have been informed in greater detail when intercourse could be safely resumed. Falicov[118] reported that a great deal of anxiety surrounded the resumption of sexual activities. In spite of high levels of sexual desire, fear of damage to the episiotomy was a major factor. Six women seemed to relive the fears that accompanied loss of virginity.

Some women view episiotomy as assault on their body, experiencing anger, especially if no immediate benefit is seen. Others may react negatively to the use of forceps. The woman may fantasize destruction to herself and the baby or feel that the use of forceps represents failure on her part as a woman. These factors may also operate in the etiology of postpartum depression.[119] Women who have had to have a cesarian section may also feel threatened and depressed because they did not have the baby "normally."

Some men have difficulty tolerating the responsibility of parenthood or the feeling of rivalry for the woman's affection engendered by the birth of the baby. The man who is essentially detached and fearful of close relationships may be threatened by the evidence of emotional union of his wife and the infant. This is sometimes expressed as loss of sexual interest following childbirth.[120]

Sociocultural Factors Affecting Sexuality

Assumption of the parent role requires a period of adjustment. The transition to fatherhood has been described as a period of stress that is influenced by many variables. The social support that men receive may help them cope with the role pressures and role conflict that they may suffer, especially for those who desire to pursue a more active role in parenting but also remain in the work world.[121] Fathers may have concerns about the responsibility of raising the child, viewing the success of these efforts as a primary function of their masculinity.[122]

More variables seem to impact on the

attainment of maternal role. These include among others, age, perceptions of child birth experience, early maternal–infant separation, support systems, self-concept, and child-rearing attitudes.[123]

The mother may have conflict between her maternal, wifely, and occupational roles. To the extent that the husband or the employer (if she returns to work) refuses to recognize her new role, internal and external conflicts will occur. Women's Liberation Movement or not, most families consider the woman the primary child caregiver, and discussion of parental detachment most frequently refers to the mother–infant attachment process.

Mothers with professional training and extensive experience in jobs suffer the most severe crisis following the birth of the first child. Working mothers must cope with fatigue and separation anxiety, while non-working mothers have their own concerns and are more disturbed by feeling trapped and inhibited.[124]

In terms of husband–wife roles, women may feel increased dependency on their husbands in the immediate postpartum period. To the degree that the dependency feeling is fully permitted and accepted, a new bond of trust is established. However, if conflicts arise over the new assignment of tasks necessitated by the infant, sexual relationships may be compromised.[125]

The sexual and sensuous aspects of the mother–baby–father relationship varies in differing cultures, in some, muted, in others, well developed. The Navahos develop erotic behavior more highly than most. The husband is reported to nurse at the wife's breast if it becomes overfull, and boy babies are observed to have erotic interchanges with the mother, who may stroke his penis while nursing. On the other hand, the Punjab are shy about nursing, covering the breast and the baby.[126]

Sexual interaction postpartum is encouraged by some societies and discouraged by others. Typical Chinese fathers of the old tradition do not even enter the room of the new mother and baby for 1 month following birth. This custom is believed to have developed from a need to protect the mother from sexual intercourse until she had recuperated from childbearing.[127]

NURSING IMPLICATIONS

Assessment

After delivery, the nurse collects data about the delivery itself; whether perineal tears occurred, the presence of stitches or an episiotomy, the condition of the infant, whether the labor and delivery experience took place as the couple planned, and whether the woman will breast feed. If complications have occurred and the couple place blame on sexual activities during pregnancy, mutual recriminations and guilt may take place, affecting the future sexual relationship.

Before discharge, the nurse determines the couple's level of knowledge about sexual activity in the postpartum period, identifying information needed, their concerns about the sexual relationship, and any myths and misconceptions that exist. When providing care in the later postpartum period, the nurse collects information about the sexual adjustment since discharge and the nature of the roles and relationship. The nurse is particularly observant for signs of depression.

The nurse's goals are similar to those of the antepartal period, only focused on problems of the postpartum.

Intervention

Biologic Aspects. Most women and men desire information about the physiologic and emotional aspects of sexual activity during the postpartum period as well as the antepartum. They may be hesitant to ask questions, so it is the nurse's responsibility to bring up these topics. Group classes in the hospital as well as after discharge can help facilitate sexual adjustment if there is limited time for individual counseling and teaching. It is again important that this be joint counseling with both sexual partners present.

Using anticipatory guidance, the nurse can provide assurance of normalcy if there are changes in erotic interest in early postpartum or if the mother experiences erotic responses to breast feeding. Suggestions to make resumption of coitus less anxiety provoking are made. If decreased vaginal lubrication exists because of steroid starvation, a water-soluble gel or contraceptive cream or jelly can be recommended to increase lubrication. If vaginal tenderness continues, the partners are instructed to rotate one or two fingers around the vagina to help it relax. The woman also identifies areas of possible discomfort.[128] The female superior position for coitus will help the women control the depth of thrusting, but the partners are urged to experiment with different positions to identify the most comfortable.

If the scar of the perineal tear or episiotomy causes pain, this can be decreased by a hot bath as well as by use of a cream or jelly. However, if this pain persists for 4 weeks after resuming sexual activity, the woman should return for treatment, at which time the vaginal opening can either be stretched digitally or with appropriate dilators.[129]

Kegal exercises are recommended. These strengthen the pubococcygeal muscle, the master muscle that controls not only bowel and bladder function, but also vaginal perception and response during intercourse. The exercise involves tightening the anal sphincter and holding for a count of ten, then relaxing. This is repeated three to four times a day.[130] The nurse also makes sure that the couple has the birth control information that they desire before discharge from the hospital.

Psychosocial Aspects. Adverse psychologic responses, especially depression, are often self-limiting, especially if the woman receives the support and love of her partner. The nurse not only provides an attentive ear, but also helps the man cope with the mother's depression while giving the love and consideration she needs. In rare cases where the depression is severe and persistent, psychiatric referral may be necessary.

Role relationship problems require mutual discussion and "working out" by the couple. The mother is reminded that she should not neglect the father because of care to the infant. Communication can be facilitated and mediated by the nurse. If seemingly irreconcilable differences exist, special counseling may be needed.

Evaluation: Pregnancy and Postpartum

The sexual partners are the best judges of the effectiveness of interventions at any stage of pregnancy and postpartum. Some may be satisfied to decrease sexual activity drastically, while others only need permission to be sexually active. Ideally, the same nurse can follow the woman during pregnancy and postpartum to provide continuity of intervention and evaluation. Increasingly, this is possible. Evidence of a warm, supportive relationship that continues and grows signifies to the nurse that her care has been successful. The following are outcome criteria indicating intervention has been successful. The couple:

1. Describes the changes in the sexual response cycle that accompany pregnancy and postpartum.
2. Identifies the changes that may or have taken place in (a) frequency of sexual activity and (b) roles and relationships.
3. States concern for and appreciation of the difficulties that the other may be experiencing in these areas.
4. Describes alternative positions for coitus or other satisfying forms of sexual activity.
5. States that they are coping with the biopsycho-social changes accompanying pregnancy or postpartum.

NOTES

1. Butler JC, Wagner NN: Sexuality during pregnancy and postpartum. In Green R (ed): Human Sexuality: A Health Practitioner's Text. Baltimore, Williams and Wilkins, 1975, pp 133–146
2. Lanahan CMC: Eroticism and orgasm in pregnancy. In McNall LK, Galeener JT (eds): Current Practice in Obstetric

and Gynecologic Nursing. St. Louis, Mosby, 1976, pp 63–69

3. Butler JC, Wagner NN: Sexuality during pregnancy and postpartum. In Green R (ed): Human Sexuality: A Health Practitioner's Text. Baltimore, Williams and Wilkins, 1975, p 133

4. Quirk B, Hassanein R: The nurse's role on advising patients on coitus during pregnancy. Nurs Clin North Am 8:501–507, 1973

5. Grimm LM: Maternity continuity clinic. Am J Nurs 73:1723–1725, 1973

6. Kowalski KE: On call staffing. Am J Nurs 73:1725–1727, 1973

7. Masters WH, Johnson VE: Human Sexual Response. Boston, Little, Brown, 1966, pp 141–168

8. Ibid, pp 143–144

9. Ibid, p 145

10. Ibid, pp 146–147

11. Ibid, p 148

12. Ibid

13. Ibid, p 149

14. Ibid, p 154–160

15. Solberg DA, Butler J, Wagner NN: Sexual behavior in pregnancy. N Engl J Med 288:1098–1103, 1973

16. Falicov CJ: Sexual adjustment during first pregnancy and postpartum. Am J Obstet Gynecol 117:991–1000, 1973

17. Holtzman LC: Sexual practices during pregnancy. J Nurse Midwife 21(1):22–38, 1976

18. Robson KM, Brant HA, Kumar R: Maternal sexuality during first pregnancy and after childbirth. Brit J Obstet Gynecol 88:882–889, 1981

19. Perkins RP: Sexuality in pregnancy: What determines behavior. Obstet Gynecol 59:189–198, 1982

20. Reamy K, White SE, Daniell WC, LeVine ES: Sexuality and pregnancy. J Reprod Med 27:321–327, 1982

21. Rosenbaum M-B: Female sexuality or why can't a woman be more like a woman. In Oaks WW, Melchiode GA, Ficher I (eds): Sex and the Life Cycle. New York, Grune and Stratton, 1976, pp 87–96

22. Mann EC, Armistead TN: Pregnancy and sexual behavior. In Sadock BJ, Kaplan HI, Freedman AM (eds): The Sexual Experience. Baltimore, Williams and Wilkins, 1976, pp 238–247

23. Falicov CJ: Sexual adjustment during first pregnancy and postpartum. Am J Obstet Gynecol 117:994, 1973

24. Ibid, p 995

25. Solberg DA, Butler J, Wagner NN: Sexual behavior in pregnancy. N Engl J Med 288:1101, 1973

26. Ibid

27. Mann EC, Armistead TN: Pregnancy and sexual behavior. In Sadock BJ, Kaplan HI, Freedman AM (eds): The Sexual Experience. Baltimore, Williams and Wilkins, 1976, p 241

28. Ibid, 239

29. Solberg DA, Butler J, Wagner NN: Sexual behavior in pregnancy. N Engl J Med 288:1101, 1973

30. Holtzman LC: Sexual practices during pregnancy. J Nurse Midwife 21(1):38, 1976

31. Mann EC, Armistead TN: Pregnancy and sexual behavior. In Sadock BJ, Kaplan HI, Freedman AM (eds): The Sexual Experience. Baltimore, Williams and Wilkins, 1976, p 241

32. Pugh WE, Fernandez FL: Coitus in late pregnancy. Obstet Gynecol 1:636–642, 1953

33. Masters WH, Johnson VE: Human Sexual Response. Boston, Little, Brown, 1966, p 148

34. Goodlin R, Keller DW, Raffin M: Orgasm during late pregnancy. Obstet Gynecol 38:916–921, 1971

35. Goodlin RC, Schmidt W, Creevy DC: Orgasm during late pregnancy. Obstet Gynecol 39:125–127, 1972

36. Solberg DA, Butler J, Wagner NN: Sexual behavior in pregnancy. N Engl J Med 288:1102, 1973

37. Perkins RP: Sexual behavior and response in relation to complications of pregnancy. Am J Obstet Gynecol 134:498–505, 1979

38. Grudzinskas JC, Watson C, Chard T:

Does sexual intercourse cause fetal distress? Lancet 2:692–693, 1979

39. Naeye RL: Coitus and associated amniotic fluid infections. N Eng J Med 301:1198–1201, 1979

40. Rayburn WF, Wilson GA: Coital activity and premature delivery. Am J Obstet Gynecol 137:972–974, 1980

41. Guttmacher AF: Pregnancy Birth and Family Planning. New York, Viking, 1973, p 102

42. Goodlin R, Keller DW, Raffin M: Orgasm during late pregnancy. Obstet Gynecol 38:920, 1971

43. Masters WH, Johnson VE: Human Sexual Response. Boston, Little, Brown, 1966, p 167

44. Ibid, p 168

45. Mann EC, Armistead TN: Pregnancy and sexual behavior. In Sadock BJ, Kaplan HI, Freedman AM (eds): The Sexual Experience, Baltimore, Williams and Wilkins, 1976, p 245

46. Grimm E: Psychological and social factors in pregnancy, delivery and outcome. In Richardson SA, Guttmacher AF (eds): Childbearing, Its Social and Psychological Aspects. Baltimore, Williams and Wilkins, 1967, pp 1–51

47. Grimm ER: Women's attitudes and reactions to childbearing. In Goldman GG, Milman DS (eds): Modern Woman. Springfield, Illinois, Thomas, 1969, pp 131–133

48. Rubin R: Cognitive style in pregnancy. Am J Nurs 70:502–508, 1970

49. Jessner L, Weigert E, Foy JL: The development of prenatal attitudes during pregnancy. In Anthony EJ, Benedek T (eds): Parenthood: Its Psychology and Psychopathology. Boston, Little, Brown, 1970, pp 210–244

50. Iffrig MC: Body image in pregnancy. Nurs Clin North Am 7:631–639, 1972

51. Jessner L, Weigert E, Foy JL: The development of prenatal attitudes during pregnancy. In Anthony EJ, Benedek T (eds): Parenthood: Its Psychology and Psychopathology. Boston, Little, Brown, 1970, p 220

52. Falicov CJ: Sexual adjustment during first pregnancy and postpartum. Am J Obstet Gynecol 117:996, 1973

53. Ibid

54. Ibid, p 997

55. Grimm ER: Women's attitudes and reactions to childbearing. In Goldman GG, Milman DS (eds): Modern Woman, Springfield, Illinois, Thomas, 1969, p 133

56. Semmens JP: Female sexuality and life situations. Obstet Gynecol 38:555–563, 1971

57. Benedek T: Fatherhood and providing. In Anthony EJ, Benedek T (eds): Parenthood: Its Psychology and Psychopathology. Boston, Little, Brown, 1970, pp 167–183

58. Rainwater L: And the Poor Get Children. Chicago, Quadrangle, 1967, pp 84–85

59. McNall LK: Concerns of expectant fathers. In McNall LK, Galeener JT (eds): Current Practice in Obstetric and Gynecologic Nursing. St. Louis, Mosby, 1976, pp 161–178

60. Rainwater L: And the Poor Get Children. Chicago, Quadrangle, 1967, p 84

61. Benedek T: The psychology of pregnancy. In Anthony JE, Benedek T (eds): Parenthood: Its Psychology and Psychopathology. Boston, Little, Brown, 1970, pp 137–151

62. McNall LK: Concerns of expectant fathers. In McNall LK, Galeener JT (eds): Current Practice in Obstetric and Gynecologic Nursing. St. Louis, Mosby, 1976, pp 168–169

63. Masters WH, Johnson VE: Human Sexual Response. Boston, Little, Brown, 1966, p 168

64. Shereshefsky PM, Yarrow LJ: Psychological Aspects of a First Pregnancy and Early Postnatal Adaptation. New York, Raven, 1973, p 239

65. Ibid, p 247

66. Block NT: Psychology of the pregnancy experience. In Dickson E, Schult MO (eds): Maternal and Infant Care. New York, McGraw-Hill, 1975, pp 139–149

67. Ibid, p 136
68. Man EC, Armistead TN: Pregnancy and sexual behavior. In Sadock BJ, Kaplan HI, Freedman AM (eds): The Sexual Experience. Baltimore, Williams and Wilkins, 1976, p 246
69. Block NT: Psychology of the pregnancy experience. In Dickson E, Schult MO (eds): Maternal and Infant Care. New York, McGraw-Hill, 1975, pp 139–149
70. Jessner L, Weigert E, Foy JL: The development of prenatal attitudes during pregnancy. In Anthony EJ, Benedek T (eds): Parenthood: Its Psychology and Psychopathology. Boston, Little, Brown, 1970, p 240
71. Mead M, Newton N: Pregnancy and outcome: A review of patterns of culture and future research needs. In Richardson SO, Guttmacher AF (eds): Childbearing: Its Social and Psychological Aspects. Baltimore, Williams and Wilkins, 1967, pp 147–241
72. Ibid, p 166
73. Ibid, p 168
74. Ibid, p 208
75. Bullough VL, Bullough B: Health Care for the Other Americans. New York, Appleton-Century-Crofts, 1982
76. Higgins PG: Pueblo women of New Mexico: Their background, culture and childbearing practices. Top Clin Nurs 4:69–78, 1983
77. Block NT: Psychology of the pregnancy experience. In Dickason E, Schult MO (eds): Maternal and Infant Care. New York, McGraw-Hill, 1975, p 148
78. Man EC, Armistead TN: Pregnancy and sexual behavior. In Sadock BJ, Kaplan HI, Freedman AM (eds): The Sexual Experience. Baltimore, Williams and Wilkins, 1976, p 244
79. Bryan-Logan BN, Dancy BL: Unwed pregnant adolescents. Nurs Clin North Am 9(1):57–68, 1974
80. Ibid, p 62
81. Ibid, p 67
82. Jensen MD, Bensen R, Bobak I: Maternity Care: The Nurse and the Family. St. Louis, Mosby, 1977, pp 148–151
83. Ibid, p 148
84. Liebenberg B: Prenatal counseling. In Shereshefsky PM, Yarrow LJ (eds): Psychological Aspects of a First Pregnancy. New York, Raven, 1973, pp 123–161
85. Lanahan CMC: Eroticism and orgasm in pregnancy. McNall LK, Galeener JT (eds): Current Practice in Obstetric and Gynecologic Nursing. St. Louis, Mosby, 1976, pp 63–69
86. Jensen MD, Bensen R, Bobak I: Maternity Care: The Nurse and the Family. St. Louis, Mosby, 1977, p 150
87. Ibid
88. McNall LK: Concerns of expectant fathers. In McNall LK, Galeener JT (eds): Current Practice in Obstetric and Gynecologic Nursing. St. Louis, Mosby, 1976, p 177
89. Smith ED: Maternity Care; A Guide for Patient Education. New York, Appleton-Century-Crofts, 1981, p 126
90. Newton N: The trebly sensuous woman. Psychol Today 5:6–71, July 1971
91. Butler JC, Wagner NN: Sexuality during pregnancy and postpartum. In Green R (ed): Human Sexuality: A Health Practitioner's Text. Baltimore, Williams and Wilkins, 1975, p 140
92. Shereshefsky PM, Yarrow LJ: Psychological Aspects of a First Pregnancy and Early Postnatal Adaptation. New York, Raven, 1973
93. Ibid
94. Ibid, p 92
95. Ibid, p 93
96. Cronewett LR, Newmark LL: Fathers' responses to childbirth. Nurs Res 23:210–217, 1974
97. Ibid, p 216
98. Bullough VL, Bullough B: Health Care for the Other Americans. New York, Appleton-Century-Crofts, 1982, p 83
99. Higgins PG: Pueblo women of New Mexico: Their background, culture and childbearing practices. Top Clin Nurs 4:73, 1983
100. Meleis AI: The Arab American in the

health care system. Am J Nurs 81: 1180–1183, 1981

101. Chung HJ: Understanding the oriental maternity patient. Nurs Clin North Am 12(1):67–75, 1977

102. Mann EC, Armistead TN: Pregnancy and sexual behavior. In Sadock BJ, Kaplan HI, Freedman AM (eds): The Sexual Experience. Baltimore, Williams and Wilkins, 1976, p 246

103. Masters WH, Johnson VE: Human Sexual Response. Boston, Little, Brown, 1966, p 150

104. Falicov CJ: Sexual adjustment during first pregnancy and postpartum. Am J Obstet Gynecol 117:997, 1973

105. Wood SO: Postpartum. In Lytle NA (ed): Nursing of Women in the Age of Liberation. Dubuque, Iowa, Brown, 1977.

106. Masters WH, Johnson VE: Human Sexual Response. Boston, Little, Brown, 1966, p 161

107. Guttmacher AF: Pregnancy Birth and Family Planning. New York, Viking, 1973, p 250

108. Jensen MD, Bensen R, Bobak I: Maternity Care: The Nurse and the Family. St. Louis, Mosby, 1977, p 418

109. Richardson AC, Lyon JB, Graham, EE, Williams NL: Decreasing postpartum sexual abstinence time. J Obstet Gynecol 126:416–417, 1976

110. Masters WH, Johnson VE: Human Sexual Response. Boston, Little, Brown, 1966, p 162

111. Falicov CJ: Sexual adjustment during first pregnancy and postpartum. Am J Obstet Gynecol 117:997, 1973

112. Robson KM, Brant HA, Kumar R: Maternal sexuality during first pregnancy and after childbirth. Brit J Obstet Gynecol 88:885, 1981

113. Masters WH, Johnson VE: Human Sexual Response. Boston, Little, Brown, 1966, p 162

114. Cronenwett L: Transition to parenthood. In McNall LK, Galeener JT (eds): Current Practice in Obstetric and Gynecologic Nursing. St. Louis, Mosby, 1976, pp 179–187

115. Kaufman C: Biologic considerations of parenthood. In Anthony EJ, Benedek T (eds): Parenthood: Its Psychology Psychopathology. Boston, Little, Brown, 1970, pp 3–55

116. Hamilton JA: Postpartum Psychiatric Problems. St. Louis, Mosby, 1962, p 102

117. Masters WH, Johnson VE: Human Sexual Response. Boston, Little, Brown, 1966, p 163

118. Falicov CJ: Sexual adjustment during first pregnancy and postpartum. Am J Obstet Gynecol 117:996, 1973

119. Daley M: Psychological impact of surgical procedures on wives. In Sadock BJ, Kaplan HI, Freedman AM (eds): The Sexual Experience. Baltimore, Williams and Wilkins, 1976, pp 308–312

120. Rubin TI: Understanding Your Man: A Woman's Guide. New York, Ballantine, 1977, pp 155–159

121. Cronenwett LR, Kunst-Wilson W: Stress, social support and the transition to fatherhood. Nurs Research 30:196–201, 1981

122. Benedek T: Fatherhood and providing. In Anthony EJ, Benedek T (eds): Parenthood: Its Psychology and Psychopathology. Boston, Little, Brown, 1970, p 170

123. Mercer RT: A theoretical framework for studying factors that impact on maternal role. Nurs Research. 30:73–77, 1981

124. Cronenwett L: Transition to parenthood. In McNall LK, Galeener JT (eds): Current Practice in Obstetric and Gynecologic Nursing. St. Louis, Mosby, 1976, p 185

125. Ibid

126. Mead M, Newton N: Pregnancy and outcome: A review of patterns of culture and future research needs. In Richardson SO, Guttmacher AF (eds): Childbearing: Its Social and Psychological Aspects. Baltimore, Williams and Wilkins, 1967, p 180

127. Chung HJ: Understanding the oriental maternity patient. Nurs Clin North Am 12(1):74, 1977

128. Jensen MD, Bensen R, Bobak I: Maternity Care: The Nurse and the Family. St. Louis, Mosby, 1977, p 150

129. Guttmacher AF: Pregnancy Birth and Family Planning. New York, Viking, 1973, p 250

130. Jensen MD, Bensen R, Bobak I: Maternity Care: The Nurse and the Family. St. Louis, Mosby, 1977, p 151

Unit V

Health Deviations and Sexuality

INTRODUCTION TO UNIT V

Three etiologic types of sexual dysfunction have been identified—constitutional, psychogenic, and organic. In the male, constitutional impotence is usually associated with weak sexual drive (libido) and responsiveness, and there is no demonstrable organic pathology. Organic impotence develops after previous sexual competency and results from some pathologic condition. Clinically, organic impotence is constant and continues unchanged irrespective of any sexual stimulation that is presented. In contrast, psychogenic impotence is selective and transient, occurring in certain situations and at certain times. In practice, however, distinction between etiologic types is not easy or always possible, since overlap among causes may occur. Thus, impotence may be predominately constitutional, organic, or psychogenic, or the three factors may coexist

and complicate each other to a greater or lesser degree. Etiology, however, must be identified so therapy can be initiated.[1]

Organic impotence may occur with any debilitating disease, metabolic disorders, disorders of the central nervous system, cardiovascular diseases, diseases of the endocrine system, and after the use of some drugs.[2]

Female sexual dysfunction, in terms of orgasmic dysfunction and failure of vaginal lubrication (the female equivalent of erection), may also result from organic or psychogenic causes and, although the literature is sparse in this area, from constitutional causes.

This unit's focus is organic causes of sexual dysfunction, with the recognition that psychogenic and constitutional factors may play an equal or greater role as causative factors. The differentiating characteristics of organic and psychogenic impotence are given in Table 1.

[1]Cooper AJ: Diagnosis and management of "endocrine" impotence. Br Med J 1:34–36, 1972

[2]Ibid, p 34

TABLE 1.   DIFFERENCES BETWEEN PSYCHOGENIC AND ORGANIC
            IMPOTENCE

Psychogenic Impotence	Organic Impotence
1. Acute onset	1. Insidious onset after previous competency (unless due to accident or injury)
2. Temporal relationship to a specific stressful event (bereavement, marriage, fatigue)	2. Develops in association with a disease
3. Selective, intermittent, and transient—present on some occasions and not on others	3. Generally persistent and worsening progressively
4. Evidence of the potential to respond erotically, e.g., to masturbation, morning erections, spontaneous erections to fantasies	4. Evidence of progressive generalized waning of sexual interest and activity; absence of use of other sexual outlets such as masturbation or spontaneous erections

Summarized from: Cooper, A. J.: "Diagnosis and management of 'endocrine' impotence." British Medical Journal 1:34–36, 1972. Kent, Saul: "Impotence as a consequence of organic disease." Geriatrics 155:157, September 1975.

Chapter 22

Sexually Transmitted Diseases

The focus of this chapter is on all sexually transmitted diseases (STD) rather than only on those that are labeled *venereal* disease. By legal definition, venereal disease includes syphilis, gonorrhea, and in some countries chancroid (soft chancre), lymphogranuloma venereum, and granuloma inguinale. However, there are many other infections that are usually or often sexually transmitted. These include nongonococcal urethritis, condylomata acuminata, herpes simplex due to type II herpesvirus, molluscum contagiosum, scabies, and pediculosis pubis.[1] The newest and most feared sexually transmitted disease is acquired immune deficiency syndrome (AIDS).

Although traditionally venereal disease was transmitted through sexual intercourse, now sexual behavior includes all types of activity—oral–oral, oral–genital, oral–anal, genital–genital, and oral–cutaneous, any of which may result in infection.[2]

PROBLEM OF SEXUALLY TRANSMITTED DISEASES

The term *venereal disease* represents a host of diseases caused by a variety of organisms. They have rather specific requirements for growth and are unstable when removed from their natural environment. Factors that encourage their growth in the genital area are not well studied, but they may include chemical and physical factors such as pH, temperature, moisture, and hormonal influences.[3]

In the past two decades, there has been a general increase in venereal disease, especially syphilis and gonorrhea. Particularly disturbing is the steeper rate of increase among adolescent women 15 to 19 years old.

Control measures for STD are the responsibility of federal, state, local health departments, private medicine, and voluntary organizations. State and localities have the legal obligation for control and most legislation for sexually transmitted disease is promulgated at the state level. County and municipal governments are primarily responsible for providing diagnostic and treatment services while a primary role of the federal government is to insure, through grant programs and technical assistance, that control activities are carried out consistently throughout the country. The federal government also develops and evaluates diagnostic tools, therapy, and control program strategies.[4]

These measures have been largely ineffective due to a combination of demographic, biologic, psychologic, and cultural factors.[5]

Demographic Factors

The increased number of young people, earlier beginning and longer lasting active sex life, and increased population per se all exacerbate the problem. Moreover, better notification procedures have resulted in increased numbers of cases recorded.[6] Young people and students are high risk groups. Other

351

high risk groups for venereal disease are the military, workers separated from families, seafarers, tourists, homosexuals, prostitutes, and convicts.[7] The increased number of women with venereal disease has resulted in similar VD rates for both sexes.

Biologic Factors

The effects of antibiotics for treatment of venereal disease have been equivocal. There is an increasing number of failures in gonorrhea treatment, and there is the possibility that less obvious signs and symptoms are appearing due to the effects of courses of antibiotics. Fortunately, reinfections are more commonly diagnosed due to better treatment facilities and better diagnostic procedures.

Side effects of new methods of contraception may contribute to increase in disease rates. Hormonal pills increase alkalinity of the vagina, and this favors growth of gonococci. The IUD, too, may favor persistent gonococcal infection by altering the endometrial barrier.[8]

Psychologic Factors

Religious and traditional attitudes have served to limit the incidence of venereal disease in many countries. However, modern and more permissive sexual attitudes, which operate in many areas, are being adapted not only by the older but the younger generations.

Although increased promiscuity is blamed for the increase, Morton[9] argues that the word is moralistic rather than scientific in implications. Rather than using the word *promiscuity*, a term that expresses behavior in kind or degree or both is needed, a new word denoting more than one sexual partner or sexual exposure. Only part of the population is represented by the word *promiscuous*, and these people are not affected because of lack of knowledge but because of special personality traits.

Morton[10] stresses that when talking about behavioral aspects of venereal disease one must look at two types of behavior—that of a mature individual who has made a mis-take in health care and the behavior of those who do not have a well-developed ego, who have failed to mature, and use venereal disease, unconsciously, as a form of self-destructive status- or attention-seeking behavior. Some individuals use venereal disease as if they are accident prone. Others know they are exposed to venereal disease before the sexual act but continue anyway.

Some young venereal disease patients express feelings of anomie, the feeling of pointlessness or purposelessness in life, not knowing where one comes from or where one is going. Their disease may be an expression of this anomie.[11] Morton[12] also feels that venereal disease, particularly among young people who are frequently infected, is an expression of a self-hostility–aggression–guilt syndrome.

Sociocultural Factors

The World Health Organization states that socioeconomic factors affect VD rates— greater independence for women, greater urbanization and industrialization, more leisure activities and greater consumption of alcohol, vast movement of workers, greater prosperity, group mobility, and rise in travel. Although a high incidence is found in deprived social groups, a larger proportion is now from middle class groups, no social category being spared.[13]

Culturally determined attitudes have contributed to the increasing exposure to sexual activity. A greater tolerance for heterosexual and homosexual activity, more frequent premarital and extramarital intercourse, and sexual freedom that permits multiple contacts now operate to increase chance of infection. Fears of illness and pregnancy have decreased due to new methods of contraception, liberalization of abortion laws, and the simplicity of venereal disease treatment. Adolescents particularly have been affected by the new permissiveness toward sexual activity. Unfortunately, young girls particularly have difficulty persuading sexual partners to take responsibility for protecting them from VD.

It is controversial whether the contraceptive pill leads to promiscuity or whether a promiscuous person seeks contraception. Gonorrhea was increasing in the United States before the pill, but there has been a notable increase since 1965, coinciding with wide pill utilization.[14]

The influence of a number of institutions on venereal disease rate, family, school, and peer groups, has not been evaluated. Questions of the relationship of home life and religious affiliation on the incidence of venereal disease are difficult to study, and the most that one could hope for is some evidence of correlation of these social factors with individual behavior.

Peer group influence is also complex. From groups that engage in mate swapping to the corner gang of "fellows," peer groups influence behavior by providing support, approval, or disapproval. If individuals take their identity from negative forces, then they will continue to take support from these forces. For example, "clap" (gonorrhea) is "good" in many subcultures.[15] One solution may be to break this cycle.

It would appear that syphilis and gonorrhea are higher in nonwhites than whites, but data may not be accurate, since public clinics report VD cases completely, while private physicians do not. Most socioeconomically deprived individuals (of whom nonwhites are a large proportion) tend to seek care at public clinics and are more likely to be reported.[16]

Darrow[17] studied infection in the black, white, and chicano populations in Los Angeles and found that gonorrhea was most likely to occur in the black male. He hypothesized that this is related to a number of factors—blacks are less likely to enter the care system for checkups, are less likely to detect symptoms, are more likely to delay treatment or to rely on self-treatment, and are less likely to follow prescribed treatment and to refer sexual partners.

The incidence of sexually transmitted diseases has risen to unprecedented levels in most countries during the last decade.[18]

After World War II and the discovery of antibiotics, especially penicillin, there was hope that the spread of VD would be contained or even that it would be eradicated. It has now reached epidemic proportions.

Some countries still view venereal disease as a moral rather than a medical problem, so that funds for control programs are limited.

The homosexual community has castigated the United States government for what gays see as delay in allocating funds to investigate acquired immune deficiency syndrome (AIDS) because of moralistic overtones. Statements such as one by a fundamentalist minister that the disease be allowed to "run its course"[19] support the "disease-as-punishment" school of thought.[20]

Tragically, the moral stigma that is still connected with venereal disease serves to discourage individuals from seeking treatment and identifying contacts. Some resort to self-treatment, particularly of gonorrhea. This stigma also contributes to lack of sex education and aversion to public discussion of sexual topics, resulting in ignorance about the disease, especially in young people. Constant vigilance is needed, for whenever society becomes complacent, disease rates increase, as was evidenced from 1950 to 1960, when the advent of simple treatment lulled everyone into believing that venereal disease would be eradicated.

SYPHILIS

Description

The name syphilis is derived from the Greek *siphlos*, which means crippled or maimed. It was first named in 1530 and is caused by *Treponema pallidum*, a spirochete (Table 22-1). It may be referred to as "syph," "old joe," "lues," or "the sore."[21] This infection, 95 percent of which is transmitted sexually, may also be transmitted by accidental direct inoculation at the operating room table, kissing, fetal exposure, and transfusion. Patients are most infectious the first year, with grad-

TABLE 22–1. SEXUALLY TRANSMITTED DISEASES

Etiology and Prevalence	Clinical Presentation	Diagnosis	Therapy	Complications
Syphilis *Treponema pallidum:* spirochete 68,832 cases were reported in 1980. Highest reported case rates are in age group 20–24. Early syphilis increasing among women of childbearing age.	Incubation—10–90 days. *Primary syphilis:* Classical chancre is painless, eroded lesion with a raised, indurated border. Atypical lesions common; multiple lesions may occur. Extragenital chancres may appear. Uni- or bilateral lymphadenopathy may accompany. *Secondary syphilis:* Highly variable cutaneous and mucous membrane lesions, alopecia, generalized lymphadenopathy, mild cold symptoms.	Demonstration of *T. pallidum* from exudate of primary or secondary lesions by dark-field microscopy is definitive. Typical lesions (with or without the presence of Treponemes) and a reactive (positive) reagent test for syphilis (VDRL or RPR). FTA/ABS or MHA-TP can confirm questionable reagent tests. If the initial reagent test is nonreactive, repeat tests 1 week, 1 month, and 3 months later.	*For early syphilis* (less than 1 year duration): Benzathine penicillin G, 2.4 million units IM at 1 visit or aqueous procaine penicillin G, 4.8 million units total; 600,000 units IM daily for 8 days or tetracycline HCl, 500 mg orally qid for 15 days; erythromycin, 500 mg qid for 15 days. (More than 1 year duration): Benzathine penicillin G 2.4 million units IM 1 time a week for 3 successive weeks	Late syphilis (Tertiary) Late syphilis: Gumma (painless lesions on mucous membranes, nose, skin, bones, viscera visceral syphilis (liver, esophagus, stomach, intestines) cardiovascular syphilis (aortic valve incompetence, aneurysms, coronary artery disease) neurosyphilis (general paresis: dementia, euphoria, mania, depression, schizoid reactions, Argyll Robertson pupils, optic nerve atrophy) Tabes dorsalis (loss of sensation, locomotor ataxia, incontinence, constipation, pain or sensory disturbance, swelling joints [Charcot's arthropathy], pathologic fractures. Congenital syphilis: fetus affected: crippling blindness, facial abnormalities, deafness Abortion, stillbirth

Disease / Epidemiology	Incubation / Signs & Symptoms	Diagnosis	Treatment	Complications
Gonorrhea *Neisseria gonorrhoeae:* 1,004,029 cases reported in 1980. Highest reported case rates are in age group 20–24. First among reported communicable diseases in United States.	Incubation—Male: 3–30 days. Female: 3–indefinite time. Men have dysuria, frequency, and urethral discharge that is usually purulent and often more severe in the morning. Women experience vaginal discharge and cystitis. 10–40% of men and about 10–80% of women have no symptoms.	Presumptive identification—Microscopic identification of typical gram-negative, intracellular diplococci on direct smear of urethral exudate from men. Because sensitivity is low in females smears *cannot* be substituted for culture or positive oxidase reaction of typical colonies from specimen obtained from anterior urethra, endocervix, anal canal, or oral pharynx and inoculated on selective media.	Aqueous procaine penicillin G, 4.8 million units IM at 2 sites with 1 g of probenecid orally or tetracycline HCl, 0.5 g orally qid for 5 days, 10 g total or ampicillin, 3.5 g or amoxicillin, 3 g, either with 1 g of probenecid orally. Test of cure should be done 3 to 5 days after therapy. (Reculture.) PPNG: spectinomycin 2.0 g IM, cefoxitin 2.0 g IM plus probenecid 1.0 g orally; single dose of 9 tablets trimethoprim sulfamethoxazole for 5 days for pharyngeal infection	epididymitis pharyngitis meningitis septicemia arthritis endocarditis neonatal conjunctivitis PID urethral stricture prostatitis bartholinitis proctitis tuboovarian abscesses skenitis
Genital Herpes (Herpes Genitalis) *Herpes simplex virus*—Types I & II: 300,000–500,000 new cases reported annually. Highest reported cases found in 20–29-year-olds. (10–50% of genital herpes infection found to be Type I.)	Incubation—virus is dormant from 3 days to years. Virus migrates along sensory nerves into dorsal root ganglia, remaining inactive, non-replicating until reactivated. Multiple shallow vesicles, lesions, or crusts occur on genital area, including buttocks and inner thighs. Inguinal adenopathy, dysuria, local pain, edema, fever are more severe with primary infections. Initial infection lasts 7–10 days; recurrent infection, 3–10 days.	Clinical appearance of herpetic lesions. Papanicolaou smears from lesions, stained to show multinucleated giant cells with intranuclear inclusion bodies (40% sensitivity). Tissue culture most definitive test.	No known cure. Symptoms may be relieved by warm baths, topical anesthetic, and systemic analgesic. Acyclovir ointment 5%. Apply sufficient quantities to cover all lesions every 3 hours 6 times a day for 7 days. Therapy should be instituted as early as possible following onset of signs & symptoms. (Note: Acyclovir has not been found to prevent recurrences and has not been tested in pregnant and lactating women.) Acyclovir IV may be prescribed.	neonatal herpes infection associated risk of cervical cancer neuralgia, meningitis ascending myelitis urethral strictures lymphatic suppuration

(continued)

TABLE 22–1. (cont.)

Etiology and Prevalence	Clinical Presentation	Diagnosis	Therapy	Complications
Nongonococcal Urethritis (Nonspecific Urethritis, NSU, NGU)				
1. *Chlamydia trachomatis*—estimated cause in 40% of cases. 2. *Ureaplasma urealyticum*—estimated as cause in 40% of cases. 3. *Other etiological agents*—(*Trichomonas vaginalis*, *Candida albicans*, HSV, coliform bacteria)—estimated cause in 10–20% of cases. Age distribution parallels other STDs, notably gonorrhea. Recurrences very common.	Incubation period—appears to exceed 10 days in half of the cases. Urethral discharge varies from profusely purulent to slightly mucoid. Dysuria may or may not be present. Some men may have asymptomatic infection; asymptomatic in women; often appears following gonorrheal infection (Postgonococcal urethritis) in 30% of treated infections. Female sexual partners of men with NGU likely to have chlamydial endocervicitis	Clinical picture of dysuria and/or urethral discharge with greater than or equal to 4 polymorphonuclear leukocytes on urethral smear negative for intracellular *Neisseria gonorrhoeae* and negative culture for gonorrhea on modified Thayer-Martin medium. *Chlamydia trachomatis* difficult to diagnose	Tetracycline, 500 mg qid for 7 days; erythromycin, 500 mg qid for 7 days. Doxycycline 100 mg PO bid for 7 days	epididymitis sterility prostatitis proctitis urethral strictures chlamydial NGU transmitted to female sexual partners results in endocervicitis and PID If pregnant, risk for spontaneous abortion, stillbirth and postpartum fever neonatal ophthalmia or pneumonia
Vulvovaginitis (Gardnerella vaginalis)				
(Formerly *Corynebacterium vaginale* or **Hemophilus vaginalis)** Cultured from 23–96% of women with vaginitis. Recovered from 0–52% of asymptomatic women.	Nondescript thick or thin, occasionally frothy vaginal discharge, usually gray-white. Punctate hemorrhages and vulvar irritation are occasionally seen. Between 10% and 40% of culture-positive patients have no symptoms. Foul, fishy amine odor.	Clinical picture, microscopic examination, or culture. Gram stain or KOH wet mount of vaginal exudate may show tiny, gram negative cocobacilli ("clue cells") adhering to vaginal epithelial cells and the presence of white cells, though specificity of this finding is low.	Metronidazole. 500 mg PO bid for 7 days Alternative regimen: Ampicillin 500 mg PO, 4 times a day for 7 days—less effective but suggested for pregnant women	none

Vulvovaginitis: Candidiasis (Moniliasis)

Candida albicans

Epidemiology	Clinical findings	Diagnosis	Treatment	Complications
Saprophytic in the oropharyngeal and gastrointestinal tracts in 25–50% of the population and in the vagina of 25–50% of asymptomatic women.	Vulva is usually erythematous and edematous. Vaginal discharge, may be thick and white, resembling cottage cheese. Occasionally discharge is thin and watery. Satellite lesions may spread to the groin. Many women have no symptoms. Sexual partners may develop balanitis or cutaneous lesions on penis.	Microscopic examination of gram-stained smears of introital or vaginal wall scrapings. Microscopic examination of KOH wet mount of vaginal discharge. Culture on Sabouraud's modified agar.	Nystatin vaginal suppositories bid for 7 to 14 days or Miconazole vaginal cream qd for 7 days.	increased risk of neonatal thrush

Vulvovaginitis (Trichomoniasis)

Trichomonas vaginalis

Epidemiology	Clinical findings	Diagnosis	Treatment	Complications
Prevalence ranges from as low as 5% of private gynecologic patients to as high as 50–75% of prostitutes. Colonization rates are higher among women than men.	Incubation period—unknown. From no signs or symptoms to excoriation, edema, and pruritis of external genitalia and frothy, foul-smelling, greenish-gray vaginal discharge. Punctate hemorrhages and granular appearance of vagina and cervix yields classic strawberry appearance of trichomonal cervicitis. Postcoital bleeding may occur. Most men are asymptomatic, though some may present with urethritis.	Microscopic examination of wet mount of vaginal discharge. Papanicolaou smears may show the parasite. Culture methods are available.	Oral metronidazole, 2 g po STAT or 250 mg tid for 7 days.	rare epididymitis prostatitis

(continued)

357

TABLE 22–1. (cont.)

Etiology and Prevalence	Clinical Presentation	Diagnosis	Therapy	Complications
Acquired Immune Deficiency Syndrome (AIDS) **Kaposi's sarcoma:** unknown etiology cytomegalovirus (CMV) infection suspected, genetic predisposition **Pneumocystis pneumonia (PCP); Pneumocystis carinii** small protozoan, highest reported groups: homosexual/bisexuals (72%), IV drug abuser (16.6%); Haitians (4.4%); hemophiliacs (17%); 94% males age 20–50, with greatest incidence in 30–39-yr-old groups 1,128 confirmed cases, 423 deaths (March 3, 1983)	Kaposi's sarcoma (KS): fatigue, malaise, lymphadenopathy, purple discrete modular skin lesions, tumors on internal organs (*not itchy or painful*) *Pneumocystis carinii* pneumonia (PCP); fever, chills, cough, headache, dyspnea on exertion, pain on inspiration, fever, weight loss, tachypnea, cyanosis, anxiety, cystic packs in lungs, hypoxemia	Presenting signs and symptoms culture or serologic evidence of CMV or *pneumocystis carinii*	No known cure for AIDS PCP: trimethoprim and sulfamethoxazole; PO or IV (Bactrim, Septra) Pentamidine isethionate (Lomidine) If no response to Bactrim; supportive measures	PCP fatality rate from 41– 85% pneumothorax rib fractures azotemia hypoglycemia liver disease severe secondary infections

Adapted from Campbell CE, Herten RJ: VD to STD: Redefining venereal disease. American Journal of Nursing 81:1629–1635, 1981; Sexually Transmitted Diseases Summary 1982. Atlanta, Georgia, U.S. Department of Health and Human Services. Public Health Service, Center for Disease Control; Sexually Transmitted Diseases Treatment Guidelines, 1982. Morbidity and Mortality Weekly Report 31:355–605, 1982; Wiesner PJ, Parra WC: Sexually transmitted diseases: Meeting the 1990 objectives—A challenge for the 1980's. Public Health Reports 97:409–416, 1982.

ual decrease until, after 4 years, the disease cannot be spread by sexual contact.

The incidence has more than tripled since 1957, when there were 3.8 cases per 100,000 population. By a 20 to 1 margin, there is less likelihood of exposure as compared to gonorrhea. Syphilitic infection occurs most commonly in the 20 to 24 year age period. However, there has been a marked increase in individuals in older age groups.[22] Twice as many men as women are infected with syphilis, but at least half of the women infected pass through the primary and secondary stages unaware that they have the disease. These silent cases may result in underreporting. Syphilis is four times more prevalent in large cities of 200,000 or over than in small towns or rural areas.

The disease appears to have changed over the centuries from a virulent form to a less rapid and more predictable infection. It is also possible that a more educated public that consults physicians sooner and improved diagnostic and therapeutic interventions have accounted for its decreased virulence.[23] With better treatment there also has been a decline in congenital syphilis and late syphilis.

Syphilis is less socially acceptable than gonorrhea, which may be viewed with amusement or indifference, partly because the consequences of untreated syphilis are better known and more dramatic.[24]

Clinical Course

Syphilis has a variable clinical picture depending on how early and if it is treated. Its course is divided into four stages: primary, secondary, latent, and tertiary. Each has its own constellation of signs and symptoms. (See Table 22-1.) Relapses can occur during the latent phase when individuals are asymptomatic. They may still be infectious in the early latent stage but are less likely to be so in late latent phase. Detection and treatment of latent syphilis are essential to prevent development of tertiary syphilis.[25]

Since syphilis is not detected in blood serum prior to onset of the primary chancre, there is no way of knowing if an individual exposed to syphilis will develop the disease. By the time the disease is discernible, it may already have been transmitted to others. Therefore, every known contact of individuals with an infectious case of syphilis is treated identically to a diagnosed case of syphilis.[26]

Congenital syphilis is passed from the infected mother to the fetus through the umbilical cord and results in crippling, blindness, facial abnormalities, deafness, abortion, and stillbirth. If the mother receives early treatment, prevention is possible. Consequently, a diagnostic blood test before the eighteenth week of pregnancy is essential, since after the eighteenth week, the spirochete can pass into the uterus and infect the fetus.[27]

Prognosis

With early treatment, syphilis is curable. The outcome of central nervous system syphilis depends on the speed of the diagnosis and establishment of treatment. Untreated, it is fatal in 3 years; with adequate treatment, one-third of those infected can resume their usual activities, one-third have partial recovery, and one-third are unchanged.[28]

The prognosis of tabes dorsalis varies. In some persons, the disease is stationary. In others, ataxia may develop slowly or progress rapidly so that walking is impossible in a few months. Treatment may arrest the disease process in some individuals, but in others it is ineffectual. Death frequently results from urinary tract infection, cardiovascular involvement, or from other diseases.[29]

Cardiovascular syphilis has a variable course. Some patients live many years after diagnosis, others have a rapid downhill course. Patients with angina and signs of heart failure usually survive less than 2 years, while those with aortic aneurysm live longer. Treatment before the onset of symptoms prolongs life, but in later stages, there is little evidence that it does.[30]

GONORRHEA

Description

Scientific interest in gonorrhea began with Hippocrates (460–355 B.C.) who identified inflamed urethras and called the condition "stangury."[31] The disease was first named by Galen in the second century A.D., although the first description is in the Bible (Leviticus 15:2–3). At the present time, it is considered the number one communicable disease in the United States.[32] (See Table 22-1.) The World Health Organization reports that gonorrhea is increasing on five continents, so that it is the most commonly reported communicable disease in many countries. In addition, the actual number of individual cases is usually higher than the number reported, so the statistics may be spuriously low.[33] It is estimated that 2.5 million cases are treated each year in the United States, where some consider it out of control.[34] Commonly used synonyms are "clap," "drip," "a dose," "a case," "strain," "whites," "morning dew," "gleet," and "G.C."[35]

Gonorrhea is spread by sexual contact.[36] but children have been known to have become infected after sleeping with an infected mother. Contagion does not occur from door knobs, towels, or toilets.[37]

The organism is usually sensitive to penicillin. One exception is the penicillinase-producing *Neisseria gonorrhoeae* (PPNG). The numbers of these penicillin-resistant cases are increasing dramatically in the United States, and may account for as many as 50 percent of all infections in other nations. The majority of cases initially arose in Southeast Asia and the Philippines. These patients are treated with spectinomycin intramuscularly. If this is ineffective, cefoxitan and probenecid are used.[38]

If women are affected at the time of delivery, the newborn is exposed to the disease during passage through the birth canal, the organism attacking the mucous membrane of the eyes and resulting in corneal ulcers or panophthalmitis (ophthalmia neonatorum).

Use of silver nitrate eyedrops or antibiotics at birth control these problems.[39]

Prognosis

Effective therapy to eradicate the disease is difficult because of the great number of asymptomatic individuals. As many as 25 percent of males with gonorrhea remain asymptomatic but infectious 2 weeks after their last exposure. The high proportion of asymptomatic women is also a major factor in the poor control. Over 80 percent remain this way throughout their entire infection.[40]

Individual cases respond well to antibiotic therapy. However, the high number of asymptomatic cases result in sterility in a large number of females. The gonococcus is slowly developing a resistance to antibiotics, although the correct dose of penicillin is still effective. Unfortunately, individuals may try to doctor themselves, and their practice of taking penicillin frequently does not ensure that it is in large enough doses to kill the gonococcus.[41]

MINOR SEXUALLY TRANSMITTED DISEASES

Lymphogranuloma Venereum, Granuloma Inguinale, Chancroid

Lymphogranuloma venereum, granuloma inguinale, and chancroid are classified as lesser or minor sexually transmitted diseases, not only because they are less frequent but because their symptoms are usually local rather than systemic and therefore not life threatening.[42]

Prognosis is usually good in these diseases especially if they are diagnosed and treated early.

Chlamydial Infections

Although the *Chlamydia trachomatis* is associated with lymphogranuloma venereum (LCV), during the past decade an increasing number of other infections have been attributed to the organism. It has been implicated in nonspecific urethritis and inclusion conjunctivitis in the newborn, endometritis, acute urethral syndrome (dysuria and frequent urination in women whose urine is sterile), and salpingitis. Long-term effects include infertility, ectopic pregnancy, possible stillbirths, and chlamydial pneumonia of the newborn.[43] It may be the most common sexually transmitted pathogen[44] with 4 to 5 percent of sexually active women carrying the organism in their cervix, the most common site of infection (see Table 22-1).

HERPESVIRUS

Description

Herpesvirus infection is increasing in incidence at epidemic rate. Two types of *Herpesvirus hominis* have been identified. Type I (HVH-1 or "oral herpes") causes the usual fever blister or cold sore, but is also involved in dermal, upper respiratory tract, and central nervous system infections. Type II (HVH-2 or "genital herpes") is most often connected with infection of the genital tract and perineum and is highly contagious and debilitating.[45]

The previous anatomic classification of viral infections above the waist as HSV-1 and those below the waist as HSV-2 has been found to be inaccurate since one-third of the genital lesions in women 25 years or younger are caused by HSV-1. Both are potentially pathogenic.[46] (See Table 22-1.)

Both types are transmitted through interpersonal contact. The lesions are highly contagious in the vesicular stage, and any break in skin or mucous membrane may be the portal of entry. Genital herpes has become the second most common venereal disease among young Americans, and 80 percent of susceptible women who come in contact with an infected male become infected with HVH-2.[47]

Socioeconomic factors seem to influence the incidence of herpesvirus infection, urban areas having a higher incidence than rural. Only 41 percent of a rural pregnant population was found to have HSV antibodies while the rate was 90 percent for inner city women.[48]

Clinical Course

Clinical signs and symptoms of herpes depend on the immune status of the individual. Three distinct syndromes have been identified: first-episode primary genital herpes in which the individual does not have circulating antibodies to HSV-1 or 2; first-episode nonprimary genital infection in which the individual has circulating antibodies, and finally, recurrent disease, an activation of latent herpes.

Recurrent disease seems to occur more frequently after primary infection with HSV-2 and is usually mild with fewer lesions, absence of systemic symptoms, and shorter duration of viral shedding from the cervix.[49] HSV reaction seems to be associated with the onset of menstruation, other infection, emotional upsets, sexual intercourse, and other nonspecific conditions.[50] Sunlight has been implicated.[51]

Other venereal diseases commonly coexist with herpes. Approximately 10 percent of women with herpes have concomitant gonorrhea.[52]

The potential for transmission is from just before sores show until the area is healed over with new skin. There is no virus in the skin between outbreaks and the virus cannot penetrate undamaged skin.

Susceptibility to cervical dysplasia and cancer occurs in women with a history of HVH-2 infection and an increased incidence of HVH-2 antibodies are found in women with cervical cancer.[53]

HVH-2 infection has negative effects on pregnancy and the newborn. A pregnant woman contacting an HVH-2 infection in the first 5 weeks of her pregnancy is five times more likely to abort. If acquired later, this does not cause increased prematurity. However, later in pregnancy, the fetus may become infected through transplacental infection, by ascending infection from the cervix to the endometrium, thence to the tubes and ovaries, or at passage of the infant through the infected birth canal, the most common means of transmission. Cesarian section may be indicated to protect the fetus from infection. It appears to be effective but infection from asymptomatic mothers is still a problem. Some physicians permit vaginal delivery with active infection of the buttocks, presacral area, and thighs providing that culture and clinical examination of the genital tract shows no infection present.

After delivery the mother with active infection is isolated although breast feeding may be permitted as long as the baby is protected from contact with the lesions. Since it appears that the virus tends to remain bound to skin surfaces during reactivation, careful handwashing and personal hygiene will reduce transmittal of the infection.[54]

The infected infant may have a wide spectrum of diseases, approximately one-half of infected newborn infants dying or suffering from neurologic or vascular problems. It has been estimated that symptomatic herpes infection occurs in 1 in 7500 deliveries. Conjunctivitis followed by keratitis may be the first abnormalities noted. These are followed by seizures, increased intracranial pressure, and bulging fontanelles. Severe mental retardation with microcephaly, microphthalmia, intracranial calcifications, and retinal dysplasia may result.[55] Treatment of newborns has not been satisfactory, and prognosis is related more to whether or not central nervous system involvement has resulted.[56]

There has not been any particularly satisfactory therapy. Local preparations such as analgesic ointment, ether, Burrow's solution compresses, and idoxuridine (Herplex) may provide some symptomatic relief. Systemic treatment with smallpox vaccine between bouts of recurrent infections has relieved some patients from frequent attacks.[57]

Topical and intravenous forms of acyclovir (Zovirax) have been approved for use in treatment of herpes infection. The ointment is used for initial genital herpes infection.

Accelerated healing in both sexes and decreased pain in men occurs with the application of topical acyclovir (Zovirax ointment), but the virus remains latent in the dorsal root ganglion and is not irradicated.[58] Acyclovir also appears to shorten the time the virus is in the sores, shortening the contagious period. The ointment is more effective against first-time than recurrent infections, although there is decreased duration of virus shedding from lesions in men with recurrent infections.[59]

Intravenous acyclovir reduces duration of viral shedding and healing times. Alterations in renal function have been observed with IV acyclovir as well as life-threatening metabolic encephalopathy so patients on the drug must be monitored carefully.[60]

Herpes has had many psychologic ramifications. Fear of infecting the sexual partner, future sexual contacts, or their babies can be devastating. Divorces, based largely on claims of infidelity, are other sequelae of infection. Some individuals choose celibacy rather than risk the guilt of infecting another.[61]

Herpes support groups have been established to help individuals cope with the disease and the sequelae. HELP is an organization sponsored by the American Social Health Association (ASHA). It promotes research, provides information, and offers self-help opportunities for herpes victims. Members receive a newsletter which provides information about the disease.[62]

NONGONOCOCCAL URETHRITIS (NONSPECIFIC URETHRITIS)

Nonspecific urethritis (NSU) is a general term applied to inflammation of the male urethra that does not have gonococci as the cause. Although several organisms have been implicated in many cases, no determining cause is found, and the relationship to sexual intercourse is shown only through epidemiologic study. (See Table 22-1.)

It has been suggested that some males are allergic to vaginal secretions or to chemicals such as soap, deodorants, or contraceptives causing symptoms.[63] Female sexual partners may also have the disease.

VULVOVAGINITIS (GARDNERELLA VAGINALIS, CANDIDA ALBICANS, TRICHOMONAS VAGINALIS)

Three types of organisms have been implicated in vulvovaginitis, the *Gardnerella vaginalis,* a small gram-negative coccobacillus (formerly identified as *Corynebacterium vaginale* or *Hemophilus vaginalis*), *Candida albicans,* a fungus which grows as budding yeast cells and chains of cells, and the *Trichomonas vaginalis,* a motile protozoan. The term nonspecific vaginitis (NSV) has been used for infections with the *Gardnerella vaginalis* which has different characteristics than the *Hemophilus* species.[64] (See Table 22-1.)

Host factors have been associated with candidiasis. Individuals with depressed cellular immunity because of pregnancy or because of immunosuppressive drug therapy are predisposed to the disorder. Diabetics are prone to the infection because elevated blood sugars favor *Candida* overgrowth.[65] (See Table 22-1.)

Trichomonas vaginalis is a sexually transmitted anaerobic parasite which frequently coexists with gonorrhea. (See Table 22-1.)

OTHER SEXUALLY TRANSMITTED DISEASES

Molluscum contagiosum is a viral disease that occurs as small pink lesions with depressed white centers anywhere on the body. It is more common in children. During the age of sexual activity, it is thought to be passed by close sexual contact, particularly if lesions occur near the genitals.[66]

Scabies is caused by the *Sarcoptes scabiei* (acarus). Scabies frequently occur with other sexually transmitted disease, so thorough clinical examination for other conditions is essential.[67]

Crabs is the name commonly used to describe pediculosis pubis or pubic lice (*Phthirus pubis*). They attach themselves to the pubic hair with strong claws or legs and then suck on the small blood vessels under the skin.[68]

Condylomata acuminata, genital warts, are caused by the papillomavirus group and have been known for centuries. They appear on the genitalia but usually start on the glans, foreskin, or urinary opening in males and the labia, vaginal walls, and perineum in females. Both sexes may have anal warts, especially if anal intercourse has taken place.[69]

HEPATITIS

Increasingly frequent sexual transmission is thought to be a major factor in the prevalence of hepatitis.[70] The hepatitis A, B, and non-A, non-B viruses have been implicated, although the evidence for sexual transmission is not as strong for A as for hepatitis B[71] which has been found in saliva, serum, urine, bile, menstrual blood, vaginal secretions, and pleural fluid.

ACQUIRED IMMUNE DEFICIENCY SYNDROME (AIDS)

In June, 1981, five homosexual males were found to have *Pneumocystis carinii* pneumonia. Twenty-six other males developed severe Kaposi's sarcoma, a rare vascular neoplasm which produces cutaneous lesions, usually in elderly males and usually with a benign course. These men, however, had unusually severe cases as well as other opportunistic infections usually seen only in severely immunosuppressed individuals. These opportunistic infections appear to be outcomes of a single problem, acquired immune deficiency syndrome (AIDS), a breakdown in the body's natural defense mechanism. (See Table 22-1.)

Early cases were confined to urban areas of California and New York State, among white males, 94 percent of whom were homosexual or bisexual.[72] In addition to a common sexual preference, these men also had evidence of infection with cytomegalovirus (CMV) which is extremely prevalent among homosexuals in America.[73]

Evidence of another unusual virus, human T-cell leukemia virus (HTLV), has also been detected in 25 to 35 percent of blood specimens of AIDS patients. Although the evidence does not directly implicate HTLV in AIDS, the findings may be important because evidence of exposure to the virus had not been detected in individuals other than those who had T-cell leukemia.

Since the first cases reported, the incidence of AIDS has increased, not only among homosexuals but among intravenous drug abusers, Haitian immigrants, and hemophiliacs.

Hemophiliacs are especially vulnerable since they depend on the blood byproducts, antihemophiliac concentrate (AHF), which in a year comes from the blood of 25,000 to 75,000 donors. There is also some evidence that AHF itself may cause immunosuppression.

Many experts believe that AIDS will enter the general population and that hospital workers, because of their contact with AIDS patients and blood, are at high risk.[74] Other vulnerable groups may be women whose husbands or lovers are drug addicts, female partners of bisexual men, and children of drug addicts and bisexuals.

Gay leaders organized health-advising services, hotlines, lobbies, and fund-raising groups. Many homosexuals radically altered life styles because of AIDS's association with promiscuity, some turning to celibacy.[75] Homosexual men and women were especially

bitter by what they saw as a delay by the National Institute of Health in awarding 4 million dollars set aside for AIDS research.[76]

Because of inaccurate and inflammatory reporting, AIDS "panic" is affecting the public and some health care professionals. There are a few who have refused to care for AIDS patients. Some individuals think AIDS may be a mutated biologic warfare strain developed by the government and being tested on gays and drug users.

VENEREAL DISEASE AND HOMOSEXUAL ACTIVITY

Homosexuals are especially prone to sexually transmitted diseases. Diagnosis is particularly difficult, because the lesions are often so well hidden that the individual is unaware of the disease. Reporting of cases is poor, since the sexually active patient may not know the names of the sexual partners or the homosexual person may hesitate to name contacts for fear of exposing his or her sexual predilection as well as the partner's.[77]

Syphilis contacted through anal intercourse may result in a lesion hidden within the anus so that the rash of the secondary stage may be the first sign of the disease. Proctitis may occur with gonorrhea but may go unnoticed for a long period. Gonorrheal pharyngitis or a syphilitic lesion of the mouth may be ignored if the person is not aware of venereal disease symptoms. Throughout the world, primary and secondary syphilis is particularly high.[78]

The oral–genital contact of some homosexuals also has resulted in the transmission of enteric pathogens, resulting in amebiasis, shigellosis, and giardiasis.[79]

Amebiasis caused by *Entamoeba histolytica* frequently is found in travelers and causes diarrhea and abdominal pain. It is transmitted in homosexuals by rectal intercourse followed by oral–genital contact,[80,81] or by fecal ingestion following analingus (oral–anal sex contact). In addition to typical gastrointestinal symptoms, amebic infection of the penis may also result.[82]

Hepatitis A and B are also increasing among male homosexuals, although not among lesbians.[83] This may be related to males' higher degree of sexual activity.[84]

It is imperative that homosexuals be informed of the danger of venereal disease. Organized homosexual groups are recommending venereal disease education, regular serology, and are organizing gay health centers.[85]

IMMUNITY

Paradoxically, Evans cites early treatment of venereal disease as preventing development of good immunity. The decline in syphilis before the advent of antibiotics was attributed to group immunity among sexually active populations. He cites the greater incidence of gonorrhea in individuals under 20 years of age and the increased resistance to syphilitic reinfection about 2 years after inoculation as possible evidence that immune status increases with age and after infection.[86]

The role of the immune system in the pathogenesis of syphilis is being investigated. In studies to confer passive immunity, rabbits were infused with massive amounts of immune serum or immunogloulin (IgG). The animals developed chancres, although they were slower to develop and atypical in appearance.

The classical hormonal immune response did not seem to be protective.[87] It may be that specific treponemocidal antibody production and synthesis may be suppressed during syphilis. Controversy continues about the value of cellular and hormonal immunity in the eradication of the disease.[88]

However, there is no vaccine that has been developed for any of the venereal diseases. The only real preventive measure is prophylaxis through the use of condoms and vaginal spermicides. Evans estimates that the use of a prophylactic that is only 50 percent efficient by only 30 percent of the population at risk could presumably reduce the gonorrhea rate to minimal level in 5 years.[89]

NURSING IMPLICATIONS

Identifying the danger of venereal disease has not provided motivation to prevent its occurrence; discovery of antibiotics has not resulted in its eradication. Whether one calls it promiscuity or indiscriminancy, as long as individuals change sexual partners, venereal disease is inevitable.

Nurses must look at their own attitudes toward venereal disease, sexual activity, and the individuals who are in their care. They need to work through their feelings and concerns and to identify their role with the patient, the physician, and the community. In dealing with adolescents, this is particularly essential so that nurses can understand and accept the nature of their behavior.[90] A nurse who conveys her prejudices, even though competently performing duties, is failing to permanently help the venereal disease patient. There must be roles of mutual understanding between both.[91]

Assessment

The nurse has a role in detection of venereal disease; the public health nurse especially is in an ideal position to do epidemiology. Ability to assess individuals' psychologic reaction is essential. Patients who suspect they have venereal disease may be experiencing guilt, anxiety, or embarrassment. Intense depression, disgust, shame, fear of relatives and friends finding out, and fear of a marriage breakup and loss of children may also be manifested. Some develop venereophobia, intense fear of venereal disease.[92] They must confide in the nurse personal intimate information. Assessment of their reactions is the first step in data gathering.[93] Patients will be more likely to confide to a nurse who is compassionate and sensitive.

Diagnosis and treatment of disease through drop-in centers and multiphasic screening centers for individuals is only the first step. If there is no followup or contact interviewing, further control of the disease is unchecked. One of the first tasks is case finding and case prevention by obtaining the names of all sexual partners through a structured interview. This is especially necessary for cases of syphilis. Case partner contacts are located and referred for treatment, and *cluster* section is identified. The patient is asked to name what are referred to as *suspects,* people with similar lesions, the same sexual partners, or those who are close friends of someone who is known to have syphilis. The next step is to interview *associates,* those designated by a noninfected contact for the same reasons.[94]

A careful social history is taken. Data about age, address, employment, and education and marital status are important sources of information for identifying contacts. The social history also gives insight into the particular patient, the willingness to share information or withhold information.[95]

Use of principles of assessment (detailed in Chapter 10) is essential to obtain needed information. In addition to the epidemiologic information, data about social behavior, patterns, and sexual attitudes are also important. For the purpose of the interview, it is assumed that the person is able to name a minimum of two contacts and an indeterminate maximum.[96]

A serologic history is established. The last known serology is a starting point to determine the length of the current infection and how far in the past to identify contacts. Use of visual aids to identify lesions and matter-of-fact discussion by the interviewer about modes of transmission may help individuals remember contacts and feel more comfortable in describing the sexual activity.

Patients may refuse to name contacts, may name only one, or may lie by saying they do not know names. When this happens, the interviewer confronts the patient in a nonhostile manner. Unfortunately, some highly sexually active individuals may not know the contacts' names. If persons are not

motivated to respond, reasons for the importance of the information to their well-being are shared—spreading of his own reinfection, late effects of the disease, lack of symptoms on reinfection, danger of penicillin sensitivity with repeated treatment, congenital transmission, and the urgent need to treat the contacts before any of these events occur.[97]

Once contacts are named, identifying data about them are obtained. All individuals will be contacted. A second interview is also scheduled so that recollection of other contacts can be communicated. Increasingly, it has been the custom to "epitreat," preventively treat, all contacts even if they do not have positive blood tests or signs of syphilis, since studies have shown that approximately 10 percent of these individuals develop syphilis later.[98]

The same principles apply to the interview with the individual with gonorrhea, although the interview is shorter and not as extensive. Contact interviewing for a gonorrhea patient often finds a female partner who has no inkling she is infected. When she is tested, about 60 to 70 percent of tests are negative, even though she has the disease. The numbers of males who are asymptomatic is also rising, so that the interview focuses on having all steady sex partners come for checkups, even if no symptoms are present. When partners do not come together for treatment, a ping-pong reinfection pattern often results, each partner reinfecting the other.

Some treatment centers are now using a self-interview form, not only to facilitate obtaining information but to decrease patient embarrassment because of the personal nature of the information. This method has been found to be effective and acceptable to the clients.[99]

A careful history is also important if a patient has had a history of infection with *herpesvirus.* In addition to recording the onset and duration of each episode, relevant factors such as employment changes,

changes in life style, psychologic stress, and changes in sexual partner should be assessed.[100]

Intervention

In spite of data collection, thorough epidemiologic approaches, serologic testing, and contact-interview tracing and drug treatment, the overwhelming increase in VD statistics shows that these methods have been ineffective.[101] Research is being done in the laboratory, but a human approach is needed to teach prevention, since without it, any patient can be and often is reinfected.

Education of the public to the mechanics, complications, and control of venereal disease is necessary. Education must also mean that people in a more sexually free society become aware of their responsibilities, not only to their own bodies but to their lovers as well, and that they are motivated to take steps to keep themselves healthy.[102]

Washing the genitals before and right after sexual activity and urinating afterward may be helpful in preventing some infections. Obviously, if any genital lesions are present on the sexual partner, they should not be touched and sexual activity should not be attempted.

The condom is one of the most effective prophylactics against venereal disease, but most individuals think of it only as a birth control measure. Some spermicidal preparations are also effective against VD. The nurse not only stresses the value of their use, but also reminds individuals that the condoms will be ineffective if oral–genital contact has been made with an infected individual before its application. The home remedies of immediate urination, douching, or external cleansing after coitus may be helpful but will not necessarily prevent venereal disease. The client with herpes is taught preventive measures and those to relieve pain (Table 22-2).

TABLE 22–2. TEACHING THE CLIENT WITH HERPES

Relief of pain:	Hot compresses to rash, 5 minutes, 2–3 times a day or ice pack; short baths in body water temperature, or with Burrows or Epsom salts added; dry with hair dryer—not too hot or too close; dab rash with plain alcohol, topical xylocaine; wear loose clothes, skirts for women instead of pants, cotton underwear.
Treatment of rash:	Keep area clean and dry (see above for relieving pain); do not break blisters with hands or pin; work on ways to reduce tension and anxiety; eat well; multivitamin supplement with B and C vitamins; get adequate rest; avoid excess alcohol, coffee, cigarettes.
Preventive measures: (genital herpes)	No intercourse when sores are present; no oral sex if oral or genital sores present; use a condom when prodromal signs are present (best *not* to have sex); avoid rough handling of tissue if early signs present; *wash hands after contact with area;* take a shower if exposed; wash with soap and water; know your partner; look and get to know your partner's body; ask.
Preventive measures: (facial herpes)	Avoid rubbing chin, licking or itching the area; playing with moustache; poking the sore; smoking so sore is touched; running chapstick over sore and the rest of lips; wash hands.
Relief of tension, anxiety, stress:	Good physical well-being; exercise; rest; reduce conflicts; utilize muscle relaxation; plan and organize time; forget about herpes—do not let it control your life.

Adapted from: Gillespie O: Herpes: What to Do When You Have It. New York, Grossett and Dunlap, 1982; The Herpes Resource Center, P.O. Box 100, Palo Alto, California, 94302
Service of American Social Health Association.

TABLE 22–3. ACQUIRED IMMUNE DEFICIENCY SYNDROME (AIDS)

Client Teaching

Select sexual partners from small group of people who are known.

Abstain from sex with persons with known infections.

Good hygiene.

Avoid combination of oral and anal sex.

Use condom during anal sex.

Take Bactrim or Septra 1 hour before or 2 hours after meals with large glass of water.

Drink at least 1 quart or more of fluids each day, report decreased urine.

Avoid exposure to sun.

Stop alcohol and drug abuse.

Good general health measures—adequate diet, sleep, exercise.

Pregnant women with herpes infection need support and counseling, particularly when spontaneous abortion has occurred or when cesarian section is likely. The physician usually discusses the need for cesarian section, but the nurse can clarify, explain, and reinforce physician's recommendations.[103]

Patients with AIDS may be frightened, angry, depressed, or denying the severity of their disease, yet they may be refused the support they need because of the nurse's fear of contacting the disease. Special precautions for blood, oral secretions, urine, and stool are instituted. Patients may be isolated to protect them from contact with those with infectious diseases, but time must be made to sit with them, listen, and show that someone cares. Teaching preventive measures is also essential (Table 22-3).

Nurses can take part in dissemination of information through clubs, telephone hotlines, workshops, and venereal disease awareness campaigns. School nurses and public health nurses have the opportunity to initiate education programs in schools, not only for the students, but for parents. Utilization of peer group members for venereal disease education has been effective. A knowledgeable member of an athletic team or the leader of a teenage group has a more willing and open audience than an adult authority figure.[104]

In the school, the National Council on Venereal Disease recommends that information be introduced in the seventh grade; the Parent–Teacher Association recommends the eighth grade. Small group discussion is more effective than large group for teaching and discussing the consequences of VD (see Chapter 11). The school nurse is the first to see the adolescents who are particularly vulnerable because of their sporadic and impromptu sexual contacts. They are more amenable than others, however, to education and discussion.

Nurses can also be instrumental in establishing social hygiene clinics in already existing treatment centers. Special sessions for adolescents are particularly effective, since counseling and the development of a trust relationship is often easier to establish with a nurse than with educators.

In the physician's office, the nurse can help the physician understand the importance of case reporting of venereal disease to the public health authorities.

The nurse in a venereal disease clinic has an especially important role. She must be able to deal with patient behavior. If VD is part of the patient's life style, the nurse helps him/her avoid it, the same way the dentist teaches how to avoid cavities. People are taught to care for their genitals and to make routine medical checkups a part of all sexually active life styles and behavior. The patient should have as part of his awareness the immediate treatment of all partners as well as himself/herself.[105] In some clinics, nurses take part in the diagnostic process by obtaining smears from the urethra, vagina, and cervix. While preparing patients for the examination, describing what is going to be done and why does much to allay fears.[106]

Worried patients include individuals from all sociocultural and economic groups and of all ages who present the opportunity to do on the spot health teaching to a receptive audience. The nurse's nonjudgmental acceptance of them and their problems, along with knowledge of venereal disease, results in an increase in their health knowledge.[107]

Evaluation

Outcome criteria that indicate that intervention has been successful include the following. The patient:

1. Identifies contacts who may have VD.
2. Follows the treatment regimen outlined.
3. Has a negative serologic or other test for a specific disease.
4. Identifies preventive measures that should be used.
5. Can state the symptoms, complications, and methods of transmission of sexually transmitted diseases.

NOTES

1. World Health Organization: Social and Health Aspects of Sexually Transmitted Diseases. Geneva, WHO, 1977, p 8
2. Taub W: Sex and infection: Venereal Disease. In Sadock BJ, Kaplan HI, and Freedman AM (eds): The Sexual Experience. Baltimore, Williams and Wilkins, 1976, pp 318–327
3. Evans TN: Sexually transmissible diseases. Am J Obstet Gynecol 125:116–131, 1976
4. STD Fact Sheet, Edition Thirty-five. U.S. Department of Health and Human Services Public Health Service, Centers for Disease Control, 1982
5. World Health Organization: Social and Health Aspects of Sexually Transmitted Diseases. Geneva, WHO, 1977, p 14
6. Ibid, p 15
7. Ibid, p 17
8. Evans TN: Sexually transmissible diseases. Am J Obstet Gynecol 125:116, 1976
9. Morton BM: VD, A Guide for Nurses and Counselors, Boston, Little Brown, 1976, p 92
10. Ibid, p 97
11. Ibid, p 98
12. Ibid, p 118
13. World Health Organization: Social and Health Aspects of Sexually Transmitted Diseases. Geneva, WHO, 1977, p 15
14. Evans TN: Sexually transmissible diseases. Am J Obstet Gynecol 125:116, 1976
15. Morton BM: VD, A Guide for Nurses and Counselors. Boston, Little, Brown, 1976, p 96
16. Ibid, p 123
17. Darrow WW: Venereal infection in three ethnic groups in Sacramento. Am J Public Health 66:446–449, 1976
18. Evans TN: Sexually transmissible diseases. Am J Obstet Gynecol 125:116, 1976
19. Frolik J: Gays finding AIDS battle is largely theirs. The Plain Dealer. 16 C, March 13, 1983
20. Singer L: A short history of sexually transmitted infection. Bulletin Cleveland Medical Library XXVII:17–23, 1981
21. Morton BM: VD, A Guide for Nurses and Counselors. Boston, Little, Brown, 1976, p 96
22. Evans TN: Sexually transmissible diseases. Am J Obstet Gynecol 125:120, 1976
23. Charles D: Syphilis. Clin Obstet Gynecol 26:125–137, 1983
24. Morton BM: VD, A Guide for Nurses and Counselors. Boston, Little, Brown, 1976, p 31
25. Catterall RD: A Short Textbook of Venereology, 2nd ed. Philadelphia, Lippincott, 1974, p 102
26. Brown WJ: Acquired syphilis: Drugs and blood tests. Am J Nurs 71:713–715, 1971
27. Morton BM: VD, A Guide for Nurses

and Counselors. Boston, Little, Brown, 1976, p 24

28. Catterall RD: A Short Textbook of Venereology, 2nd ed. Philadelphia, Lippincott, 1974, p 124

29. Ibid, p 132

30. Ibid, p 116

31. Singer L: A short history of sexually transmitted infection. Bulletin Cleveland Medical Library Association XXVII:20, 1981

32. Evans TN: Sexually transmissible diseases. Am J Obstet Gynecol 125:118, 1976

33. World Health Organization: Social and Health Aspects of Sexually Transmitted Diseases. Geneva, WHO, 1977, p 12

34. Morton BM: VD, A Guide for Nurses and Counselors. Boston, Little, Brown, 1976, p 36

35. Boston Women's Health Book Collective: Our Bodies, Ourselves, 2nd ed. New York, Simon and Schuster, 1976, pp 167–180

36. Spence MR: Gonorrhea. Clin Obstet Gynecol 26:111–123, 1983

37. Morton BM: VD, A Guide for Nurses and Counselors. Boston, Little, Brown, 1976, p 37

38. Spence MR: Gonorrhea. Clin Obstet Gynecol 26:122, 1983

39. Morton BM: VD, A Guide for Nurses and Counselors. Boston, Little, Brown, 1976, p 44

40. Evans, TN: Sexually transmissible diseases. Am J Obstet Gynecol 125:120, 1976

41. Morton BM: VD, A Guide for Nurses and Counselors. Boston, Little, Brown, 1976, p 53

42. Schwartz RH: Chancroid and granuloma inguinale. Clin Obstet Gynecol 26:138–142, 1983

43. Sweet RL, Schachter V, Landers DV: Chlamydial infections in obstetrics and gynecology. Clin Obstet Gynecol 26:142–164, 1983

44. Schachter J: Chlamydial infection. N Engl J Med 298:428, 490, 540, 1978

45. Neeson JD: Herpesvirus genitalis: A nursing perspective. Nurs Clin North Am 10:599–607, 1975

46. Grossman JH: Herpes simplex virus (HSV) infection. Clin Obstet Gynecol 25:555–561, 1982

47. Neeson JD: Herpesvirus genitalis: A nursing perspective. Nurs Clin North Am 10:600, 1974

48. Grossman JH: Herpes simplex virus (HSV) infection. Clin Obstet Gynecol 25:556, 1982

49. Baker DA: Herpesvirus. Clin Obstet Gynecol 26:165–172, 1983

50. Allergic and Infectious Disease Research. Prepared by Office of Research Reporting and Public Response. National Institute of Allergy and Infectious Diseases. National Institute of Health, Public Health Service, U.S. Department Health and Human Services, 1982

51. Bettoli EJ: Herpes: Facts and fallacies. Am J Nurs 82:924–928, 1982

52. Baker DA: Herpesvirus. Clin Obstet Gynecol 26:169, 1983

53. Dreesman GR, Burek J, Adam F, et al: Expression of herpesvirus induced antigens and human cervical cancer. Nature 283:591, 1980

54. Grossman JH: Herpes simplex virus (HSV) infection. Clin Obstet Gynecol 25:559–560, 1982

55. Evans TN: Sexually transmissible diseases. Am J Obstet Gynecol 125:124, 1976

56. Ibid, p 125

57. Neeson JD: Herpesvirus genitalis: A nursing perspective. Nurs Clin North Am 10:603, 1975

58. Bettoli EJ: Herpes: Facts and fallacies. Am J Nurs 82:926, 1982

59. Reichman RC, Badger GJ, Guinan ME, et al: Topically administered acyclovir in the treatment of recurrent herpes simplex genitalis: A controlled trial. J Infect Dis 143:336–340, 1983

60. Department of Health and Human Services. FDA Drug Bulletin 13:5, 1983

61. Bettoli EJ: Herpes: Facts and fallicies. Am J Nurs 82:929, 1982
62. STD Fact Sheet, Edition Thirty-five. U.S. Department of Health and Human Services. Public Health Service Centers for Disease Control, 1982, p 15
63. Morton BM: VD, A Guide for Nurses and Counselors. Boston, Little, Brown, 1976, p 72
64. Eschenbach DA: Vaginal infection. Clin Obstet Gynecol 26:186–202, 1983
65. Ibid, p 197
66. Morton BM: VD, A Guide for Nurses and Counselors. Boston, Little, Brown, 1976, p 71
67. Catterall RD: A Short Textbook of Venereology, 2nd ed. Philadelphia, Lippincott, 1974, p 172
68. Morton BM: VD, A Guide for Nurses and Counselors. Boston, Little, Brown, 1976, p 75
69. Ibid, p 76
70. Minkoff H: Hepatitis. Clin Obstet Gynecol 26:178–185, 1983
71. Ibid, p 181
72. Immunocompromised homosexuals. Lancet 2:1325–1326, 1981
73. Allen J, Mellen G: The new epidemic: Immune deficiency, opportunistic infections and Kaposi's sarcoma. Am J Nurs 82:1718–1722, 1982
74. Carpenter M, Thompson D: Battling a deadly new epidemic. Time, March 28, 1983, pp 53–55
75. Ibid, p 55
76. Frolik J: Gays findings AIDS battle is largely theirs. The Plain Dealer, 16 C, March 13, 1983
77. Morton BM: VD, A Guide for Nurses and Counselors. Boston, Little, Brown, 1976, p 152
78. World Health Organization: Social and Health Aspects of Sexually Transmitted Diseases. Geneva, WHO, 1977, p 18
79. Mildvan D, Gelb AM, Williams D: Venereal transmission of enteric pathogens in male homosexuals. JAMA 238:1387–1389, 1977
80. Schmerin MJ, Gelston A, Jones TC: Amebiases: An increasing problem among homosexuals in New York City. JAMA 238:1385–1387, 1977
81. Sexual transmission of enteric pathogens. Lancet 2:1328–1329, 1981
82. Mildvan D, Gelb AM, Williams D: Venereal transmission of enteric pathogens in male homosexuals. JAMA 238:1387, 1977
83. Taub W: Sex and infection: Venereal disease. In Sadock BJ, Kaplan HI, Freedman AM (eds): The Sexual Experience. Baltimore, Williams and Wilkins, 1976, pp 326–327
84. Kruger P, Pedersen NS, Mathiesen L, Nielsen J: Increased risk of infection with hepatitis A and B viruses in men with a history of syphilis: Relation to sexual contacts. J Infect Dis 145:23–26, 1982
85. VD Facts for Gay Women and Men. The Gay Health Collective of Boston, Boston, 1982
86. Evans TN: Sexually transmissible diseases. Am J Obstet Gynecol 125:130, 1976
87. Charles D: Syphilis. Clin Obstet Gynecol 26:127, 1983
88. Ibid, p 128
89. Evans TN: Sexually transmissible diseases. Am J Obstet Gynecol 125:130, 1976
90. Brown MA: Adolescents and VD. Nurs Outlook 21(2):99–103, 1973
91. Morton BM: VD, A Guide for Nurses and Counselors. Boston, Little, Brown, 1976, p 103
92. Fong R: Talking to patients in special clinics. Nurs Times 73:1648–1649, 1977
93. Schofield EM: The nurse in a special clinic. Nurs Times 72:1059–1060, 1976
94. Morton BM: VD, A Guide for Nurses and Counselors. Boston, Little, Brown, 1976, p 132
95. Ibid, p 134
96. Ibid, p 136
97. Ibid, p 140
98. Ibid, p 142
99. Van Cura LJ, Jensen N, Greist JH,

Lewis, WR, Frey SR: Venereal disease: Interviewing and teaching by computer. Am J Public Health 65:1159–1164, 1975

100. Neeson JD: Herpesvirus genitalis: A nursing perspective. Nurs Clin North Am 10:604, 1975

101. Wiesner PJ: Magnitude of the Problem of Sexually Transmitted Diseases in the United States. Reprint by U.S. Department of Health and Human Services, Public Health Service from: Sexually Transmitted Diseases/1980 Status Report 21–31

102. Morton BM: VD, A Guide for Nurses and Counselors. Boston, Little, Brown, 1976, p 105

103. Neeson JD: Herpesvirus genitalis: A nursing perspective. Nurs Clin North Am 10:606, 1975

104. Morton BM: VD, A Guide for Nurses and Counselors. Boston, Little, Brown, 1976, p 108

105. Ibid, p 111

106. Schofield EM: The nurse in a special clinic. Nurs Times 72:1059, 1976

107. Matthews R: TLC with penicillin. Am J Nurs 71:720–723, 1971

Chapter 23

Cancer and Cancer Therapy

Cancer is many diseases involving all parts of the body and often requiring complex and protracted therapy. The diagnosis of cancer and/or its medical treatment may have adverse effects on body image, sexual response, and sexual roles and relationships. Cancer is so widespread, its effects so feared and pervasive despite tremendous increase in effective therapies, that the diagnosis represents a crisis for the individual and the significant others.

Cancer and its treatment may so occupy the individual's life, so consume psychic and physical energy, that as one patient stated, "All my energy is spent in trying to get well. I have no sexual activity!" Other individuals may desire coitus, but because of fears about the disease avoid sexual activity, often unnecessarily. Consequently, at a time in life when the closeness, sharing, and pleasure of intercourse and other sexual activity can be most beneficial, they are avoided.

This chapter focuses on the bio-psycho-social changes that may accompany cancer and its therapies and that may affect sexuality. The effects of surgical treatment, radiotherapy, chemotherapy, and immunotherapy are discussed. The psychologic sequelae are also presented—anxiety, depression, body image disturbance, guilt, shame, and dependency. Sociologic factors that compromise sexuality, role changes, economic concerns, and societal attitudes are discussed. The chapter includes a brief discussion of sexuality and the dying patient. Information about nurses' role in helping the cancer patient meet sexual needs concludes the chapter.

SEXUAL PRACTICES: RELATIONSHIP TO CANCER

Some sexual practices have been identified as increasing the susceptibility to cancer, while others appear to decrease the risk of certain types of malignancy. Carcinoma of the cervix is more frequent in women who have had multiple pregnancies, but this factor decreases in importance when groups of women compared start their sex life at the same age. The development of cancer seems to be related to coitus rather than pregnancy. Cervical carcinoma is less common in virgins than in married women, higher in those who have coitus at an early age, who have had multiple sex partners, and who have had genital herpes.[1]

Among circumcised men, cancer of the penis is virtually unknown. The means by which circumcision provides better protection is unknown, but is probably related to better hygiene. There is also a lower incidence of cancer of the uterine cervix in women whose sexual partner has been circumcised and in cultures in which the men, even though not circumcised, have a high standard of genital hygiene.

The correlation with sexual experience and breast cancer is the reverse of that for

373

the uterine cervix. Breast cancer patients have usually been married and become pregnant later in life. Lactation may provide some protection against breast cancer, since women who have breast fed their infants have a lower incidence of breast malignancy. Among Eskimo women, breast cancer is reported to be unknown; among Japanese women, it is relatively rare. Both cultures practice breast feeding.[2]

BIOLOGIC EFFECTS OF CANCER AND ITS THERAPY ON SEXUALITY

The effects of cancer are legion. Untreated, the disease may result in pain, disfigurement, and malfunction of any body system, depending on its location and the presence and/or extent of metastasis. Ulcerating and other lesions of the breast, vulva, penis, face, and mouth may be particularly devastating to the body image, as well as interfering with the usual means of sexual expression. Cancer of the reproductive system and the urinary system may cause infertility, impotence, or orgasmic dysfunction. Even when the systems affected by cancer are less directly related to sexual response, the malignant tumor's higher metabolic rate and appropriation of nutrients needed for other biologic processes results in the weakness, fatigue, and cachexia that may result in decreased libido and sexual dysfunction. Treatment, especially if initiated early, has significant potential for cure. However, the therapies themselves bring their own assault on human sexuality.

Surgical Therapy
Although surgical excision of malignancy provides significant opportunity for cure, individuals must cope with changed function and disfigurement as a consequence of the procedure. Large draining incisions, new openings in and out of the body, cause negative views of self as a sexual being; of equal

portent, the sexual partner may be repulsed and shocked by these results of therapy.

Surgery is frequently anticipated with dread even if the projected operation is neither extensive nor mutilative. The patient is faced with two threats, the disease and the surgery, which often is the only definitive therapy. Both produce special problems, one related to the loss of or change in function of the body part and the other related to the meaning of the organ in the total adaptation of the individual. Because of psychic investment in some body parts, the surgical experience and the negative sequelae associated with hospitalization and convalescence may disrupt sexual performance without having any direct relationship to the part that was lost.[3] (See Chapter 24 for discussion of specific surgical procedures.)

Extensive surgical procedures for cancer may compromise sexual activity because of their outcome in terms of general loss of strength and vigor. Poor nutrition following surgery, delay or inadequate resumption of activities of daily living, inadequate rest and relaxation, and pain may adversely affect sexual response.

Radiotherapy
Radiation therapy is utilized in treatment or palliation of localized disease, alone or in combination with surgery, immunotherapy, and/or chemotherapy. Although it acts on rapidly dividing undifferentiated cells, it also adversely affects normal tissue to some degree.

Body image changes may occur as a result of change in the appearance of the skin—erythema (reddening of the skin) or more acute reactions such as desquamation, blisters that burst to form ulcers, loss of hair, and radiation burn. Burns are rare, but when they occur, they are marked by deeper blisters and slough of entire skin areas. Healing may take weeks or months due to blood vessel destruction. Skin of the axilla, groin, vulva, and anus are especially sensitive to radiation, in part due to friction and moisture. Even without the more serious side effects, sequelae to skin reaction may include ischemia, pigmentation, atrophy, thickening, telangiectasia, late ulceration, and malignancy.[4] The patient is told to avoid any irritation and friction to irradiated areas. Fear of damage to the skin may cause the individual to avoid sexual activity.

The gastrointestinal mucosa is especially sensitive to radiation because of its rapid cellular turnover. Depending on the area of the body being irradiated, oral–genital sexual activity or oral–anal activity may be limited by oral ulceration and sore throat. Vaginitis may cause dyspareunia, while diarrhea, proctitis, or tenesmus may cause pain, discomfort, and avoidance of sexual activity for esthetic reasons.

Abitol[5] reports that extensive changes in pelvic organs and tissue takes place in women treated for cervical cancer by radiotherapy or a combination of radiotherapy and surgery. With irradiation, the vagina loses its elasticity and possibility of expansion. Venus plexus and arteries, especially in the upper vagina, are also obliterated, so vaginal lubrication is eliminated. Twenty-two of 28 patients who received radiation therapy reported a complete or almost complete disappearance of orgasm. The shortened and narrowed vagina and pelvic fibrosis resulted in marked pain and discomfort during intercourse. The vagina of some women was almost completely obliterated, making coitus impossible. Even early resumption of sexual activity, mechanical dilation of the vagina, and use of topical estrogen were of little value for many women as fibrosis became established and irreversible.

Three husbands stopped intercourse because they no longer found satisfaction in the sex act and ten reported changes, but were unable to describe their feelings.[6] Fear of recurrence of the cancer that necessitated the therapy was given by many patients for sexual abstinence.

Reproductive organs may also be adversely affected. In males, sperm production can be inhibited by doses as low as 50 rad, and permanent sterility can result with 1000 rad. Production of androgenic hormones is not changed markedly, but in females, ovarian hormonal production can be reduced or abolished, leading to temporary or permanent cessation of menstruation. With low doses of radiation, genetic mutations may occur.[7] Gonick[8] reports that 30 percent of men receiving radiation therapy for early cancer of the prostate became impotent and the remainder noted diminished sexual activity.

Radiation sickness, a generalized illness, may cause nausea, fatigue, malaise and weakness, and decreasing interest and ability to function sexually.[9] Depending on the size of the area and the amount of bone marrow irradiated, patients may develop decrease in white blood cell count and platelet counts, predisposing them to infection and hemorrhage. Vaginal, oral, and/or rectal infection and bleeding may follow vaginal or anal intercourse and oral sexual activity.

When lung tissue is irradiated, an inflammatory reaction, radiation pneumonitis, may lead to fibrosis, preventing proper expansion of the lung and subsequent decrease in vital capacity. The patient's shortness of breath, either with or without exertion, makes vigorous intercourse difficult, if not impossible.

Chemotherapy

Depending on the drug given, chemotherapy may result in toxic side effects causing dysfunction.[10] Gastrointestinal toxicity with nausea, vomiting, and stomatitis; bone marrow suppression with decrease in white blood cells and platelets; and pulmonary toxicity, pneumonia followed by fibrosis, may cause sexual problems similar to those resulting from radiation therapy.

Neurotoxicity following vincristine and vinblastine administration may cause impotence in males. Alopecia, hair loss, may be devastating to body image, especially for adolescents who usually place great emphasis on appearance and peer approval[11] and who are beginning to relate to and test out their sexuality with the opposite sex. These, along with skin changes, such as increased pig mentation, acne, and urticaria, may be especially difficult to cope with for the adolescent as well as for older individuals.

Antineoplastic drugs may cause amenorrhea and aspermia[12] or severe fetal abnormalities.[13]

Many drugs used for cancer therapy also cause immunosuppression, resulting in decrease in antibody and lymphocyte production. As a result, organisms not normally pathogenic to humans may overwhelm the host and cause death. For this reason, some institutions place the patients in "reverse" isolation to protect them from infection. In others, isolation is not used, but much emphasis is placed on cleanliness and protection from visitors who have infections. The individual and the sexual partner may become fearful of resumption of sexual activity after treatment is discontinued because of fears of infection. In addition, individuals in isolation have a tendency to withdraw and to develop difficulty in communication. They may become suspicious of others and overly concerned about their condition and the care they receive from staff or loved ones. Reestablishment of the sexual relationship will be particularly difficult when the individual returns home.

Some drugs can cause change in libido, all cross the placental barrier, causing fetal abnormalities, while most of the drugs can cause abnormal sperm production. Persons receiving chemotherapy are usually urged to practice some form of birth control.

Many of the nonchemotherapeutic drugs that cancer patients take have adverse effects on sexual functioning. Alcohol, narcotics, and some of the tranquilizers may decrease libido and inhibit sexual response, especially when taken in large doses (see Chapter 30).

Immunotherapy

Body image disturbance may follow immunotherapy. The scarification technique to administer vaccines involves multiple scratches on the arm or thigh in a square to form a gridlike appearance. The scratches are deep enough to cause oozing but not frank bleeding. Side effects, ulcerations, induration, and drainage may not only cause discomfort, but also fear that in some ways the lesions may be contagious.

Pustular lesions may be as large as 10 to 15 mm deep. Drainage may be serosanguinous to purulent and may last as long as 1 to 2 months. Four to 6 months may be needed for complete healing. Sites of administration include the back, proximal, and lateral thigh and lateral hip area. Domenick[14] reports that choice of sites must be considered so that one side of the body can be free for use during sitting and sleeping. Clothes can rub or irritate unprotected treatment sites. Sleep may become difficult when drainage causes sheets to stick to the treatment area.

No research has been done to determine the individual's psychosexual reaction to immunotherapy. Although there are relatively few physical side effects, one wonders what fantasies individuals with cancer and their sexual partner may weave about treatment.

PSYCHOLOGIC EFFECTS OF CANCER AND ITS THERAPY ON SEXUALITY

The diagnosis of cancer precipitates an emotional crisis for the patient and the family.[15] At most, cancer connotes death; at least, it connotes pain and suffering. Anxiety, depression, guilt, shame, dependency or regression,[16] anger,[17] and altered body image[18] may cause altered sexual response patterns of the person with cancer and of the sexual partner.

Anxiety

Anxiety about touching and in some way causing harm to the loved one may inhibit sexual expression and sexual satisfaction. These fears plus instruction about the need for cleanliness and the danger of infection and bleeding from various therapies may in turn cause anxiety about intimate contact. Even when sexual activity is resumed, fear of failure coupled with other anxieties may set up the failure–impotence pattern in men or may result in orgasmic dysfunction in women. Uncertainty by either the individual or the sexual partner blocks free expression of sexuality.[19]

Anger

A frequent response to a diagnosis of cancer and to its therapy is anger.[20] "Why me?" The anger may be directed toward the sexual partner, who is seen as the symbol of the health and well-being denied the individual with cancer. It may be expressed in criticism, nit picking, and aversion to any signs of affection and/or sexual overtures.

Depression

Cancer and its therapies present loss—of health, beauty, youth, valued activities, and potentially life itself. Contrary to popular belief, however, Sutherland and Orbach[21] found that although fear of dying from cancer was an important factor in the emotional reaction of patients, they were just as concerned about death in surgery or injury and possible consequent disruption in their pattern of living. Fears of unacceptability and of isolation from the loved one can be greater sources of depression than fear of recurrence.[22]

Acute depression, sometimes with suicidal trends, may occur in anticipation of surgery as the individual projects into the future the effects of the limitations that will ensue. A man whose self-worth was intimately related to his sexual powers became depressed when he foresaw impotence as a consequence. Those whose sense of value is based on a body without blemish may become acutely depressed and suicidal when the diagnosis of cancer is made and therapy suggested.

After treatment, the depression persists until the individual is able to resume valued activities. Some individuals, because of real or imagined limitations, are unable to resume the activity and as a result remain depressed for an indefinite period and sometimes for a lifetime.

Individuals who lose an organ of great psychologic value are prone to develop ideas that the general health of the body has been impaired. Decreased vitality and energy is not related to the actual physiologic function of the organ, but this belief contributes to the depression. Individuals who place great value on sexual activity and body parts that they perceive essential to sexual expression may be particularly prone to depression if they perceive that therapy has removed or has altered these valued organs.

No matter what the etiology, the consequence of depression is decreased libido and sexual dysfunction, often out of proportion to the biologic effects of the cancer and its therapy. (See Chapter 29 for discussion of depression.)

Body Image Disturbance

Distortion in body image is especially prevalent in the individual with cancer. It can result from changes in size and shape of the body, changes in structure and function, and feelings of being dirty or in some way defiled. As a result of the decreased self-esteem that accompanies this disturbance, sexual activity may be avoided or decreased in frequency. The sexual partner may also hold the individual in less esteem because of his/her negative perceptions of the changed body.[23] Surgery may be particularly assaultive on body image. (See Chapter 24.)

Adolescents may suffer severe body image disturbances, since they compare their development with their peers to see "how well they are doing," while sexual concerns center on the body development and image as well as peer relationships.[24]

Guilt and Shame

Cancer may be viewed by some as punishment for past indiscretions, often sexual in nature.[25] Cancer of the reproductive system can be especially traumatic in terms of the guilt and shame generated. With the publication in the popular literature of the relationship of early sexual activity with multiple partners and cervical cancer,[26] the potential for increased guilt and shame associated with this form of cancer is even greater.[27] (See Chapter 13 for discussion of guilt and shame.)

Dependency

Regression and increased dependency on others, especially the spouse, may develop. Often this dependency is thrust upon the individual by others in a desire to protect the other person. One wife declared, "You have to treat your husband like a child, make him feel like he is loved and wanted."[28] Hospitalization brings its own forced dependency on staff and the routines that control the activities of daily living (see Chapter 13). However, the cancer patient may be especially dependent on staff for the management of complicated therapies and their negative sequelae. This forced dependency may be assaultive on individuals who equate their masculinity or femininity with self-care and decision making.

SOCIOCULTURAL EFFECTS OF CANCER AND ITS THERAPY ON SEXUALITY

Sexual Role Changes

Related to the dependency response of individuals with cancer and their sexual partners is the subtle or not too subtle change in sexual roles, especially if longer-term treatment is involved or if the cancer initiates drastic changes in the individual's strength and well-being. Even when able, employment opportunity may be denied the person with cancer because of the employers' fears about the disease or the individual's ability to function and be productive.[29]

Spouses may have to assume financial responsibilities and, of even more negative portent for sexuality, may have to assist the individual with care of an ostomy, an incision, or a draining wound. Even with subsequent recovery, the partners' conception of each other in sexual roles may be replaced by a mother or father nurturant role conception, with negative effects on sexual expression.

Societal Attitudes

One of the most prevalent reactions described by patients with cancer is a sense of isolation, of being cut off from those persons and things that are important to them. They may report that there is a gradual break in relationships.[30] In some cases, it is patient initiated,[31] in others, it may result from actions of significant others because of their negative attitudes toward the disease. Perhaps the most profound isolation is the inability to relate to and derive comfort from others.

Tragically, myths and misconceptions about the nature of cancer, its causes and its therapies may result in social and sexual isolation of the person with cancer. Sexual partners may avoid sexual activity because of the belief that sexual abstinence will prevent recurrence of the cancer.[32] The belief that cancer is in some way contagious, that others may get it from contact with the individual, may cause the sexual partner to avoid, not only sexual intercourse, but also signs of affection and sexual interest such as kissing, holding, and fondling.[33] Yet some patients express more need for touch, than intercourse.[34]

The sexual partner may view the person with cancer as somehow unclean or dirty and may be overwhelmed by fears about the chronicity of the disease and the debilitation that may result. In addition, the common belief that the illness of cancer also involves termination of sexual expression, establishes an expectation for many people that sexuality vanishes with the diagnosis. Cancer's most severe damage may be to communication between patients and loved ones.

Economic Security

Cancer's great expense in terms of time, financial outlay, and job insecurity may produce much stress on roles and relationships. Concerns about payment of bills and money for food, housing, and schooling may assume tremendous proportions, blocking out other facets of the relationship. In any chronic illness, feelings of anger that the individual is causing financial hardship to the family or the sexual partner may surface or remain hidden, but in either case may adversely affect the relationship.[35]

SEX AND THE DYING INDIVIDUAL

At the close of the movie *Love Story,* the young husband, whose wife is dying from leukemia, climbs on the bed amid the tubes and intravenous equipment and takes her into his arms. He holds her until she dies. Some may protest: "theatrical," "unrealistic," but this young man was providing the one thing that he knew would provide comfort to her and to him—closeness, touching, body to body contact.

The terminally ill person from any cause, not only cancer, and the sexual partner experience tremendous problems in trying to maintain sexual identity. Because of anxiety about death and dying and grief over anticipated loss, the sexual partner may avoid sexual contact. Yet, the dying person may desire and seek sexual closeness. The opposite may also occur, the work of the dying may decrease libido and cause the individual to isolate herself/himself, while the sexual partner desires sexual contact. A basic conflict exists between coitus and dying. The first may result in the beginning of life, the other signifies the end of life.

Burkhalter and Donley[36] conceptualize the terminally ill cancer patient's dilemma in terms of the vitality, epitomized by sexual expression, in contrast to the debilitation anticipated with dying. However, while the individual may be experiencing diminution of physical and/or psychosocial capabilities, a fundamental need may remain for sexual expression. The method of expression of this need may have to change for some. Affection, closeness, and love can be expressed by touching, holding, kissing, intimate conversation, tenderness, and consideration.

NURSING IMPLICATIONS

Assessment and Planning

Cancer patients expect the health professional to bring up the topic of sexuality.[37] The nurse's first contact with the individual may be in the home after therapy has been completed or while it is still in progress. The newly hospitalized patient may be focusing his/her attention on the disease process, so sexual concerns may not be prominent at this time.

Consequently, the assessment must be a dynamic process in which the nurse is consistantly gathering data about the bio-psycho-social affects of cancer and its therapy on the sexuality of the individual and the sexual partner with a goal of rehabilitation to the highest level of sexual function. (See Chapter 13 for assessment related to body image, shame, and guilt.)

Assessment data from client and partner include: knowledge of the disease and its therapy, readiness for sex, ability to use usual method of expression, feelings about sexual activity while ill, reactions to hair loss, or other physical changes, information needed to function sexually, and information desired about alternative methods of sexual expression.[38]

Because the cancer patient's physical and psychologic well-being may fluctuate with therapy, the nurse must be flexible in setting and changing goals and in planning care. The nurse's creativity and sensitivity to the individual's responses promote sexual well-being. Nurses should be sensitive to subtle clues that indicate something is important to the patient.[39]

There are times when sexuality and sexual problems are uppermost in the individual's mind. At other times, he/she "couldn't care less." Optimal sexual well-being as defined by the sexual partners should be the major goal.

Intervention

Anticipatory guidance can help prevent some of the negative sexual responses to cancer and its therapy. The intervention for specific surgical procedures are discussed in Chapter 24, so focus in this discussion will be on the teaching and counseling of individuals and their sexual partners when other types of therapy are contemplated or are in progress.

Counseling may take the form of on-the-spot response, focus on present concerns, questions, problems, or resolutions of a crisis. A future-oriented counseling program involves several sessions over a longer period of time.[40] The "I Can Cope Program" of the American Cancer Society provides such a support program.

Biologic Changes. Patients who are receiving chemotherapy or radiation with subsequent changes in hematopoietic tissue and/or in mucous membranes are instructed in alternate forms of sexual expression. If oral ulceration is present, oral–oral activity may be replaced by oral stimulation of the breasts or by manual stroking and fondling of the body. Contraceptive options are discussed.

Since danger of infection is great, both sexual partners should be especially meticulous in their personal hygiene before sexual activity, but especially in perineal and oral hygiene. Because of the danger of infection and damage to mucosa, excessive friction during coitus should be avoided. If the woman is having difficulty achieving adequate vaginal lubrication, a sterile water-soluble jelly should be used. Anal intercourse should be avoided, since the anus is very prone to abcess formation if breaks in the tissue occur.

After pelvic radiation and subsequent stenosis, elevation of the hips on a pillow, rear entry or lubrication of adducted thighs to simulate a deeper vaginal barrel may improve sexual response. Vaginal dilator insertion three times a day increasing in size is effective but normal sexual activity is preferred, since some women may be concerned about masturbatory implications and putting objects in their bodies. The woman is told the dilator use is temporary and part of routine rehabilitation.[41]

Vigorous manipulation of breast or other tissue may cause bleeding, so the nurse instructs the persons to use gentle stimulation. In fact, sexual partners often find this more sensuous and sexually stimulating than vigorous manipulation. Application of lotions and creams to the body by gentle stroking can be an extremely effective means of erotic stimulation.

Timing of sexual activity may need to be changed. Nausea and vomiting or pain may be more severe in the evening, so coitus or other forms of sexual activity may be more pleasurable in the early morning or soon after taking medication to relieve these symptoms. Early morning sexual activity has the additional advantage of usually finding both partners more rested, so that fatigue is minimized. Rest periods before sexual activity may be beneficial.

Individuals need information about drugs that they are taking,[42] especially those with adverse effects on sexual response. Many individuals with cancer turn to alcohol as a source of relief from their fears and anxiety, without realizing its adverse effects on sexual functioning (see Chapter 30).

If alopecia occurs, nurses remind persons to purchase wigs to help maintain sexual identity. Women's wigs are inexpensive and widely available. Men may have more difficulty in finding inexpensive hairpieces, but even they are becoming more readily available. Although baldness in men may be considered a sign of virility by some, the nurse should not assume that the sexual identity of men will be undisturbed by hair loss.

Psychosocial Changes. Intervention to maintain or decrease the psychologic responses of anxiety, depression, dependency, and anger are detailed in many nursing textbooks devoted to meeting psychologic needs. Intervention for body image disturbances, guilt, and shame are presented in Chapter

13. The nurse remembers, moreover, that most sexual activity involves a partner and mutuality of expression. Consequently, the nurse must recognize the psychologic reactions of the sexual partner as well as the cancer patient and intervene to help him/her.

The sexual partner must become a part of the treatment team if at all possible. The nurse first dispels misconceptions about the nature of cancer and the results of therapy. Rehabilitation begins in the hospital, but the sexual partner continues it at home. Klagsburn[43] graphically describes the role of a husband, and his statement could apply to any sexual partner. "A husband who is encouraged to grin lecherously at his wife on her return home from the hospital will do more for her than any occupational therapy program can."

Nurses suggest that holding and touching are forms of sexual expression that can substitute for coitus. Intimacy is more than intercourse. Some clients may be concerned about the normalcy of their thoughts and desires, such as still wanting sexual activity. Reassuring them that these are acceptable behaviors and dreams will relieve anxiety.[44]

The sexual partner can be instrumental in preventing the social isolation and affectional deprivation that may be experienced. A gift, a surprise visit at another time than usual, and expressions of affection can be tremendously therapeutic. The sexual partner should also be encouraged to allow the patient to resume the usual role activities rather than to protect her/him in the mistaken idea that this will facilitate recovery.

When a sexual partner is not available for reducing sexual tensions some individuals may substitute masturbation, looking at erotically stimulating pictures, or reading erotically stimulating books. In the institutional setting, the nurse tries to provide the privacy that the individual needs for whatever sexual expression is preferred. Privacy may be particularly difficult to achieve for the cancer patient if there is frequent need for administration of medication, adjustment of intravenous rates, etc. (See Chapter 13 for discussion of privacy and the effects of hospitalization.)

Finally, care of the cancer patient may require the help of other members of the health team.[45] If overwhelming financial burdens are disrupting the relationship, the social worker is called in to help find sources of financial support or the family members are directed to these sources. If the effects on sexuality are incapacitating and continuous, then referral for psychotherapy or to a sexual counselor may be necessary. Individuals bring their premorbid sexual problems with them, so that the nurse recognizes that in some cases, where the sexual relationship was either fragile and/or nonsupportive, any illness, but especially cancer, may cause its disruption and dissolution.

Evaluation

If the nurse's goals were consistent with those of the individual and sexual partner, the following outcome criteria can be identified:

1. The patient and sexual partner verbalize their feelings about the effects of the illness and therapy on sexuality.
2. The patient and sexual partner can identify side effects of therapy that necessitate change in sexual expression.
3. The couple state which changes should be made in sexual activity.
4. The sexual partner identifies ways in which the patient can assume usual role activities and encourages these activities.

NOTES

1. Dreesman GR, Burek J, Adam F, et al: Expression of herpesvirus induced antigens in human cervical cancer. Nature 283:591, 1980
2. Committee on Professional Education of the International Union Against Cancer: Clinical Oncology: A Manual for Students and Doctors. New York, Springer-Verlag, 1973, p 22

3. Sutherland AM, Orbach CE: Depressive reactions associated with surgery for cancer. In The Psychological Impact of Cancer. New York, American Cancer Society, 1974, pp 17–21

4. Committee on Professional Education of the International Union Against Cancer: Clinical Oncology: A Manual for Students and Doctors. New York, Springer-Verlag, 1973, pp 86–87

5. Abitol MM, Davenport JH: Sexual dysfunction after therapy for cervical carcinoma. Am J Obstet Gynecol 119:181–189, 1974

6. Ibid, p 185

7. Burkhalter PK, Donley DL: Dynamics of Oncology Nursing. New York, McGraw-Hill, 1978, p 144

8. Gonick P: Urologic problems and sexual function. In Oaks WW, Melchiode GA, Ficher I (eds): Sex and the Life Cycle. New York, Grune and Stratton, 1976, pp 191–198

9. Maguire P: The psychological and social consequences of breast cancer. Nurs Mirror 140:54–57, April 3, 1975

10. Fredette SL, Gloriant FS: Nursing diagnosis in cancer chemotherapy. Am J Nurs 81:2013–2020, 1981

11. Wilbur J: Sexual development and body image in the teenager with cancer. Front Rad Ther Oncol 14:108–114, 1980

12. Buchanan JD, Farley KF, Barrie JU: Return of spermatogenesis after stopping cyclophosphamide therapy. Lancet 2:156–163, 1975

13. Sokal JE, Lessman EM: Effects of cancer chemotherapeutic drugs on the human fetus. JAMA 172:1765–1771, 1960

14. Domenick NP: The methanol extract residue (MER) of Bacillus calmette-guérin in cancer immunotherapy. Nurs Clin North Am 13:369–380, 1978

15. George MM: Long term care of the patient with cancer. Nurs Clin North Am 8:623–631, 1973

16. Francis GM: Cancer, the emotional component. Am J Nurs 69:1677–1681, 1969

17. Shepardson J: Team approach to the patient with cancer. Am J Nurs 72:488–491, 1972

18. Klagsburn SC: Communication in the treatment of cancer. Am J Nurs 71:944–948, 1971

19. Burkhalter PK, Donley DL: Dynamics of Oncology Nursing. New York, McGraw-Hill, 1978, p 259

20. Shepardson J: Team approach to the patient with cancer. Am J Nurs 72:488, 1972

21. Sutherland AM, Orbach CE: Depressive reactions associated with surgery for cancer. In The Psychological Impact of Cancer. New York, American Cancer Society, 1974, p 18

22. Cantor RC: Self-esteem, sexuality and cancer. Front Rad Ther Oncol 14:51–54, 1980

23. Dyk RB, Sutherland AM: Adaptation of the spouse and other family members to the colostomy patient. In The Psychological Impact of Cancer. New York, American Cancer Society, 1974, pp 72–87

24. Morrow M: Nursing management of the adolescent. Nurs Clin North Am 13:319–335, 1978

25. Shepardson J: Team approach to the patient with cancer. Am J Nurs 72:491, 1972

26. Jordan JA: Sexual activity and cervical squamous carcinoma. Nurs Mirror 143(15):48–49, 1976

27. Abitol MM, Davenport JH: Sexual dysfunction after therapy for cervical carcinoma. Am J Obstet Gynecol 119:187, 1974

28. Dyk RB, Sutherland AM: Adaptation of the spouse and other family members to the colostomy patient. In The Psychological Impact of Cancer. New York, American Cancer Society, 1974, p 77

29. Burkhalter PK, Donley DL: Dynamics of Oncology Nursing. New York, McGraw-Hill, 1978, p 22

30. Davis MZ: Patients in limbo. Am J Nurs 66:746–748, 1966

31. Francis GM: Cancer, the emotional component. Am J Nurs 69:1680, 1969

32. Abitol MM, Davenport JH: Sexual dysfunction after therapy for cervical carcinoma. Am J Obstet Gynecol 119:187, 1974

33. Golden JS, Golden M: Cancer and sex. Front Rad Ther Oncol 14:59–65, 1980

34. Leiber L, Plumb MM, Gerstenzang M, Holland J: The communication of affection between cancer patients and their spouses. Psychosom Med 38:379–389, 1976

35. Spouses speak. Ostomy Review II. Los Angeles, United Ostomy Association, 1974, pp 22–23

36. Burkhalter PK, Donley DL: Dynamics of Oncology Nursing, New York, McGraw-Hill, 1978, p 259

37. Bullard DG, Causey GG, Newman AB, et al: Sexual health care, a needs assessment. Front Rad Ther Oncol 14:55–58, 1980

38. Shipes E, Lehr S: Sexuality and the male cancer patient. Cancer Nurs 5:375–381, 1982

39. What health professionals did for me and what I wish they had done. Front Rad Ther Oncol 14:115–122, 1980

40. Adams GK: The sex-counseling role of the cancer clinician. Front Rad Ther Oncol 14:66–78, 1980

41. Donahue VC, Knapp RC: Sexual rehabilitation of gynecologic cancer patients. Obstet Gynecol 49:118–122, 1977

42. Levine ME: Cancer chemotherapy—A nursing model. Nurs Clin North Am 13:271–280, 1978

43. Klagsburn SC: Communication in the treatment of cancer. Am J Nurs 71:944–948, 1971

44. Lamb MA, Woods, NF: Sexuality and the cancer patient. Cancer Nurs 4:137–144, 1981

45. Shepardson J: Team approach to the patient with cancer. Am J Nurs 72:488, 1972

Chapter 24

Mutilating Surgery

Paradoxically, that which may heal may also harm. Therapeutic measures that are directed toward health may bring increased well-being in one area of the individual's life but distress in another. This is especially true in relation to some surgical procedures. Surgical procedures are a physical assault on the person's body. The psychosocial sequelae may be diverse, since each person perceives surgery in his/her own individual way, and the emotional responses that accompany physical trauma are proportional to the intensity of threat that is perceived.[1] In surgical procedures, the individual has concerns about the effects on self and on the appearance of the body. Sometimes the person's life becomes centered around the body part, and the result may be intense emotional attachment to that part.[2]

All surgical procedures bring some degree of threat to body image and self, but none pose greater threat than those procedures that directly or indirectly affect sexual functioning or the individual's view of self as a sexual being. Any procedure, no matter how seemingly innocuous, may produce sexual disequilibrium if the person views it as an assault on the sexual self. Consequently, an uncomplicated herniorrhaphy may produce sexual dysfunction if a man believes that it makes him less of a man. This feeling, accompanied by the shock of seeing swollen and ecchymotic genitals, may produce intense anxiety and subsequent problems in the area of sexuality.

However, there are some surgical procedures that are especially assaultive on body image and sexuality. Some of the procedures may produce anatomic and physiologic changes that alter sexual response patterns, some do not. Procedures discussed include mastectomy, hysterectomy, female radical pelvic surgery, enterostomy, prostatectomy and male radical pelvic surgeries, surgery of the face and neck, and amputation.

NURSING PROCESS RELATED TO MUTILATING SURGERIES

Two principles give direction for planning nursing care and establishing realistic intermediate and long-term goals for all patients undergoing mutilating surgery. First, there is no typical pattern of response to mutilating surgery. Second, when an individual suffers radical body mutilation, he resists accepting reality and tends to persist in viewing his body in terms of his previously intact body image. Consequently, denial may operate to make intervention difficult.[3] Careful data collection is essential to identify each patient's individual responses.

Gallagher[4] suggests a patient behavioral chart to record patient's day-to-day verbal and nonverbal responses, which give some indication how he/she feels about the body and the operative procedure. Constant pre- and postoperative observation is necessary to collect data so that the nurse can recognize when denial becomes less operative and reality is faced. This may not happen until the individual returns home, so the nurse in a public health setting or industrial or office setting must be observant.

MASTECTOMY

Bio-Psycho-Social Factors

In recent years, the breast's function as a source of nourishment for the infant has received less attention than its function as a source of erotic stimulation for both sexes and as an important component of feminine identity for many women. The frequency with which the breast's size and shape are temporarily augmented by special brassieres and padding and, when desired, permanently augmented or reduced by surgical procedures attest to society's breast consciousness. In addition to its sociosexual importance, in many relationships breast stimulation plays an important role in erotic play, some women responding intensely to stroking, sucking, and manipulation of breast tissue. (See Chapter 3.)

Along with the loss of a source of erotic stimulation, removal of the breast produces obvious changes in the contour of the body, the degree of change dependent on the surgical procedure performed. This change in contour, the scar, lymphedema, and restricted motion and sensation also contribute to the third sequela of mastectomy, altered body image.

In addition to fears related to disfigurement and loss of desirability as a sexual being, most women are also confronted with the fear and anxiety associated with the diagnosis of cancer. As a result of these factors, the individual may have concerns about her identity as a woman, wife, and/or mother and about her security in these roles.[5,6]

In a poll conducted for the American Cancer Society, 1007 women 18 years and older were questioned regarding their attitudes toward breast cancer and breast surgery. Fears were expressed about disfigurement, and change in body, cancer and its cure, emotional adjustment, and loss of femininity.

Particularly threatened were middle class women, single women 18 to 34 years of age, and women who were highly sociable, tense, and more concerned with their physical appearance than the average woman.[7]

Although the younger women indicated a greater fear of loss of femininity in the Cancer Society study, Kent[8] feels that adjusting to mastectomy may be more difficult for older women than for younger ones, since older women are already having to face the implications of declining physical appearance, which will be compounded by the surgery.

The woman's response to mastectomy is predicated on different factors in her life and in her own psychologic processes. Bard and Sutherland[9] have identified five significant variables:

1. The value the woman assigns to her lost breast.
2. The response of significant others.
3. The positive reinforcement she receives from health professionals regarding her body and her rehabilitation.
4. The role models or positive identification models with whom she comes in contact.
5. The coping principles that she can learn in an environment of acceptance.

The woman who places high value on her body as a measure of self-worth and social acceptability will probably have more difficulty incorporating the loss of a breast in an altered body image than women who place greater value on their intellectual and affective qualities. Body oriented women are more likely to withdraw from sexual relationships and to either consciously or unconsciously foster rejection by the sexual partner. If the sexual partner's relationship with her is also predicated on her physical qualities, the problem is doubly compounded.[10]

Profound depression may follow mastectomy because of the emotional impact of surgery. The suffering caused by a loss of the breast far outweighs physical pain. Of 41 patients studied by Jamison et al.,[11] one in four had considered suicide. Women described loss of libido, anger, hostility, outrage, and hatred of men. Tests and questionnaires administered to the women showed they had a sense of body disfigurement and loss of feeling of femininity.

In a sample of 40 3-months postmastectomy women, Derogatis[12] found that those with a high feminine gender role identity are often at a greater risk for sexual dysfunction.

Support may be needed for an extended period of time but at least for the first 3 months after surgery.[13] Ignorance and fear are particularly destructive to adjustment. In a controlled study of 75 patients counseled by a nurse and 77 who received usual care, Maguire and associates found that even nurse counseling failed to prevent adverse reactions but her regular following of the patients enabled her to identify those who needed psychiatric help so that 12 to 18 months after surgery the counseled group had less psychiatric morbidity than the control group.[14]

The trend toward less radical procedures and breast reconstruction may account for less depression and maladjustment found in other studies.[15,16]

As sophistication in use of other therapy increases, fewer mastectomies may be done. Some physicians are using primary radiation therapy for early cancer and are reporting not only similar cure rates but excellent cosmetic results.[17]

Changes in Sexual Activity after Surgery

Women. Loss of libido in itself results in decreased sexual activity. In addition, women hesitate to resume sex, because they fear damage to the incision and the surrounding area. Fear of rejection by the sexual partner also may cause women to avoid intercourse. Others may have coitus in the dark, may refuse to take off their brassieres, or may wear clothing on their upper body.[18]

The unmarried woman usually faces more difficult problems in reestablishing her sexual life. She may dread the prospect of telling a partner about the surgery, because she fears rejection and may be completely inhibited from entering new sexual relationships.[19]

In a study of 450 women with breast cancer, Maguire[20] found that older women over 60, with decreased interest in sexual activity, with understanding husbands or close friends to confide in, and with little psychologic investment in their breasts, adjusted fairly readily to mastectomy. Younger women for whom an active sexual relationship was important, who considered bust size important for attractiveness, and who perceived husbands or friends as unsupportive had a difficult time adjusting. These women became upset when looking at themselves in the mirror or when engaging in sexual activity. They described themselves as "lopsided," "abnormal," "peculiar," "mutilated," or "below standard." Early provision for a breast prosthesis sometimes did much to restore self-confidence. If its acquisition was delayed for any reason, many women had loss of libido and enjoyment in coitus. Some marriages were put under great strain, continual arguments and disagreements leading them to consider separation.

No normative data are available regarding change in coitus or orgasmic frequency. Some women report that their sexual relationships had suffered, but interestingly and more importantly, others say that the relationships had deepened and become better as they and their sexual partners worked through their concerns and problems.[21]

Sexual Partners. In reviewing research related to social support Lindsey[22] found that the husband's or partner's reaction and behavior is important to the woman's adjustment. Some of the same fears and concerns, however, are also experienced by men.

The degree of adjustment is predicated

on whether there is a good sexual and inter-personal adjustment preoperatively. If there is concern and caring, the postoperative adjustment will be far easier. Initially, the sex partner may be as shocked by changes in the woman's body as was the woman. If they are revulsed and repulsed, they experience difficulty in hiding these feelings, which may be communicated to the woman. One husband stated, "I think I'm used to her mastectomy already, but maybe I'll wake up in the middle of the night and wonder what has happened to us."[23]

The husband may feel that his wife's sexual desirability is necessary for a successful marriage and may regard the operation as a threat to his sexual satisfaction. He may try to disguise his feelings but react with anxiety, guilt, or rage. He may be appalled by the wound because of the meaning that bodily injuries or wounds have for him, withdrawing from his wife and sexual intimacy. The husband's fear of hurting his wife if he resumes sexual activity may reinforce the wife's fear of injury and further compromise the sexual relationship and her view of her femininity. The operative site may initiate anxiety about mutilation in the husband, and if the anxiety is strong enough, he may unconsciously withdraw from the sexual relationship, reinforcing the wife's feelings of rejection. Some women have helped their husbands cope with their fears by covering the mastectomy site with a pillow to protect it.[24]

Rehabilitation for Sexual Function

Three rehabilitative approaches to confronting the woman's changed body image have proven successful—the Reach to Recovery program of the American Cancer Society, the Encore program of the YWCA, and surgical breast reconstruction.

Reach to Recovery. Reach to Recovery was begun in 1952 by Terese Lasser, who had had a mastectomy. Volunteers are women who have had the surgery and are at least 3 years postoperative. They must be cleared for

participation by two physicians who state they are physically healed and psychologically adjusted. After referral by the physician, the volunteer visits the woman, usually in the hospital, bringing a kit and manual about rehabilitative exercises, clothes and arm care. Information may also be given about resumption of sexual relations. The woman is reassured that as she begins to feel better, her desire for coitus will return. Women are told that at first, pain in the incisional area may cause some discomfort during sexual activity. They are also urged to maintain communication by sharing their feelings and concerns with their sexual partner.[25]

Of equal if not more importance is the role modeling of the volunteer, identified as one of the important factors in adaptation to mastectomy. The volunteer by her appearance and behavior helps convey to the woman that rehabilitation from mastectomy is possible.

Encore. The Encore program was developed by Helen Glines Kohut, a nurse who had had a mastectomy. The program focuses on land and water exercises that aid women in rebuilding their physical and emotional strength after mastectomy. Exercises are designed to strengthen muscles on the affected side, so full use of shoulder, arm, and chest muscles can be restored. In addition, the fellowship of the group and exchange of information is a source of support and encouragement.[26]

Reconstruction. Recently, with more early detection, and use of less radical surgery, women are better candidates for reconstruction.[27] Patients feel socially isolated, awkward, and insecure, even with well-fitted prostheses,[28] and the external prostheses give little semblance of normality in sexual relationships, since they are not a permanent part of the body.

Reconstructive surgery was described by one woman as "the miracle after the devastation of mastectomy." Another stated that "the darkness of fear and anxiety left entirely . . . life can be pursued with more vigor and joy. The change shows not only in my chest but in my face and my heart."[29]

Some surgery may be done immediately after mastectomy but most surgeons wait 3 to 6 months. There is no outer time limit. Silicone gel or silicone saline prosthesis is used.[30] Nipples have been constructed from nonhair-bearing skin of the axilla, groin, labia majora or minora.

For patients whose mastectomy scar is tight, several procedures are possible: a flap procedure involving skin from the back or lower abdomen, or the abdominal advancement technique which involves sliding some skin from the upper abdomen into the breast area.

Surgeons often do not give women a choice of mastectomy procedure for cancer. Reconstructive Education for National Understanding (RENU) has been formed to coordinate efforts to reach women before they have cancer, so they know their options. Hotlines and trained speakers are being developed and RENU is now endorsed as the Breast Reconstruction Program for the American Cancer Society in some states.[31]

NURSING IMPLICATIONS

Assessment and Planning

Preoperatively, the nurse assesses biologic variables that may affect the woman's psychosexual response to the surgery—age, type of procedure contemplated, her usual level of sexual activity, marital status, and whether she has a sexual partner. The nurse also assesses the patient's level of anxiety and depression and her feeling about change in her body appearance (see Chapter 13 for body image data). At this stage, however, she may be in a stage of shock and disbelief and may be coping by denying the implications of the surgery. The impact of the surgery on body image may not be felt for 2 or 3 months[32] and develops gradually. Rather than press her for information, the nurse interviews to establish rapport and a trusting relationship. She also uses this time to answer any questions that the woman may have.[33]

The preoperative interview may be short or a long discussion of fears about sexuality, femininity, and her sexual relationships.[34]

The nurse also involves the patient's sexual partner in the assessment process if possible to identify concerns and feelings about the proposed surgery and the degree of support that is available for the woman.

Significant objective data are the individual's commitment to her personal appearance, clothes, makeup, and hair, since this gives some clues to her degree of investment in her physical self.

Postoperatively, the nurse gathers data related to body image changes, and the patient's initial reaction to the surgery, especially as it relates to feelings of femininity and her relationship to the sexual partner.

The nurse's goals are to help the woman incorporate her changed body image into a positive view of her sexual self. She also focuses on helping the sexual partner to cope with fears and feelings about the woman as a sexual being.

Intervention

Detailed intervention for individuals with disturbance in body image are given in Chapter 13, so only specific intervention for mastectomized women are given here. Klagsburn[35] believes that there are no shortcuts to dealing with mutilating surgery and that the best way to develop a relationship with the patient is to open up a discussion about her fears. The nurse takes the initiative in beginning the conversation by a comment such as "It's a rough thing that you went through," then follows up the woman's responses so that she keeps on talking. Use of reflective techniques, open-ended statements, and validation of patient responses encourages open communication and expression of feelings.

Major questions about body changes that affect sex life must be addressed. For example, how soon should the sexual partner see the woman's scar? This answer must be individualized, since it depends in part on openness and habits in the relationship. The first step is having the patient look at her own body. However, if the wound is still draining or inflamed, it is wise to let the wound heal some before having the patient see it.[36]

Try and include the spouse or sexual partner in some teaching. Reassure the clients that feeling depressed and experiencing lack of interest in sex is normal for a while and that she should not feel rejected if the partner will not look at the scar for a while. Both are reassured that breast play and touching are without harm.[37]

The nurse assures the woman and her sexual partner that the mastectomy does not decrease her worth as a woman or her abilities as a sexual partner. Intercourse is not medically contraindicated and may be resumed as soon as the woman is discharged from the hospital. The nurse should explain that there might be some discomfort initially because of the scar but that it will be decreased as healing continues. Different positions for intercourse should be tried. If the women experiences phantom pain, massaging the area can help. In time the pain will go.[38]

The nurse helps the patient maintain and gain self-respect for her body by meticulous care and positive reinforcement of the patient's efforts to maintain her appearance. As a part of these interventions to bolster self-image, a breast prosthesis should be fitted as soon as possible after the operation. The initial prosthesis is temporary and with the newest surgical techniques can be worn as early as the second or third day after surgery.[39] At no time should the woman be forced to stuff facial tissues, sanitary napkins, or handkerchiefs into an old brassiere. The sexual partner can be reminded of the importance of complimenting the woman when she makes efforts to maintain her appearance. A little tenderness can go a long way toward fostering self-esteem.

Some institutions are initiating evening meetings in which couples who are going through a mastectomy and a volunteer couple who are postmastectomy meet to discuss topics such as handling depression and changes in the relationship. The theme of these sessions is that what is happening is a common burden, to be shared. The philosophy is that the sexual partner will hear what he can accept and screen out what he cannot tolerate.[40]

The American Cancer Society's Reach to Recovery Program also has "Men in Our Lives," group meetings for the men in the life of the mastectomy patients. Health professionals discuss mastectomy, giving men guidance for coping as well as information on how they can assist the mastectomy patient with her recovery.

At all times, the nurse promotes communication between the sexual partners, serving as an intermediary to help them work through their feelings of confusion, frustration, and threat and to help them problem solve to arrive at their own decisions. Ideally, at discharge, the nurse gives the couple a telephone number where he/she can be reached for any problem regarding surgery or the adjustment.

Evaluation

The nurse evaluates the responses of the woman and the sexual partner, since they are interdependent. The following outcome criteria are identified:

1. The woman and her sexual partner look at the scar.
2. The woman can state where to obtain a breast prosthesis.
3. The woman obtains a prosthesis.
4. The woman and her sexual partner can describe different positions for intercourse or alternate forms of sexual expression, if indicated.
5. The sexual partners communicate to each other about concerns and fears.
6. The couple show evidence of mutual support: (a) the sexual partner compliments the woman, (b) the woman verbalizes her

awareness that this is a difficult time for the sexual partner.

HYSTERECTOMY

Bio-Psycho-Social Factors

If the breast is the external confirmation of femininity, the uterus is the internal. Although its loss is not visable, the bio-psycho-social response can be devastating to the woman, to her sexual partner, and to their relationship. Postoperative depression is the most common adverse response to this perceived loss of femininity.

Budd[41] studied posthysterectomy depression related to women's concept of their femininity as reflected in perception of their sex role. Although the literature reports that women involved in the homemaker and mother role are more likely to be depressed after hysterectomy, Budd found the opposite. Those endorsing the homemaker role were less depressed than those who did not strongly endorse it.

Krouse and Krouse[42] found that womens' initial feelings of depression and body image disturbance continued even at 20 months after surgery. Ethnicity may be a factor in response. Krueger[43] and associates found that Mexican-Americans were most depressed and blacks least depressed with Anglo-Americans in between.

Women themselves give clues to their change in body image. "I was all cleaned out," "They took everything out," or "I lost my nature," "I'm all used up." The depression that follows loss of other valued body parts usually resolves itself in a few weeks, but Bunker[44] states that depression occurs at a higher than normal rate in women with hysterectomy. Those with a prior history of emotional and marital disturbances, who are without pelvic disease, and who are under 40 are more likely to experience a depressive reaction. Women who are experiencing other emotional stress, such as children's problems with adolescence, grown children leaving home, and husbands with midlife crises are also particularly vulnerable.

Much of the adverse response is predicated on misconceptions and misinformation about the role of the uterus and the effect of its removal. Drellich and Bieber[45] studied a group of 23 premenopausal women who had had hysterectomies. They viewed the uterus as a badge of femininity and perceived themselves as less attractive as women, fearing rejection by their spouses or other men. In addition to reproduction, they attributed the uterus with functions of excretion, regulation of body processes, expression of sexuality, and maintenance of strength and vitality, youth, and attractiveness.

Dennerstein and associates[46] ranked the concerns in terms of frequency in a retrospective study involving 89 women who had hysterectomies and oophorectomies. Preoperatively, the women were primarily worried about altered sexual function, followed in order by fear of weight gain, the procedure itself, cancer, loss of femininity, mental deterioration, and finally excessive hair growth. Significantly, women who were worried about sexual alteration preoperatively had the greatest deterioration of sexual relationships postoperatively.

Postoperatively, other concerns may arise. The removal of a reproductive organ has significant symbolic meaning. No matter what age, no woman ever renounces the possibility of pregnancy as long as menstruation continues, even though she desires no more children. The woman may view menstruation as indicating that she is biologically alive.[47]

The loss of a valued organ brings its own fears and disturbances. Some of the women in Drellich and Bieber's study experienced significant feelings of loss because they were no longer able to bear children. Other women view surgery as punishment for sinful, tabooed, or self-abusive activities that were sexual in nature. Some believed that there is a relationship between the uterus and gastrointestinal function and took vitamins to compensate for perceived nutritional loss after surgery. Of the group, five experienced no change in their sexual experience; others described feeling raw, tender, and vulnerable inside, even if the incision was well-healed. Some felt that the vagina had become old and useless and contained a lump or some other impediment to successful intercourse.[48] Some women report feelings of weakness, loss of strength, and easy fatigability—that when certain organs such as the uterus are lost, one is not as good anymore.[49]

The Woman: Change in Sexual Function

The uterus is also involved in the sexual response cycle. During the excitement phase, it elevates from its usual position in the pelvis, and during the orgasmic phase, it rhythmically contracts. Although some women report that they are not aware of this response, those that are may report dissatisfaction after surgery.

Biologic changes may have greater impact on sexual problems than many studies indicate. Zussman[50] and associates argue that poor methodology, retrospective studies, biased samples, lack of control groups, and failure to consider physiologic aspects of sexuality make findings of earlier studies questionable. They urge consideration of androgen loss with oophorectomy. Even in postmenopausal women the ovaries secrete some androgens which contribute to sex drive.

Other women describe loss of the feeling from cervical and broad ligament stimulation,[51] a sensation of a shortened and narrowed vagina with dyspareunia, lack of libido, and bleeding.[52,53]

If bilateral oophorectomy is also performed, the administration of estrogen can prevent the menopausal changes that follow,[54] but Dennerstein et al.[55] found estrogen therapy unsuccessful in the treatment of decreased or absent libido. However, literature concerning the effect of hormones on sexual behavior is conflicting. Although the atrophic changes in the vagina are prevented by estrogen, it is not known what effect, if

any, estrogen and progesterone have on human sexual behavior.[56]

Even with the administration of estrogen and with teaching and counseling of the 89 patients in Dennerstein[57] and associates' study, 33 (37 percent) reported decrease in frequency of sexual activity, 30 (34 percent) stated sexual relations had improved, and 26 (29 percent) reported no change. There was no relationship between giving hormones and sexual dysfunction, desire for sex, enjoyment of sex, ability to reach orgasm, and ease of vaginal lubrication. Forty-seven percent of the women had difficulty achieving vaginal lubrication. This may have been secondary to psychologic factors or to organic factors. Although Masters and Johnson demonstrated that the cervix had only a small role to play in production of vaginal lubrication in their subjects, a woman who has had a tenuous sexual adjustment and difficulty becoming aroused before surgery may not be able to tolerate the absence of cervical mucus as a source of lubrication for intercourse. There was a relationship between coital frequency before surgery and frequency afterward. Those who had intercourse less than one time per week tended to have a worse overall sexual outcome than those who had intercourse one time a week or more.[58] However, the major factor that was associated with a poor sexual outcome was psychologic.

A negative expectation of the operation was significantly associated with poor overall sexual outcome and loss of desire postoperatively, demonstrating the effectiveness of self-fulfilling prophecies. Some explanation for the woman's negative expectations may be related to lack of knowledge of the expected sexual outcome, negative comments by friends and relatives concerning the operation and its results, and change in treatment by the partner, even when positive. (The husbands of 17 women were more understanding after the operation.)[59]

In spite of negative outcomes reported in the literature, beneficial effects or no change may take place in the sexual relationship.

Some women see positive aspects of hysterectomy, expressing relief that they no longer had to practice methods of contraception. Twenty-one of 49 patients who had vaginal hysterectomy reported that they found sexual intercourse better than before surgery, 7 found it worse, and 21 saw no difference.[60] The sexual morbidity found by Dennerstein and associates was higher than in several earlier studies, but her samples were not random and representative of all women undergoing the operation, so that the proportion of women with sexual inadequacy may have been spurious.

Depression may not be inevitable. A prospective study of 60 premenopausal women before and after hysterectomy who were randomly assigned to receive placebo or estrogen replacement found no evidence of depression or sexual difficulties. From baseline both groups had improved mood, vigor, and unimpaired sexual activity.[61]

No generalizations can be made about response to the surgery. Each individual values various body parts and functions differently, and the degree of concern is in proportion to the perceived value and will differ between women.

Nevertheless, teaching to clarify myths and misconceptions might be effective in promoting better sexual health after hysterectomy. Nurse counseling was positively related to the sexual adjustment of 108 premenopausal women after hysterectomy.[62]

Physicians, moreover, did not seem to be effective in this role. Only 10 of 119 women reported being able to discuss their sexual anxieties with their doctors, and the discussion did not seem to make any difference in the sexual outcome.[63] This may indicate that women with sexual anxieties need a greater amount of counseling or supportive psychotherapy than has been available to them.

These findings also raise questions relative to the wisdom of elective hysterectomy for birth control or for prevention of cancer. On the basis of his finding of increased depression and decreased self-esteem in women, Bunker[64] states that the elective surgery is not justified.

The Sexual Partner: Responses to Hysterectomy

The response of the sexual partner may negatively or positively affect the woman's sexual response. Melody's[65] view is that women are adversely affected by societal attitudes. He found that a depressive reaction in 11 women after hysterectomy was initiated by a social event that the woman saw as an act of disapproval or rejection, real or imagined. These events ranged from desertion by husbands who considered their wives either adulterous or neuter to disinheritance by parents who believed their daughter's operation was punishment for her promiscuity and venereal disease.

Daley reports findings of a study at Temple University Medical Center. Eighteen percent of black males became impotent with a woman who had her uterus removed, although they could function sexually with other women who had a uterus. In another study, Daley[66] reports that husbands of women who received psychiatric referrals after a hysterectomy also showed disturbed behavior; about 20 percent of this behavior included impotence, suicide, irritability, promiscuity, and tormenting the wife with being half a woman.

Unfortunately, research has not focused on the changes in the partner's sexual response during coitus. Some men report that penile sensation is altered with deep vaginal thrusting when the cervix has been removed, and others report obtaining less sexual satisfaction, but no definitive study documents the prevalence of these alterations and the degree of dissatisfaction with coitus.

OTHER PELVIC SURGERY IN FEMALES

Pelvic Exenteration

Women with cancer of the pelvis may require

radical surgery removing all the pelvic organs, the vagina, and necessitating a colostomy and artificial urinary bladder (ileal conduit). This surgery is one of the most destructive performed on women but represents a choice between life and death. Life may make some of the surgery's effects acceptable.

Depression and emotional illness can be high in these women, especially if the woman does not clearly understand what will be done. Brown[67] followed 15 women with this surgery over a 3-year period. Sexual activity varied. The colostomy inhibited any type of sexual activity early after surgery. Four patients had autoerotic activity, the colostomy stoma of one becoming eroticized and providing orgasm when digitally stimulated. Others manipulated the scar tissue on the mons veneris. Thirty-eight percent said they had indulged in "unusual" sex practices and the same number reported "unusual" or "strange" experiences.

In a study of 46 women who had undergone either exenteration, radical vulvectomy or Wertheim hysterectomy, Sewell and Edwards[68] found that all had decrease in the frequency of intercourse and problems with body image. Severe relationship change was reported by 29 percent of the women. Older women with more lengthy, stable relationships tended to have fewer problems than younger women with shorter time relationships. In a small group of six patients, Fisher[69] reported similar problems.

Radical Vulvectomy

Extensive alteration of perineal anatomy and physiology results from this procedure. Effort is made to leave the vagina intact so intercourse will be possible, but if radical surgery is required, bilateral superficial and deep inguinal lymph node dissection is done, and depending on the presence of metastasis, the urethra, vagina, and bowel are altered. A large open area is left for 2 to 3 months until healing occurs. A second procedure, plastic surgery to reconstruct pelvic structure is nec-

essary in some women. Because of extensive skin retraction during surgery, the wound may be bruised, "lumpy," and "battered," and women describe themselves as "repulsive" and "disfigured."[70]

NURSING IMPLICATIONS

Assessment

Since some of the adverse response to hysterectomy results from lack of information and misinformation about the function of pelvic organs, the nurse assesses the woman's knowledge of the procedure and its effect on reproductive, menstrual, and hormone production ability. By identifying fantasies and expectations of the procedure preoperatively, the nurse can bring these in line with reality. The nurse also assesses how the individual has coped with previous surgery, illness, or serious threat; whether the woman has children and/or whether she has already completed her family. Those who have not are at a higher risk for adverse reaction postoperatively. Menstrual history will indicate whether she is pre- or postmenopausal.

Important psychosocial data includes determining what the loss of the uterus means to the woman and noting her general affect during the nursing history. Is she unusually giggly, anxious, or hostile? Is her appearance appropriate or unusual, and does she seem to rely heavily on physical attributes?

Information about social support system is also essential. The presence of other stressful events in her life, the family's ability to provide emotional support, and the attitude of the male toward surgery is assessed. The woman's attitude and investment in her feminine sex role is noted as well as her cultural and ethnic background. Some ethnic and religious groups espouse well-defined sex roles, and these women may see the uterus as more essential to their role identity (see Chapter 8 for discussion of role).

Postoperatively, the nurse watches for signs of depression, loss of interest in appearance, crying, withdrawal from interaction, loss of appetite, inability to sleep, and signs of body image disturbance (see Chapter 13).

Planning

In planning care, the nurse's goals are similar to those identified for the patient with a mastectomy. In addition, promotion of sexual knowledge and clarification of myths and misconceptions about the role of the uterus and the effects of the surgery are especially important.

When planning intervention, the nurse is aware of those patients who seem to have the greatest potential for adverse effects from surgery:

1. Those who regard the uterus and menstruation as a badge of femininity.
2. Those who have had poor sexual adjustment before surgery, with limited coital and orgasmic experiences.
3. Those who have not completed their families.
4. Those who verbalize negative expectations of the sexual outcome of surgery.
5. Those with poor understanding of the reproductive tract and its function.

Intervention

The focus of preoperative teaching and counseling is to correct misinformation, to allow the woman to verbalize her fears, and to identify the symbolic meaning of the uterus. If the symbolic meaning appears to the nurse to have only negative potential in terms of impending loss, the nurse can point out positive aspects of the procedure. If the patient sees the uterus as a source of physical strength, the nurse can point out that a diseased uterus may not be strengthening and that removal of a "sick" uterus can be strengthening.[71]

Women who think the uterus and genital areas are sensitive and slow to heal should be given an opportunity to inspect the vaginal vault pre- and postoperatively so they can see healing has taken place and

that no physical impairment to intercourse exists.[72]

If the woman views the loss of the uterus as punishment for earlier transgressions, intervention related to guilt is appropriate (see Chapter 13).

When intervening with the depressed patient, the nurse, although not agreeing that the situation is as hopeless as the patient believes it to be, empathizes with her feelings of hopelessness and unworthiness. At the same time, the nurse helps her see that these feelings are defenses, attempts to escape her sensation of being trapped. The nurse gives credence to her feelings of being trapped, rather than to the conclusion that the situation is hopeless. It is also advisable to help the woman limit the demands on herself and not do more than she is able, while encouraging activities that make her feel worthwhile and able to function in her sexual role.

Before discharge, matter-of-fact discussion must take place about the woman's ability to respond sexually and when sexual activity may be appropriate. In the case of the patient with hysterectomy, there are few changes that should negatively affect sexual function. Different positions for sexual intercourse can be discussed with both the woman and her sexual partner, if they express concern about a shortened vagina. (See Chapter 4.)

Teach the partner to take a more active role in arousing and stimulating response, encouraging more clitoral stimulation when the woman misses an internal arousal.[73]

If oophorectomy has been performed, the patient is instructed about the hormones she will be taking and is given realistic reassurance about their benefits in preventing menopausal symptoms.

Patients with radical pelvic surgery must be given an opportunity to discuss what these radical procedures mean to them and to their sexual partners. As appropriate, alternate forms of sexual stimulation can be suggested. (See Chapter 4.) Some of these patients and their sexual partners may need continued counseling and support after discharge to cope with the profound body changes.

Evaluation

The following outcome criteria should be identified. The woman and the sexual partner:

1. Describe the function of the uterus in relation to the sexual response cycle and in other female physiologic processes.
2. State when sexual activity may be resumed.
3. Describe alternate forms of sexual expression, if indicated, and positions for intercourse.
4. Identify the importance of medication that is prescribed and state the role of estrogen in preventing menopausal symptoms.
5. State that she is still valued as a woman.

ENTEROSTOMY

Although colostomy, ileostomy, and procedures for urinary diversion produce anatomically and functionally different results, the psychosocial and sexual sequelae are similar enough to warrant their discussion as a totality with identification of the differences that exist. Whether or not impotence or orgasmic dysfunction are biologic sequelae, these procedures can have devastating effects on body image, sexuality, and sexual role behavior.

Our society puts early emphasis on bowel and bladder control, and the sudden loss of this control can be one of the worst possible insults to self-esteem. In this respect, ostomies are unique among mutilating surgical procedures.[74]

Bio-Psycho-Social Factors

Preoperatively, patients' reaction to recommendation of surgery varies. Some view it as necessary, lifesaving, or as palliative from pain and suffering. Postoperatively, some describe horror and despair at first viewing the ostomy, no matter how well prepared they were. Accidents, odor, staining, and spillage were frequently described fears of most patients.[75-78]

After surgery, patients reported that they felt weaker, more fatigued, and viewed their body as being more fragile and vulnerable to harm. These feelings coupled with depression resulted in marked invalidism for some patients.[79] Some expressed disgust that feces now came from the front of their bodies.[80] Other patients reacted with excessive emotional investment in the stoma.

Patients who had colostomies because of malignancy have the additional concern that the cancer may recur. In terms of bowel control, the ileostomy is untrainable. The contents of the colostomy are more solid, and it is a more trainable organ.[81] Urinary diversionary procedures also result in uncontrollable elimination of urine.

For many reasons, the initial psychologic reaction in many patients is depression. There is the loss of highly valued body parts and a sense of being mutilated. Some men react to the surgery as castration; others unconsciously perceive any initial bleeding from the stoma as menstruation and therefore evidence of feminization. Women may be concerned that they had been violated and eviscerated.[82]

Fear of social rejection leads many patients to isolate themselves from jobs, friends, and family, although married children may be regarded as an important social resource. Dyk and Sutherland[83] found that some male patients did not allow their spouses to see the colostomy because of anticipation of rejection and feelings of degradation and shame. Later, disgust and revulsion shown by some wives was also responsible for concealment. With women, modesty, shame, and embarrassment at exposure were reinforced by the feelings of disfigurement. Yet for men, the primary source of care was their wives, while women had help from daughters, sisters, and other female relatives, as well as husbands. However, the marital partner was regarded by both wives and husbands as the most desired source of care. The marital relationship of the ostomy patient is an important force for good or evil.[84]

Change in Sexual Activity

Males. Estimates for complete loss of potency range from 15 to 90 percent for the male colostomate and from 0 to 25 percent for the ileostomate.[85] During radical rectal surgery, damage to essential nerve fibers may occur.

The stimuli for erection run along parasympathetic pathways in the sacral spinal cord. The nerves originate in the second, third, and fourth sacral segments. The parasympathetic axons, the nervi erigentes, pass through the inferior hypogastric plexus toward the pelvic viscera. These fibers are in close proximity to the lateral and anterior walls of the rectum. If sectioned during surgery, erectile ability will be destroyed.[86]

Ejaculation depends on the integrity of sympathetic enervation to the internal genitalia. The sympathetic fibers pass forward and down below the peritoneum and lie close to the rectum. Removal of tissues is confined as close to the rectal wall as possible to keep nerve damage to a minimum. Protection of nerve fibers is possible when the colectomy is done for ulcerative colitis, but more difficult when the combined abdominal–perineal resection for cancer is required.

Dlin and associates[87] studied the psychosexual response to ileostomy and colostomy. Four hundred nine respondents, 211 males and 198 females ranging in age from 17 to 87 years of age, answered 93 questions. Impotence was reported by only 15 percent of the males, far less than the previous estimates. Low incidence of impotence was also found by Druss and associates.[88] In a group of 25 male patients who had undergone colectomy for ulcerative colitis, only 5 developed potency problems.

In contrast, Dyk and Sutherland[89] found that 19 of 22 men had changes in potency or frequency of intercourse after surgery for cancer. Seven had marked impairment both in erectile strength and frequency, while 12 had been totally impotent.

In a sample of 25 men, Sutherland and associates[90] found that 14 were wholly impotent, 5 had marked impairment of erectile strength, and 7 stated they had slight or no change in potency. Three of those who were impotent did not consider it a problem, while 11 were very dissatisfied, expressing feelings of degradation and personal inadequacy. They felt that the absence of sexual relations had an adverse effect on their wives and their relationships.

In a sample of 40 patients with either colostomy, ileostomy or ileal conduit, Gloeckner[91] found that 29 percent of the males had permanent impotence, and 12 of the 24 who were not impotent reported less frequent intercourse.

Many patients see sexual performance problems primarily in the expected reactions of the partner. The spouse, particularly, determines sexual adjustment after surgery.[92,93]

Reaction of Wives. Dyk and Sutherland found that change in economic status after surgery for some men resulted in loss of esteem from their partners. One man described his wife's estimate of him as "useless," another felt that he was a "pauper."[94] Wives expressed this lowered esteem in several ways—derogatory statements about the colostomy, complaints about loss of income and curtailment of social activities, the embarrassment about spillage, and ultimately withdrawal from sexual intercourse.[95]

When esteem was maintained, negative feelings toward the colostomy were concealed and wives tried to make their husbands feel wanted. Physical care was given without complaint, and sexual withdrawal was by mutual agreement, although at times their desire to help and protect the husband reinforced, unnecessarily, feelings of vulnerability and weakness. At no time were these wives hostile and rejecting. The quality of the marriage before the surgery determined the postoperative adjustment.

Some wives continued with orgasm and satisfactory sexual relations, but others encouraged reduction of activity, fearing for their husbands' health and well-being; others avoided intercourse because of the colostomy. Some men felt that they would have been capable of more intercourse if their wives' attitudes had been different, reporting that they felt nervous and rejected by their wives.

Potency was highly valued by the men, and loss or impairment had individual meaning and outcome—feelings of humiliation, aging, nervousness, tension, and friction. Most authors agree that loving and considerate partners are essential if sexual activity is to be maintained.

Females. The majority of women in the Dyk and Sutherland[96] group saw marriage as a source of economic support and security. Few of the marriages had strong affectional ties before surgery, and only 1 of 28 women spoke of enjoying orgasm prior to surgery. Seven continued to have intercourse, but nearly all with decreased interest and frequency. Reasons given included fears of being unacceptable, degraded, or injured. In this group of women, reduction and cessation was initiated by the women, and rejection by the husband was not given as a reason for cessation of sexual activity. In the married women, it appears that the colostomy was an excuse for withdrawing from a sexual relationship that had not been a source of pleasure to them before surgery.

The women in the Sutherland and associates[97] study were reluctant to discuss sexual matters. Fourteen of 28 who did give information had ended sexual relations before surgery and 4 from the surgery on. Two continued coitus after surgery, while protesting that their health would be compromised—one infrequently with little satisfaction and

the other with some frequency and orgasm in spite of urinary incontinence at climax.

Change in sexual response may occur. Removal of the lower rectum may result in fibrous adhesions of the upper part of the posterior vaginal wall to the anterior surface of the lower rectum impairing mobility of the vaginal vault and causing dyspareunia with deep thrusting.[98]

Ten of 13 women who had proctocolectomy reported dyspareunia during intercourse and difficulty achieving orgasm. Their major concerns were the reaction of the sexual partner and in younger women, the ability to bear children. Thirty-nine of the 40 said that sexuality should be discussed pre- and postoperatively but many received no information or were upset because they received written information but no discussion.[99]

Dlin[100] found that although a large number of women expressed concern about body image, "I feel like a freak," "I find myself less attractive," sexual interest was present and pursued after surgery. Ninety percent had been able to achieve orgasm before surgery, and 87 percent continued to be orgasmic after the ostomy, although they were less able to achieve multiple orgasms.

Reaction of Husbands. Unlike the reaction of wives to husbands who had ostomies, husbands desired to resume sexual intercourse. They were more willing to contend with spillage or, in the case of one woman, incontinence of urine at orgasm. In most cases, it is the woman who initiated the decrease in or cessation of sexual activity.[101,102]

Sex and the Single Ostomate

The value of an individual is seen through the eyes of the partner. In all studies, the adaptation of the spouse became a major factor in recovery and resumption of sexual activity. The single ostomate does not have this support. Presence of an ostomy was a deterrent to remarriage or new sexual contacts for persons in the Dyk and Dlin studies, who expressed concerns about problems of courtship and acceptance. Although Dlin and associates report that colectomy did not alter habits of petting and premarital sex, the single ostomate's major concern was how and when to reveal the condition to a potential sexual partner.[103]

Rehabilitation for Sexual Function

Many persons report they have received much help from membership in ostomy clubs or societies. Members of these organizations try to see patients prior to surgery, since a patient who sees someone neatly dressed with no visible signs of a stoma is tremendously reassured. The visitor can answer pragmatically from his or her experiences such questions as how the appliance is secured, how the skin is protected, and how sexual activity may be affected.

Postoperatively, another visit can help decrease or shorten depression. Effort is made to match the type of person and sometimes the type of affliction. The groups have been able to help both married and nonmarried individuals' sexual adjustment.[104]

The United Ostomy Association is an organization open to persons with stomas and other concerned individuals and is headquartered in Los Angeles. It publishes a quarterly bulletin and helps to educate not only the individuals with ostomies, but physicians and families.[105] Ostomy clinics have been established in some areas to help disseminate information and assist ostomates to cope with problems with their conditions.[106]

New surgical procedures may facilitate rehabilitation. An improved quality of life was reported by 85 percent of 45 men and women who had an ileostomy changed to a continent ileostomy, by the construction of a low pressure reservoir from the terminal ilium. Intestinal discharge is collected and stored in the reservoir and emptied three times a day with help of a catheter. Patients felt they had regained human dignity and had feelings of almost complete social rehabilitation, since the ileostomy had resulted

in decrease in sex life which, in all but one, returned to normal.[107]

Pregnancy and the Ostomate

Women with ostomies can and do become pregnant. In the past, they have been advised against pregnancy because of fear that the enlarging uterus would compress the stoma or that the woman's intestines would be interfered with. This is not true, and the number of children is often a matter of individual preference.[108] Dlin[109] found that pregnancy occurred frequently after surgery and that childbirth was successful, in some cases only a few days after surgery. Some obstetricians recommend waiting about 2 years when possible and limiting the children to two. Some women with colitis have stated that their ostomy made possible their children.

The most commonly reported problem during pregnancy was swelling of the stoma, which became tender and protruded beginning in midpregnancy. After delivery, the stoma of colostomies returned to normal size, as did that of ileostomies. Some women with ileostomies reported their stoma was easier to care for after birth, since it would no longer retract or it increased in length, which helped prevent discharge around the faceplate. Adjustment is needed in stomal care and appliance size. Norris's[110] pamphlet *Sex, Pregnancy and the Female Ostomate* has some excellent suggestions for the pregnant ostomate.

NURSING IMPLICATIONS

Assessment

The same preoperative assessment parameters apply as those indicated for individuals undergoing other mutilating surgeries.

Postoperatively, the nurse watches for signs of depression and alteration in body image in the patient as well as in the spouse or sexual partner.

Intervention

Ostomate with a Sexual Partner. Psychologic preparation must begin in the preoperative period. The patient is given the opportunity to verbalize fears about sexuality and anxiety about the outcome of the surgery and its effects on relationships with others. Teaching about the effects of surgery is essential, although the type and amount of information given to the patient varies between individuals. The highly anxious patient will hear and/or retain little. More important than the actual information given is that the individual perceives that it is given in a protective and supportive manner.[111]

Postoperative counseling is essential. Sixteen subjects who had ostomies for cancer and who received postoperative counseling experienced positive alterations in self-concept/self-esteem as compared to 16 subjects who were not counseled. The effects of counseling were sustained 1 month after discharge.[112]

The patient's adaptation to changed body image depends to a great extent on the reaction of the nurse and those around him/her. Signs of disgust, aversion, or distaste when caring for the ostomy will be incorporated into the individual's self-image.

The topic of sexuality is discussed with the patient and his sexual partner in three areas—the stoma itself, attitudes toward it, and the anatomic changes created by surgery. The nurse gives information, but of greater importance, provides the patient and the sexual partner opportunity to verbalize feelings and fears about the surgery, the stoma, and the possible effect on sexual activity.

The initial postoperative period is too early to determine the existence of potency problems, orgasmic dysfunction, or genital anesthesia. Men should be advised that failure to attain an erection soon after surgery does not indicate failure, since some men do not recover full sexual function until several months after surgery, when their strength returns.[113] For patients with anatomic or biologic changes that are known, alternate means of sexual satisfaction are suggested.

As patients recover, regain their strength, and approach release from the hospital, concerns about sexual relationships become more intense. The patient may have questions about spillage, odors, and accidents but may be too embarrassed to bring them up. The nurse can open up the subject matter-of-factly, giving specific information about ostomy care to help psychosocial sexual adjustment.

Simmons,[114] a female ostomate, gives some practical suggestions for resuming intimacy. Approach your partner with sensitivity and newness of early romance, allowing plenty of time to ease into sexual relations. Resume sleeping in the same bed using a plastic sheet if you are concerned about leakage. Spend at least an hour a day away from the partner. Accept your body; it is the individual's choice to affirm the stoma, body, and sexuality. The individual should be open to sexual fantasies, diverting sexual feeling to the stoma may occur. Some women regard their stomas as a source of pride.

The nurse stresses communication between the individual and the sexual partner. Sexual activity does not harm the stoma. In preparing for coitus, confidence during lovemaking is achieved if the individual is sure the ostomy is free of odor and danger of smelling. Appliances can be taped on and deodorants used. It is suggested that those who use belts use them without hooks, so the sexual partner is not scratched.[115]

The nurse shares methods to decrease odor when diet and good personal hygiene are ineffective alone. Some foods are more likely to stimulate bowel activity and gas formation. Each individual must find his/her "problem" foods. Oral preparations, such as bismuth subgallate, charcoal, and 100 percent chlorophyll tablets, can be placed in the pouch to absorb odors.[116]

Opaque appliances and pouches are preferable to transparent ones.[117] However, some individuals do not require an appliance on their colostomy at any time. If desired, women can cover their ostomy with a decorative sack or a frilly cummerbund. Some make "anticipants," splitting the crotch of a pair of panties, 5 inches from the waistband, from front to rear and binding the cut edges with soft lace. Other women get a lightweight two-way stretch panty girdle (preferably black) and make a snapflap by cutting across the front horizontal seam and sewing on a strip of small snaps. These hide the appliance or colostomy covering, support it, yet allow unhampered intercourse.[118] Men can conceal their appliances, although fewer are interested in doing so. A cloth appliance cover, a cummerbund or a lightweight male girdle with the crotch removed can also be used.[119] Decorated extra-odorproof opaque pouches and pouch covers can also be purchased.

Personal cleanliness is a must. Bathing and emptying the appliance before sexual activity is important. However, when sex can occur spontaneously, individuals should go ahead, but only if sexual activity can be done safely.

Different positions for intercourse should be tried. If the appliance or stoma seems to be in the way, the partners can experiment to find the positions that are the most satisfying to both sexual partners. (See Chapter 4 for description of positions.) The inferior position may result in leakage if the partner compresses the pouch.

Of greatest importance, the nurse helps the ostomate and the sexual partner become more relaxed about sexual activity. Ostomates and their lovers need to develop a good sense of humor.[120]

Having a rehearsal response for occasions when there is leakage makes the situation less embarrassing. Simply acknowledging that there is a leak and that the appliance needs changing is probably the best approach.

If coitus is not possible because of male impotence, the couple communicates to each other what pleases them the most, what parts of the body are most sensual, what really is the most sexually stimulating. Sexual techniques and forms of physical love play can be enjoyable and satisfying. Noncoital stimulation by manual or oral stimulation of the clitoris, vulva, and vagina can lead to orgasm and sexual satisfaction for the female partner. The woman in turn can caress and manipulate her partner to the maximum satisfaction he is capable of achieving. A survey by the United Ostomy Association indicated that many ostomates who cannot have erections can obtain a great deal of sexual satisfaction.[121]

For those who have difficulty getting a full erection or sustaining one, a rubber band placed around the base of the penis helps maintain erection. However, the nurse emphasizes that its use requires caution and that the patient should discuss its use with the physician.[122]

The nurse stresses the importance of good health practices to get the maximum desire and sexual performance. Adequate rest and exercise and good nutrition contribute to sexual well-being, especially in the ostomate.

When teaching and counseling the sexual partner, the nurse stresses allowing the patient to resume the usual role activities. Spouses have a tendency to overprotect the ostomate, which will deter rehabilitation and interfere with the development of self-esteem. Since spouses provide most of the assistance with care at home, the nurse encourages expression of their feelings about providing this care and how it may affect the sexual relationship. If the spouse feels much aversion and distress about giving care, to minimize stress in this relationship, it is preferable that the ostomate assume self-care as soon as possible. When this is not possible, ideally, someone other than the spouse should help with irrigation until the individual can do it himself/herself.

Single Ostomate. Counseling the single ostomate demands sensitivity and concern.

Single ostomates have many concerns about sexual intimacy and marriage. In addition to teaching discussed earlier, they want information about how and when to tell about the ostomy. It is important that the nurse stress that the individual be free, open, and honest about the stoma. An explanation about the ostomy should take place at the latest when it seems that sexual intimacy of any type is possible. If marriage is anticipated, the time to tell is when the relationship appears to be developing in that direction and at the latest as soon as discussion of marriage begins.[123]

A simple explanation might be "I was ill with a disease that needed surgery to correct it. Now I have an alternate opening for eliminating waste and wear a collective pouch so I can go about my normal activities." At first, the explanation does not have to be too detailed or technical. A partner who is interested will ask questions, and the individual should answer them honestly without trying to elicit sympathy and admiration for all that has been endured. By giving explanations clearly, confidently, and with self-assurance, stressing that the ostomy does not interfere with activities and enjoyment of life, the partner will be reassured and accepting of the explanation.[124] Individuals with ostomies can use their judgment about showing the stoma or its covering. At first, just showing a spare appliance, pouch or pad, may be all that is necessary.

Single ostomates may fear rejection by partners who are "turned off" by the appliance. The nurse can remind them that someone who is turned off by the ostomy is not accepting them as individuals, that it is not their fault or anything to be ashamed of. People have different values, and some cannot accept an ostomy. There are others who will accept the ostomates for what they are.

Some partners may express need to "think about" the ostomy. Many have to get used to the idea of the ostomy and need time to sort out their feelings. The nurse urges the ostomate to be calm, patient, and understanding. A potential spouse may also want information from a physician's point of view,

and this should be encouraged to help allay myths and misconceptions.[125]

Unfortunately, physicians have been found remiss in the teaching and the counseling that they give to ostomates.[126–128] Nurses cannot only share information but also give all ostomates a chance to share their fears, concerns, and their hopes.

Evaluation

The following outcome criteria are identified. The patient (and the sexual partner):

1. Identifies and verbalizes concerns about changes in sexual function, care of the ostomy, and changes in the relationship or in forming new relationships.
2. States how to care for the ostomy to decrease chances of spillage or odors.
3. Cares for the ostomy.
4. Identifies alternate positions for coitus and methods of sexual expression.
5. Describes how to prepare for sexual activity by ostomy care.
6. Resumes sexual activity if it has been a part of the presurgical life style or describes how he/she would tell a perspective partner about the ostomy.
7. Resumes usual role activities commensurate with general health and well-being.

PELVIC SURGERY IN THE MALE

Prostatectomy

Removal of the prostate for benign prostatic disease theoretically should not cause sexual dysfunction; neither transurethral, retropubic, nor suprapubic enucleation of a prostate adenoma should result in potency problems. However, in practicality, 10 to 66 percent of men become impotent. Some of the procedures are not overtly mutilating (transurethral prostatectomy leaves no scar), but surgical procedures of the genitals bring their own problems. Gonick[129] gives three reasons for the difficulty. First, the operation may provide an excuse for some men to terminate intercourse in the face of previously decreasing desire, ability, and performance. Second, impotence may be iatrogenic in origin due to the physician's attitude that suggests it is a frequent sequela. Finally, the man may be concerned that coitus will in some way weaken the wound or endanger his health.

Retropubic, suprapubic, and transurethral prostatectomy cause retrograde ejaculation into the bladder, because the bladder neck is resected, resulting in loss of the urethral phase of orgasm. The man should retain potency but will become infertile. After retrograde ejaculation, the urine will be milky in color due to the presence of semen.

Radical prostatectomy, by either the perineal or retropubic approach, almost invariably results in impotence. In one study, only 10 percent of the men were potent after surgery. In addition to the prostatic capsule, the surrounding fascial layers, seminal vesicles, and the autonomic nerves to the penis are removed. An additional sequela may be loss of urinary control.[130]

Cystectomy, Perineal Biopsy

Cystectomy involves removal of the pelvic plexus of nerves necessary for erection and results in impotence. "Open" perineal biopsy of the prostate has an impotence rate of 29 percent and diminished levels of sexual activity in another 37 percent of the patients.[131]

Carcinoma of the Penis, Urethra, or Testes

These conditions necessitate amputation of the penis and dissection of the surrounding lymph nodes. If a partial penectomy is done, phallic size may be enough for coitus and orgasm may occur from stimulation of the stump, stimulation of the perineum or the mons pubis.

A radical inguinal orchiectomy is done for cancer of the testes. There may be psychologic trauma but no impairment of fertility or endocrine function occurs if the contralateral testis is spared. If there is retroperitoneal dissection of lymph nodes, there may be impairment of emission of seminal fluid and sperm with decreased ejaculate.[132]

Plastic reconstructive surgery has been used, but most men are ashamed of the altered genitals and feel they have lost social face and masculinity. The incidence of suicide is high in these patients.[133]

Surgery on the penile part of the urethra may cause scarring that restricts the extensibility of the inferior surface during erection resulting in a chordee or downward curving.[134]

Psychologic Factors

Men experiencing radical pelvic surgery may become extremely depressed, even with the best of preparation for the procedure. The self-esteem of the man is severely threatened either by change in appearance or function of the genitals. If urinary incontinence also occurs, lack of dignity and shame will result. "Gallows humor" acting out may be some men's response. Silicone implants have been used by some men as a solution to impotence, and testicular prostheses have been implanted in some men so that the sexual partner believes the man is intact. (See Chapter 3 for information about implants.)

NURSING IMPLICATIONS

Assessment, intervention, and evaluation for body image disturbance and problems with sexual self-esteem are indicated for most men (see Chapter 13).

SURGERY TO THE FACE AND NECK

Bio-Psycho-Social Factors

In a society that values youth and beauty, the threat of radical facial surgery, with its potential for mutilative outcomes, presents tremendous problems in developing and for continuing relationships. The face is what people see, react to, and respond to.[135,136] It is through the mouth, lips, and tongue that communication takes place, that relationships are begun. The person who undergoes surgery for cancer of the face, lips, tongue, throat, or larynx is faced with problems in communication and with cosmetic and other defects.

In addition to removal of specific organs, sacrifice of nerves during the operative procedure may result in functional defects postoperatively. During parotid gland surgery, the seventh cranial nerve may be removed, resulting in paralysis of the muscles of facial expression. Surgery of the tongue may produce difficulty in speech and deglutition.[137] Laryngectomy removes the ability to speak until rehabilitation provides esophageal or other types of speech, which, although providing a means of communication, alters its pattern and quality. The sexual partner, or potential sexual partner, may be repulsed by the individual's appearance or patterns and quality of verbalization.

None of these procedures affects genital response per se, but the individual whose concept of masculinity or femininity is damaged by body image changes may be as sexually compromised as the individual who has genital surgery.

Of forty-eight members of a Lost Cord Club, 75 percent men, 25 percent women, 16 (33 percent) said their sex life had changed and 49 percent wished "things" were different. Only one patient's physician discussed possible effects on sex life.[138]

Rehabilitation of the individual with facial surgery is frequently overlooked. External prosthesis, that is, ears, noses, or eyes, may be needed and aid in maintaining self-esteem.[139]

NURSING IMPLICATIONS

Assessment intervention and evaluation for body image changes and shame are indicated.

After tracheostomy, rapid shallow breathing at orgasm causes coughing and the neck breathing can take away the partner's pleasure. The stoma should be suctioned and covered with a porous stoma shield before intercourse. If the missionary position causes problems, rear or leg over leg side entry can be used. Pelvic thrusting can be increased to compensate for lack of body support when breath cannot be held. Oral–genital activity may serve as a substitute for some couples.[140]

AMPUTATION

To lose a body part and function is to be threatened with loss of self. The patient who has had an amputation is faced with loss of self-esteem and feelings of helplessness. Loss of control of and inability to move the body from place to place at will contribute to feelings of worthlessness and vulnerability.[141] Some male patients may see amputation as a castrating procedure.[142] Others may experience feelings of guilt and shame, viewing the surgery as punishment for past indiscretions. (See Chapter 13.)

The loss of a leg means less control of the body during coitus. If the individual has been accustomed to take the more active role in coital activity, the need to change may be threatening, not only to sexual expression, but to the individual's view of the sexual role. Change in other role activities at home or at work may threaten masculinity or femininity. The sexual partner may have an equal, if not greater, difficulty accepting and coping with changed appearance and function.

NOTES

1. Grundemann BJ: The impact of surgery on body image. Nurs Clin North Am 10:635–643, 1975
2. Ibid, p 635
3. Gallagher AM: Body image changes in

the patient with a colostomy. Nurs Clin North Am 7:669–676, 1972

4. Ibid, p 671

5. Owen ML: Special care for the patient who has a breast biopsy or mastectomy. Nurs Clin North Am 7:373–382, 1972

6. Harrell HG: To lose a breast. Am J Nurs 72:676–677, 1972

7. Women's attitude regarding breast cancer. Occup Health Nurs 22:20–23, 1974

8. Kent S: Coping with sexual identity crises after mastectomy. Geriatrics 30:145–146, 1975

9. Bard M, Sutherland AM: Psychological impact of cancer and its treatment. Cancer 8:656–672, 1955

10. Bard M, Sutherland, AM: Adaptation to radical mastectomy. In The Psychological Impact of Cancer. New York, American Cancer Society, 1974, pp 55–71

11. Jamison KR, Wellisch DK, Pasnau RO: Psychosocial aspects of mastectomy. Am J Psychiatry 135:432–436, 1978

12. Derogatis LR: Breast and gynecologic cancers. Front Rad Ther Oncol 14:1–11, 1980

13. Lindsey AM, Norbeck JS, Carrieri VL, Perry E: Social support and health outcomes in postmastectomy women: A review. Cancer Nurs 4:377–383, 1981

14. Maguire P, Tait A, Brooke M, et al: Effect of counseling on the psychiatric morbidity associated with mastectomy. Brit Med J 281:1454–1455, 1980

15. Krouse HJ, Krouse JH: Psychological factors in post-mastectomy adjustment. Psychol Rep 48:275–278, 1981

16. Krouse HJ, Krouse JH: Cancer as crises: The critical elements of adjustment. Nurs Research 31:96–101, 1982

17. Harris JR, Levine MB, Hellman S: Primary radiation therapy for early breast cancer. Front Rad Ther Oncol 14:83–89, 1980

18. Bard M, Sutherland AM: Adaptation to radical mastectomy. In The Psychological Impact of Cancer. New York, American Cancer Society, 1974, pp 65–67

19. Kent S: Coping with sexual identity crises after mastectomy. Geriatrics 30:146, 1975

20. Maguire P: The psychological and social consequences of breast cancer. Nurs Mirror 140:54–57, 1975

21. Donnie PA: Rehabilitation of the patient after mastectomy. Nurs Mirror 140:58–59, 1975

22. Lindsey AM, Norbeck JS, Carrieri VL, Perry E: Social support and health outcomes in postmastectomy women: A review. Cancer Nurs 4:383, 1981

23. Talking together. Am J Nurs 72:682, 1972

24. Bard M, Sutherland AM: Adaptation to radical mastectomy. In The Psychological Impact of Cancer. New York, American Cancer Society, 1974, p 68

25. Puhaty HD: Confronting one's changed image, two rehabilitative approaches. Am J Nurs 77:1437, 1977

26. Ibid

27. Thomas SG, Yates MM: Breast reconstruction after mastectomy. Am J Nurs 77:1438–1442, 1977

28. Asken MJ: Psychoemotional aspects of mastectomy: A review of the literature. Am J Psychiatry 132:56–59, 1975

29. Harvey RA: Breast reconstruction following mastectomy. Front Rad Ther Oncol 14:90–103, 1980

30. Ibid, p 92

31. RENU's Letter IV:1–2, March, 1983, Cleveland, Ohio

32. Carroll RM: The impact of mastectomy in body image. Oncol Nurs Forum 8:29–32, 1981

33. Owen ML: Special care for the patient who has a breast biopsy or mastectomy. Nurs Clin North Am 7:375, 1972

34. Chow A: Mastectomy. In Smith D (ed). Women's Health Care: A Guide to Patient Education. New York, Appleton-Century-Crofts, 1981, pp 136–154

35. Klagsburn SC: Don't make nice, make real. Am J Nurs 77:1432, 1977

36. Ibid

37. Frank DI: You don't have to be an expert to give sexual counseling to a mas-

tectomy patient. Nursing 81 11:64–67, 1981

38. Dulcey MP: Addressing breast cancer assault on female sexuality. Top Clin Nurs 1:61–68, 1980

39. Kent S: Coping with sexual identity crises after mastectomy. Geriatrics 30:145, 1975

40. Talking together. Am J Nurs 72:682, 1972

41. Budd KW: Variations in response to hysterectomy. In Lytle NC (ed): Nursing of Women in the Age of Liberation. Dubuque, Iowa, Brown, 1977, pp 187–204

42. Krouse HJ, Krouse JH: Cancer as crises: The critical elements of adjustment. Nurs Research 31:98–99, 1982

43. Krueger JC, Hassell J, Goggins DB, et al: Relationship between nurse counseling and sexual adjustment after hysterectomy. Nurs Research 28:145–150, 1979

44. Bunker J: Elective hysterectomy: Pro and con. N Engl J Med 295:264–268, 1976

45. Drellich MG, Bieber I: The psychologic importance of the uterus and its functions: Some psychoanalytical implications of hysterectomy. J Nerv Ment Dis 126:332–336, 1958

46. Dennerstein L, Wood C, Burrows GD: Sexual response following hysterectomy and oophorectomy. Obstet Gynecol 49:84–96, 1977

47. Cornish J: Psychodynamics of the hysterectomy experience. In McNall L, Galeener JT (ed.): Current Practice in Obstetric and Gynecologic Nursing. St. Louis, Mosby, 1976, pp 223–232

48. Drellich MG, Bieber I: The psychologic importance of the uterus and its functions: Some psychoanalytical implications of hysterectomy. J Nerv Ment Dis 126:328–333, 1958

49. Drellich MG, Bieber I, Sutherland AM: Adaptation to hysterectomy. In The Psychological Impact of Cancer. New York, American Cancer Society, 1974, pp 88–94

50. Zussman L, Zussman S, Sunley R, Bjornson E: Sexual response after hysterectomy-oophorectomy: Recent studies and reconsideration of psychogenesis. Am J Obstet Gynecol 140:725–729, 1981

51. Ibid, p 728

52. Craig GA, Jackson P: Sex life after hysterectomy. Br Med J 3:97, 1975

53. Dennerstein L, Wood C, Burrows GD: Sexual response following hysterectomy and oophorectomy. Obstet Gynecol 49:95, 1977

54. Daley MJ: Psychological impact of surgical procedures in women. In Sadock BJ, Kaplan HI, Freedman AM (eds): The Sexual Experience. Baltimore, Williams and Wilkins, 1976, pp 308–312

55. Dennerstein L, Burrows GD: Oral contraception and sexuality. Med J Aust 1:796–798, 1976

56. Bancroft J: Endocrinology of sexual function. Clin Obstet Gynecol 7:253–279, 1980

57. Dennerstein L, Wood C, Burrows GD: Sexual response following hysterectomy and oophorectomy. Obstet Gynecol 49:95–96, 1977

58. Ibid, p 95

59. Ibid

60. Craig GA, Jackson P: Sex life after hysterectomy. Br Med J 3:97, 1975

61. Coppen A, Bishop M: Hysterectomy hormones and behavior: A prospective study. Lancet 1:126–128, 1981

62. Krueger JC, Hassell J, Goggins DB, et al: Relationship between nurse counseling and sexual adjustment after hysterectomy. Nurs Research 28:145–150, 1979

63. Dennerstein L, Wood C, Burrows GD: Sexual response following hysterectomy and oophorectomy. Obstet Gynecol 49:95, 1977

64. Bunker J: Elective hysterectomy: Pro and con. N Engl J Med 295:268, 1976

65. Melody GF: Depression reactions after hysterectomy. Am J Obstet Gynecol 83:410–413, 1962

66. Daley MJ: Psychological impact of surgical procedures in women. In Sadock BJ, Kaplan HI, Freedman AM (eds): The Sexual Experience. Baltimore, Williams and Wilkins, 1976, p 310

67. Brown R, Haddox V, Posada A, Rubio A: Social and psychological adjustment following pelvic exenteration. Am J Obstet Gynecol 114:162–171, 1972

68. Sewell HH, Edwards DW: Pelvic genital cancer: Body image and sexuality. Front Rad Ther Oncol 14:35–41, 1980

69. Fisher SG: Psychosexual adjustment following total pelvic exenteration. Cancer Nurs 2:219–225, 1979

70. Servatius D: Easing the shock of radical vulvectomy. Nursing 75(5):27–31, 1975

71. Cornish J: Psychodynamics of the hysterectomy experience. In McNall L, Galeener JT (eds): Current Practice in Obstetric and Gynecologic Nursing. St. Louis, Mosby, 1976, p 230

72. Ibid, p 232

73. Zussman L, Zussman S, Sunley R, Bjornson E: Sexual response after hysterectomy-oophorectomy: Recent studies and reconsideration of psychogenesis. Am J Obstet Gynecol 140:729, 1981

74. Winkelstein C, Lyons AS: Insight into the emotional aspects of ileostomies and colostomies. Reprinted from Medical Insight. New York, Insight, December 1971

75. Druss RG, O'Connor JF, Stern L: Psychologic responses to colectomy. Arch Gen Psychiatry 20:419–427, 1969

76. Dlin BM, Perlman A, Ringold E: Psychosexual response to ileostomy and colostomy. AORN J 10(5):77–84, 1969

77. Dyk RB, Sutherland AM: Adaptation of the spouse and other family members to the colostomy patient. In The Psychological Impact of Cancer. New York, American Cancer Society, 1974, pp 72–87

78. Druss PG, O'Connor JF, Prudden JF, Stern LO: Psychologic response to colectomy. Arch Gen Psychiatry 18:53–59, 1968

79. Dyk RB, Sutherland AM: Adaptation of the spouse and other family members to the colostomy patient. In The Psychological Impact of Cancer. New York, American Cancer Society, 1974

80. Druss PG, O'Connor JF, Prudden JF, Stern LO: Psychologic response to colectomy. Arch Gen Psychiatry 18:59, 1968

81. Druss RG, O'Connor JF, Stern L: Psychologic responses to colectomy. Arch Gen Psychiatry 20:424, 1969

82. Ibid, p 425

83. Dyk RB, Sutherland AM: Adaptation of the spouse and other family members to the colostomy patient. In The Psychological Impact of Cancer. New York, American Cancer Society, 1974, p 77

84. Druss PG, O'Connor JF, Prudden JF, Stern LO: Psychologic response to colectomy. Arch Gen Psychiatry 18:58, 1968

85. Dlin BM, Perlman A, Ringold E: Psychosexual response to ileostomy and colostomy. AORN J 10(5):78, 1969

86. Williams JT, Slack WW: A prospective study in sexual function after major colorectal surgery. Brit J Surg 67:772–774, 1980

87. Dlin BM, Perlman A, Ringold E: Psychosexual response to ileostomy and colostomy. AORN J 10(5):80–81, 1969

88. Druss PG, O'Connor JF, Prudden JF, Stern LO: Psychologic response to colectomy. Arch Gen Psychiatry 18:53, 1968

89. Dyk RB, Sutherland AM: Adaptation of the spouse and other family members to the colostomy patient. In The Psychological Impact of Cancer. New York, American Cancer Society, 1974, p 79

90. Sutherland AM, Orbach CE, Dyk RB, Bard M: Adaptation to dry colostomy. In The Psychological Impact of Cancer. New York, American Cancer Society, 1974, pp 1–15

91. Gloeckner MR, Starling JR: Providing

sexual information to ostomy patients. Dis Colon Rectum 25:575–579, 1982

92. Druss PG, O'Connor JF, Prudden JF, Stern LO: Psychologic response to colectomy. Arch Gen Psychiatry 18:58, 1968

93. Dyk RB, Sutherland AM: Adaptation of the spouse and other family members to the colostomy patient. In The Psychological Impact of Cancer. New York, American Cancer Society, 1974, p 79

94. Ibid, p 78

95. Ibid, p 82

96. Ibid, p 81

97. Sutherland AM, Orbach CE, Dyk RB, Bard M: Adaptation to dry colostomy. In The Psychological Impact of Cancer. New York, American Cancer Society, 1974, p 77

98. Myerscough PR: Sexual function in illness. Clin Obstet Gynecol 7:387–400, 1980

99. Gloeckner MR, Starling JR: Providing sexual information to ostomy patients. Dis Colon Rectum 25:578, 1982

100. Dlin BM, Perlman A, Ringold E: Psychosexual response to ileostomy and colostomy. AORN J 10(5):81, 1969

101. Sutherland AM, Orbach CE, Dyk RB, Bard M: Adaptation to dry colostomy. In The Psychological Aspects of Cancer. New York, American Cancer Society, 1974, p 7

102. Dyk RB, Sutherland AM: Adaptation of the spouse and other family members to the colostomy patient. In The Psychological Impact of Cancer. New York, American Cancer Society, 1974, p 81

103. Dlin BM, Perlman A, Ringold E: Psychosexual response to ileostomy and colostomy. AORN J 10(5):81, 1969

104. Winkelstein C, Lyons AS: Insight into the emotional aspects of ileostomies and colostomies. Reprinted from Medical Insight. New York, Insight, December 1971

105. Ibid

106. Yahle M-E: An ostomy information clinic. Nurs Clin North Am 11:457–467, 1975

107. Nilsson LO, Kock NG, Kylberg F, et al: Sexual adjustment in ileostomy patients before and after conversion to continent ileostomy. Dis Colon Rectum 24:287–290, 1980

108. Norris C: Sex, Pregnancy and the Female Ostomate. Los Angeles, United Ostomy Association, 1972, p 12

109. Dlin BM, Perlman A, Ringold E: Psychosexual response to ileostomy and colostomy. AORN J 10(5):81, 1969

110. Norris C: Sex, Pregnancy and the Female Ostomate. Los Angeles, United Ostomy Association, 1972, p 14

111. Sutherland AM, Orbach CE, Dyk RB, Bard M: Adaptation to dry colostomy. In The Psychological Aspects of Cancer. New York, American Cancer Society, 1974, p 15

112. Watson PG: The effects of short-term postoperative counseling on cancer/ostomy patients. Cancer Nurs 6:21–29, 1983

113. Rush AM: Cancer and the ostomy patient. Nurs Clin North Am 11:405–415, 1976

114. Simmons KN: Sexuality and the female ostomate. Am J Nurs 83:409–411, 1983

115. Gambrell E: Sex and the Male Ostomate. Los Angeles, United Ostomy Association, 1973

116. Bosten A, Litman L: Controlling colostomy odor. Am J Nurs 77:444, 1977

117. Gambrell E: Sex and the Male Ostomate. Los Angeles, United Ostomy Association, 1973, p 9

118. Norris C: Sex, Pregnancy and the Female Ostomate. Los Angeles, United Ostomy Association, 1972, p 10

119. Gambrell E: Sex and the Male Ostomate. Los Angeles, United Ostomy Association, 1973, p 10

120. Ibid, p 11

121. Ibid, p 14

122. Ibid, p 18

123. Binder DP: Sex, Courtship and the Single Ostomate. Los Angeles, United Ostomy Association, 1973, p 8

124. Ibid, pp 9–10

125. Ibid, p 10

126. Dlin BM, Perlman A, Ringold E: Psychosexual response to ileostomy and colostomy. AORN J 10(5):81, 1969

127. Dyk RB, Sutherland AM: Adaptation of the spouse and other family members to the colostomy patient. In The Psychological Impact of Cancer. New York, American Cancer Society, 1974, p 14

128. Druss RG, O'Connor JF, Prudden JF, Stern LO: Psychologic response to colectomy. Arch Gen Psychiatry 18:58, 1968

129. Gonick P: Urologic problems and sexual function. In Oaks WW, Melchiode GA, Ficher I (eds): Sex and the Life Cycle. New York, Grune and Stratton, 1976, pp 191–192

130. Ibid, p 192

131. Ibid, p 193

132. von Eschenbach AC: Sexual dysfunction following therapy for cancer of the prostate testes and penis. Front Rad Ther Oncol 14:42–50, 1980

133. Zinsser HH: Sex and surgical procedures in the male. In Sadock BJ, Kaplan HI, Freedman AM (eds): The Sexual Experience. Baltimore, Williams and Wilkins, 1976, pp 303–307

134. Myerscough PR: Sexual function in illness. Clin Obstet Gynecol 7:387, 1980

135. Curtis TA, Zlotolow IM: Sexuality and head and neck cancer. Front Rad Ther Oncol 14:26–34, 1980

136. Welty MJ, Graham WP, Rosillo RH: The patient with maxillofacial cancer. Nurs Clin North Am 8:137–151, 1973

137. Ibid, p 146

138. Meyers AD, Aarons B, Suzuki B, Pilcher L: Sexual behavior following laryngectomy. Ear, Nose Throat J 59:327–329, 1980

139. Rosillo RH, Welty MJ, Graham WP: The patient with maxillofacial cancer: Psychological aspects. Nurs Clin North Am 8:153–158, 1973

140. Larsen GL: Rehabilitation for the patient with head and neck cancer. Am J Nurs 82:119–121, 1982

141. Leonard BJ: Body image changes in chronic illness. Nurs Clin North Am 7:687–694, 1972

142. Brown FL: Knowledge of body image and nursing care of the patient with a limb amputation. J Psychiatr Nurs 2:397–409, 1964

Chapter 25

Impaired Neurologic and Musculoskeletal Function

Although many illnesses and surgical procedures may cause sexual dysfunction as a result of their biologic or psychosocial sequelae, none produces more pervasive and devastating effects than diseases that effect neuromuscular function. The words *handicapped* or *disabled,* with their negative connotations, are most often used. Yet there is a difference between disability and handicap. A handicap is the result of all the barriers a disability puts between an individual and optimal function. There are many degrees of optimal function and the degree to which a disability becomes a handicap is relative to each individual situation, social role,[1] and person.

These individuals are the most discriminated against minority. A cultural bias exists in a society that values strength and beauty, wholeness and independence. Tragically, sexual activity, one of the important means of obtaining pleasure, experiencing feelings of closeness and love, and of confirming sexual identity, is frequently denied them. In fact, sexual activity may be seen as a perversion.[2]

Individuals with neuromuscular disabilities bring their own myths, taboos, and biases regarding sexuality to the interpersonal relationship. They may also have feelings that sex is bad, dirty, and perverted when a disability is present. These feelings

may result, sometimes unnecessarily, in sexual dysfunction and marital conflict. More tragically, these distortions and myths may be passed on to their children.[3]

The problems experienced are not all biologic and psychologic. The disabled person's opportunity to meet with and to socialize with other persons of both sexes is severely compromised. Lack of transportation, inaccessible public bathroom facilities, and other architectural barriers may prevent them from learning to socialize and to relate to others, from making friendships and falling in love.[4]

Attitudinal barriers raised by others can limit expression of sexuality. Many people avoid relationships with those with obvious physical disability because of fear, pity, or ignorance. When the individual with a handicap already has concerns about femininity or masculinity, these attitudinal barriers may be doubly threatening.[5]

This chapter will focus especially on the effect of spinal cord injury on sexuality. The effects of other neurologic diseases will be discussed in less detail. These include multiple sclerosis, cerebral vascular accident, and less common disorders such as amyotropic lateral sclerosis and temporal lobe lesions. This chapter closes with a brief discussion of diseases that affect muscular and skeletal

409

movement and strength—arthritis and the muscular dystrophies.

ANATOMY AND PHYSIOLOGY OF MALE SEXUAL RESPONSE

Erection and Ejaculation

Erection takes place on a purely segmental reflex basis in paraplegic patients. In the normal male, erection may be activated by psychic stimuli as well as physical stimuli, although the response is the same. In the spinal cord-injured, the afferent sensory impulses that initiate the reflex are caused by tactile stimuli of the glans and travel to the second, third, and fourth sacral segments by way of the internal pudendal nerves. Efferent impulses leave these segments by way of the parasympathetic supply and cause dilation of the arterioles of the penis, with distention and congestion of the corpora cavernosa and spongiosum. Efferent impulses also leave some segments over the internal pudendal nerves to cause contraction of the periurethral muscles, resulting in compression of the venous channels. Blood is trapped in the penis and erection results.[6]

Ejaculation is a complex, purely spinal, segmental reflex mediated by pathways and centers in the lower thoracic and upper lumbar segments of the spinal cord (T12 to L2). The first part of the reflex is controlled by sympathetic response, which releases semen from the seminal vesicles. The second stage of ejaculation is also reflex initiated by sensory impulses set up by the presence of semen in the posterior urethra, which set up efferent impulses that cause contraction of the periurethral muscles and result in actual ejaculation of semen from the urethra. These efferent and afferent impulses travel over the internal pudendal nerves by way of the second, third, and fourth sacral segments. The final release of semen is facilitated by contraction of striated muscles of the pelvic floor.

In normal men, higher cortical centers control these reflexes, and psychic stimuli may either inhibit or excite them.[7] Psychogenic erections result when stimuli travel from the brain to the sacral cord area. The brain sends out messages because of stimuli received through the senses of sight, sound, and smell, as well as imagination and memory.

The scrotum has a rich nerve supply, the skin from the sacral cord segments and the testes from the sympathetic system. Consequently, in a patient with a lesion at T12, the scrotal skin may be denervated but testicular sensation preserved.[8]

Diseases or injuries of the nervous system produce alterations in sexual response by interfering with the cortical centers, peripheral nerves, and autonomic and spinal cord pathways.

SPINAL CORD INJURY

Problems related to sexuality and injury to the spinal cord have been investigated, analyzed, and followed up for almost 30 years. Individuals with other diseases of the spinal cord or other parts of the nervous system have been less well studied. However, the experiences and problems of cord-injured persons may be extrapolated to other neuromuscular disorders.[9]

Spinal cord injury affects 30 persons per million population. Males in the 15 to 29 year age group are the most frequent victims. The cervical (30 percent) and the lumbar (70 percent) areas are the most frequent sites of injury, because they are relatively more flexible than the rest of the spine.

Persons with injury to the cervical cord (C1–7) become paralyzed in all extremities (quadriplegic), while those with thoracic or lumbar cord injury become paralyzed in the lower extremities (paraplegic). The extent of disability depends on the level of injury and completeness of the cord lesion. Trauma of the cord is the major cause of neurologic deficit, but cord diseases may cause similar effects.[10]

Biologic Factors: Male Sexual Response

Degree of Cord Injury. Although erection and ejaculation are purely spinal reflexes, they may be inhibited or stimulated by higher psychic stimuli. These are extremely important factors, since the first symptom of cord injury may be loss of libido. In general, if there are some connecting fibers remaining with even a little retention of sensation or motor function, the cord lesion is incomplete and there is greater possibility that the individual will retain sexual function. If all fibers are severed or irreversibly damaged, the lesion is said to be complete, and sexual response will be even more severely compromised, if not lost.

If the spinal cord is transected or severely damaged between the brain and the area controlling sexual response, the man usually will be unable to obtain a psychogenic erection. Some spinal cord-injured men, however, are able to obtain psychogenic erections, because the stimuli from the brain may bypass the injured portion of the cord via the autonomic nervous system.[11]

Level of Transection. Erection is a reflex, and if necessary pathways in the lumbar and sacral parts of the cord are intact, erections can take place. Therefore, individuals who have a clear-cut transection of the cord in the cervical or thoracic region will be able to have erections, providing the damage does not extend longitudinally down the cord to impair pathways in the lumbar and sacral sections. These erections may easily occur during spasm or during penile manipulation during a spasm. Patients with lesions in the lower part of the cord with destruction of the pathways are less likely to have erections. A much smaller percentage of patients can ejaculate.

An intact lumbar cord and its motor connections are not necessary for ejaculation. To ejaculate, the periurethral muscles must be innervated at least reflexly and be activated by way of the internal pudendal nerves. Paradoxically, individuals with cauda equina lesions are unable to have an erection, but because the testes and seminal vesicles are innervated by the sympathetic nervous system, they may have emissions.[12]

Male Fertility. There is loss of fertility in men with complete cord transection of the lumbar and sacral segments. Even if the men can ejaculate, sperm are not mobile and are fewer in number. Infertility may also be due to retrograde ejaculation, recurrent bladder infections, or possibly change in temperature regulation in the scrotum as a result of autonomic denervation or hormonal abnormalities.[13]

Sexual Capability in the Male. Sexual capability has been identified on the basis of neurologic classification and by statistical studies and review.

Neurologic Classification. Comarr and Gunderson[14] have classified sexual function among spinal cord-injured patients depending on the presence or absence of reflex activity from the second through the fourth sacral segment of the spinal cord. The diagnosis is made by digital rectal examination. They define an upper motor neuron lesion as one occurring above the sacral segments of the cord and a lower motor neuron lesion as one either in the sacral segments or in the sacral nerves.

The presence of tone in the external (striated) rectal sphincter, a positive bulbocavernosus reflex, or both indicate that the patient has an upper motor neuron lesion and is capable of reflex sexual function. If the rectal sphincter tone or a bulbocavernosus reflex or both are absent, the patient has a lower motor neuron lesion and is capable of areflexic sexual function.

To identify whether the lesion does or does not transect the cord at S_2 through S_4

segments, the penile skin, scrotal skin, and saddle area are tested bilaterally with a pinprick to determine whether spinothalamic (sensory) and posterior (motor) column pathways are intact. Findings may indicate one of four types of lesions—complete or incomplete upper motor neuron lesions, complete or incomplete lower motor neuron lesion. In general, the higher the cord lesion the more likely that erection is possible.[15]

Studies of Sexual Function. Studies and reviews have contributed information. Munro[16] and associates, Guttman,[17] Talbot,[18,19] and Comarr[20] have reported varying degrees of function depending on level and completeness of lesion. Some men are fertile and potent, could ejaculate, experience orgasm, and have intercourse, but more had varying degrees of difficulties.

Comarr and Gunderson summarize sexual capabilities. The majority of men with upper motor neuron lesions have reflexogenic erections (produced by reflex activity) either spontaneously or in response to external stimulation of the penis by manual massage, pulling the catheter or the external urinary receptacle, fellatio, etc. Those men who can attain only spontaneous reflexogenic erections are unfortunate, since these can occur at any time of the day or night but may not be attainable when wanted and may be of such short duration that coitus is impossible. Even those who obtain erections by external stimulation may not be able to achieve intromission, since the erection may be so brief. Still others with upper motor neuron lesions never have an erection.

Approximately 70 percent of men with complete lesions can achieve coitus compared to 85 percent of those with incomplete lesions, that is, successful coitus involving not only intromission but bringing the woman to orgasm.

The great majority of men with complete upper motor neuron lesions cannot sire children, since they cannot ejaculate or have an orgasm. There are a few exceptions, but possibly these patients' lesions, which appear clinically complete, are not anatomically complete. It is also possible that these men may not have told the truth during interviews or that the autonomic nervous system played a role in these exceptions.[21]

Those with incomplete upper motor neuron lesions may achieve psychogenic erection, but the ability to ejaculate varies with the extent of the lesion. The smaller the lesion, the greater the possibility for erection and ejaculation.

Seventy-five percent of men with complete lower motor neuron lesions are unable to have erections of any kind and therefore are unable to have coitus, ejaculate, reach orgasm, or sire children. About 25 percent of those men with segmental lesions below T12 can have psychogenic erections produced by mental or mental and physical stimuli. Only a smaller number of the 25 percent will be able to have coitus because of nonfirm or too brief erections, and even fewer can ejaculate.[22]

As many as 83 percent of men with incomplete lower motor neuron lesions may have psychogenic erections, with 90 percent of these achieving coitus. Fifty to 70 percent may be able to ejaculate, and 10 percent of these may sire children. (See Table 25-1 for summary of sexual capability and type of lesion.)[23]

Orgasmic Experience. Variation in orgasmic responses occur. Some individuals have complete anesthesia, while others have what is described as normal orgasmic response. Some describe "paraorgasms," pleasurable sensations derived from stimulation of various parts of the body. Some paraplegics with upper motor neuron lesions reported flexor and extensor spasticity before and during ejaculation, while others with complete upper motor neuron lesions experienced pleasurable sensations from the skin of the back above the level of the lesion. Those with sacral cord lesions report voluptuous sensations in the lower abdomen, groin, and inner thighs.[24]

TABLE 25–1.   SEXUAL CAPABILITY AND TYPE OF LESION

Type of Lesion	Percent Achieving Erection and Coitus	Percent Achieving Ejaculation	Percent Achieving Orgasm
Upper motor neuron			
Complete	72% reflexogenic erections and coitus	Rare	Absent
Incomplete	85% reflexogenic erection and coitus; psychogenic erection possible with small lesion	29% (67% of these can sire children)	29%
Lower motor neuron			
Complete	26% psychogenic erections (only a few can achieve coitus)	17% (5.6% can sire children)	17%
Incomplete	83% psychogenic erection only (90% of these achieve coitus)	60% (10% can sire children)	60%

Based on data from Comarr, A.: "Sexual Concepts in Traumatic Cord and Cauda Equina Lesions." Journal of Urology 106:375–378, 1971.

Biologic Factors: Female Sexual Function

Female Sexual Response.   The nerve supply to the female genital organs is similar to that of the male. The clitoris is innervated by the pudendal nerve and the vagina by the sacral segments. It is doubtful, however, that there are reflex centers in the spinal cord that serve sexual function in the same way as in the man. Women with complete lesions and those with incomplete lesions with bilateral section of the spinothalamic tracts have no orgasmic sensation. However, it may be present in complete lesions below T5–6 in response to tactile stimulation, especially of erogenous zones of the breast.[25]

Thirty-one spinal cord-injured women interviewed by Bregman and Hadley[26] reported on their sexual response. Three women with high injuries who could not move or feel below their shoulders frequently enjoyed sexual stimulation in their ears, mouth, and other parts of the body where they had partial feeling. The majority enjoyed breast stimulation, and five experienced great pleasure in body massages as a preliminary to sexual encounters. Most of the women's descriptions of orgasm were similar to those of able-bodied women as reported by Masters and Johnson. The orgasms ranged from a wide variety of psychologic experiences (good mental feelings, close and affectionate feelings for their mate) to a wide variety of physiopsychologic experiences (pleasant, relaxful, glowing, tingling feelings, release). Only three, however, stated that orgasm was unchanged from before injury. Since the investigators did not report on the level and extent of the injuries except in general terms, it is not possible to compare their sexual response to that reported in other literature.

Pregnancy.   Although women with complete denervation of sacral centers have little sensation during intercourse, in contrast to males, they are fertile and able to have children. Denervation of the ovaries does not seem to decrease their fertility.

The woman with paraplegia or quadriplegia may suffer from amenorrhea soon after the injury. Durkan[27] reported that six of seven women with high spinal cord transection had abrupt amenorrhea and a hypogonadotropic state. However, most regain menses, and nearly 50 percent do not miss a single period.[28]

Problems are attendant upon pregnancy and delivery. Urinary tract infections, especially pyelonephritis, are frequent. Unattended delivery may occur if the woman is not observed, since she may not be aware that she is in labor.[29] An occasional complication of labor and delivery is autonomic dysreflexia, characterized by high blood pressure, chills, headache, and diaphoresis.[30] However, whether suffering from cervical, thoracic, lumbar, or sacral injury, if their pelvic measurements are adequate, women can deliver vaginally. They usually carry their babies to full term, but may deliver prematurely if the lesion is above T10.

Unfortunately, research is inadequate in relation to female sexual function and fertility. In addition to the smaller number of studies, females also seem less willing to share information about sexual function. Banek and Mendelson[31] found that the female paraplegics in counseling sessions did not wish to discuss their sexual problems, if any. They had a tendency to hold back when sexual problems were discussed and were less direct in identifying problems when they did exist than men. However, since these were group sessions, it is possible that cultural prohibition against discussing sexual topics may have been operating.

Other Impediments to Coitus in Males and Females

The effects of spinal cord injury on sexual function do not solely revolve around innervation of sexual organs. Other side effects of the disease process—incontinence, loss of power and sensation in the muscles, severe spasticity, pressure sores, and infections—may all serve to limit coitus or at least make it distasteful to the individual and the sexual partner. The cord-injured person may have difficulty positioning or flexing the legs for coitus because of severe muscle spasm. If poor care has resulted in contractures, abil-

ity to assume positions for intercourse may also be compromised.

Some individuals have bladder neck resection to enable them to empty the bladder completely. This will result in retrograde ejaculation and sterility. External sphincterotomy may temporarily limit ability to erect, probably because of damage to the blood supply of the penis. Cordotomy or an alcohol block of the cord will also impair erection.[32] Drugs used for the treatment of spasticity, such as diazepam and barbiturates, may also inhibit erection (see Chapter 30).

In addition to the complex biologic changes that accompany spinal cord injury, profound psychosexual changes can further compromise sexuality.

Psychologic Factors

Some individuals may feel dirty, degraded, and inadequate after spinal cord injury. Loss of bowel and bladder control and mobility evoke highly charged reactions within the individual and in society, arousing feelings of shame and guilt.[33] (See Chapter 13 for discussion of shame and guilt.) Anxiety may accompany the perceived loss of masculinity and femininity[34] that usually accompanies loss of functional abilities. Muscle spasms, vasomotor disturbances, infections, and skin breakdown all contribute to fear about life itself.

As the patients move out of the acute phase, sexual concerns may begin to surface. The patient now must come to accept the loss or "death" of the previous self-image and must develop a new self-image. Working through the grieving process is a major task associated with recovery. The person moves through stages of denial and then despair when he/she realizes the implications of the loss. With help, the individual can come to accept the disability and develop a self-image that emphasizes essential worth and capabilities rather than the status of a "disabled" person.[35]

The dependent position that the person

experiences has a devastating effect on self-concept, and the change in function and appearance may initiate body image disturbance.[36,37] Conomy[38] studied the disturbances of body image occurring in 18 patients with spinal cord injury. He found that body image disorder involved hallucinatory disturbances, including (1) disordered perception of the body in space (proprioceptive body image), (2) disordered perception of posture and movement, and (3) disorders of perception of somatic bulk, size, and continuity. The individuals were hesitant to talk about these phenomena with physicians but often mentioned them to the nurses and other ward attendants. Well-kept nurses' notes were often the best index of the severity of the phenomena.[39] The patients found the experiences terrifying, fearing they were becoming mentally unbalanced. Conomy[40] questions if these patients in addition to experiencing a distortion of their own bodies may also have an altered perception of other persons.

Because of the hospitalization and immobility at an age when able-bodied young adults are actively coping with problems of life, many individuals may experience severe depression, frustration, and anxiety expressed as acting out behavior involving aggression, hostility, and anger. Sexually oriented jokes and flirting with staff members may produce severe patient–staff conflict.[41] (See Chapter 14 for discussion of aggressive sexual behavior.)

Sociologic Factors

Sexual role behavior is precipitously interrupted by spinal cord injury. Interpersonal and vocational skills are altered or terminated. The role relationship with the sexual partner may be reversed or significantly damaged, with the partner assuming employment and financial responsibilities, and of even greater portent, actual physical care of the cord-injured person. A parent–child role rather than a husband–wife role relationship can easily develop.

Other persons may be uncertain about proper behavior with the individual, and the return home may be particularly stressful. Cogswell[42] studied 36 young adult paraplegics, males and females, whites and blacks, from lower to upper middle class. All experienced marked reduction in (1) social contacts with others, (2) frequency in entering community settings, and (3) the number of roles they played. Only 6 of 26 followed regularly were able to assume the work role.

It is at home that self-esteem suffers as the social stigma of disability reaches its height. Unfortunately, the spinal cord-injured may have to become their own socializing agents. However, they are quick to withdraw from interactions if they perceive any response as derogatory, fearing that the attention of others is focused on the disability and that other aspects of self will be considered irrelevant.[43]

Individuals must be mobile in some way to assume social activities. Introduction may also be difficult, since able-bodied persons may hesitate to approach someone in a wheelchair. Consequently, the person with a disability will usually have to open up the conversation. This may be more difficult for a woman with spinal cord injury, although the greater equality of social roles that now exists makes it more acceptable for women to ask men for a date and assume more assertive behavior.[44]

As spinal cord-injured resume social relationships, they seldom resume relationships with pretrauma friends, but associate with individuals of lower class status, decidedly younger or older, or less attractive in other ways. They may break up old relationships because of their difficulty in assisting others to adjust to their new status as disabled. By forming new relationships with those of lower status, the spinal cord-injured are able to project themselves as persons of worth. However, as their self-esteem grows, they eventually form relationships with those of equal status.[45]

Conflict may exist over the resumption of sexual activity. In a permanent relationship, one of the partners may wish to resume or attempt sexual activity, while the other may fear injury or harm in some way.[46] Sexual adjustment may be difficult.

Sexual Adjustment

One of the most pervasive fears of the cord-injured is that the spouse or sexual partner may reject them because they cannot function satisfactorily.[47] In some cases, the injury has been the cause of termination or considerable decrease of sexual activity. Others, although having less frequent sexual relations, agree that their marriage has many compensations and enjoyments other than sex.[48]

Berkman and associates[49] gathered information from 148 spinal cord injured outpatients by use of the Index of Sexual Adjustment, which measured factors such as adaptation to sexual limitations, partner satisfaction, sexual self-concept, and regularity of sexual contact. They found that high scores on the index were positively correlated with better physical function, higher level of income, role of worker and community participant, higher morale, injury at earlier age, younger current age, and positive attitudes of self-acceptance and independence. It was evident that psychologic and social as well as physical factors were relevant for sexual rehabilitation.

Of the 148 individuals, 33 reported no sexual relations since injury. Forty-one percent of the persons rated their sex relations as satisfactory, 36 percent said they were somewhat satisfied, and 23 percent stated they were unsatisfactory. In contrast, 76 percent thought their partners were satisfied. Since sexual partners were not interviewed, the accuracy of these reports cannot be verified.[50] However, the findings of this study are especially significant, since they refute the myth that individuals cannot engage in sexual activity after cord injury. Ninety-seven percent of the group had sexual experience and 79 percent felt they were desirable partners.[51]

Each of the 31 spinal cord-injured women interviewed by Bregman and Hadley[52] had at least one sexual experience since the injury not necessarily involving intercourse; however, 27 reported they had intercourse. Sexual adjustment scores were computed on the basis of each subject's stated degree of adjustment, the subject's and her mate's satisfaction with the frequency of the sexual encounters, and the woman's stated degree of pleasure derived from the sexual encounter.

Seven women reported their sexual adjustment and satisfaction improved over time; however, the correlation between sexual adjustment scores and time since injury was near zero. Fourteen women who had received some information about sexual ability were not adjusting any better than the 17 who had not received information. However, the women were told only that they could have intercourse, would have normal menstrual cycles, and would be able to have children. They were not told how they could go about having intercourse, and most were not given sexual counseling while in the hospital.[53]

The first sexual experiences after injury were psychologically uncomfortable, and much time was needed to get over fear of rejection experienced especially by divorced and single women. As women began to feel like themselves again and feel good about themselves, their social and sexual relationships improved. Those with poor self-images had more difficulty adjusting sexually. All stressed the importance of being open and honest with sexual partners, that communication was the key to a healthy relationship.[54]

The quality of the relationship between the sexual partners is of greatest importance in adjusting to other modes of sexual behavior. Empathic understanding on the part of a spouse or sexual partner plays a vital role in the nature of any sexual relationship, but even more so if one has a physical disability.[55] Many of the newly disabled are not married and do not have lovers. Their greatest concern is finding mates who are willing to work their problems through with them. The issue of sexual incompatibility is secondary to the social problem of meeting and developing a relationship.

Even though men and women whose lesions are complete have no sensations below the level of injury, most indicate that the general bodily responses and stimulation above the injury are satisfying. The most significant satisfaction is probably not physiologic but that of participating, even in a more limited way, in what is one of the most important social experiences.

Marriage. Comarr[56] studied 858 patients with spinal injuries; 20 percent were unmarried before and remained so after injury, 48 percent were married before injury, and 26 percent were married for the first time after injury. Of those married after injury, 20 percent were later divorced. Smith and Bullough[57] suggest that marriage and satisfactory sexual adjustment can take place, especially among couples with no previous sexual experience who are willing to experiment and who are supportive of each other.

Motivation for marriage may vary. Love and affection, as in any marriage, are the major reasons, but some women marry cord-injured out of loyalty to the person to whom they had been engaged before the cord injury. Some women also have a highly developed mothering instinct and a need to care for others.[58]

Not all spinal cord-injured seek sexual partners or a marriage relationship. Some young and unmarried persons with no sexual experience may tend to feel that finding a mate is not worth the effort.[59]

Divorce. The divorce rate of spinal cord-injured is less in those who were married before injury than in those who were married after. Those who have already been married have had experience with the companionship

and loyalty involved in the relationship. Guttman[60] reports that 52 of 1505 spinal cord-injured persons (5.1 percent) were divorced after injury. There was a higher rate of divorce among those who had military service-connected disabilities (24 percent) than among those whose injury was not service connected (10 percent). Guttman speculates that some of these marriages were hastily entered into and were not based on love and affection, but may have been for purposes of financial security, since high disability pensions are paid to service persons.

NURSING IMPLICATIONS

Only a small part of sex relates to physical factors and intercourse. The greater part involves being a man or woman, husband or wife, sexual roles that constitute a way of life more than a periodic experience with sexual activity. The main reason for living may be to love and be loved. Nurses caring for spinal cord-injured individuals, as well as for all persons with diseases of the neuromuscular system, help the individual cope with profound changes in all aspects of sexuality, not just the physical. Baxter and Linn[61] describe the nurse's role as a specific one, with nurse counseling and teaching effective in giving patients something to live for. However, one of the most pervasive problems that the nurse faces is the individual's lack of knowledge about sexuality and sexual function.[62]

Assessment
Biologic Factors. The level and extent of spinal cord injury is determined. The method used by Comarr and Gunderson[63] and described earlier in this chapter is effective and not difficult to carry out. Other biologic data to be collected include the presence of complications, degree of bowel and bladder control, mobility, spasticity or flaccidity of muscles, and sensory losses. Within 6 months of spinal cord injury, the person should know how much sexual function will return.

The length of the disability is significant. The sexual concerns of the individual soon after the injury may be minimal,[64,65] but as other physical problems are corrected and as rehabilitation takes place, they surface and may become paramount.

Psychologic Factors. If the individual is still going through the grieving process and is depressed, little energy will be mobilized for interest in sexual activities. Some patients continue to deny that loss of sexual function is permanent and are not interested in discussing or learning about alternate sexual life styles. Other concerns, such as incontinence or financial difficulties, may occupy most of the individual's attention. Identification of the correct time for intervention is essential, but early after injury two-thirds of patients may have sexual concerns.[66]

Persons with cord injury, like others, are not usually direct in their request for information or their expression of concerns about sexuality. The nurse notes nonverbal behavior indicating signs of depression, or sexual acting-out behavior may be the first sign that help is needed (see Chapter 14). General statements such as, "I'm not good for much, anymore," "I wonder why my girlfriend bothers to visit me," may be the first indication that the individual has sexual concerns. The nurse also assesses the individual's degree of interest in sex (libido). Some become obsessed with sexuality, while others sublimate it completely.[67]

Sociologic Factors. These include marital status, presence of a girlfriend or boyfriend, and the nature of these relationships. The nurse also considers the potential for resumption of usual role activities, at home or at work, and the extent of mobility of the individual. The fears and concerns of the patient and the sexual partner about sexuality, their attitude about the disability, and alternate forms of sexual activity other than penile–vaginal intercourse are also important data that the nurse obtains. Religious and sociocultural beliefs about "normal" sexual

activity are also assessed. Financial problems should also be identified, since these may be paramount among concerns.

The reaction of the sexual partner as well as that of the patient is important. Hostility to questions may be evidence of serious problems that need further exploration.[68] The nurse should not get defensive but plan to return to the topic later.

Planning

It is essential that the nurse consider the concerns and the goals of the spinal cord-injured individual and the spouse or sexual partner when planning care. The nurse is also aware that the interest in and concern about sexuality may vary with time and the emergence of complications. If urinary or respiratory tract infections occur, sexual needs may be superseded by concerns about life itself.

The nurse's goals are to enable the individual and partner to develop a satisfying sexual life style and to maintain positive sexual self-concept and sexual identity.

Intervention

Biologic Factors. Reflex arc activity as evidenced by erections can be expected in most spinal cord-injured patients, and these are important diagnostic signs. The patient lying on his back may have no idea that he is having an erection. Rather than being shocked or embarrassed, the nurse meets the situation with equanimity, reassurance, and, if appropriate, humor, so the stage is set for the patient to feel comfortable to ask questions about sexual function and sexuality.[69] By acknowledging that sexuality is an appropriate topic for discussion, the nurse gives the patient tacit approval to bring up sexual concerns.

Nurses stress the positive aspect of the individual's sexuality at all times. When they do not, patients question their ability to perform, become apathetic, and do not pursue relationships. The patient must maintain or attain human relationships before sexual relationships can be reestablished or established. The same is true for the sexual partner. Hohmann[70] has advice for those who care for persons with disabilities:

> In general, the cord injured person should be encouraged to engage in whatever types of sexual activities are physiologically possible, pleasing, esthetic, gratifying and acceptable to him and his partner. The counselor should begin by assuming that some genital functioning is possible until experience, time and careful neurological examination demonstrate the contrary.

Although Hohmann refers to "he," his words are equally applicable to the cord-injured female.

Teaching includes information about sexual response of the male and female, different techniques of sexual arousal, and the effects of thoughts, memories, and fantasies on arousal and response. The nurse stresses the importance of the physical setting and mood setting as well as indicating what factors can inhibit sexual response. (See Chapters 3 and 4.)

Various types of conception control are discussed with female patients although all types present some problems. Birth control pills are contraindicated because of the danger of phlebitis. Intrauterine devices are a good choice, although the woman may not feel signs of pelvic inflammatory disease. Weakened pelvic muscles may not maintain a diaphragm which may have to be inserted by the partner. Foam and condoms are effective but again the partner may have to insert the foam and an indwelling catheter, if not removed, may tear the condom. The woman and her partner[71] together make a decision about the suitable type.

Eisenberg and Rustad[72] give useful information to guide interventions. The nurse continually stresses open communication between the sexual partners as to what is pleasurable and what is not. The patient is reassured that sex can be a meaningful dimension of life, even without erection and orgasm, that through sexual activity they can express affection and love; that a person can be attractive in a wheelchair if he/she is self-confident

and aware of his/her worth. The nurse stresses that masculinity is more than maintaining an erection or how many times one can have intercourse in an evening. The ability to make commitments, accept responsibility, and to give love and receive it are also important qualities that contribute to masculinity (or to femininity).[73] Satisfying the sexual partner can be by other techniques than coitus, and the psychologic aspects of love can be more important than the physical.[74]

Information about coital techniques and how to prepare for coitus will be sought and accepted when the patient is ready. The first step should be one-to-one counseling without use of explicit pictures of sexual activity and without emphasis on the physical acts of intercourse. Rather, the nurse tells the patient about some alternatives—the importance and pleasure of caressing, kissing, fondling, and touching, especially if the relationship is new. However, with an established relationship or one that has developed to a point where coitus is desired, further information is desired and needed to decrease anxiety and to insure a satisfying sexual experience no matter what its form.

Preparation for Intercourse. The nurse conveys information to help the cord-injured individual solve common problems. Many have catheters. These can be left in place, lubricated with K-Y jelly, and either taped to the penis or covered with a condom. However, it is probably best to remove the catheter. External catheters are usually removed. If the bladder is empty, it is safe to be without the catheter for 3 to 6 hours.[75] Avoiding fluids a few hours before sexual intercourse is helpful to insure that the bladder is empty. Although there is no published evidence to date that urine in the vaginal tract causes pathology (perhaps because the woman is usually in the dominant position),[76] some women may find it esthetically offensive. Those who have an ileoconduit pouch leave it in place and tape it to the abdomen.

It is probably safest for cord-injured

women to remove the catheter, but this depends to a great extent on size of the vagina and position during intercourse. If the man enters from behind (dog-fashion) it is usually unnecessary to remove the catheter.

Some women use K-Y jelly or other water-soluble lubricant before engaging in sexual activity. Petrolatum should not be used, since it is not water soluble and can be a vehicle for vaginal infection. Others prepare for sexual activity by reading erotic material with their husband or sexual partner, telling each other descriptive sexual stories while listening to soft background music.

Effective physical stimulation for cord-injured women includes body massages with cream or oils, rubbing each other's backs with tongue and hands, manual genital stimulation of each other, oral–genital intercourse, and sucking the woman's breasts.[77]

Mood setting is equally important for the spinal cord-injured male. A vibrator along with manual stimulation may serve to make erection firm enough for intromission.[78] A warm shower or bath or a drink can further enhance sexual response.[79]

Bowel care should be practiced to minimize the possibility of fecal incontinence.

Intercourse and Its Alternatives. Experimentation to discover effective means of sexual arousal is important to discover areas of sensitivity and types of stimulation that are especially pleasing. Stimulation of the lips, nipples, and ears can be just as erotic as penile or genital stimulation. Many men with midthoracic lesions find they have a sexually responsive area just above the point where their loss of sensation begins.[80] The nurse stresses that the individual should try to "feel" the surface of the partner's body and not be so concerned about stimulating the partner so that the personal experience and sensations are overlooked.

Positions for intercourse may vary, but most frequently the spinal cord-injured male assumes the bottom position with the female superior. From this position, the partners can roll over to either side. Cord-injured women usually use the male superior ("missionary") position. Some lie on their backs with pillows under their knees and buttocks. Others use a side-lying position, either facing the partner or with the back toward him.[81] Some couples face each other while she sits on his lap and they move in a rocking position.[82] When erection cannot be attained or maintained, the "stuffing" technique may help some couples. The man assumes the bottom position with the woman on her knees above him. She then gently "stuffs" his penis into her vagina and rotates her pelvis.[83] Some sustain an erection by the "rubber band technique," placing a rubber band or tying a soft condom around the base of the penis to maintain turgidity. Care must be taken not to damage the penis.[84] Some males may decide to have penile prosthetic implants[85] (see Chapter 3). (See Chapter 4 for information about positions for intercourse.)

Other forms of sexual stimulation, such as fellatio and/or cunnilingus, may be extremely pleasurable.[86] However, before giving any suggestions, the nurse counselor gains insight into the personalities of the individuals being counseled.[87] Some may have religious convictions that some types of sexual activity, oral–genital or manual stimulation, for example, are immoral and "unnatural." Any activity must be mutually acceptable to both.[88]

Eisenberg and Rustad[89] identify the factors that should be considered in any sexual relationship.

1. Sex has many meanings. There is more to making a sexual relationship work than penile intromission.

2. Do not expect too much too soon from your partner. Give her (him) time to adjust and to acquaint herself (himself) with you. Keep the doors of communication open.

3. It is difficult for a spouse to see the spinal cord-injured person as a sexually desirable partner when she (he) must provide bowel and bladder care and other health

needs. If this is the case, try to get outside help in performing these tasks—a visiting nurse, welfare aid, or part-time attendant.

4. The most important things for the cord-injured individual and the partner to develop are mutual trust, willingness to discuss each other's needs, and a desire to discuss how they can mutually satisfy each other. Sexual relationships enhance life if they grow out of feelings of mutual respect, love, and tenderness and concern.

Psychologic Factors. Nurses and other personnel may have difficulty in responding in a helpful way to the spinal cord-injured person's acting-out behavior. Personnel may view the patients as sexually nonfunctional, "bad," or dirty, and may respond to provocative remarks made to test sexuality with antitherapeutic attitudes. Staff or group meetings can give them an opportunity to ventilate their feelings and examine their sexual attitudes and beliefs, as well as enable them to obtain more information about sexual response so they can answer the patient's/client's questions adequately.[90] (See Chapter 14 for discussion of acting-out behavior and aggressive sexual behavior.)

The spinal cord-injured individual must also work through the grieving process and overcome any feelings of shame or guilt (see Chapter 13). The nurse remembers that although sexual dysfunction may be caused by the injury, the medication, psychologic reactions of fear, anxiety, and depression, or a combination of factors may also be operating.[91]

Social Factors. A motorized wheelchair with adaptations for the specific person provides needed mobility and greater independence. Automobiles can be adapted with hand controls to decrease dependence on others. The nurse can supply encouragement and positive feedback that the individual is sexually attractive.

When caring for the woman with a spinal cord injury, the nurse can also share some methods used by other spinal cord-injured women to increase physical and social attractiveness.[92] Clothes that cover a catheter leg bag (long dresses or full skirts) are important, but slacks may be preferred for style, comfort, and transferring from the wheelchair. Some prefer to transfer to a chair or couch from the wheelchair and to cross their legs at the ankle, not only to help with back support, but to improve their appearance. Some wear clothes that draw attention to their upper torso, wear a hook and wire girdle to support their upper torso, and short jackets or ponchos instead of long coats.[93]

Obtaining a job and becoming financially independent may do more for sexual self-concept than any words of praise. State and local departments of vocational rehabilitation can provide job retraining if the individual does not have the physical capacity to return to the former occupation.

If a couple desires children and the woman is unable to conceive, adoption may be the solution. There has been a shortage of children in recent years, but children who are difficult to place because of age, race, or physical or emotional problems are available.

The nurse also encourages the individual to maintain personal appearance, personal hygiene, and good grooming, since inadequacies in any of these areas will impede socialization. Realistic and appropriate compliments do much to enhance self-esteem. The spouse or sexual partner should also give realistic compliments and positive feedback about the individual's efforts to improve appearance.

At all times in the rehabilitative process, the spouse or friend should be part of the team effort. The nurse answers their questions, listens to their fears and concerns, and serves as an intermediary to maintain channels of communication.

Mixing sexes in the same rooms in a rehabilitation unit has been suggested as a possible therapeutic tool. Sixty-one patients,

39 men and 22 women (not all spinal cord-injured), shared rooms with someone of the opposite sex. Nurses scrupulously observed privacy needs. Almost 82 percent of the patients liked the arrangement stating that it "deinstitutionalized" the setting.[94]

Teaching and Counseling. In addition to one-to-one counseling and teaching, sessions with a small group of patients may be extremely effective. Some rehabilitation institutions offer broadly focused group sessions. Some are more structured, others are less so. Eisenberg and Rustad[95] use a didactic presentation, with movies and audiovisual materials followed by group discussion over a period of 8 weeks. Most individuals participating are at least 3 to 6 months postinjury, by which time they have made an initial adjustment to their injury. In addition to films, slides, books, and other visual aids, prosthetic devices such a vibrators, sheaths, and artificial phalluses are available for inspection.[96] Content includes information about anatomy and physiology of normal male sexual functioning and effects of cord injury; a discussion of communication skills to facilitate building of relationships and of factors that may interfere with satisfactory sexual adjustment; female sexual response, presented in terms of similarities and differences between male response; techniques for preparation for coitus, relaxation, and arousal; and marriage, divorce, and children. The sessions are closed with a film *Touching,* which portrays a C6 quadriplegic and his girlfriend engaging in sexual activity. The film is useful as a stimulus for discussion, and by the final meeting, the participants are generally able to discuss the contents freely. The film may also serve to summarize previous sessions and to allow the group leaders to assess participants' understanding of the material that has been discussed.[97]

This is just one program. Depending on the setting, teaching and counseling may be structured in different ways, but content should contain more than "how tos" of sexual activity. Flexibility and creativity to initiate a program that is suitable for the particular setting is essential.

Sexual rehabilitation takes the combined efforts of all members of the health team—the nurse, the physician, social worker, vocational rehabilitation worker, at times the psychiatrist or clinical psychologist, and most important, the patient and the spouse or sexual partner.

Evaluation

The following outcome criteria indicate that interventions were effective. The patient and sexual partner:

1. Identify the changes in sexual response that accompany his/her injury.
2. Identify alternate types of sexual expression and their acceptability for them.
3. Describe preparatory steps to sexual activity.
4. Discuss sex openly with each other.
5. Interact socially with others.
6. Express satisfaction with employment status or make efforts to increase economic independence.
7. Express satisfaction with role as male or female.
8. Engage in whatever sexual activity is mutually satisfying.

OTHER DISORDERS RESULTING IN IMPAIRED NEUROLOGIC OR MUSCULOSKELETAL FUNCTION

Multiple Sclerosis

Bio-Psycho-Social Factors. The etiology of this disease continues to be an enigma, despite widespread research. This disease of adults (incidence peaks at 30 to 35 years) is more common in women than in men. Its etiology has been attributed to an autoimmune disorder and/or to slow viruses, but these theories are yet unproven.[98]

The neurologic dysfunction consists of both motor and sensory dysfunction and at times disturbances in personality and mentation. Symptoms are variable, but one common manifestation of the disease is interference with bowel and bladder control marked by frequency, urgency, and slight incontinence, followed later by retention and severe incontinence. This results from involvement of efferent suprasegmental pathways in or adjacent to the pyramidal tracts of the cord and to lesions in the posterior funiculi.[99] In men, impotence[100] and ejaculatory difficulties occur.[101] Spasms of adductor muscles may make positioning for intercourse difficult.

The disease affects the individual during the most productive years, restricting pattern of daily living, employment, marriage, and parenthood. The person suffers a drastic change in life style, ability to carry out usual role activities, and degree of independence.[102]

NURSING IMPLICATIONS

The nurse focuses care on the capabilities rather than disabilities, involving both the individual with multiple sclerosis and the family. Careful psychosocial evaluation concerning attitudes and temperament of each individual is essential.[103] Teaching about the effects of the disease and measures to prevent complications may help maintain the individual's independence and well-being. As the disease progresses, the nurse helps the patient/client and others accept change in sexual functioning, personality, and role. (See interventions in Chapter 13 to promote sexual self-esteem.) Different positions for intercourse and alternative methods of sexual expression are suggested.

Cerebral Vascular Accident and Brain Injury

Any interruption of the blood supply to the brain may result in sexual problems, depending on the areas affected and the extent of damage. Cerebral vascular accident (CVA), the most common problem, causes varying degrees of paralysis to one side of the body (hemiplegia). In addition, infarction in the brain can affect central centers for libido or the communicating tracts between the brain and spinal cord, adversely affecting sexual response.[104]

It appears that libido may be increased or decreased depending on the side of the brain that is damaged. Interviews with 25 post-CVA patients suggest that libido increases if the nondominant hemisphere is damaged and decreases if the dominant hemisphere is affected. The patients did not perceive change in sexual interest, although it appeared that there was considerable anxiety about sexuality.[105] Bray[106] and associates also found no significant changes in sex interest in 35 male and female subjects. However, all the men had significant decrease in ability to achieve erection and to ejaculate; the 5 women who were premenopausal had major change in menses and only 1 of the 11 women attained orgasm.

Other changes in function adversely alter ability to carry out sexual roles. Paralysis of one side of the body, visual, perceptual,[107] and communication problems, especially aphasia,[108] may make reestablishment of a sexual relationship difficult. Body image disturbances may be profound.

Changes in tactile sense and proprioception may make self-care difficult. In addition, the hemiplegic individual is burdened with decreased attention span, poor memory for recent and sometimes past events, and a difficulty in processing directions.[109] Families and sexual partners may tend to overprotect the individual instead of fostering independence. Sexual roles and relationships are severed, and the decreased ability to communicate may further place the stroke patient in a childlike position. Relearning activities of daily living that the individual has performed independently and automatically are frustrating and humiliating for the stroke patient. Little energy or interest may be left for sexual activity.

Damage to the frontal lobes may cause loss of fantasy life and moral and ethical restraints. During early recovery from brain damage, the patient's sexual behavior may be shown through autoerotic activity.

Some stroke patients may use exhibitionism to disprove what is feared, that they are no longer men or women. Frankel[110] describes a woman who would lie in bed nude or stand at the sink in her hospital room after removing her clothes to wash herself. Exposure of her genitals proved she was a woman.

NURSING IMPLICATIONS

Assessment parameters identified for the spinal cord-injured individual are applicable for the stroke patient. Sexual intercourse may be facilitated by use of a footboard or hand lever for moving.[111] Interventions to increase sexual self-esteem and correct body image disturbances are applicable (see Chapter 13). The nurse helps the family of the aphasic patient see that the patient can still mentate and needs to be allowed to express thoughts and ideas.

When stroke patients use exhibitionism to prove sexual identity, staff should be helped to see what being a woman (or man) means to the patient. In one patient's case, it meant being taken care of. With her perceived body disfigurement, she feared loss of this nurturance, and her exhibitionism was a plea for care. With a great deal of attention from the nursing staff, the behavior disappeared.

Sympathectomy
Sympathectomy may interfere with male sexual response. Impotence, interference with erection, sterility, and interference with ejaculation may occur. Whitelow and Smithwick[112] questioned 183 men who had the procedure. In the bilateral transthoracic procedure, there was no permanent loss of ejaculation, but difficulty with erection occurred in 57 percent of the men, although this was not complete and did not seriously interfere with intercourse. After bilateral lumbodorsal procedure, 26 of 116 patients reported disturbance of erection and 24 reported permanent loss of ejaculation. White-

low and Smithwick[113] stress that the possible secondary effects of sympathectomy on sexual functions should be discussed and the patient allowed to make the decision about the surgery. There appear to be fewer problems with function in women, but there are no careful studies to support the conclusion.[114]

Nervous System Diseases Resulting in Impotence
Some diseases affect the motor system, causing impotence, but few sensory changes. These include amyotrophic lateral sclerosis[115] (loss of motor cells), tabes dorsalis (demyelinization of posterior ganglia), syringomyelia[116] (formation of a cavity or syrinx in the center parts of the spinal cord), and herniated lumbar disc.[117] Patients with Alzheimer disease[118] (diffuse cerebral atrophy) may become impotent later in the disease. Increased interest in sexual activity may occur in the early stages.

TEMPORAL LOBE LESIONS

The terms *psychomotor seizures* and *seizures arising in the temporal lobe* have been applied to all seizures that involve primarily one temporal lobe, although commissural transmission to both temporal lobes and the limbic system often follows. These seizures may not include a generalized tonic and clonic aspect. They may involve disturbance of thinking, language, affective disturbances, and antisocial behavior.[119]

The most common sexual abnormalities in temporal lobe lesions in the male are loss of libido and genital arousal. Of 15 married men studied by Hierons and Saunders,[120] 12 had temporal lobe epileptic attacks. In three, impotence preceded the development of the epilepsy by 6 to 9 months. In four cases, increased medication brought the epilepsy under control and at the same time, potency improved.

Experimental and clinical evidence indicates that the limbic portion of anterior temporal lobes and their connections are in control of sexual function. The impotence occurs in association with organic disease of the temporal lobe.[121,122]

After treatment, Blumer[123] describes occurrence of hypersexual behavior in 50 temporal lobe epileptics; 42 had temporal lobe lobectomy. Twenty-nine were hyposexual before surgery. The hypersexual behavior after the lobectomy was characterized by quantitative change in sex drive, sexual arousal, and response that was abnormal in intensity and frequency for the individual.

LOSS OF MUSCULAR AND SKELETAL MOVEMENT AND STRENGTH

Arthritis

Juvenile Rheumatoid Arthritis. Individuals with juvenile rheumatoid arthritis are presently living longer and maintaining better functional capacity, so they are now better able to explore and develop their sexuality than were earlier victims of the disease. Juvenile arthritis is a constitutional disease in which there are inflammatory changes in the connective tissues of the body. The disease may affect only one or nearly all of the joints, with or without involvement of other systems. Consequently, individuals may be mildly or severely handicapped by the disease. Herstein and associates[124] examined and interviewed 58 adults, 37 females, and 21 males at an average of 14.5 years from the onset of juvenile rheumatoid arthritis (JRA). Thirty-nine patients were capable of near normal physical activity, and 19 had JRA that prevented them from carrying out many normal activities. Forty-one patients (70 percent) were financially independent.

Those who develop arthritis later in life have a sexual behavior pattern prior to onset of the disease, but these patients went through puberty and sexual development while their arthritis was in varying degrees of activity.

Of the 58 patients, 38 (73 percent) were having coital activity and all married patients were sexually active. Thirteen of 19 unmarried females and 4 of 12 unmarried males were sexually active. Masturbation was used as a sexual outlet by some, and oral sex was used by 16 of 33 of the females. Coital positions were limited by the JRA because of pain, fatigue, and functional joint disability for 24 of 38 patients.

Twenty persons indicated a need for sexual counseling, a two to one ratio of women to men. Almost all indicated that when they were adolescents they particularly needed sexual information. The counseling requests included need for information about birth control, the effect of the pill on arthritis, effects of medication on libido, and how to cope with intimacy when in pain or fatigued. Those who had knee or hip disability were particularly anxious for information about coital positions.[125]

Patients' comments indicated that the arthritics' inability to be as sexually receptive as their spouses can produce marital tension. The women who desired sexual counseling wished information about ways to improve their sexual responses, and many felt their sexual adjustment would improve if their partners attended the session. They saw the partners' contribution as essential, especially if they expressed interest, concern, and desire to help the affected person.[126]

Adult Rheumatoid Arthritis and Osteoarthritis. Adult rheumatoid arthritis has joint inflammation as its chief manifestation and occurs three times more often in women than in men. With pathologic changes, joints become contracted and stiffened, usually in a dysfunctional position. The patients may have depressed production of red blood cells by bone marrow followed by anemia, fatigue, anorexia, weight loss, and weakness. Spasm and pain lead to disuse and atrophy.[127]

Osteoarthritis is a condition in which there is deterioration of articular cartilage and overgrowth of adjacent bone without the joint inflammation of rheumatoid arthritis.

It is most common after age 50, but may occur after joint injury.[128] In all types of arthritis, the fatigue, malaise, limitations of joint mobility, pain, and stiffness that characterize the disease decrease interest in sexual activity or decrease the energy and the physical mobility needed for satisfying intercourse, or for stroking, caressing, and genital manipulation.

NURSING IMPLICATIONS

The nurse emphasizes the importance of rest before sexual activity and of taking prescribed medication so that pain is minimized and the person is more sexually responsive. Sexual activity in the early morning when the arthritic individual is rested and is experiencing less pain may be more satisfying and pleasurable for both partners. The couple can be urged to experiment with different and more comfortable positions for sexual intercourse (see Chapter 4). Though specific positions may be described, the couple is urged to experiment to find out which are most comfortable for them. To coordinate care a team approach involving occupational therapy, physical therapy, social worker and nurse is usually needed.[129]

Although further research is needed, it is interesting to note that sexual activity and especially intense sexual stimulation provides 4 to 6 hours of pain relief according to Ehrlich and Patten. Their conclusions are based on a survey of 220 rheumatoid arthritis patients, 70 percent who had pain reduction after sexual stimulation, although not necessarily intercourse. They theorize that sexual stimulation stimulates the adrenal gland to produce cortisone which in turn decreases pain.[130]

Muscular Dystrophies
These diseases affect voluntary muscles and the neuromuscular junction. They are a group of genetically determined, progressive diseases characterized by degeneration and wasting of muscle fibers, without involve-

ment of the peripheral or central nervous system. Children with the Duchenne type usually die by the age of 20.[131]

The disease occurs predominately in males; the female is the carrier and is usually unaffected clinically. When the female is a definite carrier or where other signs of the disease are present, genetic counseling is given, and the family is informed that the condition is a sex-linked recessive form of genetic inheritance. Theoretically, in any pregnancy, 50 percent of the male offspring will probably develop the disease and 50 percent of the female offspring will be carriers.[132]

Parents will need much support as they face the decision to limit their family. Choosing a form of conception control that will be effective is essential. In addition, the couple will need support to work through their feelings and to maintain a satisfying sexual relationship in the face of fears of pregnancy and the burden of caring for a child with the disease. (See Chapter 27 for a discussion of genetic counseling.)

SENSORY CHANGES AND SEXUALITY: BLINDNESS, DEAFNESS, PAIN

The blind have difficulty developing social skills often because of overprotection as children. Often their sex education is minimal and they have no accurate model of the human body.[133] Not only may they have difficulty developing relationships but they have a lack of emotional feedback from the visual responses of a sexual partner. They may fear intercourse, fear being watched during sex play, and fear exploitation. The married blind may have conflict between their desire to have children and fear of the responsibility of child raising.

The deaf are also socially isolated, have less knowledge of sexuality and are more accepting of myths and misconceptions. (See Chapter 15 for discussion of child and deafness.) If marriage occurs, there may be difficulty because of immaturity, dependency, low self-image and self-confidence. Shaul[134] found, however, that their sexual problems are similar to those of the hearing populations.

Pain affects sexual response. Del Bene[135] and associates found that 10 percent of 362 individuals with migraine reported sexual arousal during the attack. They believe that supersensitivity of central nervous system centers which control sexual behavior is the cause of the response. Pain syndrome may develop as an accompaniment of chronic marital problems with sexual maladjustment as a consequence. Fifty patients with pain and their spouses reported decrease in frequency and quality of sexual activity. The patients had no malignancy, arthritis or other conditions for which medical, surgical or psychiatric interventions were applicable. Before pain there was no difference in rating of overall marital adjustment of patient and spouse group. After pain a significant number of spouses rated the marriage below average while the patients rated it average or above average. It is difficult to sort out what is primary or secondary: decrease in sexual activity could be due to pain; it could be due to the response of the spouse to pain behavior or a combination.[136]

NOTES

1. Cole TM, Cole SS: Rehabilitation of problems of sexuality in physical disability. In Kottke FJ, Stillwell GK, Lehmann JF (eds). Krusen's Handbook of Physical Medicine and Rehabilitation. Philadelphia, Saunders, 1982, pp 889–905
2. Glass DD: Sexuality and the spinal cord injured. In Oaks WW, Melchiode GA, Ficher I (eds): Sex and the Life Cycle. New York, Grune and Stratton, 1976, pp 179–190
3. Ibid, p 179
4. Romano MD: Sex and the handicapped. Nurs Care 10:18–20, 48, 1977
5. Ibid, p 20
6. Silver JR: Sexual problems in disorders of the nervous system: Anatomical and physiological aspects. Br Med J 3:480–482, 1975
7. Ibid, p 480
8. Ibid
9. Ibid
10. SCI—Incidence and cost. Am J Nurs 77:1340, 1977
11. Eisenberg MG, Rustad LC: Sex and the Spinal Cord Injured: Some Questions and Answers, 2nd ed. Washington, D.C., U.S. Government Printing Office, 1975
12. Silver JR: Sexual problems in disorders of the nervous system: Anatomical and physiological aspects. Br Med J 3:481, 1975
13. Ibid
14. Comarr AE, Gunderson BB: Sexual function in traumatic paraplegia and quadriplegia. Am J Nurs 75:250–255, 1975
15. Ibid, p 250
16. Munro D, Horne HW, Paull DP: The effect of injury of the spinal cord and cauda equina on the sexual potency of men. N Engl J Med 239:903–911, 1948
17. Guttman L: Spinal cord injuries: Comprehensive management and research. Oxford, England, Blackwell's, 1973, pp 446–478
18. Talbot HS: A report on sexual function in paraplegics. J Urol 61:265–270, 1949
19. Talbot HS: Sexual function in paraplegics. J Urol 73:91–100, 1955
20. Comarr AE: Sexual concepts in traumatic cord and cauda equina lesions. J Urol 106:375–378, 1971
21. Comarr AE, Gunderson BB: Sexual function in traumatic paraplegia and quadriplegia. Am J Nurs 75:250, 1975
22. Ibid, p 251
23. Ibid, p 252
24. Bors E, Comarr AE: Neurological disturbances of sexual function with special reference to 529 patients with spinal cord injury. Urol Surv 10:191–222, 1960

25. Guttman L: The sexual problem. In Guttman L (ed): Spinal Cord Injuries. Oxford, England, Blackwell's, 1976, pp 474–505

26. Bregman S, Hadley RG: Sexual adjustment and feminine attractiveness among spinal cord injured women. Arch Phys Med Rehabil 57:448–450, 1976

27. Durkan JP: Menstruation after high spinal cord transection. Am J Obstet Gynecol 100:521–527, 1966

28. Comarr AE: Observations on menstruation and pregnancy among female spinal cord injury patients. Paraplegia 3:263–272, 1966

29. Guttman L: The sexual problem. In Guttman L (ed): Spinal Cord Injuries. Oxford, England, Blackwell's, 1976, p 488

30. Ibid, p 493

31. Banek SN, Mendelson MA: Group psychotherapy with a paraplegic group with an emphasis on specific problems of sexuality. Int J Group Psychother 28:123–128, 1978

32. Silver JR: Sexual problems in disorders of the nervous system: Anatomical and physiological aspects. Br Med J 3:481, 1975

33. Crigler L: Sexual concerns of the spinal cord injured. Nurs Clin North Am 9:703–715, 1974

34. Lindh K, Richerson G: Spinal cord injury: You can make a difference. Nursing 74(4):40–45, 1974

35. Larrabee JH: Physical care during early recovery. Am J Nurs 77:1320–1329, 1977

36. Pepper G: Psychological care: The person with a spinal cord injury. Am J Nurs 77:1330–1335, 1977

37. Evans JH: On disturbance of body image in paraplegia. Brain 85:687–700, 1962

38. Conomy JP: Disorders of body image after spinal cord injury. Neurology 23:842–850, 1973

39. Ibid, p 849

40. Ibid

41. Banek SN, Mendelson MA: Group psychotherapy with a paraplegic group with an emphasis on specific problems of sexuality. Int J Group Psychother 28:124, 1978

42. Cogswell BE: Self-socialization, readjustment of paraplegics in the community. J Rehabil 34(3):11–13, 35, 1968

43. Ibid, p 12

44. Smith J, Bullough B: Sexuality and the severely disabled person. Am J Nurs 75:2194–2197, 1975

45. Cogswell BE: Self-socialization, readjustment of paraplegics in the community. J Rehabil 34(3):13, 1968

46. Frankel A: Sexual problems in rehabilitation. J Rehabil, September–October 1967, pp 19–20

47. Banek SN, Mendelson MA: Group psychotherapy with a paraplegic group with an emphasis on specific problems of sexuality. Int J Group Psychother 28:127, 1978

48. Comarr AE, Gunderson BB: Sexual function in traumatic paraplegia and quadriplegia. Am J Nurs 75:254, 1975

49. Berkman AH, Weissman R, Frielich MH: Sexual adjustment of spinal cord veterans living in the community. Arch Phys Med Rehabil 59:29–33, 1978

50. Ibid, p 31

51. Ibid, p 33

52. Bregman S, Hadley RG: Sexual adjustment and feminine attractiveness among spinal cord injured women. Arch Phys Med Rehabil 57:448, 1976

53. Ibid, p 449

54. Ibid, p 450

55. Banek SN, Mendelson, MA: Group psychotherapy with a paraplegic group with an emphasis on specific problems of sexuality. Int J Group Psychother 28:126, 1978

56. Comarr AE: Proc 11th Annu Clin Spinal Cord Conf. New York, Veterans Administration, 1962, pp 163–215

57. Smith J, Bullough B: Sexuality and the severely disabled person. Am J Nurs 75:2197, 1975

58. Guttman L: The sexual problem. In Guttman L (ed): Spinal Cord Injuries. Oxford, England, Blackwell's, 1976, p 502

59. Lindh K, Richerson G: Spinal cord injury: You can make a difference. Nursing 74(4):44, 1974

60. Guttman L: The sexual problem. In Guttman L (ed): Spinal Cord Injuries. Oxford, England, Blackwell's, 1976, p 502

61. Baxter RT, Linn A: Sex counseling and the SCI patient. Nursing 78(8):46–52, 1978

62. Banek SN, Mendelson MA: Group psychotherapy with a paraplegic group with an emphasis on specific problems of sexuality. Int J Group Psychother 28:126, 1978

63. Comarr AE, Gunderson BB: Sexual function in traumatic paraplegia and quadriplegia. Am J Nurs 75:376, 1975

64. Pepper G: Psychological care: The person with a spinal cord injury. Am J Nurs 77:1332, 1977

65. Cole T, Glass D: Sexuality and physical disabilities. Arch Phys Med Rehabil 58:585–586, 1977

66. Miller S, Szarz G, Anderson L: Sexual health care clinician in an acute spinal cord injury unit. Arch Phys Med Rehabil 62:315–320, 1981

67. Pepper G: Psychological care: The person with a spinal cord injury. Am J Nurs 77:1335, 1977

68. Cole TM, Cole SS: Rehabilitation of problems of sexuality in physical disability. In Kottke FJ, Stillwell GK, Lehmann JF (eds). Krusen's Handbook of Physical Medicine and Rehabilitation. Philadelphia, Saunders, 1982, p 894

69. Crigler L: Sexual concerns of the spinal cord injured. Nurs Clin North Am 9:713, 1974

70. Hohmann GW: Considerations in management of psychosexual readjustment in the cord injured male. Rehabil Psychol 19(2):54, 1972

71. Hale G: Source Book for the Disabled. Philadelphia, Saunders, 1979

72. Eisenberg MG, Rustad LC: Sex and the Spinal Cord Injured: Some Questions and Answers, 2nd ed. Washington, D.C., U.S. Government Printing Office, 1975, p 13

73. Ibid, p 14

74. Baxter RT, Linn A: Sex counseling and the SCI patient. Nursing 78(8):51, 1978

75. Eisenberg MG, Rustad LC: Sex and the Spinal Cord Injured: Some Questions and Answers, 2nd ed. Washington, D.C., U.S. Government Printing Office, 1975, p 16

76. Comarr AE, Gunderson BB: Sexual function in traumatic paraplegia and quadriplegia. Am J Nurs 75:255, 1975

77. Bregman S, Hadley RG: Sexual adjustment and feminine attractiveness among spinal cord injured women. Arch Phys Med Rehabil 57:449, 1976

78. Smith J, Bullough B: Sexuality and the severely disabled person. Am J Nurs 75:2197, 1975

79. Eisenberg MG, Rustad LC: Sex and the Spinal Cord Injured: Some Questions and Answers, 2nd ed. Washington, D.C., U.S. Government Printing Office, 1975, p 19

80. Ibid

81. Ibid, p 20

82. Bregman S, Hadley RG: Sexual adjustment and feminine attractiveness among spinal cord injured women. Arch Phys Med Rehabil 57:449, 1976

83. Eisenberg MG, Rustad LC: Sex and the Spinal Cord Injured: Some Questions and Answers, 2nd ed. Washington, D.C., U.S. Government Printing Office, 1975, p 20

84. Silver JR: Sexual problems in disorders of the nervous system: Anatomical and physiological aspects. Br Med J 3:481, 1975

85. Wood RY, Rose K: Penile implants for impotence. Am J Nurs 78:234–238, 1978

86. Baxter RT, Linn A: Sex counseling and the SCI patient. Nursing 78(8):52, 1978

87. Comarr AE, Gunderson BB: Sexual function in traumatic paraplegia and quadriplegia. Am J Nurs 75:255, 1975

88. Eisenberg MG, Rustad LC: Sex and the Spinal Cord Injured: Some Questions and Answers, 2nd ed. Washington, D.C., U.S. Government Printing Office, 1975, p 26

89. Ibid, p 27

90. Eisenberg MG, Rustad LC: Sex education and counseling program on a spinal cord injury service. Arch Phys Med Rehabil 57:135–140, 1976

91. Whitley M, Bush MT, Williams RA: Human sexuality and the spinal cord injured person. Imprint 24(2):50–52, 1977

92. Bregman S, Hadley RG: Sexual adjustment and feminine attractiveness among spinal cord injured women. Arch Phys Med Rehabil 57:450, 1976

93. Ibid

94. Gibson CJ: Mixing sexes in a rehabilitation unit. Arch Phys Med Rehabil 63:386–387, 1982

95. Eisenberg MG, Rustad LC: Sex education and counseling program on a spinal cord injury service. Arch Phys Med Rehabil 57:136, 1976

96. Ibid

97. Ibid, p 138

98. Dean G: The multiple sclerosis problem. Sci Am 223:40–46, 1970

99. Schumacher GA: Multiple sclerosis. J Chronic Dis 8:465–485, 1958

100. Thorn GW, Adams R, Braunwald E, Isselbacher KJ, Petersdorf RG (eds): Harrison's Principles of Internal Medicine, 8th ed. New York, McGraw-Hill, 1977, p 1903

101. Myerscough PR: Sexual function in illness. Clin Obstet Gynecol 7:387–400, 1980

102. Dillon AM: Nursing care of the patient with multiple sclerosis. Nurs Clin North Am 8:653–664, 1973

103. Alden JH: Rehabilitation of multiple sclerosis patients. J Rehabil 33(2):10–12, 1967

104. Mills LC: Sexual disorders in the diabetic patient. In Oaks WW, Melchiode GA, Ficher I (eds): Sex and the Life Cycle. New York, Grune and Stratton, 1976, pp 163–174

105. Goddess E, Wagner NN, Silverman DR: Poststroke sexual activity and CVA patients. Med Aspects Hum Sex 13:16–30, 1979

106. Bray GP, DeFrank RS, Wolfe TL: Sexual functioning in stroke survivors. Arch Phys Med Rehabil 62:286–288, 1981

107. Burt MN: Perceptive deficits in hemiplegia. Am J Nurs 70:1026–1029, 1970

108. McCartney VC: Rehabilitation and dignity for the stroke patient. Nurs Clin North Am 9:693–701, 1974

109. Burt MN: Perceptive deficits in hemiplegia. Am J Nurs 70:1029, 1970

110. Frankel A: Sexual problems in rehabilitation. J Rehabil September–October 1967, p 19

111. Renshaw DC: Sexual problems in old age, illness and disability. Psychosomatics 22:975–985, 1981

112. Whitelow GP, Smithwick RH: Some secondary effects of sympathectomy. N Engl J Med. 245:121–128, 1951

113. Ibid, p 129

114. Myerscough PR: Sexual function in illness. Clin Obstet Gynecol 7:398, 1980

115. Thorn GW, Adams R, Braunwald, E, Isselbacher KJ, Petersdorf RG (eds): Harrison's Principles of Internal Medicine, 8th ed. New York, McGraw-Hill, 1977, p 1931

116. Ibid, p 1829

117. Amelar RD, Dubin L: Low back pain and impotence. JAMA 216:520, 1971

118. Thorn GW, Adams R, Braunwald E, Isselbacher KJ, Petersdorf RG (eds): Harrison's Principles of Internal Medicine, 8th ed. New York, McGraw-Hill, 1977, p 1920

119. Gilroy J, Meyer JS: Medical Neurology. New York, Macmillan, 1975, p 321

120. Hierons R, Saunders M: Impotence in

patients with temporal-lobe lesions. Lancet 2:761–763, 1966

121. Ibid, p 762

122. Blumer D: Hypersexual episodes in temporal lobe epilepsy. Am J Psychiatry 126:1099–1106, 1970

123. Ibid, p 762

124. Herstein A, Hill RH, Walters K: Adult sexuality and juvenile rheumatoid arthritis. J Rheumatol 4:35–39, 1977

125. Ibid, p 39

126. Ibid

127. MacRae I: Arthritis. Nurs Clin North Am 8:643–652, 1973

128. Ibid, p 647

129. Figley BA, Ferguson KJ, Bole GG, Kay DR: A comprehensive approach to sexual health in rheumatic disease. Top Clin Nurs 1:69–74, 1980

130. Kirkham D: Doctors report sex dims arthritis pain. The Cleveland Press, October 25, 1979, p 6

131. Gilroy J, Meyer JS: Medical Neurology. New York, Macmillan, 1975, p 693

132. Ibid, p 696

133. Chigier E: Sexuality of physically disabled people. Clin Obstet Gynecol 7:325–343, 1980

134. Shaul S: Deafness and human sexuality: A development review. Am Ann Deaf 126:432–439, 1981

135. Del Bene E, Conti C, Poggioni M, Sicuteri F: Sexuality and headache. Adv Neurol 33:209–214, 1982

136. Maruta T, Osborne D, Swanson DW, Halling JM: Chronic pain patients and spouses. Marital and sexual adjustment. Mayo Clinic Proc 56:307–310, 1981

Chapter 26

Impaired Hormonal Function

Hormonal influences on human sexuality begin at the moment of conception and continue throughout life. Specific hormonal changes that affect sexual development are discussed in Unit III. The focus of this chapter is on disturbances of endocrine function that adversely affect sexual response; one of the most insidious of these is diabetes. The incidence of diabetes and its adverse affects on sexuality are probably equal if not greater than those of all other endocrine disorders combined. Consequently, the emphasis of this chapter will be on this disease, without neglecting, however, discussion of pituitary, thyroid, adrenal, testicular, and ovarian dysfunction and their effects on sexuality.

DIABETES MELLITUS

Shagan[1] suggests that diabetes mellitus is a model for aging. It is a chronic, debilitating, degenerative disease, which, like aging, may have as its concomitants peripheral arterial disease, arteriosclerotic heart diseases, premature loss of a limb, neuropathy, and nephropathy. In addition, changes in sexual function, which sometimes accompany aging, may also be one of its sequelae—impotence and female orgasmic dysfunction, loss of libido, and infertility.[2] Most of the research and interest regarding the effects of diabetes on sexuality has been directed toward male diabetics and their impotence and ejaculatory incompetence, while the effects of diabetes

on females has received much less attention. The changes in sexual function that accompany diabetes may be considered the prototype for those that occur in other endrocrine disorders; with few exceptions, they are identical.[3]

Diabetes and Impotence

The association between diabetes and impotence was first recognized in 1798,[4] but in the past 20 years, it has received increased attention.

Frequency. Schöffling and associates[5] found that of 314 diabetic patients, 160 (51 percent) had disturbances of sexual function. The problems varied in quality and severity, the predominate ones being periodic or constant impotence. Among patients 31 years or younger, 29.4 percent had decreased potency. This percentage increased for older diabetics, reaching 72.6 percent for diabetics 60 years of age or older. Rubin and Babbitt[6] had similar findings in a group of 198 diabetics. Seventy percent of the males with diabetes of less than 1-year duration had potency problems. Among those who had diabetes from 1 to 5 years, the rate dropped to 43 percent; among those with diabetes for over 5 years, it was 45 percent. The authors theorize that the generally high rate of impotence in the newly diagnosed diabetic may be the result of poor control of the disease, since the problem often disappeared once the disease was well controlled. However, when impotence developed among those more or less well controlled, it was usually more permanent.[7]

In a later study, Kolodny and associates[8] found that 49 percent of 175 randomly selected male diabetics were impotent and 2 percent had ejaculatory difficulty. It is estimated that between 30 and 60 percent of all diabetic men will develop impotence of varying degrees at some time in their lives.[9]

Onset of Impotence. The onset of impotence is usually gradual over a period of 6 months to 1 year. There may be a gradual loss of firmness of erection. During early stages of impotence, the man may be able to experience orgasm and ejaculate. If changes continue, total impotence may occur. Libido persists, and patients may have normal or increased sexual interest and drive despite loss of erectile ability.[10–12]

Biologic Factors and Impotence. The precise etiology of diabetic impotence is unclear, but it has been postulated that four mechanisms are possible: (1) a type of diabetic neuropathy; (2) vascular changes, arteriosclerotic changes in penile blood vessels that impair pooling and trapping of blood in the corpora of the penis; (3) a disruption of biochemical or hormonal balance; (4) psychogenic factors. It is also possible that two or three of these conditions may exist together.

Neuropathy. Diabetic neuropathy has been identified as a possible cause of impotence. Stimulation of the second, third, and fourth sacral segments of the parasympathetic nerves is needed to obtain erection. There is evidence that innervation of the penis is also supplemented by sympathetic vasodilator fibers (although the sympathetic fibers primarily control ejaculation). Involvement of the parasympathetic system by diabetic neuropathy leads to failure of erection; damage to the sympathetic system interferes with ejaculation or both ejaculation and erection.[13]

There are several diabetic neuropathies rather than one single entity. The scope of

the involvement includes every system. Peripheral neuropathy and visceral neuropathy as well as direct autonomic neuropathy may occur. Pathophysiologic changes include (1) thickening of the walls of the vasa vasorum, progressing to complete occlusion; (2) mononeuropathies; (3) motor end plate alterations in juvenile diabetics; and (4) segmented demyelination of peripheral nerve fibers and of some myelin sheath.[14]

Neuropathy may be related to many factors. In the past, it was believed to be related to poor diabetic control, but it is now believed that (1) it may occur with good control; (2) it may occur simultaneously with the symptoms of uncontrolled glycosuria due to factors such as sorbitol and water accumulation in nerve fibers;[15] (3) it may be related to the severity and the duration of the diabetes; (4) it may be the initial clinical manifestation of diabetes, without symptoms of hypoglycemia and glycosuria; (5) it may occur paradoxically following initiation of good control; (6) it may follow stress situations. Moreover, neuropathy may already be present in the newly diagnosed diabetic.[16]

In a routine survey of 200 diabetic men, Ellenberg[17] found that 59 percent were impotent and 82 percent of these had evidence of neuropathy. Of the 41 percent who were potent, only 12 percent had neuropathy.

In a study involving 45 impotent diabetic men with an average age of 43.2 years, 37 had neurogenic bladder abnormalities (indicative of autonomic neuropathy), and 38 had other signs of peripheral neuropathy. All of the men had normal testosterone levels and did not respond to the therapeutic use of testosterone, indicating that the neuropathy was the significant factor in the etiology of the impotence.[18]

Vascular Aspects of Impotence. Vascular insufficiency has been implicated but not confirmed as a cause of impotence. Endarteritis affecting the vascular mechanism of erection has been suggested as a cause of impotence. Atherosclerosis and arteriosclerosis are known to occur more extensively in the diabetic than the nondiabetic. Diabetics may also develop proliferation of endothelial cells of arterioles and thickening of the basement membranes in many vascular areas (diabetic microangiopathy).[19]

Schöffling and associates found angiopathy in 20.6 percent of patients with impotence and in only 6.2 percent of those without impotence.[20] The involvement of penile blood vessels has not received wide investigation, but Koncz states that it may be possible that obliteration of the arteries of the penis or microangiopathy involving the small vessels leading to the corpora cavernosa could disrupt the blood flow needed for erection, while libido and further ability for orgasm may be retained.[21]

Endocrine Aspects of Impotence. Endocrine factors have been investigated as a cause of diabetic impotence with equivocal findings. Some report decrease in urinary steroids (17-ketosteroids) in diabetics with sexual dysfunction, but Schöffling and associates[22] found the 17-ketosteroids of impotent diabetics were elevated. However, they explained this by demonstrating that one fraction of androsterone with low effectiveness for virilization was increased, while the alpha steroid fraction, which includes testosterone, was significantly decreased. They also found that pituitary gonadotropin was reduced or absent in 28 out of a group of 30 impotent diabetics, while in 12 diabetics without potency difficulties, 20 of 26 determinations were in the normal range.[23]

In contrast to these findings, others have found that plasma testosterone levels in a group of inpotent diabetics were normal and concluded that androgen deficiency did not seem to be a causative factor[24,25] and that endocrine factors did not seem implicated.[26] Cooper[27] speculates about the role of testosterone in potency. He feels that, provided a certain minimum level exists at receptor sites, potency is not specifically dependent on testosterone, which is more concerned with fertility and anabolism. Moreover, he believes that it is more likely

that blood level of testosterone is secondary to sexual arousal and response, describing a feedback role in facilitating and/or maintaining sexual arousal and response after they are initiated by the central nervous system. Clinically, then, decreased testosterone level probably indicates sexual disinterest, rather than being the cause of it. This helps explain the generally poor results of androgen therapy for impotence. Once potency has been established in men, it does not depend on testosterone.

Histologic Findings. Faerman and associates[28] found that the morphology of interstitial tissue and the Leydig cells was normal. The most frequent finding by Schöffling and associates after biopsies of the testes of 24 diabetic men with sexual disturbances was atrophy of the tubules. The basal membranes of the canaliculi were thickened, and the number of spermatocytes was reduced. Frequently, there were no mature spermatozoa in the lumen of the tubules.[29] Physical examination of 60 male diabetics with impotence showed 14 patients with testes that were decreased in size and 39 who had testes of reduced consistency. Decreased prostate size, a fairly reliable indication of gonadal insufficiency, was also present.[30]

Psychogenic Factors. Fear of failure, with accompanying decrease in erectile strength, may operate to cause impotence, even though pathophysiologic problems are not extensive. It is possible that in the diabetic, fear of transmitting the disease to children may be an additional factor.[31] (See Chapter 3 for discussion of psychogenic impotence.)

In general, however, organic causes are implicated, rather than or in addition to psychogenic. Using penisplethysmography, Kockett[32] and associates compared sexual response of a control group and 10 diabetic men who viewed an explicit sexual film. The men had slower response and decreased amplitude and duration of erection, although they were sexually stimulated. The change in erection parameters supports an organic cause of impotence.

Retrograde Ejaculation

Retrograde ejaculation in the diabetic occurs as a result of neuropathy involving the autonomic nervous system, but it also occurs in the nondiabetic after transurethral prostate resection (see Chapter 24) and bilateral sympathectomy (see Chapter 25). In order for retrograde ejaculation to occur, the male must have maintained his libido, potency, and erectile ability. However, it can be one of the causes of sterility in the male diabetic.[33,34]

Fertility and Sterility in Male Diabetics

More attention has been paid to the unfavorable effects of diabetes on female reproduction; less has been written on its influence on male reproductive capacity. Rubin studied 198 diabetic men in relation to their reproductive histories. Of these, 168 were or had been married. One hundred sixty-eight nondiabetic married male dental patients served as a control group.[35] There was no statistical difference in the level of fertility between the diabetic and the control group, and there was no statistical difference in the incidence of sterility (defined as 2 years of cohabitation without conception) prior to age 45 for the husband and 40 for the wife.[36]

The wives of diabetic men had a significantly higher incidence of abortions than the control population. The abortion incidence before and after the clinical evidence of diabetes did not differ significantly. Moreover, offspring that were born did not significantly differ in weight than those of nondiabetic fathers, and no differences were found in incidences of premature births, stillbirths, malformation, and sex of offspring.[37]

Schöffling and associates[38] studied sperm counts, motility, and morphology in 38 diabetic men. Slight reduction in fertility was found in six patients, severe reduction in eight, and infertility in three patients. One

had complete aspermia. They questioned 500 male married diabetics of all ages regarding fertility. Wives of impotent diabetics conceived less frequently than those with normal potency. In addition, similar to the findings of Rubin, healthy wives of diabetics, particularly those with disturbed potency, had more miscarriages than did wives of healthy nondiabetic men.

Diabetes and Female Sexual Function

The same reflex neurogenic control of sex organs is present in the male and female. Consequently, the development of turgidity in the erectile tissue of the clitoris is identical with that of the penis. Krosnick and Podolsky[39] speculate that female dysfunction may be caused by neuropathy of the clitoris and vagina or inadequate vaginal lubrication because of microangiopathy of the vaginal mucosa and thickening of capillaries that would inhibit flow of secretions into the vagina.

Surprisingly, there are little data to indicate a change in sexual response in the female diabetic comparable to that experienced by the male. Ellenberg[40,41] reports there is no diminution in female libido or fulfillment of sex drive with or without presence of diabetic neuropathy. Kolodny,[42] however, reports that 44 of 125 (35.2 percent) diabetic women experienced complete orgasmic dysfunction, while only 6 of 100 nondiabetic women (6 percent) in a control group were nonorgasmic. Moreover, none of the nonorgasmic women in the control group had ever experienced orgasm, while 40 of the 44 nonorgasmic diabetic women had previously been orgasmic.

The onset of dysfunction occurred gradually, over a period of 6 months to 1 year, and in all cases followed the onset of diabetes. There was also a striking correlation between the duration of the diabetes and the frequency of sexual dysfunction. There was no significant relationship between the sexual dysfunction and other complications of diabetes. In addition, only 6 of the 44 nonorgasmic women reported difficulty with vaginal lubrication (the female equivalent of erection). Two became orgasmic after use of a water-soluble lubricant and instruction to both partners. One of two additional women became orgasmic after treatment of painful monilial vaginitis.[43]

Kolodny[44] speculates about the causes of the dysfunction, suggesting that neuropathy, increased susceptibility to infection, microvascular changes, and psychosocial adaptation to chronic illness may be implicated. Unfortunately, there is a paucity of information about changes in sexual response of female diabetics. Their problems have essentially been ignored.

Fertility and Pregnancy in Female Diabetics

Diabetic women may suffer from irregular menses and when achieving pregnancy bear larger babies than nondiabetic women.[45] Pregnancy itself may precipitate diabetes (class A diabetes), which for some women continues only through the period of gestation and is controllable by diet.[46] Many feel that pregnancy may accelerate the metabolic difficulty of diabetes, but there is less unanimity of belief regarding pregnancy's effects on neuropathy and microangiopathies. Oral contraceptives may also cause changes in metabolism that may be diabetogenic, so it has been suggested that women who develop class A (gestational) diabetes not be given oral contraceptives as a conception control method after delivery.[47]

The development of gestational diabetes does not seem to result in a significantly different perinatal mortality rate than that of the regular population. However, birth weights of babies of 38 class A mothers were higher than those of nondiabetic mothers, especially in those who were obese.[48] Most of these mothers, however, could safely be delivered at term. In contrast, women with more severe diabetes (classes B to F) may require delivery by cesarian section or induction of labor at 37 weeks of gestation. Those

whose diabetes is difficult to control may be delivered at 34 to 35 weeks.[49]

Kučera[50] investigated the rate and type of congenital anomalies of children of diabetic women from nine geographic and ethnic areas of the world compared with a control group. Although there were some variations in reporting and in classification, the findings suggest a higher incidence of anomalies in children of diabetic women. The perinatal mortality rate among fetuses of diabetic women was five to seven times that of the control population. Of particular interest was an extremely low incidence of anomalies reported in the data from the United States. However, further investigation is needed to determine which factors are responsible for anomalous development in offspring of diabetic women.[51]

Although fetal mortality rate is high, maternal mortality rate is only slightly increased in diabetics. Stillbirth or neonatal deaths have been attributed to poor diabetic control, placental insufficiency, respiratory distress syndrome, and congenital defects.[52]

Genetic Counseling

Diabetes is familial in character. Geneticists indicate that the inheritance of diabetes is a polygenic or multifactorial type, rather than a simple Mendelian dominant or recessive gene.[53] If both parents are diabetic, 60 percent of the offspring will have the disease; if one parent has diabetes and the other is a carrier, 50 percent; and if one parent has diabetes, 25 percent.[54]

Couples contemplating marriage in which one or both are diabetic should be told of the problem that may accompany reproduction so they can plan to deal beforehand with possible problems that may occur. (See Chapter 27 for discussion of genetic counseling.)

Psychosocial Effects of Diabetes

The emotional reaction to diabetes can be severe. Anxiety and fear of disability and death may adversely affect sexual function. Individuals whose disease is poorly controlled may experience continued stressful incidents of hypo- and hyperglycemia and may be chronically apprehensive.[55] Difficulty in obtaining an erection by the male or the development of orgasmic dysfunction in the female diabetic contributes to this anxiety.

Impotence may become a source of marital friction and distrust, eventually leading to separation and divorce.[56] Even if the etiology is psychologic some men may rationalize their sexual dysfunction as due to diabetes, preferring to blame it on the disease process.[57] Disturbances in the interpersonal relationship between the diabetic and the sexual partner may also occur with problem pregnancy or with difficulty in achieving conception.

Diabetes, if well controlled, should not disturb usual roles and relationships. However, if neuropathy or vascular or endocrine complications affect many systems, the diabetic individual may have to curtail or alter many sexual role activities, with subsequent threat to sexual identity.

Adolescents, in particular, may have difficulty accepting the limitations posed by the disease when these limitations seem to conflict with their sociosexual activities. Their need to restrict diet and to take insulin may cause them to feel "different" from their peers at a time when conformity is important. Body image disturbances and problems with esteem and identity may occur (see Chapter 13).

Therapy to Correct Male Sexual Dysfunction and Infertility

In spite of evidence of biologic cause of dysfunction, Fairburn[58] feels that there is a complex interaction of physical and psychologic influences and believes a modified form of sex therapy is needed with special emphasis on the couple's enjoyment of nongenital sexual activities. No matter what the etiology, control of diabetes, malnutrition, and weakness may restore potency.[59] If an endocrine basis exists, hormonal therapy is used by some, although others emphasize that once potency is established, testosterone therapy is ineffective.[60]

Schöffling[61] argues, however, that the cause of diabetic impotence is hypogonadotropic hypogonadism and treats younger diabetics by combined therapy of chorionic gonadotropin and testosterone. Diabetics over 45 years old who are less interested in fertility are given testosterone only for 2 to 24 months.

However, in most instances, the cause of diabetic sexual dysfunction appears to be neurogenic. There is yet no specific prophylaxis or therapeutic intervention, and the prognosis is poor. Surgical implantation of a silicone prosthesis to maintain erection may be an acceptable solution to some males and their sexual partners (see Chapter 3). In patients with partial impotence, a rubber band may be used at the base of the penis to help maintain erection. It serves as a tourniquet to prevent the return flow of blood and detumescence.[62] Care must be taken, however, that circulation is not interrupted for long periods.

Bourne and associates[63] have successfully used artificial insemination in a diabetic with retrograde ejaculation. The man voided immediately after ejaculating, the specimen was centrifuged and used to inseminate his wife.

If no signs of vascular, endocrine, or neuropathic damage are evident, sexual counseling is indicated. In some anxious individuals, relaxation techniques have been used[64] (see Chapter 12).

Therapy to Correct Female Sexual Dysfunction

Therapeutic interventions to obtain good diabetic control may be successful in restoring sexual function in diabetic women. Treatment of vaginal infections reduces the discomfort associated with intercourse. Sexual counseling may also be indicated for her and her sexual partner if psychogenic etiology is identified. As with the male, when the dysfunction is due to pathophysiologic changes, no effective therapy exists.[65]

NURSING IMPLICATIONS

Assessment

Biologic Factors. The sexual history is obtained, including information about fertility and pregnancies. The nurse also obtains information about the circumstances attending the onset of the sexual dysfunction and the nature of the problem and reviews the medical history and laboratory studies to determine if a differential diagnosis has been made that identified pathophysiologic changes as a cause of the dysfunction. Data about the types of medications the individual is taking are important, since diabetics may be taking antihypertensives and other drugs that have impotence as a side effect (see Chapter 30).

Psychologic Factors. It may be that the reason diabetic women have lower reported incidence of sexual dysfunction is their reluctance to bring up the topic.[66] The same reticence may exist in men, so it is important that the nurse initiate the subject and not wait for the diabetic individual to do so. The nurse is especially sensitive to psychologic factors such as feelings of sexual inferiority and poor self-esteem, fear, and anxiety.

Sociologic Factors. The nurse assesses the nature of the relationship with the sexual partner. Is the partner supportive, understanding, and knowledgeable about the diabetes and its effects? Are both aware of genetic transmission of the disease? If infertility exists or if previous pregnancies have been problematic, has the result been interpersonal friction? Has the diabetic been able to carry out usual role functions and activities?

Planning

The nurse's goals are to assist the diabetic and the sexual partner to obtain a satisfying level of sexual function and to cope with sexual changes that are irreversible as well as to increase their knowledge of the effects of diabetes on sexuality.

Intervention

Biologic Factors. If poor control of diabetes is evident, the nurse can provide diabetic and other health teaching to help the individual attain maximal health status. Referral to a physician may be indicated for necessary changes in medical management of the disease. If hormonal therapy is prescribed, the expected action of the drugs is communicated. For all diabetic individuals, explanation of the causes of the impotence and the pathophysiology that results may do much to alleviate the diabetic person's feelings of failure.

Impotence in some diabetics seems to be associated with early morning hypoglycemic reactions. Myers[67] reports that two or three Life Savers taken before sexual activity make a great difference. Of 10 patients aged 25 through 50 who complained of impotency, 8 were able to resume sexual activity after the "Life Saver therapy."

Alternate forms of sexual expression such as manual stimulation of the sexual partner can be suggested as appropriate (see Chapter 4). In the man who is not completely impotent, the rubber band and "stuffing" techniques may be helpful (see Chapter 25).

In the female, dyspareunia may result from vaginal infections and irritations, so the nurse teaches the importance of good perineal hygiene as well as the importance of adequate foreplay. If the diabetic woman still complains of a dry vagina, the nurse suggests a water-soluble lubricant. Persistent infections require referral to a physician.

Premarital genetic counseling about the effects of the disease include information about the genetic transmission of the disease; its side effects on fertility in both sexes; the increased evidence of stillborn children; and the problems related to sexuality, impotence, and orgasmic dysfunction. Often a decision for marriage has been made long before the nurse has an opportunity to do genetic counseling, so although the potential problem areas are discussed, the nurse stresses the positive aspects—that not all children are diabetic, not all diabetics develop these complications, and that the disease can be controlled. (See Chapter 27 for discussion on genetic counseling.)

In family planning, the duration and severity of the disease must be considered. Women with long-standing diabetes with vascular complications experience more difficulty with pregnancy. The IUD (intrauterine device) should be avoided because of increased incidence of infection, morbidity, mortality, and neonatal complications. Oral contraceptives are contraindicated because of increased glucose intolerance and increased cardiovascular risk.[68]

Psychologic Factors. When organic factors are identified, it is vital that the nurse communicate this to the diabetic male and female. Males have been found to benefit from the information that the problem was organic and not a reflection on their virility and manhood.[69] The nondiabetic partner is also reassured that the disability is not caused by her. Interventions to promote sexual self-esteem may be necessary for both the male and the female diabetic (see Chapter 13). If severe emotional reactions occur, referral may be necessary.

The nurse may also have to intervene to relieve guilt and depression if problems related to fertility or pregnancy surface, or if a stillborn infant or one with an anomaly is born (see Chapter 13).

Adolescent diabetics may have difficulty adjusting to the limitations imposed by the disease. Eating together is a social event and a time for establishing relationships among peers, and the dietary restrictions may seem insurmountable. Adolescents need compassionate listeners so they can verbalize their concerns. The nurse can suggest food substitutes that are permitted or, if necessary, refer the adolescent to a dietician who can construct a diet that will include some of the foods especially important to them.

Evaluation

The nurse's interventions have been effective if the following outcomes have been achieved. The diabetic and/or sexual partner can:

1. State the effects of the disease on sexual response.
2. State the importance of good diabetic control and optimal health status for optimal sexual function.
3. Describe the effects of diabetes on fertility and identify its genetic component.
4. Describe alternate forms of sexual expression when impotence exists.
5. Utilize good hygiene measures to decrease the potential for vaginal infection.
6. State that they are satisfied with their level of sexual function.
7. Identify sources of counseling when psychologic stress associated with sexual dysfunction continues.

OTHER HORMONAL DISORDERS

In addition to their direct effects on sexual function, many hormonal imbalances cause changes in body appearance and in the function of other body systems which can indirectly affect sexuality. Even if biologic sexual function is maintained, society reacts negatively to deformity and the body less than beautiful, so the individual with altered appearance may have difficulty establishing relationships.

In discussing the changes resulting from over- or underproduction of these hormones, only those sequelae that directly or indirectly affect sexuality will be described. The reader is urged to consult a textbook of endocrinology for a complete discussion of these hormones.

Anterior Pituitary Gland

The anterior pituitary gland produces seven hormones, all of which directly or indirectly affect sexual function: growth hormone (GH); corticotropin (ACTH) and melanocyte-stimulating hormones (α- and β-MSH); the gonadotropins, follicle-stimulating hormone (FSH), and luteinizing hormone (LH) [which is named interstitial cell-stimulating hormone (ICSH) in the male]; prolactin; and finally, thyroid-stimulating hormone (TSH).[70]

Growth hormone is necessary for growth of bone, viscera, and soft tissue. Corticotropin (ACTH) acts on the adrenal gland to promote synthesis of corticosteroids, mainly cortisol (hydrocortisone) and some corticosterone.[71] β-melanocyte-stimulating hormone affects skin pigmentation.[72] Under the action of follicle-stimulating hormone (FSH), the primary follicle, the ovary develops to the vesicular stage. FSH also stimulates granulosa cell proliferation, has a role in estrogen biosynthesis, and increases estrogen production. In the male, FSH increases spermatogenesis and seminiferous tubule development.[73]

LH in the female induces ovulation, stimulates estrogen production, and initiates and maintains the corpus luteum. In the male, ICSH stimulates the interstitial or Leydig cells to produce androgen, and it consequently has a secondary role in maturation of sperm and in the development of secondary sex characteristics.[74]

Blood gonadotropin levels increase after the gonad failure that results in menopause. The gonadotropin is excreted in the urine and is extracted for therapeutic use. One (Pergonal) has been used to stimulate ovulation.[75]

Chorionic gonadotropin (HCG) is produced by the human placenta and by ovarian, testicular, and uterine tumors of trophoblastic origin. It is closely related to LH and has similar function. One pregnancy test is based on the presence of HCG in urine of pregnant women. Peak levels occur about the ninth week of pregnancy, followed by low levels in midpregnancy and a second smaller peak in the third trimester. In some cases of threatened abortion, a fall in level of HCG may be warning of impending failure of the placenta.[76]

Prolactin is the lactogenic hormone whose main action is to initiate and sustain lactation, its secretion probably maintained by the stimulus of suckling.[77]

Thyroid-stimulating hormone (TSH) controls the enzymatic reactions in which iodine is trapped and converted to thyroid hormones.[78] (See Table 26-1 for effects of hormonal disorders on sexuality.)

Effect of Hypophysectomy on Sexual Function in Women. Removal of the pituitary gland may be done to control metastatic breast cancer. Schon and Sutherland[79] investigated the affects of hypophysectomy on sexual function in 20 women by interviewing them to obtain information about sexual desire, activity, and satisfaction. Another group of 30 women, 23 of whom had had mastectomy and 7 who also had had an oophorectomy were also interviewed. Neither mastectomy nor oophorectomy had a significant influence on sexual function, but hypophysectomy influenced desire, activity, and gratification. It appears that absence of the tropic pituitary hormones that activate adrenal androgens accounted for the decrease in sexual function. Although removal of the pituitary also affects the thyroid and the gonads, administration of thyroid did not cause increase in sexual function, and absence of the ovarian hormone did not necessarily influence sexual behavior.

Thyroid Gland

The thyroid gland secretes the hormones thyroxine (T_4) and triiodothyronine (T_3).[80] Thyroid hormones are essential for normal growth and development and metabolism.[81] (See Table 26-1.)

Adrenal Glands

The adrenal glands secrete glucocorticoids (principally cortisol and small amounts of corticosterone), mineral corticoids (primarily aldosterone and small amounts of deoxycor-

TABLE 26–1. SEXUALITY AND HORMONAL DISORDERS

Organ and Hormone	Effects of Increased Hormone	Effects of Decreased Hormone
Anterior Pituitary Growth hormone	Gigantism (child) acromegaly (adult) → hypogonadism, ↓ libido, impotence, gynecomastia, galactorrhea in males, infertility, ↓ frequency of menstruation in females	Dwarfism → decreased gonadotropins → partial or complete failure of sexual development
Corticotropin (ACTH) and melanocyte-stimulating hormones (β-MSH)	Cushings disease, change in body habitus (see adrenal gland)	Addison's disease (see adrenal gland)
Gonadotropins, follicle-stimulating hormone (FSH) Interstitial cell-stimulating hormone (ICSH) in the male Luteinizing hormone (LH) in the female		In men: see testes In women: see ovaries ↓ libido, atrophy of genitalia, ↓ body hair, sometimes ↓ breast size In both sexes characteristic fineness and facial skin wrinkling
Prolactin	Inappropriate lactation (galactorrhea)	↓ Milk production
Thyroid-stimulating hormone (TSH)	Hyperthyroidism (see thyroid gland)	Hypothyroidism (see thyroid gland)
Thyroid Gland	Hyperthyroidism: no direct effect but, palpitation, weight loss, fatigability, loss of hair, irritability, symptoms of anxiety, may compromise sexual function, exophthalmos → body image problems	Hypothyroidism: primary or secondary amenorrhea in younger women, menorrhagia in middle-aged women, fatigue, depression, hair loss, puffiness of face Child: cretinism, growth retardation, adult facial features, delayed puberty, changed body proportions: trunk is larger than area from symphasis pubis to ground, span is less than the height

(continued)

TABLE 26–1. *(cont.)*

Organ and Hormone	Effects of Increased Hormone	Effects of Decreased Hormone
Adrenal Gland Cortisol	Cushing's disease: obesity, striae, bruising, hirsutism, muscular weakness, amenorrhea or irregular menstruation, impotence in men, hyperpigmentation of skin	Addison's disease: increased skin pigmentation, vitiligo (patchy depigmentation, surrounded by pigmentation), loss of body hair, especially axillary and pubic in women, infertility
Androgens: Testosterone	Pseudoprecocious puberty in boys In women: virilism, hirsutism of face, chin, upper lip, between breasts, around areola, on extremities and abdomen, extension upward of pubic hair (male escutcheon), temporal hair recession, deepening of voice, skeletal muscle hypertrophy, acne, ↑ in clitoral size, oligomenorrhea or amenorrhea	Decreased libido especially in women
Testes Testosterone		In boys: delay onset of puberty, eunuchoidal signs (infantile penis, small, soft testes, fine muscles, weak muscle strength, fine body hair, immature bone age, high-pitched feminine voice) In adult men: ↓ libido, regression of secondary sex characteristics over time, loss of pubic hair, facial, body hair
Ovaries Estrogens		Primary amenorrhea: small uterus, no breast development, pubic or axillary hair growth, no menstruation, tall height Secondary amenorrhea: failure of menstruation

ticosterone), and androgens [dehydroepiandrosterone (DHA), androsterone, and testosterone]. In addition, small amounts of estrogens and progesterone are produced.[82]

Cortisol, a glucocorticoid has profound effects on inflammatory reactions; carbohydrate, protein, fat, and water metabolism; hemopoiesis; and on the immunologic, gastrointestinal, cardiovascular, skeletal, and neuromuscular systems.[83]

Infertility in women, however, may be a side effect of untreated Addison's disease although the menstrual cycle is reasonably well maintained for such a debilitating disease. Morbidity has declined since steroids were introduced, and successful pregnancy can take place if women are treated.[84]

Androgens are produced by the adrenal cortex, but also by the testes, and the ovary under stimulation from the pituitary gland. The most powerful androgen is testosterone, which is secreted mainly by the testes. In the normal female, most of the testosterone is derived from conversion of androstenedione to testosterone in the tissues. Levels rise sharply at puberty in boys and decline in old age, but in women there is little variation with age or the menstrual cycle.[85]

Loss of adrenal androgens by the female appear to adversely affect sexual functioning. Twenty-nine women with a mean age of 51 years had bilateral oophorectomy and adrenalectomy for metastatic breast cancer. They were interviewed to identify changes in sexual desire, activity, and responsiveness. Of the 17 women with some sexual desire preoperatively, 14 experienced decrease after surgery. All reduced the frequency of intercourse postoperatively, and about half stopped sexual activity entirely. Of the 12 women who were responsive during intercourse preoperatively, 11 experienced decrease postoperatively, almost all being totally unresponsive. Sexual feeling and activity declined in all but two of the women who were not already at zero levels of functioning even though they had remission of symptoms of metastatic disease.[86]

Mineral corticoids have no direct effect on sexual functioning. (See Table 26-1.)

Testes

During fetal life, the interstitial cells of the testes (Leydig cells) develop early and reach a maximum size at 14 to 16 weeks, then largely disappear by the time of birth. At puberty, interstitial cell-stimulating hormone from the pituitary causes the Leydig cells to develop and secrete androgens, especially testosterone. Under the influence of the hypothalamus, gonadotropin secretion also increases. The high concentration of androgens stimulates spermatogenesis as well as causing secondary sex changes at puberty. Follicle-stimulating hormone (FSH) is necessary for the final stages of spermatogenesis after puberty.[87] (See Table 26-1.)

Hypogonadism in the Male. The effects of testosterone deficiency depend on the age of the individual. (See Table 26-1.) Etiology of hypogonadism varies and may be due to disease, genetic abnormalities or environmental and local changes (Table 26-2).

Ovaries

The ovaries produce ova and secrete estrogens, progesterone, and androgens. These are steroid hormones that cause maturation of the female genitalia and secondary sex characteristics, as well as affecting metabolism of other body tissues.[88]

Estrogens are responsible for initiating and maintaining maturity of the genitalia and secondary sex characteristics. Along with progesterone, they are also responsible for maintenance and control of normal menstruation. Estrogen stimulates growth (although excessive amounts cause premature fusion of the epiphyses and short stature); antagonizes the effects of androgens on the skin, resulting in sebaceous gland activity; and causes deposition of subcutaneous adipose tissue, resulting in the characteristic distribution of fat in the mature female.[89]

Estrogens are used for controlling the complications of menopause. In high doses,

TABLE 26-2. ETIOLOGY OF MALE HYPOGONADISM

Diseases:	Testicular agenesis (absence of testes); bilateral torsion; orchitis (mumps) and cryptoorchidism (undescended testes); Klinefelter's syndrome.
Environmental and Local Changes:	Increased testicular temperature; varicoceles; radiation; drugs.
Mechanical Disorders:	Duct lesions; congenital absence of vas deferens; obstruction of epididymis; absence of seminal vesicles.

they are effective in treating menorrhagia, although combinations of estrogen–progesterone are preferable. Combined regimens are also effective in treating endometriosis. Secondary sex characteristics can be induced or restored in females with ovarian failure, and osteoporosis can also be decreased or avoided in women with a premenopausal oophorectomy.[90]

The main action of progesterone is preparation of the endometrium for implantation of the ova and the maintenance of pregnancy. During pregnancy, it is responsible partly for inhibition of ovulation and for further development of breasts. It is used for treatment of dysfunctional uterine bleeding, and it may be used alone or in combination with estrogen as oral contraceptives.[91]

The stoma cells of the ovary are able to synthesize different steroids than those produced by the ovarian follicle and the corpus luteum, and these appear to be androgens. A very small amount of androgens, especially androstenedione is secreted. The physiologic significance of these androgens is uncertain,[92] although they may help maintain sex drive.

Hypogonadism in the Female. Hall and associates suggest classifying hypogonadism into failure of sexual maturation (primary amenorrhea) and failure of established sexual function (secondary amenorrhea). (See Table 26-1.) Causes may be diseases, environmental or local changes (Table 26-3).

Treatment of failure of sexual maturation is directed first toward the causative condition. In other cases, when the cause is

not amenable to therapy (castration, ovarian hypoplasia, or aplasia), treatment focuses on producing normal feminization and growth. Estrogens are prescribed to produce feminization and the psychologic affects of regular menstruation, but ovulation is not possible, and the menstrual bleeding is due to estrogen withdrawal. Care is taken, if the child is small, to prevent premature fusion of the epiphyses and therefore cessation of growth.[93]

The principles of treatment of failure of established sexual function (secondary amenorrhea) are essentially the same as for primary amenorrhea, though it may not be necessary to give replacement therapy to an older woman. Therapy of secondary amenorrhea and infertility resulting from hypothalamic–pituitary dysfunction by administration of the drug clomiphene has been effective, while others are helped by administration of human gonadotropins.

Prostaglandins

Prostaglandins (PGs) are a group of neuroregulatory agents, a class of hormonelike substances compromising over 20 distinct compounds widely distributed in the body. They probably function as modulators or mediators of humoral and other stimuli to neurons. They were first isolated in the 1930s in the semen of man and sheep. Certain PGs are found diffusely throughout central nervous tissues, which are able to synthesize and metabolize distinct types of prostaglandins. In the central nervous system, their action is varied and includes effects on behavioral regulation of food intake, body temperature reg-

TABLE 26–3. ETIOLOGY OF FEMALE HYPOGONADISM

Diseases:	Congenital hypoplasia; absence of ovaries; pituitary diseases (adenomas, hemorrhage, trauma); congenital adrenal hypoplasia; ovarian tumors; diabetes; renal failure; Turner's syndrome.
Environmental and Local Changes:	Surgery; radiation; drugs (administration of androgens, steroids); obesity; malnutrition (anorexia nervosa); functional disturbance in the normal hypothalamic–pituitary–ovarian relationship.

ulation, cardioregulation, and motor functions.[94]

They also have a role in human reproduction. It is somewhat uncertain, but amniotic fluid collected during labor contains high concentrations of one, PG $F_2\alpha$, which causes uterine contractions, but fluid collected earlier contains no PG $F_2\alpha$. This prostaglandin has also been found in maternal venous blood immediately before uterine contractions in normal spontaneous labor, but not before the onset of labor. The placenta may be the source of PGs found in amniotic fluid and maternal circulation.[95] Because of the apparent activity in induction of labor, prostaglandins are being used as abortifacients (see Chapter 20). They have also been implicated as the cause of dysmenorrhea.

Liver Disease

Liver disease may cause a decrease in total plasma testosterone and an increase in sex hormone binding globulin so that free active testosterone level is decreased. Males develop hypogonadism with decreased libido, impotence. There may be feminization, gynecomastia, and change in body hair. Women have amenorrhea or oligomenorrhea, infertility, and decreased libido.[96]

NURSING IMPLICATIONS

The nursing history will elicit information about sexual dysfunction. Assessment of body image disturbances and level of sexual self-esteem should also be included (see Chapter 13). The nurse's goal is to help the patient cope with changes in appearance and function. Teaching about the medication that the individual will have to take for the rest of his/her life is essential. Intervention to alleviate body image disturbances and decreased sexual self-esteem may also be indicated.

NOTES

1. Shagan BP: Is Diabetes a Model for Aging. Med Clin North Am 60:1209–1210, 1976
2. Mills LC: Sexual disorders in the diabetic patient. In Oaks WW, Melchiode GA, Ficher I (eds): Sex and the Life Cycle. New York, Grune and Stratton, 1976, pp 163–174
3. Cooper AJ: Diagnosis and management of "endocrine impotence." Br Med J 1:34–36, 1972
4. Ibid, p 34
5. Schöffling K, Federlin K, Ditschuneit H, Pfeiffer EF: Disorders of sexual function in male diabetics. Diabetes 12:519–527, 1963
6. Rubin A, Babbitt D: Impotence in diabetes mellitus. JAMA 168:498–500, 1958
7. Ibid, p 499
8. Kolodny RC, Kahn CB, Goldstein HH, Barnett DM: Sexual dysfunction in diabetic men. Diabetes 23:306–309, 1974
9. Cooper AJ: Diagnosis and management

of "endocrine impotence," Br Med J 1:34, 1972

10. Ellenberg M: Diabetic neuropathy: Clinical aspects. Metabolism 25:1627–1655, 1976

11. Ellenberg M: Diabetes and sexual function. NY State Med J. 82:927–930, 1982

12. Koncz L, Balodimos MC: Impotence in diabetes. Med Times 98(8):159–169, 1970

13. Ibid, p 163

14. Ellenberg M: Diabetic neuropathy: Clinical aspects. Metabolism 25:1627, 1976

15. Krosnick A, Podolsky S: Diabetes and sexual dysfunction: Restoring normal ability. Geriatrics 36:92–100, 1981

16. Fraser BM, Campbell TW, Ewing DJ, Murray A, Neilson JMM, Clarke BF: Peripheral and autonomic nerve function in newly diagnosed diabetes mellitus. Diabetes 27:546–550, 1977

17. Ellenberg M: Impotence in diabetes: The neurologic factor. Ann Intern Med 75:213–218, 1971

18. Ibid, p 217

19. Koncz L, Balodimos MC: Impotence in diabetes. Med Times 98(8):167, 1970

20. Schöffling K, Federlin K, Ditschuneit H, Pfeiffer EF: Disorders of sexual function in male diabetics. Diabetes 12:520, 1963

21. Koncz L, Balodimos MC: Impotence in diabetes. Med Times 98(8):167, 1970

22. Schöffling K, Federlin K, Ditschuneit H, Pfeiffer EF: Disorders of sexual function in male diabetics. Diabetes 12:525, 1963

23. Ibid, p 522

24. Kolodny RC, Kahn CB, Goldstein HH, Barnett DM: Sexual dysfunction in diabetic men. Diabetes 23:307, 1974

25. Faerman I, Vilar O, Rivarola MA, Rosner JM, Jadzinsky MN, Fox D, Lloret AP, Bernstein-Hahn L, Saraceni D: Impotence and diabetes: Studies of androgenic function in diabetic impotent males. Diabetes 21:23–30, 1972

26. Ellenberg M: Diabetic neuropathy: Clinical aspects. Metabolism 25:1649, 1976

27. Cooper AJ: Diagnosis and management of "endocrine impotence." Br Med J 1:35, 1972

28. Faerman I, Vilar O, Rivarola MA, Rosner JM, Jadzinsky MN, Fox D, Lloret AP, Bernstein-Hahn L, Saraceni D: Impotence and diabetes: Studies of androgenic function in diabetic impotent males. Diabetes 21:23, 1972

29. Schöffling K, Federlin K, Ditschuneit H, Pfeiffer EF: Disorders of sexual function in male diabetics. Diabetes 12:523, 1963

30. Ibid, p 521

31. Koncz L, Balodimos MC: Impotence in diabetes. Med Times 98(8):168, 1970

32. Kockett G, Feil W, Ferstt R, et al: Psychophysiological aspects of male sexual inadequacy: Results of an experimental study. Am J Psych, 138:490–91, 1981

33. Kelbanow D, MacLeod J: Semen quality and certain disturbances of reproduction in diabetic men. Fertil Steril 11:255–261, 1960

34. Ellenberg M: Diabetic neuropathy: Clinical aspects. Metabolism 25:1649, 1976

35. Rubin A: The influence of diabetes mellitus in men upon reproduction. Am J Obstet Gynecol 76:25–29, 1958

36. Ibid, p 28

37. Ibid

38. Schöffling K, Federlin K, Ditschuneit H, Pfeiffer EF: Disorders of sexual function in male diabetics. Diabetes 12:521, 1963

39. Krosnick A, Podolsky S: Diabetes and sexual dysfunction: Restoring normal ability. Geriatrics 36:95, 1981

40. Ellenberg M: Diabetic neuropathy: Clinical aspects. Metabolism 25:1650, 1976

41. Ellenberg M: Diabetes and sexual dysfunction. NY State Med J 82:929, 1982

42. Kolodny RC: Sexual dysfunction in diabetic females. Diabetes 20:557–559, 1971

43. Ibid, p 558

44. Ibid, p 559

45. Mills LC: Sexual disorders in the diabetic patient. In Oaks WW, Melchiode GA,

Ficher I (eds): Sex and the Life Cycle. New York, Grune and Stratton, 1976, p 171

46. Tyson JE: Obstetrical management of the pregnant diabetic. Med Clin North Am 55:961–963, 1971

47. Tyson JE, Felig P: Medical aspects of diabetes in pregnancy and the diabetogenic effects of oral contraceptives. Med Clin North Am 55:947–959, 1971

48. Posner NA, Silverstone FA, Pomerance W, Weiss H, Weinstein H: The outcome of pregnancy in class A diabetes mellitus. Am J Obstet Gynecol 111:886–895, 1971

49. Shea MA, Garrison DL, Tom SK: Diabetes in pregnancy. Am J Obstet Gynecol 111:801–803, 1971

50. Kučera J: Rate and type of congenital anomalies among offspring of diabetic women. J Reprod Med 7:66–64, 1971

51. Ibid, p 63

52. Hall R, Anderson J, Smart GA, Besser GM: Clinical Endocrinology, 2nd ed. Philadelphia, Lippincott, 1974, p 352

53. Ibid, p 316

54. Mills LC: Sexual disorders in the diabetic patient. In Oaks WW, Melchiode GA, Ficher I (eds): Sex and the Life Cycle, New York, Grune and Stratton, 1976, p 172

55. Shafer KN, Sawyer JR, McCluskey AM, Beck EL, Phipps WJ: Medical-Surgical Nursing. St. Louis, Mosby, 1975, p 748

56. Ellenberg M: Diabetic neuropathy: Clinical aspects. Metabolism 25:1650, 1976

57. Cooper AJ: Diagnosis and management of "endocrine impotence." Br Med J 1:36, 1972

58. Fairburn C: The sexual problems of diabetic men. Brit J Hosp Med 25:487, 489–491, 1981

59. Ellenberg M: Diabetic neuropathy: Clinical aspects. Metabolism 25:1650, 1976

60. Teter J: Treatment of endocrine impotence. Br Med J 4:114, 1972

61. Schöffling K, Federlin K, Ditschuneit H,

Pfeiffer EF: Disorders of sexual function in male diabetics. Diabetes 12:525, 1963

62. Ellenberg M: Impotence in diabetes: The neurologic factor. Ann Intern Med 75:218, 1971

63. Bourne RB, Kretzchmar WA, Esser JH: Successful artificial insemination in a diabetic with retrograde ejaculation. Fertil Steril 22:275–277, 1971

64. Cooper AJ: Diagnosis and management of "endocrine impotence." Br Med J 1:36, 1972

65. Kolodny RC, Kahn CB, Goldstein HH, Barnett DM: Sexual dysfunction in diabetic men. Diabetes 23:309, 1974

66. Ellenberg M: Diabetic neuropathy: Clinical Aspects. Metabolism 25:1650, 1976

67. Myers SA: Diabetes management by the patient and a nurse practitioner. Nurs Clin North Am 12:415–426, 1977

68. Van Son A: Diabetes and Patient Education: A Daily Nursing Challenge. New York, Appleton-Century-Crofts, 1982

69. Ellenberg M: Diabetic neuropathy: Clinical Aspects. Metabolism 25:1650, 1976

70. Hall R, Anderson J, Smart GA, Besser GM: Clinical Endocrinology, 2nd ed. Philadelphia, Lippincott, 1974, p 4

71. Ibid, p 12

72. Ibid, p 13

73. Ibid, p 18

74. Ibid

75. Ibid

76. Ibid

77. Ibid, p 11

78. Ibid, p 71

79. Schon M, Sutherland AM: Changes in female sexuality after hypophysectomy. J Clin Endocrinol Metab 20:833–841, 1970

80. Hall R, Anderson J, Smart GA, Besser GM: Clinical Endocrinology, 2nd ed. Philadelphia, Lippincott, 1974, p 100

81. Ibid, p 101

82. Ibid, p 139

83. Ibid, p 147

84. Khunda S: Pregnancy and Addison's disease. Obstet Gynecol 39:431–433, 1972

85. Hall R, Anderson J, Smart GA, Besser GM: Clinical Endocrinology, 2nd ed. Philadelphia, Lippincott, 1974, p 208

86. Waxenberg SE, Drellich MG, Sutherland AM: Changes in female sexuality after adrenalectomy. J Clin Endocrinol Metab 19:193–202, 1959

87. Hall R, Anderson J, Smart GA, Besser GM: Clinical Endocrinology, 2nd ed. Philadelphia, Lippincott, 1974, p 245

88. Ibid, p 181

89. Ibid, p 183

90. Ibid, p 185

91. Ibid, p 186

92. Ibid, p 187

93. Ibid, p 196

94. Gross HA, Fieve R: Prostaglandins. In Sacher EJ: Hormone Behavior and Psychopathology. New York, Raven, 1976, pp 159–160

95. Hall R, Anderson J, Smart GA, Besser GM: Clinical Endocrinology, 2nd ed. Philadelphia, Lippincott, 1974, p 237

96. Myerscough PR: Sexual function in illness. Clin Obstet Gynecol 7:387–400, 1980

Chapter 27

Impaired Cardiovascular-Pulmonary Function

Although most disorders of the cardiovascular and pulmonary systems do not directly compromise the sexual response cycle, their psychosocial sequelae may drastically alter sexual activity, roles, and relationships. Cardiovascular disease is the major cause of death and disability in the world, yet relatively little information exists in the literature providing specific guidelines for health professionals and patients with these disorders to help them make rational decisions about sexual behavior.

The major focus of this chapter will be on the sexual problems of cardiac patients and especially those who have had myocardial infarction. However, problems affecting sexuality that accompany other vascular diseases, sickle-cell anemia, and chronic obstructive pulmonary disease will also be presented.

MYOCARDIAL INFARCTION

In fiction, the heart is closely related to love, feelings of affection, tenderness, and passion or, conversely, with feelings of rejection and sorrow ("I'm heartbroken; you broke my heart"). Pragmatically, the heart is simply a pump whose function is to oxygenate the tissues of the body, but any change in its function, more than change in any other organ, brings fear of death, anxiety about the future, and often, unnecessary restriction of sexual activity.

Physiologic Responses to Coitus in Health

Masters and Johnson[1] have reported the changes in pulse, respiration, and blood pressure during coitus. These measurements were obtained from healthy subjects during orgasm and the period immediately preceding it and indicated marked heart rate, blood pressure and respiratory elevations, followed in a few seconds by return to normal levels. (See Chapter 3.)

However, even in well individuals, the physiologic reactions during intercourse may vary in intensity from mild to extreme. In some individuals, muscle spasm and change in vital signs may be minimal. In others, the reactions are intense, and orgasm may be accompanied by muscle spasms, shudders, moaning, dizziness, and fainting.[2]

Position for coitus influences cardiovascular response. One group of investigators has shown that cardiac output is greater by 2.2 liters per minute in the supine than in the sitting position. They also indicate that the atrioventricular oxygen difference is greater in the sitting position. These same physiologic changes occur not only in heterosexual intercourse, but also during masturbation and homosexual activity.[3]

449

Oliven[4] points out that these changes are greater than those that accompany other physical exercise for several reasons. An intense orgasm represents a tremendous autonomic response, and this, along with the sexually induced emotional stress, results in overproduction or rapid release from storage of catecholamines, which are potentially cardiotoxic. They increase the heart rate by direct myocardial stimulation and increase peripheral vascular resistance, with resultant increase in blood pressure. (There is also release of adrenocortical steroids during orgasm. These are not released during the stimulation of physical stress.) These physiologic responses, and especially the increased heart rate, result in increased demand for oxygen by the myocardium. In the individual with inadequate perfusion to the myocardium because of occluded coronary vessels, this oxygen demand cannot be met, and anginal pain may result.

Physiologic Responses to Coitus in Heart Disease

Little quantitative research had been done on the effects of sexual activity in the individual with heart damage until the research of Hellerstein and Friedman[5] of Case Western Reserve University. Their study involved 91 participants in a physical fitness evaluation program. The subjects were white, middle-aged, middle and upper class predominately Jewish business and professional men. Fifty-eight of the men had had an acute myocardial infarction three or more months previously. Forty-three had never had a heart attack, but were identified as coronary prone by evidence of high serum cholesterol, hypertension, obesity, smoking, and sedentary life style.

In addition to a detailed cardiovascular history, physical examination, and psychologic evaluation, each subject's electrocardiogram was monitored continuously for 24 to 48 hours by means of a Holter monitor. Heart rate changes and electrocardiogram changes associated with sexual activity were compared with those occurring during other activities in the 24- to 48-hour monitoring period. These heart rates were then compared to those obtained during bicycle ergometer exercise performed within several weeks of the study.[6]

Objective Data. Fourteen postcoronary patients had sexual intercourse while being monitored. The mean maximal heart rate corresponding to the orgasmic phase was 117.4 (range 90 to 144), with the average heartbeat for the 2 minutes before and 2 minutes after orgasm being 97.5 (range 85.0 to 102.2). The mean maximal heart rate during usual work (walking, climbing stairs, and doing paper work) was 120.1 (range 101 to 130). Of the 14 patients on the monitor, 6 had a maximum heart rate during sexual activity of 110 and at work of 120.[7] Symptomatic evidence gathered by Kavanagh and Shephard[8] also supports this evidence that the peak pulse rate of a middle-aged man during sexual activity is unlikely to be much higher than 120 beats per minute.

Electrocardiogram changes were noted during sexual activity. Four men had ST-T depression (three showing similar changes during work), three had ectopic heartbeats. During work, four had ST-T changes and five patients had ectopic heartbeats.

Subjective Data. Eighteen of 43 subjects (41.9 percent) with arteriosclerotic heart disease reported that they experienced symptoms during sexual activity; the most common was awareness of a rapid heart rate. This was accompanied by angina pectoris in four subjects. Nine additional subjects also experienced angina. Symptoms appeared more commonly during the resolution phase of the sexual response cycle but in most cases were not severe enough to cause curtailment of sexual activity.[9]

Summary. The monitoring showed that the physiologic cost of sexual activity was relatively low. The oxygen uptake was one-half that which occurred during a Masters two-step test. The oxygen intake equivalent to the maximal heart rate during intercourse was equal to that recorded for climbing a flight of stairs or walking briskly. Hellerstein and Friedman[10] concluded that the cardiovascular responses during coitus and normal occupational activities were comparable in frequency and severity.

Coital Death. Coital death has been celebrated in the literature and discussed by the lay public. Statistics about coital death are difficult to gather, since physicians may hesitate to ask the surviving spouse, and if death occurred during extramarital activity, the surviving partner will probably give little information.[11] To obtain objective data, a Japanese pathologist performed autopsies on 5559 cases of sudden death over a 4-year period. He found that only 34 of these had died during sexual intercourse. Twenty-five died in their hotel rooms and another five outside their homes. In most cases, the sexual relationship was extramarital and the men were an average of 20 years older than their female partner. The women who died were 3 years younger than their sexual partners. Three deaths occurred during masturbation, and most of the individuals who died had a history of serious heart damage.[12]

It is documented that acute coronary insufficiency may result from coitus, but the causal relationship, if it exists, is still a matter of conjecture. Some physicians believe that coitus may aggravate a condition or accelerate the evolution of the disease. In addition to the physical exertion that may be involved in coitus, the emotional stress may be excessive for a particular individual.[13] These factors increase the cardiac work load and may tax the already diseased heart.[14] Coitus in unfamiliar surroundings with a strange and perhaps younger partner appears to be more stressful for the coronary prone individual than coitus with a spouse in the usual locale, and under the usual circumstances.

Significance of Findings for Sexual Activity. Contrary to the popular conceptions of sexual activity gleaned from articles, movies, and fiction, sexual activity in middle-aged men is not excessive when compared with other physical activities.[15] This factor is significant in terms of the workload placed on the heart.

Although the heart rate is a crucial determination of myocardial oxygen demand, the duration of the increased heart rate is also important.[16] The average middle-aged man engaging in sexual activity two times a week expends a minimal amount of time, less than 0.3 percent of his leisure time. Hellerstein and Friedman[17] found the average time for achieving maximum heart rate after retiring to bed was 16.3 minutes (range 10 to 30 minutes). Seventy-four percent of the men averaged less than 10 minutes from beginning of intromission to male orgasm. If a cardiac patient can walk a treadmill at 3 to 4 miles per hour, climb stairs or pass a Masters test without undue strain, he is above the work requirement time of sexual activity.[18]

Larsen[19] and associates also determined that the response to sexual activity can be predicted by monitoring the response to stair climbing. A small sample of nine men without heart disease and eight with coronary artery disease (CAD) had ambulatory ECG monitored with a Holter monitor, measurement of blood pressure and heart rate at home. Measurements were done at rest, intromission, orgasm, and selected intervals after orgasm. Any position could be used for intercourse. The heart rate response to stair climbing and sexual activity was similar in both groups, although the subjects with CAD had a lower heart rate than the normal for both activities. The findings support use of a two-flight stair climbing test: 10 minutes of rapid walking followed by a climb of two flights of stairs in 10 seconds as a physiologic test of readiness to resume sexual activity. Satterfield[20] disagrees with this conclusion, stating that equivalency of the two activities is a myth. However, he does not present evidence to support the arguments.

Metabolic equivalent or METS (one MET is the energy expenditure per kilogram of body weight per minute of an average individual at rest) have been used in comparing cardiovascular cost of sexual activity with that of other activities. The average man who has recovered from an uncomplicated myocardial infarction has a maximum capacity of 8 to 9 METS. Five METS is the activity during coitus, 3.7 METS during the pre- and postorgasm time.[21] Sexual activity should not be contraindicated.

Hellerstein and Friedman recognized that differences existed between the heart rate response of their study subjects and that of other subjects who had greater increments in heart rate during coitus. They attributed these differences to differences in their subjects. They were older, had been married longer, and had heart disease. In addition, the locale of the sexual act, in the privacy of the home, and the mode of monitoring, which was indirect rather than by human or photographic observation, would tend to be less stressful than other types of data gathering.[22]

Considerations in Counseling

In spite of the limitations of this study, investigators indicate that most individuals who had had a myocardial infarction can tolerate sexual activity after consideration of several factors—the general health of the patient, the extent of recovery from the coronary attack, the physical activity level, fatigue threshold, the physiologic costs of sexual activity, emotional characteristics and involvement in sexual activity, and most important, the extent of precoronary activity. The last factor is important, since there are great variations in what may be considered normal and optimal activity between individuals.

However, not all patients can resume sexual activity. Patients with congestive heart failure or a general debilitated condition are advised to avoid strenuous physical activity, including sexual activity, until heart failure is controlled and rehabilitation has taken place.[23]

The effect of sexual activity on the younger coronary patient, who may engage in more vigorous and prolonged coitus has

not been investigated, so that no judgments can be made about their responses.

Unfortunately, despite findings that indicate that sexual activity can be resumed, this may not be the case for many coronary patients, and changes in sexual activity patterns are found due to fear, lack of information, or misinformation.

Changes in Sexual Activity Patterns

Male Patterns. All too often the return to sexual relationships is left to the judgment of the sexual partners. Two-thirds of patients who have had myocardial infarction received no advice from the physician, while the other one-third received advice that was vague with few specific guidelines.[24] Lacking specific information, the patient and the sexual partner must make their own decisions. Other patients may hesitate to ask for advice because of fear of restrictions,[25] while a third group of patients may be fearful of sexual relations despite assurances that it is medically permissible.

The most common misconceptions of the coronary patient are the beliefs that mild exertion kills, that sexual intercourse should never again be attempted, and that repeat infarctions tend to occur at orgasm.[26]

Fear may result not only in decreased sexual interest and frequency of coitus, but also impotence or paradoxically in some cases, hypersexuality. In some, fear response may become a phobia.[27] In others, anxiety may exist at a preconscious level for years.[28]

Studies of cardiac patients demonstrate that the sequelae in terms of sexual behavior include significant decrease in frequency or complete abstinence from sexual activity for as long as 4 years postinfarction.[29–31] Reasons given for change are impotence, apprehension of the patient or of the wife, loss of desire or a combination of these factors.

Hellerstein and Friedman[32] found that sexual activity decreased with age in 227 male subjects with coronary artery disease and even more so after a myocardial infarct.

After the heart attack, the resumption of sexual activity was influenced by symptoms. In the total group, the mean interval before resumption of sexual activity was 13.7 weeks, in those with symptoms, 16.4 weeks, and in the asymptomatic group, 11.7 weeks.[33]

Resumption of sexual activity was also influenced by sexual drive and occurred earlier in the subjects who were more sexually active before the coronary infarct. The overall frequency of orgasm per week also decreased in 20 of 48 subjects with arteriosclerotic heart disease (ASHD) from 2.1 1 year before the attack to 1.6 at 6 months after the attack. Decreased frequency of orgasm was attributed to change in sexual desire (11 subjects), wife's decision (7 subjects), feelings of depression (6 subjects), fears (5 subjects), symptoms of coronary disease (6 subjects). No subjects reported impotence as a problem.[34] In contrast to these findings, Weiss and English[35] found that 10 of 31 coronary subjects identified impotence as the most prevalent problem.

In a later study, questionnaires on sexual activity were completed by 161 patients attending an exercise-centered rehabilitation program an average of 3 years after myocardial infarction. In almost half the group (80), activity was unchanged or increased compared to the preinfarction period. In the remaining 81, sexual activity was reduced. Most (121 of 161) had made no change in patterns of foreplay or positions during coitus. Of the group reporting a change, 29 of those with reduced sexual activity had adopted a more passive position. Most patients (135 of 161) found intercourse as enjoyable as before infarction.[36]

Patients who develop complications during hospitalization appear to return to sexual activity more slowly. Kushnir and associates[37] investigated the effects of primary ventricular fibrillation on driving, return to work, and on resumption of sexual activity of 32 patients, comparing them to 95 patients whose myocardial infarction was less complicated. The patients were initially more slowly rehabilitated than the control group, but ultimately it did not affect either the return to work, driving, or resumption of normal sexual activity.

When sexual activity decreases, psychologic factors seem primarily implicated. In a sample of 88 male and 12 female postcoronary patients, Bloch and associates[38] found that in spite of high physical fitness, some patients had halted sexual activity, while others with poor fitness but less anxiety had frequent intercourse. Fear and apprehension can achieve more damage to sexual life than a blocked coronary vessel.

Female Patterns. Unfortunately, research has focused on changes in sexual activity of the male patient with little attention paid to the female. This may be due to the fact that female coronary patients are in an age group where sexual activity is supposedly less (postmenopause), at least by traditional beliefs.[39] With the increasing evidence that women are and can be sexually active postmenopause (Chapter 18), and with indications that they are taking a more active role during coitus, much more research is needed to identify their responses to cardiac disease.

Abramov[40] studied the sexual life of 100 female patients aged 40 to 60 with acute myocardial infarction. In comparison with a control group of 100 female patients of the same age, sexual frigidity and dissatisfaction were found among 65 percent of the coronary patients as compared with 24 percent of the controls. However, this frigidity existed for many years preinfarction and was not a sequela to heart disease. Interestingly, the author feels that frigidity may be an important part of the coronary profile.

Masturbation and the Coronary Patient

Wagner[41] indicates that masturbation in the hospital can be seen as a positive event for many patients from the point of view of a continuing sex life. Masturbation has advantages over coitus for the resumption of sexual activity, but it has not been studied or discussed. Masters and Johnson do not provide explicit data on the cardiac cost of masturbation. In addition to the possibility of lessened cardiac cost, there is not the concern about the interpersonal interaction attendant with the resumption of coitus with a former partner.

In a study by the University of Washington School of Medicine, the cardiac cost of masturbation was measured. In ten young males, it was found that at the time of orgasm by masturbation, the heart rate does not go above 130, and it rises to the 110 to 130 level for only brief moments. This is in contrast to a cardiac rate of up to 180 for coital activity of individuals in this same age and health group.[42]

Watts[43] stresses the advantage of masturbation for reentrance into sexual activity. Masturbatory activities, ranging from partial erections to full tumescence and ejaculatory release, are controlled by the patient. The development of a full erection is visible proof that masculinity is intact prior to resumption of more stressful coitus.

Effects of Drugs on Male Response

Some drugs prescribed for cardiac patients have adverse effects on male sexual response by impairing the libido or the erectile and orgasmic phases of sexual responses. Antihypertensive agents such as reserpine, methyldopa, propranolol, and guanethidine may cause difficulty. Excessive alcohol consumption may also interfere with male sexual function. (See Chapter 30 for detailed discussion of pharmacologic agents.)

Psychologic Factors

Denial, anxiety, fear, and depression are frequent responses to heart attack.[44] Other responses identified include decreased resumption of responsibility, neuroticism, and general deterioration in quality of life.[45] Lowered self-esteem, hypochondriasis, hysteria, and psychasthenia have also been reported in proportion to the severity of ar-

teriosclerotic heart disease.[46] These responses begin in the hospital and result from a combination of the threat to self, the heart disease, and the effects of environmental and iatrogenic factors.

Effects of Hospitalization. Problems begin in the hospital. The patient is connected to cardiac monitors, watched closely by nurses, and restricted in many of the usual activities of daily living. Some can comply with this regimen, but others are unable to do so. Threat to life and uncertainty of the future may produce anxiety, fear, and depression. In order to cope, some patients may need to deny the seriousness of the threat. In one psychologic evaluation of 50 hospitalized male coronary patients 30 to 50 years old, nurses consistently described them as overly cheerful, jovial, manic, flirtatious, and seductive; their conversation frequently centering on their masculine attractiveness.[47] Depression can be especially deleterious to sexual response. The depressed patient lacks the energy or motivation to think about or participate in sexual activity[48] (see Chapter 29).

Changes in Sexual Self-Esteem and Identity. In many patients, the heart muscle has healed, but the trauma of the experience is so great the individual is not able to function. To many males, cardiac damage means loss of courage, love and manliness. The heart attack portends dependency, incapacity, and inactivity,[49] with resulting threat to sexual self-esteem and identity. Fear of sexual inadequacy or of impotence may lead to aggressive sexual behavior (see Chapter 14). This behavior may be especially prevalent in 50- to 60-year-old male patients and may be related to the crisis that men in their 50s experience. There is conflict from youth orientation, which values autonomy, virility, and external achievement to the more passive activities of later years (see Chapter 17). It is possible that the heart attack intensifies the man's need to prove he is still virile.[50]

Cardiac patients may also see themselves as less effective spouses, parents, and workers. If the damaged self-concept does not improve, the individual may become a cardiac cripple, frightened to return to work, leisure activities, sex, and society.[51] Sexual activities are also affected; with poor self-esteem comes fear of sexual performance and "spectatoring" about sexual capabilities.[52]

Body Image Disturbances. To the lay person, the heart may be considered the body's hub and the lifeline with all the other organs functioning around it and because of it. When infarction occurs, there is no chance for the individual to prepare for altered function, since the heart attack occurs suddenly. Although there is no physically visible change in the body, barring the development of congestive heart failure and edema, the knowledge that the heart is damaged may cause severe body image disturbance. A view of the body as damaged may cause the individual to unnecessarily restrict activities and to view himself/herself as less than the person he/she was before.[53]

Sociologic Factors

The interaction with the spouse, family, friends, and employer may all affect sexual self-esteem and identity. The patient may be seen as unable or incompetent to perform usual activities and may be relegated to a more dependent position.

Iatrogenic factors may also operate. Inadequate, misinterpreted, or forgotten communication between the physician and the patient may cause anxiety in the patient and unwillingness to return to normal activity. Communication may be particularly difficult if the patient is from a different sociocultural background. Insufficient and vague information given about sexual activity,[54] plus the physician's reluctance to let the individual return to full physical activity may compound the problems. The response of cardiac patients' wives has been studied. Many fear for their partner's health and avoid sexual activity. They may also be overprotective or resistive to sexual overtures, leading to mar-ital disharmony that may be more destructive to the relationship than the disease process.[55,56]

Papadopoulos[57] and associates found that wives often receive little information. One hundred wives were interviewed at home; all were concerned about sexual activity, especially of coital heart attack. Forty-five of the 100 had received some information, but only 6 were given information by the physician. Ninety-two stated that they would have liked sex teaching with their husbands. Paradoxically, however, wives who did receive instruction had greater fear than those who did not. The investigators concluded that an important variable that influenced return to sexual activity was the quality of the relationship before the coronary event.

Spouses must be flexible so they can adapt to changing relationships and overcome sex role stereotypes.[58] They may be counseled to take a more active role in sexual activity, which in itself may be threatening to someone who views himself/herself as a passive recipient of sexual attention.

Many patients can return to pre-illness occupations, but others cannot, because the potential of sudden death causes risk to the public. Some individuals are uneager to return to work because physical and/or emotional stresses cause cardiovascular symptoms or because of fear of these symptoms. Others, even when eager to return, are restricted because of employer or union biases.[59]

Rehabilitation for Sexual Functioning

It must be recognized that the physiologic complications of coronary artery disease may be a significant barrier to rehabilitation and full recovery. The patient with congestive heart failure or one who experiences shortness of breath with minimal to mild exertion may not be able to maintain the same functional level as one whose heart function is not severely compromised.[60] However, the prolonged depression and continued sick role behavior can be prevented by proper education, which can override the worry about recurring myocardial infarct and minimize the mythology about heart disease.[61]

Although patients seldom initiate discussion of sex,[62] it is on the minds of many coronary patients from the onset of illness, so its discussion should be initiated as soon as the patient's condition has stabilized. Blue collar patients, particularly, ask few questions about planning for convalescence and rehabilitation, so the responsibility for bringing up the topic of sexuality rests with the health professional.[63] In addition, most physicians give general advice, shifting the decision to their patients. This is especially difficult for patients who are looking for rules to follow.[64]

Cardiac Fitness Programs. In order to pursue sexual activity safely, the heart must be trained to tolerate a specific workload. A physically fit individual can perform a given level of work at a lower heart rate and a lower systolic blood pressure than the unfit. Sexual activity is favorably influenced by enhancement of fitness by systematic physical training.

Stein[65] reports that after a physical fitness program consisting of individual 40-minute sessions 3 times a week for 16 weeks, cardiovascular fitness of 16 men, 12 to 14 weeks after a first attack, improved significantly. In addition, a physical fitness program improves blood pressure at rest and during exercise, aerobic capacity, serum cholesterol level, mood, and the frequency and quality of sexual activity.[66]

How does fitness training help cardiac function? It is believed that exercise results in changes in skeletal musculature, nervous control of the heart, and stroke volume and decreased catecholamine uptake by the trained heart. Contrary to popular belief, it is rare that improved cardiac function results from grossly visible changes in coronary circulation per se.[67] Prescription of activity is done by the physician, and a supervised exercise program can be begun for many patients while still in the coronary care unit. The activity begins with passive range of motion and progresses to ambulation.[68] After discharge and before an initiation of a fitness program, the patient's activity tolerance is assessed by the Masters two-step bicycle ergometry or treadmill. During and after testing, the patient is watched for exercise-induced S-T segment depression, conduction or rhythm disorders, chest symptoms during the stress of exercise, and quantitative patient tolerance for exercise.[69] Exercise testing has additional benefits. In addition to identifying the degree of cardiac impairment, active exercise has the effect of reducing the fear of physical activity harbored by many patients.[70]

Most individuals with known coronary artery disease are at least 2 months postinfarct before starting a long-range conditioning program, but walking can be started earlier and is extremely beneficial. The patient is taught to check the radial or carotid pulse and to limit walking to that producing a pulse rate of less than 120 per minute. They are instructed to wait at least 2 hours after meals, to avoid walking in extreme weather, and to stop if chest pain occurs.[71]

Johnston and associates[72] also found that 87 cardiac patients who took part in an exercise program had a greater frequency of coital activity than those who did not. They speculated that the more frequent sexual activity may be related to a positive self-concept derived from such programs.

NURSING IMPLICATIONS

Cardiac patients and their sexual partners have many questions about sexual activity but often are too embarrassed to ask. They have concerns about coitus, how soon and how often. They wonder about the danger of the exertion required for activity and about the effects of the drugs they take. They are concerned about their sexual partner's reaction to the problem and how to talk together about the subject of sex.[73] The nurse who is caring for the patient is in an ideal position to provide sexual teaching and counseling in the coronary care unit, the convalescent division, or the outpatient setting, since individuals find it easier to discuss sexuality with someone who is familiar.[74] Counseling begins as soon as the patient is admitted to the coronary unit, when he/she is told that most individuals are able to resume usual or modified activities after convalescence. Sexual activity is included in the activities listed by the nurse.[75]

Assessment

The physician should give the patient and sexual partner specific instructions regarding resumption of sexual activity. The nurse identifies what the patient has been told and, if the patient does not recall any specific instructions or is unclear about the details, contacts the physician to clarify or obtain information.

Biologic Data. Before sexual counseling is begun, the nurse determines the physical status of the patient. This includes the individual's general health and tolerance for physical activity before the infarction, the extent of cardiac damage, the frequency and severity of angina and/or arrhythmias, and the individual's ability to tolerate progressive activity.[76] The nurse also collects information about the patterns of sexual activity before the coronary—problems that existed, positions used, usual time of day, coital frequency, and duration. If the nurse is following the patient in the home or other outpatient setting after discharge, she/he collects data about postinfarction sexual activity, its frequency and quality and the occurrence of tachycardia, shortness of breath, angina, or other adverse symptomotology. Medications used and other disease conditions that affect sexual functions are also identified.

The nurse also assesses the patient's level of knowledge about the physiology of sexual response as it relates to the heart,[77] since anxiety based on myths and misinformation may further compromise sexual function. A stress test (treadmill or Master's two-step) may provide more information.[78]

Psychologic Data. The nurse identifies the presence of anxiety, the fears, and the concerns of both the patient and the sexual partner that may severely compromise sexual rehabilitation and cause an anxiety–impotence response. Assessment of levels of depression, body image disturbance, and change in self-image are also indicated (see Chapter 13).

Sociologic Data. The nurse identifies whether the cardiac patient has been able to assume usual roles and relationships and whether the sexual partner is understanding of changes that are necessary and willing to aid in the patient's resumption of permitted role tasks. Is the partner supportive of the patient without being overly protective? Will the patient be able to return to the former occupation, or has the patient already done so? What changes will be necessary? What anxiety does the sexual partner have about the patient's recovery?

Planning

The nurse's goals are to help the individual return to pre-illness levels of sexual activity or to adapt to necessary changes in sexual expression. When changes in body image and sexual self-esteem are identified, the nurse plans intervention in these areas while at the same time identifying when referral to other health professionals is needed to promote psychosocial and physiologic rehabilitation. At all times the goal is to facilitate communication between the sexual partners to help them arrive at a personal choice in regard to sexual activity and a life style that is satisfying for them.

Intervention

Biologic Factors. The nurse teaches about the effects of coitus on the cardiovascular system, giving information about possible alterations that will be needed in the pattern of sexual expression. This information is given in a clear, direct manner. The time when resumption of sexual activity is safe may be uppermost on some patients' minds. Based on physiologic research, intercourse should not be hazardous when the individual is able to climb two flights of stairs and walk several blocks at a brisk pace.[79] However, some changes in technique of coitus and avoidance of certain high-risk situations may be indicated.

Techniques of Coitus. Positions that impose less strain on the male patient can be suggested, although there is not unanimity of agreement about preferred positions. Some believe that physiologically, the male supine (inferior) position has the advantage of requiring slightly less oxygen consumption,[80] since the male superior position may cause sustained isometric arm and shoulder muscle contraction. If this occurs, blood pressure changes may be elevated in central aortic pressure or left ventricular afterload, which is important in determining myocardial oxygen consumption. Marked increases may cause angina, myocardial infarction, and serious or fatal arrhythmias. Because of the adverse effects of isometric exercise, coronary patients are cautioned against lifting heavy objects. For the same reasons, male patients should adopt coital positions that do not necessitate use of the arms for sustained periods.[81] Sexual intercourse in the male inferior position is also less demanding if the sexual partner kneels so he does not have to bear her full weight.[82]

A more recent study reports no significant difference in cuff and central aortic blood pressure between positions using sustained isometric arm and shoulder muscle contraction and those that do not use isometric exercise.[83] If questions about appropriate positions exist, the nurse consults with the patient's physician to determine if use of a specific position is contraindicated for the particular individual. Moreover, if anxiety results with assumption of a new coital position, less cardiac stress may be experienced by continuation of familiar positions.

Other positions that appear to require less cardiac work include rear entry and side-by-side in the face-to-face position. The cardiac patient can also sit on a wide, low, armless chair with feet resting supported or on the ground. The partner sits on his lap, facing him with her feet also on the ground.

For female cardiac patients, the male superior, female superior, and side-by-side positions do not cause isometric muscle contraction, so the question of coital positions is not so crucial as for males.[84] (See Chapter 4 for drawings of coital positions.)

Foreplay is especially important for the cardiac patient, since it serves as a form of "warm-up," facilitates neural pathways, and reflexly helps to reduce or close down the visceral vascular bed. This reduces the workload on the heart during intercourse.[85]

Environment and Atmosphere. Coitus should be resumed in usual surroundings, since a strange environment places more stress on the heart. Extremes of room temperatures, especially a hot or humid atmosphere[86] and hot or cold showers or baths produce physiologic stress and should be avoided.

Emotional stress, tension, and fear have negative effects by causing increased workload on the heart and circulatory system. Coitus should take place in a gentle, relaxed atmosphere. The nurse instructs the cardiac patient to avoid sexual relations under furtive and anxious conditions that may involve guilt, time restrictions, and a younger sexual partner or one toward whom there is resentment (coitus with a prostitute or an extramarital liaison, for example).

Hazardous Situations. The patient is cautioned to wait 3 hours after eating a heavy meal or drinking an excessive amount of alcohol. Alcohol tends to dilate vessels and increase the heart rate.[87]

Fatigue is hazardous. Sex is activity, and the workload may be excessive. The ear-

TABLE 27–1. REGIMEN FOR RESUMPTION OF COITUS

1. Week 3 postinfarct: hall walking 2–3 times a day, masturbation to partial erection; contraindications: faintness, dyspnea, diaphoresis, tachycardia.
2. Weeks 4–6 posthospital: continue earlier activity, add 3 times a week for 20 minutes, pleasure sharing by couple (stroking of back, arms, face, legs, excluding the genital area); contraindications: same as week 3 plus fatigue, emotional upset.
3. Weeks 7–9: continue earlier activities, masturbate to full erection, 3 times a week for 20 minutes, couple stroke each other's pelvic area, attention in the other rather than self; contraindication: same as before.
4. Weeks 10–12: daily walks, moderate exercise, work to tolerance, climbing two flights of stairs, masturbation to ejaculation, manipulative play, oral–genital sex (if usual practice), coitus in comfortable positions.

ly morning after a night's sleep is an optimal time for coitus, which is then followed by another rest period. However, any time that the individual feels rested may be optimal and coitus does not have to be restricted to the morning.

Anal intercourse can result in stress to the heart. Stimulation of the branches of the vagus nerve can result in potentially fatal decrease of heart rate or in cardiac arrest.

Other Types of Sexual Expression. If the sexual partners have used oral–genital sex, they may continue, since it does not place undue strain on the heart. However, if this is not a usual method of obtaining sexual satisfaction, anxiety arising from the use of a new technique may be cardiac stressful.

Masturbation may be a method of reentrance into sexual activity. However, the health professional must be aware of and sensitive to the individual's religious beliefs and feelings about autoeroticism. The suggestion can be made that if they do not find masturbation wrong from an ethical or moral

viewpoint, there is no contraindication to masturbation as a way of resuming sexual activity. If a heart rate of 130 beats per minute is not contraindicated, masturbation may be suggested.[88] Manual stimulation of the sexual partner may also be used to satisfy the sexual partner without the stress of intercourse.

Many patients with uncomplicated myocardial infarction and their spouses may benefit from a sexual activity program outlined by Watts.[89] It necessitates the use of masturbation, so the program should not be implemented until the nurse has assessed whether it is an acceptable form of sexual activity for the patient. If guilt and anxiety are associated with its use, additional stress will be placed on the heart. In Watts's program, the patient progresses from noncoital activity to coitus, corresponding with general activity increase (Table 27-1).

Warning Signs. The nurse identifies warning signals which should be reported to the physician. These include anginal pain that occurs during or after intercourse and palpitation that continues for 15 minutes or more after intercourse.[90] Sleeplessness caused by the sexual exertion and marked fatigue during the day following intercourse should also be noted.

Medications, such as nitroglycerin or isosorbide dinitrate (Isordil), may be taken prophylactically before intercourse to prevent chest pain,[91] but this should be checked with the physician. Propranolol can control tachycardia or transient hypertension.

Instructions must be tailored to the individual patient after careful assessment has been made of physical abilities. Instructions that go beyond the usual sexual activity of the patient may only serve to unnecessarily alarm the patient and the sexual partner.[92]

Role of the Sexual Partner. Partners who are accustomed to each other in a loving relationship and whose techniques are habituated can achieve sexual satisfaction without great strain on the heart. Tenderness and cooperation result in rest, relaxation, and relief of tension after coitus. The nurse communicates these facts to the sexual partner. The noncardiac sexual partner must be aware of, accepting of, and adherent to the instructions given to the cardiac patient. There may be a psychologic and physiologic advantage of the female superior position for the female sexual partner. This gives her the opportunity to express her sexual abilities as well as assume a protective role for the man.[93]

Fear on the part of the sexual partner, as well as the patient, negatively affects frequency of sexual activity.[94] Often, a wife does not know how to respond when her husband returns to bed. The nurse helps both to discuss their feelings and their concerns, since this in itself helps to relieve anxiety. Although communication with the sexual partner may be problematic, few cardiac patients recognize it as such. Individual counseling and interviewing by the nurse may be helpful to uncover feelings or problems that partners may be too embarrassed to discuss. This is followed by joint counseling to explore means of meeting each other's needs.[95]

This regimen may be considered a conservative one, since some physicians allow coitus of limited frequency and duration 8 weeks postinfarction for the asymptomatic patient. Green[96] questions if a limit of even 8 weeks is necessary, suggesting that each patient must be evaluated on the basis of his activity response.

Psychologic Factors. Intervention to restore or promote sexual self-esteem is often indicated (Chapter 13). Kavanagh and Shephard[97] suspect that some patients do not complete an exercise program because of low self-esteem and believe that resumption of sexual activity is important in generating this esteem.

If the patient is exhibiting aggressive sexual behavior, intervention is usually indicated (Chapter 14). However, the nurse recognizes that this behavior stems from anxiety about sexual adequacy and potency or life itself. The behavior is a plea for help.[98]

Simple explanations of what is happening to the patient, the effects of the various medications, and clarifying of misconceptions are major means of reducing the patient's perceived threat to self.[99]

The nurse also intervenes as appropriate when body image disturbance, anxiety, depression, and sexual identity problems surface (see Chapter 13). These patient reactions are "normal," considering the threat imposed by myocardial infarction. If they do not subside as physical recovery continues, referral to a psychiatric nurse clinician or other psychiatric help is indicated.

Sociologic Factors. The nurse intervenes to help the sexual partner cope with the anxiety about the patient's recovery and her/his role in promoting or hindering it. The nurse helps prevent role reversal and the tendency to baby the patient by teaching the spouse or sexual partner measures to help maintain the patient's sexual identity (Chapter 13). Group sessions with wives of patients may be effective in reducing their sexual fears, although one-to-one sessions may be more appropriate for some women.[100]

Referral to work evaluation programs available in some communities may assure patient evaluation and job placement.[101] Nurses' own sense of optimism about patients and their efforts to instill this feeling in the patient will do much to insure rehabilitation not only for sexual functioning but for optimal feelings of sexual self-worth and return to role function.

Nurses recognize, moreover, that sexual problems may become more acute after discharge from the acute care setting when the individual is ready to return to work and to consider resumption of the role of lover and husband. It is then that fear of impotence and death may surface, that angina, tachycardia, and dyspnea may develop during the initial postcoronary coitus. It is then that the sexual partner may discourage sexual activity because of fears for the individual's health and safety.[102] Consequently, nurses in primary practice, clinics, offices, and occupational health settings should be especially sensitive to sexual concerns and problems.

Evaluation

The following outcome criteria indicate that interventions were effective. The patient and/or spouse (sexual partner):

1. Explain the effects of sexual activity on cardiac function.
2. Identify alternate techniques of coitus and sexual expression.
3. Identify hazardous situations to be avoided during coitus.
4. List warning signs that indicate the physician should be notified.
5. Resume premorbid role activities commensurate with the cardiac status.
6. Identify ways that he/she can promote sexual self-esteem.
7. State that they are satisfied with their sexual relationship.
8. (The patient) takes part in an exercise program as prescribed.

OTHER CARDIOVASCULAR AND PULMONARY CONDITIONS

Hypertension

Biologic Factors. Masters and Johnson[103] demonstrated that blood pressure is elevated in normal individuals and hypertensives throughout all phases of intercourse leading to orgasm. However, little research has been done related to hypertension and sex. Oaks and Moyer[104] studied 50 male and female hypertension patients to obtain information about three areas of sexual function and practices: (1) before hypertension became evident, (2) practices during the time it was known the individual had hypertension, and (3) abnormalities in sexual function that could be associated with drug therapy. In

Oaks' experience, the patient with undiagnosed hypertension does not usually have specific sexual problems arising from the hypertension itself, which in early stages has no significant effect in the sexual practices of either male or female.[105]

Analysis of their questionnaires indicated that drug therapy had more frequent and more adverse effects in men than in women, who experienced few untoward effects with regard to frequency of sexual activity, ability to achieve orgasm, or overall sexual relationship. In addition, the overall sexual adjustment of women did not seem to be altered whether the blood pressure was controlled or not controlled.

The male patient suffered more adverse effects. Paradoxically, when the blood pressure was carefully controlled, some did not feel as well generally and believed that at times their sexual powers suffered.[106] The investigators did not feel that this was of overriding importance to patient care, since this response was a means of adjusting to that level of blood pressure.

The drugs used to treat hypertension—sympathetic blockers, peripheral vasodilators, and diuretics—may produce five abnormalities in sexual function. Some drugs cause (1) true impotence, (2) delayed or missed ejaculation, (3) difficulty in maintaining an erection, (4) a general diminution of sexual activity caused by toxicity of the sympathetic nervous system, or (5) decreased libido due to the sedative and depressive effects.[107] (See Chapter 30 for specific information on drugs.)

Psychosocial Factors. Oaks and Moyer[108] state that although there is no specific hypertensive personality, the female hypertensive often appears to be a dominant, aggressive kind of personality who may be the initiator of sexual activities. In general, however, it is the woman rather than the man who makes a good sexual adjustment. Generally, the man may have a driving personality, oriented toward goals, success, and achievement, including sexual success. If he begins to lose his sexual power he may suffer severe disturbance of his self-image.

NURSING IMPLICATIONS

After the initial sexual history information, questions directed specifically at changes in sexual function should be asked periodically in the lifelong course of drug therapy.[109] The nurse and patient decide what are realistic goals of therapy.[110]

The possibility of decreased sexual function and impotence should be mentioned when patients are started on drugs with these side effects. The nurse reassures the patient that most people do not have these side effects, but if he should, there are other medications available.[111] Some physicians feel that it is more important to control the blood pressure than to be concerned about these side effects and do not give information about changes in sexual function. However, failure to comply with antihypertensive therapy is most often related to side effects, and therefore, counseling is essential.[112]

The nurse teaches each patient the effects of sustained elevated arterial pressure but reassures them that no impairment of sexual function occurs as blood pressure becomes normalized.

CARDIAC SURGERY

Meyer and Latz[113] interviewed 50 open heart patients between 1 and 9 months after surgery. The patients had an outpouring of anxiety, uncertainty, and needs, especially in regard to activity, including when to resume sexual relations.

There is little information about effects of coronary bypass on sexual activity. The patient may complain of soreness when the spouse's body is against the chest wall. These pains may feel like anginal or coronary pain when it is from surgical trauma.[114] Side-by-side position may prevent this pain. They may have the same fear of coital death and

sexual problems of individuals with myocardial infarction. Women who have bypass procedures may have feelings of disfigurement similar to mastectomy patients. Because many bypass patients feel they have been given a "second chance" in life, they are often unwilling to settle for masturbation or oral sex as a substitute for intercourse or to tolerate dysfunction from the past.[115]

VASCULAR DISEASE AND SURGERY

Erectile dysfunction may be due to penile arterial disease when the triad of insufficient erection, feeling of cold in the penis, and ejaculation with the penis flaccid occurs. If there is venous disease, the patient can maintain an erection more easily when standing and loses it when moving to the missionary position. These problems cannot be treated by medical or surgical therapy, although prosthesis may be used with arterial diseases.[116]

In the male, impotence is often found with aortoiliac obstruction (Leriche syndrome), which causes decreased blood flow to the pelvic viscera,[117] so it is important to inquire about this symptom in the nursing history.[118] Surgery for aortic or iliac occlusive disease or for aneurysm may also result in sexual disturbance, although surgical techniques are now being refined to save nerves that are often damaged during surgery. Impotence or lack of ejaculation develops from surgical interference with the autonomic nervous system—the lumbar sympathetic ganglia, rami communicantes, and aortic and hypogastric plexus.[119,120] May and associates[121] investigated sexual function in 70 patients who had aortic reconstruction from 6 months to 9 years after surgery. More men had ejaculatory failure than erective failure. Those with extensive occlusion who had aortofemoral bypass grafting had a higher incidence of erective failure than those who had only thromboendarterectomy. Hallböök[122] reports that some patients describe changes in orgasmic response in terms of either a disappearance of orgasms or a painful orgasm.

IMPAIRED PULMONARY FUNCTION

Chronic Obstructive Pulmonary Disease (COPD)

COPD usually occurs during the productive years of life. The individual gradually notes that energy level and ability to perform accustomed work has decreased. Usual roles and relationships, including sexual, must be modified or given up.[123] The individual's self-concept is inevitably threatened and changed.

With a chronic respiratory problem, coitus becomes difficult. Masters and Johnson[124] have shown that hyperventilation is a constant late plateau phase reaction for both sexes. Respiratory rates have peaked at rates as high as 40 per minute for both sexes, and these were in healthy individuals. The individual with chronic lung disease must often drastically reduce, if not cease, sexual activity because of respiratory insufficiency.

One hundred and twenty-eight adults with COPD reported negative effects on physical sexual expression, employment, and income. Interestingly, 60 percent stated that the emotional aspects of marriage were better because of the increased need for each other and slower life style. Forty percent felt the increased dependency on the spouse was pleasant and led to increased feelings of worth.[125] No data were obtained from the spouses.

NURSING IMPLICATIONS

The individual with respiratory failure must assume a more passive role during coitus. Shortness of breath can be avoided by the use of pillows to maintain a sitting position. The chair position suggested for the patient with myocardial infarction can be helpful. Some individuals report that a waterbed can provide movement without excessive muscular activity.

Intervention to maintain sexual self-esteem and role identity are usually indicated, but the single most important factor in adjustment is the presence of a supportive spouse or significant other.[126]

SICKLE-CELL ANEMIA

Biologic Factors

Sickle-cell diseases are the most common genetic disorders.[127] Four major types have been identified—sickle-cell hemoglobin C disease, sickle-cell hemoglobin D disease, sickle-cell B-thalassemia, and sickle-cell anemia (SS), the most common form. Sickle-cell anemia is a chronic hemolytic type and is complicated by painful crisis resulting from the tissue infarction due to blood vessel obstruction by tangled sickled cells.[128] Many body systems may be affected, and morbidity and mortality are high.

Sickle-cell anemia is a genetically transmitted disease primarily of black people, approximately one in ten carrying the sickle-cell trait. If both partners have the sickle-cell trait, the odds are 25 percent that each child will have sickle-cell anemia, 50 percent that each will have sickle-cell trait, and 25 percent that each child will be normal. About 1 out of every 600 black children at birth should have sickle-cell anemia, although the incidence has not been accurately measured.[129]

Effect on Sexuality. Priapism occurs infrequently in children, but the frequency increases with age and becomes more severe in intensity and duration (see Chapter 28). In the young child, priapism generally lasts from hours to days to weeks and ultimately leads to decreased fertility.[130]

In women, the beginning of puberty is delayed and the development of other secondary sexual characteristics is retarded. There may be delayed appearance of estrogen-mediated changes in vaginal epithelium, sparse axillary and pubic hair, small sex organs, and delayed menarche.[131]

The adult males may exhibit signs of hypogonadism, including genital hypoplasia or atrophy, and a high-pitched voice.[132]

Pregnancy. Painful sickle-cell crises are more common in pregnancy, especially in the last trimester and postpartum period. Conclusive data on fertility of patients with sickle-cell anemia are not available, but some believe that infertility is higher than in the normal population, possibly due to the anemia and chronic poor health that accompany the disease.[133] When pregnancy occurs, there is increased incidence of hypertension, albuminuria, edema, pyelonephritis, pulmonary infarction, pneumonia, and antepartum hemorrhage.[134]

Normal vaginal delivery is usually possible because of low birth weight of infants. In the postpartum period, however, fever and crises may be frequent. Although some report a higher incidence of maternal death, this may be attributable to poor antepartal care. Infant mortality is higher; there is increased abortion, prematurity, and fetal death due to intrapartum anoxia.[135,136]

Genetic Counseling

This process may be indicated for any disease that is genetically transmitted, not only sickle-cell diseases. It is a process in which the counselor must be sensitive to and concerned about the feelings of and the anxiety attendant upon a diagnosis that may produce much threat and/or damage to the individual's sexual self-concept and identity—a threat to the very ability to reproduce oneself. It involves intense feelings, motivations, adaptive and nonadaptive defense mechanisms, the issue of right to life, conception control, and abortion. These factors overlap counseling and interfere with the client's ability to hear, integrate, and make decisions.[137]

Genetic counseling can be defined as the process of communicating all the factors that relate to the disease or condition, including the signs and symptoms, the prognosis, the genetics, and the alternatives. The total picture of the condition, rather than its isolated parts, is dealt with.[138] Genetic counseling is an education process that helps families understand the risks their future children might bear of inheriting a genetic problem.[139]

Communication is the heart of the counseling process, but frequently there is no specific idea of how much information has been communicated from counselor to counselee and of how much the counselee understands. Too often, the bulk of genetic information and communication flows from the counselor or nurse to the counselee. If the situation is to be effective, there must be increased feedback from the counselee in the form of questions and comments. Murray[140] suggests the statement, "Please feel free to ask any questions at all that come to mind. There is no such thing as a silly question. This time is yours and must be used to your best advantage."

A major factor in the success of genetic counseling is the motivation of the counselor and counselee. One who has sought out information about sickle-cell disease, for example, will be more receptive to information than one who has been sought out by the health professional and given information. Another important factor in the counseling process is the educational background of the counselor as well as the counselee. There is a positive correlation between educational background and the amount of information received and understood.

The emotional states of the counselor and counselee are important. If counselors are upset for any reason and are not able to focus on the process of counseling, it is better if they excuse themselves from any session. The counselees are usually already anxious and depressed and it is difficult if not impossible to help them when the counselor is also upset.[141]

Ethical issues and questions also must be faced by all who are involved in genetic counseling; Hsia[142] has identified seven:

1. Does genetic counseling threaten to intrude upon areas of privacy, on divine predestination, or individual rights of self-determination?
2. Is there ever a time when a counselor has a right or even an obligation to withhold information that might be harmful to the individuals being counseled or to the family partnership?
3. Should the genetic counselor ever impose his or her value system on the counselees to dictate their decisions about future children?
4. Among the options for many genetic problems are artificial insemination and selective abortion of fetuses after diagnostic testing. The counselor is obliged to offer information about these options. However, in doing so, is endorsement implied of procedures that are controversial and not universally acceptable?
5. Having received counseling, is the couple obliged to utilize information in a socially responsible way in planning for future children?
6. Will genetic counseling affect the genetic endowment of future generations?
7. What are the public's responsibilities in learning about genetics and in determining support or limitations that genetic counseling should receive?

These are questions that concern all health professionals. Answers that are universally acceptable do not yet exist—if they ever will. Nurses should be aware of these issues and identify their values and beliefs about this sensitive area that may affect the lives of millions.

Psychosocial Factors

Couples who are at risk to give birth to children with sickle-cell disease go through a prolonged period of agonizing over decisions they have to make, and it is not unusual to have them change their minds several times in the course of a year.[143] Parents who have given birth to a child or children with sickle-cell disease may be overwhelmed by guilt when they realize they "gave" the disease. They may blame each other, as one father stated, "right out of a marriage."[144] (See Chapter 13 for discussion of guilt.) In addition, their sexual identity may be threatened if having children is important to masculinity or femininity.

School-aged children may have difficulty developing a positive self-image because pain or crisis limits their interaction with peers. Since they may be shorter in stature than peers, they may be teased by classmates.[145]

The adolescent with delayed sexual development due to sickle-cell disease, may suffer body image disturbance and decreased sexual self-esteem. If frequent illness and sickle-cell crises occur, the teenager will have difficulty developing sociosexual relationships with peers and becomes increasingly socially isolated. Depression is a common reaction and the adolescent may blame parents for the disease.[146]

NURSING IMPLICATIONS

Assessment

The nurse identifies educational level, the patient's/client's knowledge about the disease, and the genetic factors involved in its transmission. The nursing history elicits information about significant others, including the presence of a spouse or sexual partner. The nurse is sensitive to the individual's desire for children or, if the children have already been born, their desire for more children. The nurse also assesses the relationship between sexual partners, especially if they have children with sickle-cell disease, identifies medical complaints or problems the individual thinks may be caused by sickle-cell trait and whether there is a family history of sickle-cell disease.[147]

Planning

The nurse's goals are to provide information, assess whether the counselee has understood the information, and then assist the counselee to make the decisions that are in his or her best interests. The nurse also seeks to help families accept the social as well as the genetic realities of their situation, resolve misunderstanding and confusion,[148] and relieve anxiety and depression. When planning interventions, the nurse recognizes that the decisions of the counselees are those that meet their needs rather than the needs of medicine or mankind in general. Some couples who both have sickle-cell trait may choose to take the 25-percent risk of having a child with the disease. Even if the counselee makes no decision (which in itself is a decision) counseling has not been a waste of time, since by giving information the individuals have been helped to make a decision based on their life situation.

Intervention

The educational phase may involve group or individual teaching and counseling, both of which can be effective. (Principles and methods of teaching and learning are detailed in Chapter 11.) Educational programs should begin for children 8 to 12 years old and should motivate them to learn about sickle-cell disease.

Teenagers are a critical target group for sickle-cell education and screening, since they have reached childbearing status,[149] while adult audiences comprise the largest and most diverse of all target audiences.[150] Not only lay persons, but health professionals will benefit from conferences. The nurse also directs the individual to sources of education and counseling in the community.

The nurse who is involved in organizing an education and counseling program can obtain specific guidelines from excellent resources.*

*National Sickle Disease Program. Division of Blood Disease and Resources. National Heart, Lung, Blood Institute, National Institutes of Health, Sickle Cell Disease Branch, Room 4 A-27, Building 31, Bethesda, Maryland, 20014; or Sickle Cell Center, Howard University College of Medicine, 2121 Georgian Ave. N.W., Washington, D.C., 20059.

Family planning options should be discussed. The diaphragm with spermicidal jelly is safe. Intrauterine devices (IUDs) are risky because untoward effects such as pelvic infection may precipitate a crisis. Women with sickle-cell disease are at higher risk for thrombosis and vascular accidents so they may be more adversely affected by the pill. Rhythm method may be ineffective since many women have irregular menstrual cycles. Condoms cause no problems and may be a good choice for males.[151] Sterilization may be a choice for some women; any choice is ultimately the patient's.

The nurse may also intervene to help parents of children cope with guilt, anxiety, and depression. Adolescents with delayed sexual development or unusual body habits may need help to cope with body image disturbance and decreased sexual self-esteem. Between acute phases, children and adolescents with sickle-cell disease should be encouraged to attend school and associate with peers.

Evaluation

Evaluation of teaching–learning is easier than evaluation of the psychologic and emotional outcomes of the counseling process. Paper and pencil tests or questioning to determine understanding may show whether the counselee has obtained information. Evaluation of the emotional aspects of the counseling process is done by asking the counselees about their reactions to the counseling or by noting their behavior and response.[152] Followup programs are essential, not only because the initial session may have been emotionally charged, but also because the information and medical concepts are unfamiliar. Reinforcement of information and correction of misconceptions are carried out in one or more subsequent counseling sessions.

Outcome Criteria. After teaching and counseling, the individual and the sexual partner

1. Identify the relation of genetics to the inheritance of sickle-cell disease.
2. Identify the manifestations of and complications of the disease that affect sexuality.
3. State where services are obtainable for further counseling and for care.
4. Make a decision about having children that is in their own best interest.

NOTES

1. Masters WH, Johnson VE: Human Sexual Response, Boston, Little, Brown, 1966, pp 34–36, 174–175
2. Griffith GG: Sexuality and the cardiac patient. Heart Lung 2:70–73, 1973
3. Ibid, p 71
4. Oliven J: Clinical Sexuality, 3rd ed. Philadelphia, Lippincott, 1974, pp 233–237
5. Hellerstein HK, Friedman EH: Sexual activity and the postcoronary patient. Arch Intern Med 125:987–999, 1970
6. Ibid, p 988
7. Ibid, p 993
8. Kavanagh T, Shephard RJ: Sexual activity after myocardial infarction. Can Med J 116:1250–1253, 1977
9. Hellerstein HK, Friedman EH: Sexual activity and the postcoronary patient. Arch Intern Med 125:991, 1970
10. Ibid, p 998
11. Griffith GG: Sexuality and the cardiac patient. Heart Lung 2:71, 1973
12. Ueno M: The so-called coition death. Jpn J Legal Med 17:333–340, 1963
13. Viewpoints: "Sudden death during coitus—fact or fiction." Med Aspects Hum Sexuality 3:22–26, June 1969
14. Wolf S: Emotional stress and the heart. J Rehabil 32(2):42–45, 1966
15. Hellerstein HK, Friedman EH: Sexual activity and the postcoronary patient. Arch Intern Med 125:999, 1970
16. Eliot RS, Miles R: What to tell the cardiac patient about sexual intercourse. Resident-Intern Consultant 2:14, 1973
17. Hellerstein HK, Friedman EH: Sexual activity and the postcoronary patient. Arch Intern Med 125:999, 1970
18. Eliot RS, Miles R: What to tell the cardiac patient about sexual intercourse. Resident-Intern Consultant 2:14, 1973
19. Larsen JL, McNaughton MW, Kennedy JW, Mansfield LW: Heart rate and blood pressure responses to sexual activity and a stair-climbing test. Heart Lung 9:1025–1030, 1980
20. Satterfield SB: Sexual rehabilitation for the post coronary patient. Top Clin Nurs 1:85–89, 1980
21. Green AW: Sexual activity and the postmyocardial infarction patient. Am Heart J 89:246–252, 1975
22. Hellerstein HK, Friedman EH: Sexual activity and the postcoronary patient. Arch Intern Med 125:997 1970
23. Koller R, Kennedy JW, Butler JC, Wagner NN: Counseling the coronary patient on sexual activity. Postgrad Med, April 1972, pp 133–136
24. Rubin I: Sex after forty and after seventy. In Brecher R, Brecher E (eds): An Analysis of Human Sexual Response. New York, New American Library, 1966, p 263
25. Bilodeau CB, Hackett TP: Issues raised in a group setting by patients recovering from initial myocardial infarction. Am J Psychiatry 128:73–77, 1971
26. Hackett TP, Cassem NH: Psychological adaptation to convalescense in myocardial infarction patients. In Naughton J, Hellerstein HK (eds): Exercise Testing and Exercise Training. New York, Academic, 1973, 253–262
27. Ibid, p 253
28. Bilodeau CB, Hackett TP: Issues raised in a group setting by patients recovering from initial myocardial infarction. Am J Psychiatry 128:73, 1971
29. Klein RF, Dean A, Willson M, Bogdonoff MB: The physician and postmyocardial invalidism, JAMA 194:143–148, 1965

30. Tuttle WB, Cook WL, Fitch E: Sexual behavior in postmyocardial infarction patients. Am J Cardiol 13:140, 1964

31. Mann S, Yates E, Raftery EB: The effects of myocardial infarction on sexual activity. J Card Rehabil 1:187, 1981

32. Hellerstein HK, Friedman EH: Sexual activity and the postcoronary patient. Arch Intern Med 125:990, 1970

33. Ibid, p 992

34. Ibid

35. Weiss E, English OS: Psychosomatic Medicine, 3rd ed. Philadelphia, Saunders, 1957, p 216

36. Kavanagh T. Shephard RJ: Sexual activity after myocardial infarction. Can Med J 116:1251, 1977

37. Kushnir B, Fox KM, Tomlinson IW, Portal RW, Aber CP: Primary ventricular fibrillation and resumption of work, sexual activity, and driving after the first acute myocardial infarction. Br Med J 4:609–611, 1975

38. Bloch A, Maeder J-P, Haissly J-C: Sexual problems after MI. Am Heart J 90:536–537, 1975

39. Green AW; Sexual activity and the post-myocardial infarction patient. Am Heart J 89:246–252, 1975

40. Abramov LA: Sexual life and sexual frigidity among women developing acute myocardial infarction. Psychosom Med 38:418–425, 1976

41. Wagner NN: Sexual activity and the cardiac patient. In Green R (ed): Human Sexuality: A Health Practitioner's Text. Baltimore, Williams and Wilkins, 1975, pp 173–179

42. Ibid, p 177

43. Watts RJ: Sexuality and the middle-aged cardiac patient. Nurs Clin North Am 11:349–359, 1976

44. Woolley AS: Excellence in nursing in the coronary-care unit. Heart Lung 1:785–911, 1972

45. Kavanagh T, Shephard RJ: Sexual activity after myocardial infarction. Can Med J 116:1253, 1977

46. Hellerstein HK, Friedman EH: Sexual activity and the postcoronary patient. Arch Intern Med 125:997, 1970

47. Rosen JL, Bibring GL: Psychological reactions of hospitalized male patients to a heart attack, Psychosom Med 28:808, 1966

48. Watts RJ: Sexuality and the middle-aged cardiac patient. Nurs Clin North Am 11:355, 1976

49. Woolley AS: Excellence in nursing in the coronary-care unit. Heart Lung 1:786, 1972

50. Scalzi CC: Behavioral responses following acute M.I. Heart Lung 2:62–69, 1973

51. Needs and Opportunities for Rehabilitating the Coronary Heart Disease Patient: Report of the Task Force on Cardio-Vascular Rehabilitation of the National Heart and Lung Institute. Bethesda, Maryland, National Institutes of Health, 1974

52. Watts RJ: Sexuality and the middle-aged cardiac patient. Nurs Clin North Am 11:359, 1976

53. Smith CA: Body image changes after myocardial infarction. Nurs Clin North Am 7:663–668, 1972

54. Hott JR: Sex and the heart patient: A nursing view. Top Clin Nurs 1:75–84, 1980

55. Lewis L: Convalescence. A positive approach. J Rehabil 32(2):35–38, 1966

56. Kavanagh T, Shephard RJ: Sexual activity after myocardial infarction. Can Med J 116:1253, 1977

57. Papadopoulos C, Larrimore P, Cardin S, Shelley SI: Sexual concerns and needs of the post-coronary patient's wife. Arch Intern Med 140:38–41, 1980

58. Needs and Opportunities for Rehabilitating the Coronary Heart Disease Patient: Report of the Task Force on Cardio-Vascular Rehabilitation of the National Heart and Lung Institute. Bethesda, Maryland, National Institutes of Health, 1974, p 55

59. Ibid, p 71

60. Ibid, p 4

61. Ibid, p 6

62. Pinderhughes CA, Grace EB, Anderson RT: Interrelationships between sexual functioning and medical conditions. Med Aspects Hum Sexuality 6:52, October 1972

63. Needs and Opportunities for Rehabilitating the Coronary Heart Disease Patient: Report of the Task Force on Cardio-Vascular Rehabilitation of the National Heart and Lung Institute. Bethesda, Maryland, National Institutes of Health, 1974, p 14

64. Tuttle WB, Cook WL, Fitch E: Sexual behavior in postmyocardial infarction patients. Am J Cardiol 13:140, 1964

65. Stein RA: The effect of exercise training on heart rate during coitus in the post myocardial infarction patient. Circulation 55:738–740, 1977

66. Hellerstein HK, Friedman EH: Sexual activity and the postcoronary patient. Arch Intern Med 125:997, 1970

67. Hellerstein HK: Heart disease and sex: Response to questions. Med Aspects Hum Sexuality 5:24–35, 1971

68. Garcia RM: Rehabilitation after Myocardial Infarction. New York, Appleton, 1979, pp 39–52

69. Fletcher GF: Exercise and Coronary Artery Disease. Springfield, Illinois, Thomas, 1974, p 74

70. Needs and Opportunities for Rehabilitating the Coronary Heart Disease Patient: Report of the Task Force on Cardio-Vascular Rehabilitation of the National Heart and Lung Institute. Bethesda, Maryland, National Institutes of Health, 1974, p 36

71. Ibid

72. Johnston BL, Cantwell JD, Watt EW, Fletcher GT: Sexual activity in exercising patients after myocardial infarction and revascularization. Heart Lung 7:1026, 1978

73. Moore K, Folk-Lighty M, Nolen MJ: The joy of sex after a heart attack. Nursing 77(7):53–55, 1977

74. Puksta NS: All about sex . . . after a coronary. Am J Nurs 77:602–605, 1977

75. Scalzi C, Dracup K: Sexual counseling of coronary patients. Heart Lung 7:840–845, 1977

76. Ibid, p 841

77. Moore K, Folk-Lighty M, Nolen MJ: The joy of sex after a heart attack, Nursing 77(7):55, 1977

78. Scalzi CC: Sexual counseling and sexual therapy for patients after myocardial infarction. Cardio-Vasc Nurs 18:13–17, 1982

79. Wagner NN: Sexual activity and the cardiac patient. In Green R (ed): Human Sexuality: A Practitioner's Text. Baltimore, Williams and Wilkins, 1975, p 178

80. Naughton J: Preferred coital position after coronary. Med Aspects Hum Sexuality 7:177, 181, 1973

81. Koller R, Kennedy JW, Butler JC, Wagner NN: Counseling the coronary patient on sexual activity. Postgrad Med, April 1972, p 135

82. Scalzi CC: Behavioral responses following M.I. Heart Lung 2:68, 1973

83. Nemec E, Mansfield L, Kennedy JW: Heart rate and blood pressure responses during sexual activity in normal males. Am Heart J 92:274–277, 1974

84. Wagner NN: Sexual activity and the cardiac patient. In Green (ed): Human sexuality: A Practitioner's Text. Baltimore, Williams and Wilkins, 1975, p 175

85. Oliven J: Clinical Sexuality, 3rd ed. Philadelphia, Lippincott, 1974, p 236

86. Griffith GG: Sexuality and the cardiac patient. Heart Lung 2:73, 1973

87. Ibid

88. Wagner NN: Sexual activity and the cardiac patient. In Green R (ed): Human Sexuality: A Practitioner's

Text. Baltimore, Williams and Wilkins, 1975, p 177

89. Watts RJ: Sexuality and the middle-aged cardiac patient. Nurs Clin North Am 11:357, 1976

90. Scalzi CC: Behavioral responses following M.I. Heart Lung 2:68, 1973

91. Koller R, Kennedy JW, Butler JC, Wagner NN: Counseling the coronary patient on sexual activity. Postgrad Med, April 1972, p 136

92. Green AW: Sexual activity and the postmyocardial infarction patient. Am Heart J 89:251, 1975

93. Naughton J: Preferred coital positions after coronary. Med Aspects Hum Sexuality, 7:177, 1973

94. Kavanagh T, Shephard RJ: Sexual activity after myocardial infarction. Can Med J 116:1253, 1977

95. Moore K, Folk-Lighty M, Nolen MJ: The joy of sex after a heart attack. Nursing 77(7):55, 1977

96. Green AW: Sexual activity and the postmyocardial infarction patient. Am Heart J 89:250, 1975

97. Kavanagh T. Shephard RJ: Sexual activity after myocardial infarction. Can Med J 116:1253, 1977

98. VanBie NS: Sexuality, nursing practice and the person with cardiac disease. Nurs Forum 14:397–411, 1975

99. Wooley AS: Excellence in nursing in the coronary-care unit. Heart Lung 1:787, 1972

100. Harding AL, Morefield M-A: Group intervention for wives of myocardial infarction patients. Nurs Clin North Am 11:339–347, 1976

101. Smith CA: Body image changes after myocardial infarction. Nurs Clin North Am 7:666, 1972

102. Hellerstein, HK: Heart disease and sex: Response to questions. Med Aspects Hum Sexuality 5:33, 1971

103. Masters WH, Johnson VE: Human Sexual Response. Boston, Little, Brown, 1966, pp 35–36, 174–176

104. Oaks WW, Moyer JH: Sex and hypertension. Med Aspects Hum Sexuality 6:128–137, 1972

105. Ibid, p 133

106. Ibid, p 129

107. Ibid, p 136

108. Ibid, p 132

109. Carver JR, Oaks WW: Sex and hypertension. In Oaks WW, Melchiode GA, Ficher I (eds): Sex and the Life Cycle. New York, Grune and Stratton, 1976, pp 175–178.

110. Jones LN: Hypertension: Medical and nursing implications. Nurs Clin North Am 11:283–295, 1976

111. Ibid, p 289

112. Carver JR, Oaks WW: Sex and hypertension. In Oaks WW, Melchiode GA, Ficher I (eds): Sex and the Life Cycle. New York, Grune and Stratton, 1976, p 178

113. Meyer RM, Latz PA: What heart surgery patients want to know. Am J Nurs 79:1558–1560, 1979

114. Waxberg JD: Sex after coronary bypass surgery: A physician's personal account. Sex Med Today 4:18–19, 1980

115. Ibid, p 19

116. Tordjam G, Thierrée R, Michel JR: Advances in vascular pathology of male erectile dysfunction. Arch Sex Behav 9:391–398, 1980

117. May AG, DeWeese JA, Rah CG: Changes in sexual function after operation on the abdominal aorta. Surgery 65:41–47, 1969

118. Taggart E: The physical assessment of the patient with arterial disease. Nurs Clin North Am 12:109–117, 1977

119. Abramovici H, Weisz GM, Timor-Tritsch I, Schramek A: Male infertility following aortic surgery. Int J Fertil 16:144–146, 1971

120. Miles JR, Miles DG, Johnson G: Aorto-iliac operation and sexual dysfunction. Arch Surg 117:1177–1181, 1982

121. May AG, DeWeese JA, Rah, CG: Changes in sexual function after operation on the abdominal aorta. Surgery 65:41, 1969

122. Hollböök T, Holmquist B: Sexual disturbance following dissection of the aorta and the common iliac arteries. J. Cardiovasc Surg 4:255–260, 1970

123. Barstow RE: Coping with emphysema. Nurs Clin North Am 9:137–145, 1974

124. Masters WH, Johnson VE: Human Sexual Response. Boston, Little, Brown, 1966, p 78

125. Hanson EI: Effects of chronic lung disease on life in general and on sexuality. Heart Lung 11:435–441, 1982

126. Barstow RE: Coping with emphysema. Nurs Clin North Am 9:142, 1974

127. Rooks Y, Pack B: A profile of sickle cell disease. Nurs Clin North Am 18:131–138, 1983

128. Lehmann H. Huntsman RS, Casey R, Lang A, Lorkin PA, Comings DE: Sickle cell diseases and related disorders. In Williams WJ (ed): Hematology, 2nd ed. New York, McGraw-Hill, 1977, pp 495–507

129. Rucknagel DL: The biochemical genetics of sickle cell anemia and related hemoglobinopathies. In Levere RD (ed): Sickle Cell Anemia and Other Hemoglobinopathies. New York, Academic, 1975, pp 1–23

130. Robinson MG: Clinical aspects of sickle cell disease. In Levere RD (ed): Sickle Cell Anemia and Other Hemoglobinopathies. New York, Academic, 1975, pp 87–112

131. Sergeant GR: The Clinical Features of Sickle Cell Disease. Amsterdam, North-Holland, 1974, p 222

132. Ibid, p 223

133. Ibid, p 230

134. Ibid, p 231

135. Luff J: Pregnancy and sickle cell disease. Nurs Clin North Am 18:164–170, 1983

136. Lehmann H, Huntsman RS, Casey R, Lang A, Lorkin PA, Comings DE: Sickle cell diseases and related disorders. In Williams WJ (ed): Hematology, 2nd ed. New York, McGraw-Hill, 1977, p 503

137. Tishler CL: The psychological aspects of genetic counseling. Am J Nurs 81:732–734, 1981

138. Murray RF: Unsolved mysteries in genetic counseling. In Levere RD (ed): Sickle Cell Anemia and Other Hemoglobinopathies. New York, Academic, 1975, pp 113–137

139. Hsia YE: Are we an endangered species? Genetic counseling and man. In Hogan TW (ed): Redesigning Man—In Search of an Ethic. Honolulu, Chaminade University and UNESCO, 1977, pp 50–53

140. Murray RF: Unsolved mysteries in genetic counseling. In Levere RD (ed): Sickle Cell Anemia and Other Hemoglobinopathies. New York: Academic, 1975, p 116

141. Ibid, p 117

142. Hsia YE: Are we an endangered species? Genetic counseling and man. In Hogan TW (ed): Redesigning Man—In Search of an Ethic. Honolulu, Chaminade University and UNESCO, 1977, p. 53

143. Murray RF: Unsolved mysteries in genetic counseling. In Levere RD (ed): Sickle Cell Anemia and Other Hemoglobinopathies. New York, Academic, 1975, p 120

144. Jackson DE: Sickle cell disease: Meeting a need. Nurs Clin North Am 7:727–741, 1972

145. Williams I, Earles AN, Pack B: Psychological consideration in sickle cell disease. Nurs Clin North Am 18:215–229, 1983

146. Ibid, p 223

147. Murray RF: Unsolved mysteries in genetic counseling. In Levere RD (ed): Sickle Cell Anemia and Other hemoglobinopathies. New York, Academic, 1975, p 118

148. Hsia YE: Are we an endangered species? Genetic counseling and man. In Hogan TW (ed): Redesigning Man—In Search of an Ethic. Honolulu, Chaminade University and UNESCO, 1977, p 51

149. Department of Health, Education, and Welfare: Model Protocol for Sickle Cell Education. Rockville, Maryland, Department of Health, Education, and Welfare, 1976, p 41

150. Ibid, p 86

151. Myrie J: Family planning and genetic counseling. Nurs Clin North Am 18:174–184, 1983

152. Murray RF: Unsolved mysteries in genetic counseling. In Levere RE (ed): Sickle Cell Anemia and Other Hemoglobinopathies. New York, Academic, 1975, p 119

Chapter 28

Impaired Urogenital Function

Chronic and acute diseases of the reproductive and the urinary systems may have adverse biologic effects on sexual function by causing changes in sexual response patterns or may have adverse psychologic effects by causing the anxiety that accompanies malfunction of a system intimately related to sexuality. Individuals with chronic diseases of these systems may have to adapt to pathophysiology that may be difficult, if not impossible, to reverse.

Renal failure may adversely affect the sexual functioning of both sexes. Prostate disease and urinary infections may plague the male, while diseases and anomalies of the reproductive tract and urinary tract may cause problems for the female. The major focus of this chapter will be on the effects of kidney disease and its therapy on sexuality, with briefer discussion of genitourinary infections and disorders.

RENAL FAILURE: BIO-PSYCHO-SOCIAL FACTORS

Individuals with renal failure, whether treated by dialysis and/or transplantation, are especially prone to alteration in their sexuality because of the profound bio-psycho-social consequences of the disease and its therapy. The effects of severe chronic renal failure affect every body system and may compromise the individual's ability to meet all the basic needs.

In women, end-stage renal failure results in the changes in menstrual cycle, with the menses more widely spaced and with bleeding that may be heavier or lighter in flow than normal or that may cease completely. Ovulation may occur normally or only a few times a year. Pregnancy in uremic women is less frequent than in the normal population. In males, gonadal dysfunction, Leydig cell atrophy[1], impotence, and decreased libido are frequently seen. Low testosterone and elevated luteinizing hormone levels have been reported. Individuals may be infertile due to low sperm counts (azoospermia) or may have few viable sperm.

In addition to the hormonal changes that accompany renal disease, vascular and neuropathic changes may contribute to decreased sexual capacity. However, there is variation in response, and some patients with chronic renal failure may retain normal sexual response, even though changes in fertility are present.[2]

Psychologic responses are those often seen in chronic illness—anxiety and depression. Changes in life style invariably occur, and the usual roles of the patient often have to be assumed by the sexual partner, with serious threat to the sexual identity and esteem of both.[3] Untreated renal failure usually ends in death, but with the advent of hemodialysis and kidney transplantation, the outcome, in terms of life and return of fertility and sexual function, becomes somewhat more optimistic.

473

RENAL DIALYSIS

Biologic Factors

Studies have found varying degrees and types of sexual dysfunction in males on dialysis. These include low or absent sperm counts, low plasma testosterone, germinal cell[4,5] and Leydig cell dysfunction; these were not corrected by dialysis.

Elstein and associates[6] reported different and more optimistic findings. Of ten female patients, six had return of menstruation with dialysis, although none became pregnant. Three wives of 15 men undergoing dialysis for terminal renal failure became pregnant, suggesting that the men's fertility was not impaired.

Impotence and diminished sexual interest appears to be more frequent in chronic dialysis patients than in the general population.[7] Fifteen couples taking part in group discussions established for hemodialysis patients reported varying changes in sexual functioning, but potency problems were frequent. Some males experienced more difficulty achieving and maintaining an erection and longer refractory periods between erections. Erections were also described as "not as hard as before." Both males and females reported lack of interest in sex when they were fatigued or emotionally upset. Although not all complained of sexual problems, most admitted that there were changes in sexual activity that required adjustments in attitudes, expectation, and practice.[8]

Thirty-two male uremic patients before receiving maintenance hemodialysis described a decrease in frequency of sexual intercourse, from a frequency of 10.4 to 5.7 times per month. While on dialysis, the frequency further decreased to 4.0. Of the 32 men, only 7 had no decrease in function at any time. Fourteen patients had reduced potency after the onset of uremia, while 11 had reduced potency only while receiving hemodialysis.[9]

Cummings[10] also reports that disruption of sexual function is an almost universal phe-

nomenon among the patients seen in a Washington, D.C., dialysis unit.

Autonomic neuropathy and diabetes have been implicated. Penile vascular insufficiency with decreased penile blood pressure may explain the impotence since chemically hemodialyzed patients often have accelerated atherosclerosis. Venous vascular problems may also contribute to the problem.[11] Use of Doppler technology gives measurement of penile blood pressure to differentiate vascular and nonvascular causes.[12,13]

Measurement of nocturnal penile tumescence (NPT) also helps distinguish between organic and psychologic causes of impotence. In healthy men three to five erections occur during the night with REM (rapid eye movement) sleep. Transducers are placed at the base and tip of the penis to measure changes associated with erection. If organic changes exist NPT is abnormal.[14]

Some believe that gonadal failure is the primary cause of decreased potency and libido in males and of amenorrhea in females. Dalla Rosa and associates[15] also found cases of hypothalamic–hypophyseal insufficiency in male hemodialysis patients. They did not find any correlation between impotence and other clinical and laboratory conditions related to uremia (anemia, degree of neuropathy, osteopathy). Women with amenorrhea had abnormal prolactin levels, which the investigators felt were more important in determining amenorrhea than gonadotropins whose level did not vary in women with or without amenorrhea.

General debilitation and fatigue related to the uremia may also be implicated in sexual response problems. Renal patients describe themselves as never "feeling really well," "not having enough energy."[16]

Sexual dysfunction in female patients has not been investigated as systematically as that of males. Levy's[17] general impression is that female patients as a group have less difficulty adjusting to maintenance hemodialysis than males.

Psychologic Factors

Despite biologic changes that take place, if data from various studies are accurate, Levy[18] feels that psychologic factors must be incriminated as a contributing cause of diminished potency in the majority of dialysis patients. Impotence has also been attributed to the men's response to therapy and to their new role in life as an emasculation. One man revealed that he felt like "half a man" due to his inability to urinate normally and because of his dependence on the dialysis machine. He had been impotent for 6 months and feared that he would "lose his wife and thus his life" if he could not function sexually as before his illness.[19]

Describing the many hours a week on a dialyzing machine as physically exhausting, patients also describe it as even more psychologically exhausting, a constant need "to deal with the simple act of surviving."[20] Patients respond to this constant struggle with anxiety, depression,[21] decreased self-concept,[22] resentfulness, and bitterness,[23] all of which may adversely affect sexuality. Although overt psychosis does occur among some, Cummings[24] argues that intense patient reactions should be distinguished from neurotic and psychotic symptomatology found in those with diagnosed mental disease.

In a 3-year evaluation of 24 patients, Greenberg and his associates[25] also found little evidence of gross emotional maladjustment. However, the individuals had experienced organic loss in intellectual function and, of greater import for sexuality and the maintenance of relationships, they had limited affective responsivity; most of the individuals had resigned themselves to their problem while withdrawing from investment in the world around them. Half of the 24 did not respond to affective stimuli, and 8 had difficulty handling feelings when stirred up. Only 4 of 24 responded appropriately. In many, if affect appeared, it took the form of either depression or anger.

Autoerotic activity may be utilized by some patients to relieve tension. Levy[26] notes that 7 of 11 male patients masturbated relatively openly and frequently during hemodialysis. This was viewed primarily as a manifestation of anxiety to the stress of the procedure. Patients who chose to masturbate less openly were left alone while those whose behavior was particularly exhibitionistic were warned that such activity would not be tolerated.

Sociologic Factors

Change in role relationships and economic concerns are also implicated as particularly important sources of stress affecting the sexual relationship. Role disturbance is especially problematic for men whose roles of breadwinner, disciplinarian, and decision maker are particularly vulnerable to encroachments by kidney disease and dialysis. Wives may have to leave home to work, make major decisions around the home, and become the dispenser of rewards and punishments.[27,28] Men describe themselves as "househusbands" who cannot do much work.[29] Levy[30] has hypothesized that the problems of potency may be related to the effects of reversal of family role upon the tenuous masculine identity of these patients. If the spouse resents having to take over responsibilities, the relationship will doubly suffer.[31]

The cost of dialysis engenders tremendous economic pressures, and the individual's decreased ability or inability to work provides further economic stress. Concerns about finances may contribute to feelings of rejection, resentment, and worthlessness.[32]

Although most of the literature focuses on the reaction of the male patient, a woman may be just as devastated if her role as homemaker and mother is altered or if advancement in her career is interrupted by kidney disease and dialysis. Diminished sexual desire and capability go beyond the matter of simple erotic pleasure. More significant is the strain on the whole fabric of the relationship between sexual partners.[33]

Home Dialysis

Sexual dysfunction is also associated with home dialysis. Of 32 male veterans with end-stage renal disease, 72 percent (23) had some erectile or ejaculatory difficulty.[34]

The sexual partners may experience even greater strain on their relationship from the psychosexual effects of home hemodialysis. The spouse is taught the fundamentals of care, the patient becoming dependent on the spouse for life itself. Hassett[35] reports psychologic responses of anxiety, anger, and guilt and fear for the patient and fear of the responsibility of dialysis.

Home dialysis, however, may not be so devastating to some relationships. In a study of 32 men with end-stage renal disease, Berkman and associates found that although the patients had decreased genital function, they rated their marriage relationships slightly better than did a random sample of healthy men.[36]

Strong family support is an essential factor in sexual adjustment. Other significant factors that positively affect adjustment include favorable response to therapy, a strong marital bond and mutual trust and acceptance, and preexisting presonality assets such as high self-esteem and ability to have dependency needs met by others.[37]

Although the focus of most attention is the patient and spouse relationship, children may also be affected. Some develop bizarre ideas about the sexes. Kossoris[38] reports that younger children of a parent who has an external shunt may believe that all adults of the same sex as the ill parent have a "tube" in their arm or leg. One can also speculate that children may grow up with other misconceptions about or problems in the area of sexuality. Since much of what is appropriate gender behavior is learned from early childhood experience, it is possible that the often negative relationships and role reversals of the parents may result in the children's sexual conflict and problematic behavior (see Chapter 15).

NURSING IMPLICATIONS

Nurses caring for individuals with renal failure and/or dialysis are in a different position than nurses who work in other aspects of critical care, since the relationship with patients and their families is both intense and long-term.[39] Most patients do not bring up the topic of sexuality.[40] Patients in dialysis and their families are especially hesitant to talk to nurses and physicians about concerns related to hemodialysis, since they are afraid to antagonize the people who are literally responsible for their lives. They have a tendency to keep their fears to themselves.[41] Consequently, they may be hesitant to bring up sexual concerns.

Assessment

Information about sexuality obtained in the initial history gives baseline data that will need continual update as the patient and his family progress through renal failure and/or dialysis, since changes in sexual function, sexual relationships, and roles may fluctuate with the changes in the individual's condition. When the individual is to begin hemodialysis, the nurse collects data from the patient and the family about their knowledge of the procedure, feelings about the dialysis, and expectations of its effects on physical and social well-being. The family can also provide significant information about the patient.

The level of communication that exists between family members and the patient and the adequacy of social support that the patient receives is also assessed.[42] Since the family may be so intimately involved in the dialysis, it is essential that the nurse ascertain their perceptions and problems as well as those of the patient.[43]

Planning

The nurses' goals may include teaching about the biologic effects of renal disease and/or dialysis on sexual function and counseling patient and family to help them cope with the effects of the disease and/or therapy on roles and relationships. Just as data must be continually obtained, the planning must be a dynamic process. To identify a care plan early after the first patient contact and to continue interventions on the basis of the early plan will almost insure that patient and family's sexuality needs will be unmet.

Intervention

Principles of teaching–learning are discussed in Chapter 11 and counseling in Chapter 12, but some general ideas need restatement.

Empathic listening may seem an overworked intervention, but it is one of the most effective means of helping the dialysis patient and the family.[44,45] Sitting down for 10 to 15 minutes with the patient and the family is time well spent, since the nurse can communicate desire to help and willingness to listen.

At times, nurses may have to set limits on sexual behavior. If masturbation is a frequent sexual outlet, but it is done where other persons can observe the activity, the nurse tries to provide the privacy the patient needs or else set limits on the behavior if the time and place are inappropriate (see Chapter 14).

The family of the patient receiving home hemodialysis needs special attention. The nurse may become so involved with teaching the procedure that the feelings of the spouse, parent, or significant others about taking responsibility for the care may be neglected. Sexual relationships may be fractured if all concerned do not have an opportunity to verbalize their anxiety, anger, and guilt. Overt coercion is never used to force a spouse or significant other to do dialysis, but one can wonder about subtle pressures that may be brought against family members to comply. A wife who insisted that she could not do dialysis for her husband settled the matter by attempting suicide.[46] Families have come close to divorce, children have become difficult to manage, and the patient may repeatedly threaten or attempt suicide by over-

reacting, overdrinking, and omitting treatment.[47] Some patients, at least covertly, choose death to the disruption in the relationships. Someone to listen and help in problem solving is essential. Crisis-oriented group meetings may provide the support that all need when their coping devices are not effective.[48] (See Chapter 11 for discussion of group teaching and Chapter 12 for group counseling.) These groups may also help nurses who care for dialysis patients work through their concerns and feelings.

Referral to a psychiatric nurse, psychiatrist, clinical psychologist, or psychiatric social worker may be necessary if there are severe psychologic problems. Patient and family members should be given sources of emotional support or counseling that are available if necessary.

Evaluation

In determining whether interventions have been effective, the nurse uses the following outcome criteria. The patient and family:

1. Describe the effects of kidney disease and/or dialysis on sexual function.
2. Are able to express their concerns about changing roles and relationships.
3. Can identify resources where further counseling is available.

KIDNEY TRANSPLANT

Biologic Factors

After months or years on dialysis, kidney transplant offers individuals the chance for the normal life that dialysis does not by freeing them from the days and hours spent connected to a dialysis machine. Although transplant procedures have improved, however, the patient is still faced with the problems of rejection and the therapy directed toward its prevention. Dietary management, fluid allowances, and medication doses continue to be a vital part of the person's existence.[49]

The surgical procedure may cause erectile difficulties. If the internal iliac artery is used for arterial anastomosis of the renal allograft, diminished penile blood flow occurs. Burns[50] and associates showed that the occlusion of distal ends of both iliac arteries causes absence of a palpable penile pulse while unilateral occlusion decreased flow, but a pulse is still discernible. Because of these findings, Waltzer[51] suggests use of the external iliac artery, especially if a second transplant is to be done.

Although general well-being is usually improved from that of the dialysis period, patients may complain of pain and the prolonged immunosuppression to prevent rejection may result in infection, aseptic necrosis of the femoral or humoral heads, or generalized myopathy.[52] The side effects of steroid therapy, truncal fat, acne, bruising, striae, and moon facies may produce body image disturbance, especially if the individual is not aware that they can occur.[53] Some or all of these factors may compromise sexual response.

In spite of the side effects of transplantation, the procedure, on the whole, results in increased biologic sexual well-being. Lim and Fang[54] reported that transplant resulted in complete reversal of the azoospermia and low levels of plasma testosterone that had been present in 13 male hemodialyzed patients, and testicular biopsy showed normal tissue posttransplant. Resumption of menses and pregnancy may occur in women even with immunosuppressive therapy with corticosteroids and azathioprine.[55]

Psychologic Factors

Nelson describes the psychologic responses of patients who were at least 1 year postrenal transplant. Patients described depersonalization, and closely related or possibly as a result of it, communication difficulties. Some patients even expressed surprise that anyone was interested in their concerns.[56] Signs of psychologic decompensation that have implication for sexuality include guilt, loss of self-esteem, fear, grief, hostility, withdrawal, and depression. Fear of transplant

rejection was pervasive and foreboding, and the dread all too frequently might prove accurate. Eight of 11 patients who died following transplant, had experienced panic and sense of pessimism about the outcome.[57]

Some patients indicated that the kidney had not been incorporated into the body image. Nelson[58] describes four stages of transplant internalization. In the first, or foreign body stage, patients describe the organ as feeling "funny" and seeming to "stick out." Thus they conceive their body configuration as changed. They feel that the kidney is fragile and they must take care to avoid being jostled. Data are not available, but one can speculate that patients would change both the usual amount and types of sexual activity or suspend it completely if they perceive that the kidney might be harmed. The adolescent has particular difficulty adjusting to body image changes.

In the second stage, partial internalization, patients tend to feel less uneasy about the organ and are less in awe of it. In the third stage, complete internalization, patients report the acceptance of the kidney to the point of being unaware of it. This tends to occur between 1 and 2 years after transplantation. Concern never disappears completely, since anxiety and revived feelings of separation and nervousness occur whenever routine investigative procedures are performed. Patients reportedly also experience sexual fantasies concerning rebirth, pregnancy, and renewed virility that at times involves the donor.[59]

Sociologic Factors

After successful transplant, some individuals may be able to resume many of the former sexual role activities, but problems continue for many.[60] The patient's withdrawal from affective relationships early in the disease may make communication with the sexual partner difficult. In addition, the family may expect the individual to assume all the usual role activities, which the patient may find difficult to do. Other families may find it difficult to allow the individual to be independent again. If there is transplant rejection, the adjustment of the patient and the family may be even more traumatic and devastating to roles and relationships.[61]

The patient is very dependent, and the family support in the recovery from transplant and its role cannot be minimized; 8 of 11 patients who died after transplant were noted to have suffered a sense of abandonment by their families.[62] Yet spouses may have difficulty adjusting to the patient's mood swings.[63] At times, it is the family member who experiences anxiety, guilt, and depression far greater than that experienced by the patient.[64]

Economic insecurity may continue. Obtaining work after transplantation may be difficult, since most places of employment require acceptance into insurance plans, and most insurance companies are reluctant to accept the individual with a history of transplantation.[65] Some patients and their families have to go on welfare, with subsequent loss of self-esteem.

The Donor

Kidney donors may experience adverse sexual response. Unfortunately, after they are subjected to long periods of medical study and discomfort, they may be forgotten, their only reward self-satisfaction.[66] Usually spouses are most willing to donate when an adult is involved, but they are not biologically related. Consequently, their role may be to solicit appropriate donors as part of the marital obligation.[67]

After the transplant surgery, donors may experience mourning and anger at the loss of a body part.[68] Commonly they suddenly become aware of their risk and their own fear. Some seem slowed down, withdrawn, and sad, and for others, body functions take an exaggerated importance. Kemph[69] investigated donor fears by use of projective tests. He found that donors believed nephrectomy might cause castration or sexual impairment.

NURSING IMPLICATIONS

After transplant, it may be fruitless for the nurse to concentrate her efforts on the patient in the hospital, since concerns are not so pressing in this environment but surface after discharge.[70]

Assessment

The candidate for renal transplant may be well known to the dialysis nurse. To promote continuity of care, the nurse shares information on a written care plan with the staff of the surgical unit. Even if surgery is done in a different hospital, patient data will help the staff better meet the patient's sexual needs. This data should include information about roles and relationships, previous concerns about sexual function and specific sexual dysfunctions, the quality of family support systems, and family attitudes. Although the patient's attention may be focused on "is the kidney working?" nurses will be better able to supply empathic support if they have this background data. If this information is not available, data should be collected on an admission nursing history (see Chapter 10). The same data collected from the patient undergoing dialysis are also needed from the transplant patient in order to plan care.

After surgery, the nurse assesses for body image disturbances, changes in the sexual relationship and role activities, and improvement in potency or orgasmic ability. If the patient had hopes for improvement that do not materialize, the nurse is alert for signs of depression and anger.

Assessment of the reaction of the donor should be done to determine if he/she is having body image disturbances or concerns about the effect of the surgery on his/her sexuality.

Planning

Since patients believe that in some way their mental attitude influences organ rejection,[71] the nurse should plan to offer realistic encouragement and hope while enhancing interpersonal and social relationships. The long-term goals include helping the patient assume usual roles and relationships, providing emotional support to cope with altered body image and anxiety, and teaching and counseling about the effects of continued therapy on physical appearance and sexual function.

Intervention

Realistic information is given to the patient who has questions about return of potency or orgasmic response. If individuals question the possibility of pregnancy, they should be told that men with transplants fathered children and women with transplants have become pregnant and had normal children. If children are not desired, birth control information is given (see Chapter 19). The nurse also describes and explains the effects of other drug therapy, especially the altered sexual drive that accompanies steroid administration (see Chapter 30). Fear of transplant rejection may be pervasive, resulting in anxiety and guilt (see Chapter 13). Interventions to help the patient cope with these responses will increase well-being. The nurse also initiates appropriate interventions for body image disturbances. Information about alternate forms of sexual expression and different positions for intercourse may help relieve concerns about injury to the kidney, although a well-healed incision and good renal function should indicate that danger of injury is past.

The nurse may have to help the patient and family adjust to new roles and relationships, intervening either to help encourage independence for the individual who is having difficulty leaving the sick role or to counsel the overly protective family so that the patient can assume his/her usual sexual role.

If economic problems persist, the nurse suggests vocational rehabilitation agencies or obtains social work consultation and assistance for the family.

Evaluation

Since the patient and family's reaction to transplantation is variable with time and with the severity of problems that arise, evaluation must be a continual process as the plan of care is revised and updated. The following outcome criteria indicates the nurse's interventions have been successful. The patient and family:

1. Describe the effect of transplantation on sexual function.
2. Identify the action and side effects of drug therapy.
3. Express the satisfaction with their level of sexual activity and relationships.
4. Identify and carry out important role activities or satisfying substitutes.

DISORDERS OF THE MALE UROGENITAL SYSTEM

Sexual dysfunction and urogenital problems are closely related in men. Sexual difficulties may be sequelae of urogenital disorders, while inadequate sexual experiences or function may motivate individuals to present with urologic complaints.

Urethritis and Prostatitis

These disorders can impair sexual function by producing dysuria, frequency of urination, and painful ejaculation. They may be bacterial or nonbacterial in origin. In men over 50, the bacterial infection may seem to disappear only to reappear weeks or months later, and this pattern can continue for years. However, impotence will result only if pain is acute.[72] When sexual dysfunction can be traced directly to urinary infection, cure will usually result in return to normal sex life.[73]

In many men, inflammation occurs without apparent infection, a condition called noninfectious prostatitis. It may be caused by a bacterium or virus that cannot be detected with present culture methods. There is no effective treatment (see Chapter 22).

Some investigators theorize that marked decrease in sexual activity can be the etiology of prostatitis by causing congestion of the prostate. When the man becomes sexually aroused, the fluid secreted from the prostate increases considerably. If arousal occurs frequently without an ejaculation, the prostate can become congested with fluid and, presumably, inflamed. This theory may partly explain the occurrence of noninfectious prostatitis among older men who have fewer opportunities for coitus than younger men.[74]

Benign Prostatic Enlargement (BPH) and Prostatic Malignancy

Benign prostatic hypertrophy, BPH, is the most common male genitourinary problem. It has been estimated that 60 percent of North American men over 60 years of age have measurable enlargement, with the incidence increasing to 95 percent in men over 80. In many men, the enlargement is not sufficient to cause symptoms, but some have symptoms ranging from mild discomfort to sexual impotence.[75] Surgical treatment is effective. Contrary to popular belief, its usual side effects do not include impotence.

Prostatic cancer is the third-ranking cause of death from cancer in men. Its therapy, by surgery and/or radiation, can produce impotence or ejaculatory incompetence while bringing cure (see Chapters 23 and 24).

Peyronie's Disease

This is a deformity of the penis due to fibrous plaque in the corpora cavernosus. The lesion interferes with erections by decreasing the blood supply to one or both of the corpora. A severe deflection of the penis occurs along with partial or complete impotence. The discomfort that accompanies the condition may be relieved by anti-inflammatory agents, but the fibrosis is permanent. In severe cases, the plaque may be excised followed by skin graft to the corpora to correct the severe deflection. Penile prosthetic implants may also be used[76,77] (see Chapter 3).

Phimosis

Tightness of the foreskin, preventing it from being drawn back from the head of the penis, may cause infection and irritation. Fibrous tissue forms between the foreskin and the glans so that the foreskin can no longer be moved, causing pressure on the glans and extreme pain with erection. Circumcision is the only treatment.[78]

Priapism

This disorder is a state of sustained erection of the penis not accompanied by sexual desire. It occurs most frequently in the 30s and 40s and is usually accompanied by pain. There are two types—sustained and recurrent nocturnal. Priapism may result from urethral inflammation, from new growth involving the corpora cavernosa, or from systemic disease such as leukemia or sickle-cell anemia. Disease of the spinal cord may be accompanied by penile erection for long periods of time. Recurrent nonsustained priapism is extremely painful and is often of unknown etiology, although it may be associated with prostatitis.[79]

Priapism may be a surgical emergency. Restoration of the venous drainage from the corpora may be needed to prevent permanent damage to erectile ability. A needle aspiration with a large-gauge needle inserted in the base of the corpora will relieve pressure. The man who is untreated will develop a fibrotic, painful, distorted penis. Some surgeons anastomose the saphenous vein to the corpora spongiosum in an attempt to gain decompression.[80] Other treatment has involved evacuating the corpora cavernosa of the penis and performing an end-to-side shunt of the saphenous vein to the corpora. This procedure results in impotence unless pressure is applied to the shunt. Some positions in intercourse will supply the pressure, or minimal pressure can be used to restore erection in all positions.[81]

Dyspareunia in Males

Poor hygiene may be a cause of painful intercourse. If the foreskin is not retracted and the head of the penis washed well to remove smegma, inflamation, irritation, and infection make thrusting or even vaginal entry painful.

Hypersensitivity reactions of the penis

caused by allergic reaction to contraceptive creams, jellies, and foams, and douching preparations may cause inflammation and blistering of the penis. If the blisters break, intercourse can be extremely painful for the man. Change in contraceptive method or in douche preparation or elimination of douching will usually result in relief of symptoms.[82]

Infections of the vaginal canal can also cause infection of the penis. As in women, burning and itching after intercourse result. Gonorrhea, particularly, can cause severe pain during and right after ejaculation. The inflammatory process results in narrowing of the urethra, making urination and ejaculation painful (see Chapter 22).

Abnormal sensitivity of the glans in some men results in the head of the penis becoming so exquisitely tender right after ejaculation that they cannot keep it in the vagina and must withdraw immediately after ejaculating. Men who are not circumcised may get relief occasionally by pulling the foreskin well back over the head of the penis.[83]

Venereal Disease

Problems associated with venereal disease are discussed in Chapter 22.

Psychosexual Factors and Urogenital Problems

Men may mask their sexual problems by presenting with urologic complaints such as difficulty in urination or pelvic pain. The patient may be convinced that the physical disability is the only cause of sexual impairment, or he may be so ashamed of his decreasing sexual capacity that he does not even mention it when discussing his symptoms. In most of these cases, there is no reason for the urogenital changes to prevent a satisfactory sex life. Anxiety about decreasing sexual function, however, may have more devastating effects.

NURSING IMPLICATIONS

When giving information for the nursing history, the man may casually make some comment about sex, but more often he does not, and the subject is only raised if specific questions are included.

Intervention may be as simple as teaching proper hygiene or suggesting change in contraceptive methods to as complex as providing emotional support to a man facing permanent sexual dysfunction. (See Chapter 11 on teaching and Chapter 12 on counseling.)

DISORDERS OF THE FEMALE URINARY SYSTEM

Kent[84] reports that the incidence of urinary tract infections in women is directly related to sexual activity. Only 1 percent of school-age girls have these disorders compared to 3 to 5 percent of adult women. The incidence in women who do not engage in sexual intercourse is lower than 1 percent. Older women who are sexually active are particularly susceptible to urologic problems because of atrophic changes that take place in genital mucous membranes.

Cystitis, Urethritis, and Cystourethritis

These conditions are the most common cause of sexual dysfunction in women. The symptoms of infection of the bladder and urethra may make sexual intercourse painful because of their close proximity to the vagina. In addition, these syndromes are most commonly caused by mechanical irritation and transmission of bacteria during intercourse.[85]

Organisms may also be introduced into the urethra by manual or oral stimulation of the vagina or clitoris during foreplay. The vulva, urethra, or bladder may be irritated during intercourse. An anterior "high-riding" position of the male partner during intercourse may increase clitoral stimulation but can also cause urethral irritation. In some women, the urethra is located intravaginally and may be pushed into the vagina during intercourse causing irritation.[86]

Postmenopausal women are predisposed to trauma during intercourse and to urinary tract infection, since they tend to have weakened urethral walls because of estrogen deprivation. Their diminished vaginal lubrication and more constricted, shorter vaginal barrel also predispose them to mechanical irritation (see Chapter 18). As women grow older, sexual intercourse is usually less frequent and some degree of atrophy of genitourinary structures results, so urinary infections are more likely to occur after intercourse. Older women may also be more disposed to urologic problems because of the tendency of their partners to engage in extended intercourse with delayed ejaculatory response. This may make the sexual experience more pleasurable, but this extended intercourse may enable infecting bacteria to be "massaged" into the paraurethral glands from which they can be transported into the bladder to cause cystitis.[87]

In addition to dysuria and frequency of urination, women may complain of increased sensitivity and discomfort during intercourse. These symptoms may be present before an infection occurs or remain after it has been treated. The causes of inflammation without infection are not clear but may be due to mechanical trauma, vascular incompetence, parasitic organisms, or even allergy.[88]

Noninfectious Urologic Disorders

Those that can cause sexual dysfunction include urethral caruncle, urethral diverticulum, or abcess formation anywhere along the urethra. These may respond to estrogen therapy but sometimes require surgical treatment.[89]

Urinary incontinence may cause dysfunction. Ninety (43 percent) of 208 women attending incontinence clinics reported less frequent intercourse because of dyspareunia and leakage during coitus. Those with bladder instability had a significantly higher incidence than those with stress incontinence.[90]

Psychosexual Factors and Urinary Disorders

The discomfort of urinary disorders can be an impediment to sexual pleasure, but it usually causes only temporary sexual abstinence. As with some men, urologic problems may be a convenient excuse to forego sex entirely. The nurse must be sensitive to possible psychosocial factors that may operate to cause a desire for sexual abstinence such as problems in the interpersonal relationship of the sexual partners.

NURSING IMPLICATIONS

The factors in assessing problems identified for male patients apply to the female patient. Medical intervention for urinary tract infections is directed toward eradicating bacteria from the urinary tract. However, it is common for these infections to recur regularly, despite antibacterial therapy. Organisms may migrate into periurethral structures, and when sexual activity resumes, they are dislodged to begin the cycle again. Long-term therapy may be required. The nurse helps relieve the concern of the individual by explaining the importance of continued therapy to obtain cure. Some women believe that after symptoms are relieved, medication can be discontinued or "saved" for another episode, so it is essential that they be told the importance of taking "all the pills" as directed.

Teaching various hygiene practices may be effective in preventing recurrent infection. It can be helpful if the patient flushes the urinary tract by urinating as soon as possible after intercourse. Increasing intake of fluids will increase output and facilitate removal of bacteria. A shower or bath for both the man and the woman before and after coitus helps to decrease the organisms in the periurethral area. The male superior position should be avoided, because this position exerts extra stress on the urethra.

DISORDERS OF THE FEMALE REPRODUCTIVE SYSTEM

Gynecologic problems may not be a deterrent to sexual intercourse until the ages of 30 to 40 but may cause fear and concerns about sexuality at any age. It is after the 20s that more overt problems prevent normal sexual activity.[91]

Vaginal Changes

In the adult woman, vaginal bleeding, discharge, and pelvic pain may affect sexual function.[92] Vaginal discharge in the absence of pathogens may be a sign of sexual disturbance; a complaint may be overlubrication of the vagina during intercourse, which may be accompanied by a widened vaginal opening. Complaints may come from the sexual partner who believes these changes are the result of childbearing and age. Surgery may be performed for minor vaginal relaxation, but afterward, the man may have difficulty penetrating the tighter vagina, especially if his erections are less firm because of age. Often, psychologic problems may require counseling of the couple.[93]

Other women may complain of inadequate vaginal lubrication. If not due to decreased estrogen because of age or pathology, it may occur from inadequate foreplay or problems in the woman's relationship with the man.

Vulvovaginitis

Infection is the most common cause of burning, itching, and aching in the vagina. The sources of vaginal infection are generally intercourse or contamination from the rectum, hands, clothing, or a foreign substance pushed into the vagina. The most common infections are caused by bacteria, but trichomonal (caused by a protozoan) and monilial (by a fungus) infections also occur frequently.

The most common bacterial invaders come from the colon and rectum. This occurs if the couple is using rectal intercourse, in which the man inserts his penis in the rectum, thrusts through the plateau stage, and then at the stage of inevitability withdraws and inserts his penis in the vagina to ejaculate. The penis has been contaminated with *Escherichia coli,* and this organism is introduced into the vagina.[94] (See Chapter 22 for other causes.)

Pelvic and Vaginal Pain

After childbirth, pelvic pain and dyspareunia may be due to trauma from an episiotomy or descent of the child through the birth canal. Levator muscle spasm or pelvic blood vessel engorgement may also cause pelvic discomfort. Vaginal sensitivity to contraceptives or douche products may cause itching and burning. Frequent douching is a major offender.[95] Tears in the broad ligaments that support the uterus may occur during childbirth, criminal abortions, or rape. Pain during penile thrusting, increased pelvic congestion, throbbing, a "tired feeling," and dysmenorrhea may be frequent symptoms. Surgical repair has been successful in relieving the symptoms.[96]

Endometriosis produces deep pelvic pain. Irritation of the pelvic organs causes fibrous tissue to grow between them, resulting in tissues that are hard and inelastic. The increase in vaginal size that occurs during sexual excitement and the movement during the thrusting put tension on these tissues, causing extreme discomfort.

When intercourse is painful, there is a possibility that the hymen is still intact or that injured parts of it are still present. An enlargement of the small glands in the labia minora can also cause pain on entry. Material may sometimes collect under the hood of the clitoris and irritate the area. Intense burning results with vaginal penetration by the penis, and any movement of the clitoral foreskin during foreplay or entry may be painful. In some cases, surgical treatment is necessary.[97]

Cancer of the Reproductive Organs

The diagnosis of cancer itself may cause sexual dysfunction. The pathophysiologic changes resulting from surgery and other therapy may require numerous changes in the sexual life style (see Chapters 23 and 24).

Increased sexual activity among adolescents and young adults has been suggested as a cause of cervical abnormality and sexual activity early in life with many partners has been connected with incidence of cervical cancer (see Chapter 23). Roddick[98] found a high percentage of cervical epithelial abnormality in 1594 sexually active young women of primarily middle and upper socioeconomic backgrounds, higher than in the so-called high-risk groups. Changes ranged from mild dysplasia to carcinoma in situ. The women also had a high incidence of vulvovaginitis and abdominal pain and bleeding.

Psychosexual Factors and Disorders of the Female Reproductive System

Psychologic factors may operate to cause dyspareunia (see Chapter 3). Fear of coitus for whatever reason is the most frequent psychologic etiology. However, before attributing sexual dysfunction to psychosomatic factors, the nurse must be sure that careful medical investigation has ruled out any pathology. A diagnosis of pelvic disease itself may cause anxiety and fear, resulting in sexual dysfunction without biologic basis.

NURSING IMPLICATIONS

Many women delay or avoid seeking health care when they know it may involve a pelvic examination until symptoms of the disorder are untenable. They may have heard stories about the discomfort of the examination and may fear the embarrassment.[99] Nurses can do much to alleviate these fears. After assessing the woman's attitudes toward and knowledge about the examination, the nurse, when necessary, explains about the examining table and the lithotomy position, shows the speculum, and describes what the examination usually feels like.

In all settings, nurses also take an active role in preventing gynecologic problems by teaching the importance of yearly or more frequent pelvic examinations and Pap test, especially to sexually active young women who may think they are too young to worry about cancer. The nurse should emphasize, however, that the Pap test does not provide insurance against cancer of other reproductive organs, but that early detection of other pelvic pathology may prevent more serious sequelae.

These contacts with women also give the nurse an opportunity to teach about the anatomy and physiology of the reproductive system and of reproduction itself. The visit for a gynecologic problem may also provide the nurse with opportunity to assess the woman's desire for conception control and, when indicated, to provide information about various methods (see Chapter 19).

Many women consider any vaginal discharge abnormal. Education about the reasons for vaginal secretions and the difference between the normal and those of sexually transmitted diseases helps clarify misconceptions (see Chapter 22).

The nurse also teaches about the dangers of frequent douching. One of the most widely held misconceptions about feminine hygiene is that routine douching is necessary after intercourse or at other periods during the menstrual cycle. The nurse explains that the vagina returns to its normally protective acid condition within a few hours after intercourse. Douching removes the residual acid and makes the vagina vulnerable to bacterial or fungal growth. Women need only wash their external genitalia with soap and water if they wish to remove seminal fluid or vaginal secretions outside the vaginal canal. The woman is also warned that she may develop sensitivity to the substances used in the douching solution.

Infections follow rectal–vaginal intercourse, so the nurse explains to the couple that the penis must be washed after rectal intromission and before vaginal intromission or vaginal infections may become a chronic problem. If pelvic infection is recurrent, teaching of the importance of hygiene measures, such as bathing and washing of hands before sexual activity is essential.

INFERTILITY

Approximately 5 million couples in the United States have infertility problems. The male is as frequently at fault as the female when infertility is present. Factors on the male side are solely responsible for about 33 percent of cases; in about the same number, both the husband and wife contribute problems and in the remainder, problems of the wife are the cause of infertility. Infertility can present a serious life crisis.[100]

Feelings of the infertile couple range from shock and surprise with news of infertility to denial, anger, isolation, guilt, and grief.[101]

It damages sexual self-worth and body image, a man or woman feeling damaged or defective. Women describe themselves as "hollow" or empty. Men describe feeling like castrates, or talk about intercourse as "shooting blanks." They worry about sexual performance and desirability. During the fertility studies, many people may have decrease in desire or orgasm and impotence. Their life is focused around ovulation time when they are "supposed" to have sex. The menstrual cycle is watched and the woman may be preoccupied with looking for signs of pregnancy. When menstruation begins, there is despair and depression.[102]

Infertile spouses may have guilt about past events they feel are responsible for infertility. Anger may be directed at physician or staff, parents or spouse. The professional helps the couples communicate and empathize with each other, facilitating their growth in self-awareness. Clear, concise information can do much to decrease anxiety.

Male Infertility

Male infertility may be caused by stress, alcohol, marijuana, heroin and methadone use,

increased scrotal temperature, chemicals and radiation, mechanical obstruction and varicoceles, as well as numerous diseases. The role of the immune system is unclear, but there may be antibodies present in cervical mucus that attack the sperm, cause decreased fertility.[103]

During the history, the man is questioned about his libido, frequency of coitus, and the occurrence of ejaculation. A history of previous illness, injury, or surgery, such as prostatectomy or sympathectomy, may give clues to etiology. Examination is made for evidence of secondary sexual characteristics and for evidence of eunuchoidism or gynecomastia. Palpation of the testes and scrotum is performed. A semen specimen is obtained for sperm count, motility, and abnormal forms. Four semen analyses are also done, one each month, to determine the sperms' response to the woman's midcycle cervical mucus,[104] since some mucus may be destructive to sperm.[105] Testicular biopsy may be necessary when the cause of azoospermia or oligospermia is not obvious.[106]

Treatment of male infertility depends on the cause. If absence of sperm is due to mechanical obstruction, surgery is rarely possible. Varicoceles can be treated by high ligations. Testosterone therapy has been used as well as therapy with human chorionic gonadotropin (HCG) and follicle-stimulating hormone (FSH), but on the whole, gonadotropin therapy has not been successful.[107] (See Chapter 26 for discussion of various hormones.) Unfortunately, there may be no demonstrable cause for oligospermia or aspermia.

Female Infertility

In the presence of ovulation, infertility is often due to interference with the ascent of sperm. Congenital malformation of the vagina, infection, or dyspareunia may interfere with normal coitus. Sperm may be prevented from ascending higher by chronic cervicitis or estrogen deficiency, both of which cause qualitative or quantitative disturbances in cervical mucus production. Abnormalities in the uterus, retroversion, fibroids, endometritis, and functional progesterone deficiency may also be problematic. The fallopian tubes may be partially or completely obstructed by congenital narrowing, inflammation, or tumors in the adnexae. Adhesions due to endometriosis or inflammation may prevent the ovum from reaching the fallopian tubes.[108]

The role of emotional factors in infertility is not well understood. In the female, they may interfere with normal coitus and may also interfere with normal hormonal balance, causing failure of ovulation. It has been postulated that psychogenic factors may cause tubal spasms and interfere with the normal transport of the ovum or ascent of the sperm.

Examination of the vagina, tests for tubal patency, endometrial biopsy, culdoscopy, or laparoscopy may be indicated. Evaluation of ovulation is made by recording basal temperatures. Cervical mucus is examined 8 to 12 hours after coitus for the number of viable sperm. The contents of the cervical canal are also aspirated and examined under a microscope. An even distribution of at least five motile sperm per high-power field indicates a satisfactory test.[109]

Treatment of physiologic problems may correct the infertility. Vaginal and cervical infections are treated by antibiotics. Patency of fallopian tubes may be restored by insufflation. Plastic repair of tubes may be helpful, but surgery may be more effective when the ovaries are fixed by adhesions or endometriosis and are still functioning and when the fallopian tubes are relatively normal. Myomectomy for fibroids and appropriate treatment for ovarian cysts may be effective in restoring fertility.[110]

Hormonal therapy, the use of clomiphene, FSH, HCG, and LH/FSH may restore ovulation (see Chapter 26). The woman who ovulates but has inadequate progesterone release from the corpus luteum can be given small doses of progestational compounds such as norethisterone.[111]

When the woman has irreversible blockage of the fallopian tubes, couples are increasingly seeking procedures such as fertilization of the ova by husband's sperm outside the uterus and reimplantation into the womb, the in vitro, "test tube" baby. The long-term effects on the sexual relationship of this and other procedures still needs to be evaluated.

ARTIFICIAL INSEMINATION

Infertility may be treated by artificial insemination (AI). There are two types: artificial insemination by husband (AIH) and artificial insemination by donor (AID). The first is used in retroversion of the uterus, impotence, premature ejaculation or apareunia. It is not effective if there is reduced semen quality or if an analysis of mucus obtained at midcycle indicates a low number of sperm have been able to penetrate (cervical mucus hostility). AID is used in this case, or when sperm are abnormal or genetic disorders exist.[112]

AID may be accomplished using fresh or frozen sperm. Using fresh spermatozoa, in a 12-year experience of AID, of 381 women treated 230 became pregnant at least once. When frozen sperm are used, the frequency of pregnancy is approximately two-thirds that expected of fresh. The advantage of using fresh sperm is that the donor is known. Opinions differ as to how often one donor should be used. Some limit it to 6 times, others 15, and one physician used the same donor for 15 pregnancies.[113]

The procedure is increasingly becoming accepted. Both infertile couples and medical students favored use of AID for infertility and where risk of genetic disease and inheritable retardation exist, but 143 of 147 said they would not tell the child.[114] The Catholic, the Lutheran Church, and Orthodox Jewry, however, prohibit all types of artificial insemination.

Careful counseling and screening of couples who have elected the procedure are essential. Adverse responses occurred in 11 of 16 husbands who had a period of impotence after insemination. Berger[115] concluded that men need to resolve conflict and mourn the loss of fertility before donor insemination takes place. Longitudinal studies of the effects of AID (artificial insemination by donor) on the sexual relationship need to be done.

Husbands may participate in the procedure by being present. Even with counseling, couples may have to work through fears that because of a mistake in the donor the child will be incongruous in racial or physical appearance, or that the baby's health, intelligence or attractiveness may not meet expectations.[116]

Legal implications involve the mother, husband, biologic father, physician, and AID child; every country and state has its own legal interpretation. Some states have found the AID child legitimate providing there is written consent between the husband and wife. In England, the child is illegitimate.[117]

NOTES

1. Lim VS, Fang VS: Gonadal dysfunction in uremic men. Am J Med 58:655–661, 1975
2. Thorn GW, Adams R, Braunwald E, Isselbacher KJ. Petersdorf RG (eds): Harrison's Principles of Internal Medicine, 8th ed. New York, McGraw-Hill, 1977, pp 1433–1435
3. Kossoris P: Family therapy: An adjunct to hemodialysis and transplantation. Am J Nurs 70:1730–1733, 1970
4. Lim VS, Fang VS: Gonadal dysfunction in uremic men. Am J Med 53:655, 1975
5. Schein PS, Winokur SH: Immunosuppressive and cytotoxic chemotherapy. Ann Intern Med 82:84–93, 1975
6. Elstein M, Smith EKM, Curtis JH: Reproductive potential of patients treated by maintenance hemodialysis. Br Med J 1:734–736, 1969
7. Sherman FP: Impotence in patients with chronic renal failure in dialysis. Fertil Steril 26:221–223, 1975
8. Hickman BW: All about sex . . . despite dialysis. Am J Nurs 77:606–607, 1977
9. Levy NB: The psychology and care of the maintenance hemodialysis patient. Heart Lung 2:400–405, 1973
10. Cummings JW: The pressures and how patients respond. Am J Nurs 70:70–76, 1970
11. Waltzer WC: Sexual and reproductive function in men treated with hemodialysis and renal transplantation. J Urology 126:713–716, 1981
12. Furlow WL: Diagnosis and treatment of male erectile failure. Diabetes Care 2:18, 1979
13. Two news reports: Which penile prosthesis? Study provides some guidelines. Doppler probe technique reveals physiologic basis for impotence. Hospital Practice 14:19, 1979
14. Waltzer WC: Sexual and reproductive function in men treated with hemodialysis and renal transplantation. J Urology 126:715, 1981
15. Dalla Rosa C, Cascone C, Antonucci F, Foresta C, Mastrogiacoma I: The hypothalamic-hypophyseal-gonadal axis in patients undergoing chronic hemodialysis. Proc Eur Dial Transplant Assoc 14:565–567, 1977
16. Oag D: The nurse's role in the dialysis unit. Nurs Times 72:926–928, 1976
17. Levy NB: The psychology and care of the maintenance hemodialysis patient. Heart Lung 2:404, 1973
18. Ibid
19. Hickman BW: All about sex . . . despite dialysis. Am J Nurs 77:607, 1977
20. Oag D: The nurse's role in the dialysis unit. Nurs Times 72:927, 1976
21. Sherman FP: Impotence in patients with chronic renal failure in dialysis. Fertile Steril 26:222, 1975
22. Cummings JW: The pressures and how patients respond. Am J Nurs 70:72, 1970

23. Oag, D: The nurse's role in the dialysis unit. Nurs Times 72:926, 1976

24. Cummings, JW: The pressures and how patients respond.Am J Nurs 70:72, 1970

25. Greenberg RP, Davis G, Massey R: The psychologic evaluation of patients for a kidney transplant and hemodialysis program. Am J Psychiatry 130:274–277, 1973

26. Levy NB: The psychology and care of the maintenance hemodialysis patient. Heart Lung 2:404, 1973

27. Kossoris P: Family therapy: An adjunct to hemodialysis and transplantation. Am J Nurs 70:1730, 1970

28. Cummings JW: The pressures and how patients respond. Am J Nurs 70:72, 1970

29. Chaney P: Surviving. Nursing 76(6): 46–49, 1976

30. Levy NB: The psychology and care of the maintenance hemodialysis patient. Heart Lung 2:403, 1973

31. Chaney P: Surviving. Nursing 76(6):47, 1976

32. Cummings JW: The pressures and how patients respond. Am J Nurs 70:72, 1970

33. Ibid.

34. Berkman AH, Katz LA, Weissman R: Sexuality and life-style of home dialysis patients. Arch Phys Med Rehabil 63: 272–275, 1982

35. Hassett M: Teaching hemodialysis to the family unit. Nurs Clin North Am 7:349–362, 1972

36. Berkman AH, Katz LA, Weissman R: Sexuality and the life-style of home dialysis patients. Arch Phys Med Rehabil 63:274, 1982

37. Hickman BW: All about sex . . . despite dialysis. Am J Nurs 77:607, 1977

38. Kossoris P: Family therapy: An adjunct to hemodialysis and transplantation. Am J Nurs 70:1733, 1970

39. Levy NB: The psychology and care of the maintenance hemodialysis patient. Heart Lung 2:404, 1973

40. Hickman BW: All about sex . . . despite dialysis. Am J Nurs 77:607, 1977

41. Chaney P: Surviving. Nursing 76(6):48, 1976

42. Cummings JW: The pressures and how patients respond. Am J Nurs 70:75, 1970

43. Chaney P: Surviving. Nursing 76(6):48, 1976

44. Levy NB: The psychology and care of the maintenance hemodialysis patient. Heart Lung 2:404, 1973

45. Oag D: The nurse's role in the dialysis unit. Nurs Times 72:927, 1976

46. Hassett M: Teaching hemodialysis to the family unit. Nurs Clin North Am 7:359, 1972

47. Ibid, p 360

48. McClellan MS: Crisis groups in special care areas. Nurs Clin North Am 7:363–371, 1972

49. Willey M: Care of the patient with a kidney transplant. Nurs Clin North Am 8:127–135, 1973

50. Burns JR, Houttuin E, Gregory JG, et al: Vascular-induced erectile impotence in renal transplant patients. J Urology 121:721–724, 1979

51. Waltzer WC: Sexual and reproductive function in men treated with hemodialysis and renal transplantation. J Urology 63:715, 1982

52. Nelson B: A practical application of nursing theory. Nurs Clin North Am 13:157–169, 1978

53. Kobrzycki P: Renal transplant complications. Am J Nurs 77:641–643, 1977

54. Lim VS, Fang VS: Gonadal dysfunction in uremic men. Sm J Med 58:559, 1975

55. Schein PS, Winokur SH: Immunosuppressive and cytotoxic chemotherapy. Ann Intern Med 82:89, 1975

56. Nelson B: A practical application of nursing theory. Nurs Clin North Am 13:160, 1978

57. Eisendrath RM: The role of grief and fear in the death of kidney transplant patients. AORN J 11:77–78, 1970

58. Nelson B: A practical application of nursing theory. Nurs Clin North Am 13:166, 1978

59. Ibid, p 162

60. Kossoris P: Family therapy: An adjunct to hemodialysis and transplantation. Am J Nurs 70:1730, 1970

61. Ibid, p 1731

62. Eisendrath RM: The role of grief and fear in the death of kidney transplant patients. AORN J 11:71, 1970

63. Nelson B: A practical application of nursing theory. Nurs Clin North Am 13:161, 1978

64. Kossoris P: Family therapy: An adjunct to hemodialysis and transplantation. Am J Nurs 70:1731, 1970

65. Nelson B: A practical application of nursing theory. Nurs Clin North Am 13:163, 1978

66. Schumann D: The renal donor. Am J Nurs 74:105–110, 1974

67. Ibid, p 106

68. Ibid, p 110

69. Kemph JP: Observations of the effects of kidney transplants on donors and recipients. Dis Nerv Syst 31:323–325, 1970

70. Kossoris P: Family therapy: An adjunct to hemodialysis and transplantation. Am J Nurs 70:1730, 1970

71. Abram HS: The psychiatrist, the treatment of chronic renal failure and the prolongation of life—III. Am J Psychiatry 128:1534–1539, 1972

72. Gonick P: Urologic problem and sexual dysfunction. In Oaks WW, Melchiode GA, Ficher I (eds): Sex and the Life Cycle. New York, Grune and Stratton, 1976, pp 191–198

73. Kent S: The intimate relationship between the urinary system and sexual function. Geriatrics 30:138–143, 1975

74. Ibid

75. Ibid, p 143

76. Gonick P: Urologic problem and sexual dysfunction. In Oaks WW, Melchiode GA, Ficher I (eds): Sex and the Life Cy-

cle, New York Grune and Stratton, 1976, p 193

77. Malloy TR, Wein AJ, Carpiniello VL: Advanced Peyronie's disease treated with inflatable penile prosthesis. J Urology 125:327–328, 1981

78. Masters WH, Johnson VE: Human Sexual Inadequacy. Boston, Little, Brown, 1970, p 290

79. Thorn GW, Adams R, Braunwald E, Isselbacher KJ, Petersdorf RG (eds): Harrison's Principles of Internal Medicine, 8th ed. New York, McGraw-Hill, 1977, p 246

80. Ryan JJ: Surgical intervention in the treatment of sexual disorders. In Meyers JK (ed): Clinical Management of Sexual Disorders. Baltimore, Williams and Wilkins, 1976, pp 226–252

81. Zinsser HH: Sex and surgical procedures in the male. In Sadock BJ, Kaplan HI, Freedman AM (eds): The Sexual Experience. Baltimore, Williams and Wilkins, 1976, pp 303–307

82. Belliveau F, Richter L: Understanding Human Sexual Inadequacy. New York, Bantam, 1970, pp 203–205

83. Ibid, p 205

84. Kent S: Urinary tract problems in women are linked to sexual activity. Geriatrics 30:145–146, 1975

85. Ibid, p 145

86. Ibid

87. Ibid

88. Ibid, p 146

89. Ibid

90. Sutherst J, Brown M: Sexual dysfunction associated with urinary incontinence. Urologia Internationalis 35:414–416, 1980

91. Eskin BA: Sex and the gynecologic patient. In Oaks WW, Melchiode GA, Ficher I (eds): Sex and the Life Cycle. New York, Grune and Stratton, 1976, pp 199–212

92. Ibid, p 206

93. Ibid, p 207

94. Belliveau F, Richter L: Understanding

Human Sexual Inadequacy. New York, Bantam, 1970, p 197

95. Ibid, p 199

96. Ibid, p 201

97. Ibid, p 200

98. Roddick JW: Gynecologic disease in young sexually active women. Am J Maternity Gynecol 126:880–889, 1976

99. Roznoy MS: Taking a sexual history. Am J Nurs 76:1279–1281, 1976

100. Buongiovani E: Infertility. In Smith ED (ed). Women's Health Care: A Guide for Patient Education. New York, Appleton-Century-Crofts, 1981

101. Menning BE: Psychosocial impact of infertility. Nurs Clin North Am 17:155–163, 1982

102. Mazor MD: Barren couples. Psychology Today 12:101–107, 1979

103. Alexander NJ: Male evaluation and semen analysis. Clin Obstet Gynecol 25:463–479, 1982

104. Smith KD: Endocrine problems and treatment. Clin Obstet Gynecol 25:483–494, 1982

105. Levin R: The physiology of sexual function in women. Clin Obstet Gynecol 7:213–249, 1980

106. Hall R, Anderson J, Smart GA, Besser GM: Clinical Endocrinology, 2nd ed. Philadelphia, Lippincott, 1974, p 259

107. Ibid, p 260

108. Hall R, Anderson J, Smart GA, Besser GM: Clinical Endocrinology, 2nd ed. Philadelphia, Lippincott, 1974, p 199

109. Ibid, p 200

110. Ibid, p 201

111. Ibid

112. Thompson W, Boyle DD: Counseling patients for artificial insemination and subsequent pregnancy. Clin Obstet Gynecol 9:211–225, 1982

113. Foss GL: Artificial insemination by donor: A review of 12 years experience. J Biosoc Sci 14:253–262, 1982

114. Leiblum FE, Barbrack C: Artificial insemination by donor: A survey of attitudes and knowledge in medical students and infertile couples. J Biosoc Sci 15:165–172, 1983

115. Berger DM: Couples reactions to male infertility and donor insemination. Am J Psych 137:1047–1049, 1980

116. Menning BE: Psychosocial impact of infertility. Nurs Clin North Am 17:162, 1982

117. Thompson W, Boyle DD: Counseling patients for artificial insemination and subsequent pregnancy. Clin Obstet Gynecol 9:218, 1982

Chapter 29

Sexuality and the Mentally Retarded and the Mentally Ill

MENTAL RETARDATION AND SEXUALITY

For many years, mentally slow individuals were often relegated to back wards of mental institutions or secluded in their families' homes, where their activities were restricted and closely supervised. Sexuality of the mentally retarded was neither discussed nor considered other than to make sure that they were not sexually victimized or did not sexually victimize someone else. At the present time, the philosophy of care of the retarded is changing and the normalization principle guides persons who are responsible for their care.

The normalization principle in the care of mentally retarded persons means making available to all a pattern of life and conditions of everyday living that are as close as possible to the regular circumstances and ways of life of society. Consequently, it means experiencing the normal rhythm of the day, with privacy, activities, and responsibilities; the normal rhythm of the week, with a home to live in, a school to go to, and leisure time with social interactions; the normal rhythm of the year, with changing ways of life, of the family, and of the community during the different seasons.[1] Unfortunately, many mentally retarded individuals still do not live in the larger society, but in the restrictive society of an institution, so they are

unable or poorly able to experience patterns of life that are so important for human development.

In recent years, many mentally retarded either have been returned to the community or have never been admitted to institutions, and nurses' involvement with the retarded will probably increase.[2] It is essential that nurses and others accept the unique individuality of the retarded, recognizing their strengths and their areas of need.

If retarded persons are to experience normal development, experiences of the life cycle from infancy through old age, and live life as fully as possible, the relationships between the sexes should also follow the regular pattern and variations of society. This does not make them "normal," but it will make their life conditions as normal as possible.[3]

This section of the chapter will give an overview of the development of sexuality in the mentally retarded and of the teaching and counseling that they and their families need so the retarded can experience their sexuality to the fullest and can avoid the sexual problems that may confront them.

Relation to Sexuality

The American Psychiatric Association has identified the levels of retardation as profound, severe, moderate, mild, and borderline. At the one end of the continuum are individuals whose handicap is so extreme that they may never learn the simple tasks of self-care, while at the other end are individuals who are barely distinguishable from so-called normal persons. Kempton[4] divides the retarded into two descriptive categories—the trainable and the educable. Only 1 in 30 is so seriously retarded that he/she needs nursing care in an institution.[5]

Mentally retarded persons share with all of mankind a desire for closeness, physical contact, affection, and being "in on things." Like the so-called normal person, the so-called mentally retarded person is likely to have but does not necessarily have a strong interest in sex. Also, like the normal person, the retarded person will have great difficulty in finding ways to express sexual interest, since many forms are defined by society as immoral, unacceptable, and illegal. Since retarded persons are also observed and supervised more closely than others, they have less privacy and are more likely to behave in ways that because of visibility, are regarded as a symptom of retardation rather than of the "goldfish in a bowl" life of the retarded.[6]

Mentally retarded people, like many other persons, are interested in sex primarily for sensual pleasure. Sexual gratification usually has little to do with desire to procreate, desire to establish a permanent or long-term relationship, or occurrence within love or marriage.

Mentally retarded also share with the "normal" population a language barrier when confronted with terms related to sexuality, lack of knowledge of sexuality, and lack of training in child-rearing practices. It seems apparent that the mentally retarded individual is in most ways not readily distinguishable from the rest of the population in relation to sexuality.[7]

Psychologic Factors Affecting Sexuality.
Slogans used to describe mentally retarded are unsupported and largely incorrect. They have been called dependent, anxious, impulsive, and immature. They are in a minority status and a stigmatized group[8] and as a consequence suffer severe assault on self-esteem. (See Chapter 7 for discussion of self-concept, esteem, and minority groups.) The individual learns to remain silent and becomes sensitive to the idea of not knowing, trying to hide ignorance because it upsets parents and causes laughter in others. Retarded individuals may try to mask defects and hide their deficiency.[9]

The child has a major identity problem. Self-concept is also diminished because the retarded individual is constantly reminded of unworthiness and weakness and is filled with feelings of futility and rejection.[10]

Moreover, in a comprehensive review of literature and research on all aspects of sexuality and mental handicap, Craft and Craft[11] found that there is little research devoted to the attitudes of retarded people toward sexuality in general and their sexuality in particular.

Society and the Retarded.
The social system, especially in education, reinforces the sense of self-abasement. The retarded come largely from the poor and suffer the additional handicap of poor family structure, physical disease, and language disability. Blacks are heavily overrepresented in classes for the retarded, and once the individual is marked as defective, he/she is formed into a deficient adult by the social system.

Society has always had difficulty coping with the sexuality of its members and even more so with the sexuality of the retarded. To develop normal sexuality, the retarded individual needs human experiences. However, it is difficult to develop or build a pattern of support for mentally retarded individuals so they can live in the community. Money and jobs are less available, as are the necessary human support systems.[12]

Living in a heterosexual world, where boys and girls, men and women are desegregated, helps the retarded person develop normal patterns of living and better patterns of behavior, since the motivation for sociosexual learning is increased.[13] Knowledge of sexuality also seems to be increased. Although Hall and Morris[14] found no differences in the total score of sexual attitudes and self-concept of 61 institutionalized and 61 noninstitutionalized adolescents; the noninstitutionalized group was more knowledgeable about sexuality. Further, as the adolescents remained in the institution, the amount of knowledge appeared to decrease.

Until relatively recent times, institutions focused more on attempting to prevent sexual experiences than providing instruction. As the focus has turned to deinstitutionalizing retarded persons, more attention is being paid to not only vocational adjustment, but also to social, sexual, and emotional competence, since studies have shown that deficits in sociosexual functioning may quickly lead to loss of job and rejection by the community.[15] In addition, teaching acceptable sexual behavior is important, because the mentally retarded person may be very suggestible and willing to follow others,[16] giving rise to deviant behavior and subsequent incarceration in an institution.

Throughout the life cycle, retarded persons must cope with the social stigma and misconceptions that society often has about them. Development of normal sexuality is problematic to say the least.

Sexual Development and Sexual Problems of the Mentally Retarded

There are three developmental tasks or precursor experiences that are needed to alleviate or to prevent problems and conflicts when physical sexual maturation with its need to express sexual impulse occurs: (1) the development of an appreciation of sensuality, (2) the development of the ability to make responsible and fulfilling choices, and (3) the development of the ability to handle feelings in a socially acceptable manner.[17] Achievement of these tasks is facilitated when the child experiences them in early life. Retarded children, however, are handicapped, since they rarely have the opportunity to experience these tasks.

Childhood. Little attention has been paid in the literature to the sexual development of the retarded child, and scientific knowledge of psychosexual development based on research done on early developmental phases is lacking. The majority of research studies reviewed by Saunders[18] indicate that physical growth and secondary sexual development are delayed coinciding with the degree of retardation, but there is little explanation for this relationship.

Morgenstern's[19] postulations based on Freudian concepts rely on the general principle that the retarded require more time to go through normal developmental phases. He describes the child as never as capable of love as the normal child. Others strongly disagree with Morgenstern's inferences that the retarded have a "weak ego," are unable to form personal relationships, and are unable to understand both the expression and reception of affection.[20]

Although Freud's latency period is a time of relative sexual inactivity, Bernstein[21] describes problems in the latency period of retarded children as those of hyperactivity, masturbation, and a variety of fears, hypochondriasis, and phobias. Unfortunately, retarded children have difficulty identifying and then handling their feelings and can only describe them in limited ways.[22]

Adolescence. Pubescence is late in the retarded. The severely or profoundly retarded have few opportunities for sex and for peer contact. For the mildly retarded, the sexual impulse is normal but their personality may not be. Some fear the future and are made apprehensive by people around them. They may be regarded permanently as children and, as such, asexual, perhaps reflecting the parents' wishes that puberty never come.[23,24]

They have few outlets to sublimate sexual feelings, since they tend to be passive, with a limited repertoire of social skills. The kinds of feelings that adolescents can express are limited and they often talk only of love and hate, not of happiness, sadness, all of which influence the young person's ability to relate meaningfully to others. Adolescents and young adults may act out their feelings in bizarre ways that further alienate them from others.[25]

They are frightened by masturbation, excited and guilty about homosexual play. They yearn to enjoy themselves, but efforts to plan parties or to arrange dates between retarded adolescents are sometimes useful, at other times, disturbing, depending largely on the often conflicted attitudes of adults arranging the events and the resulting false social atmosphere that prevails.[26]

Sexual Problems. The impression is that retarded adolescents show normal sexual interest but are met with suppression and disapproval. Masturbation continues in more childlike form and may be associated with thumbsucking, rocking, and other mannerisms. Fantasies associated with masturbation in the few cases studied appear to be a combination of oral concerns and usual adolescent imagery for both adolescent boys and girls.[27]

Homosexual Experiences. Homosexual experiences of institutionalized adolescents are not much different than those of deprived and institutionalized adults. Passive and retarded adolescents appear to be the ideal passive, intimidated partner.[28]

Pregnancy. Hysterectomy may be used to solve problems of menstrual hygiene and pregnancy. Retarded girls are more likely to become involved with men in the hope of attracting attention and positive regard in social interactions. If pregnancy occurs, the retarded girls do not always have access to therapeutic abortion and are either unaware of or too embarrassed to ask for birth control information. Many parents are willing to approve sterilization procedures to avoid the alternative of pregnancies.[29]

Legal counsel must be sought before sterilization procedure even with parental permission since the courts are now ruling that the mental retardate's constitutional rights be protected. Federal funds are no longer available for this purpose.

If the patient has an IQ over 70, most authorities feel she can give informed consent for sterilization, but only after psychologic testing, social evaluation, and interviews to identify understanding.

Rationalizations favoring abortion for the retarded include overpopulation of the world with retardates, endangering the genetic pool, and increasing economic cost to society. Findings of research related to the IQ of children of the retarded are equivocal and the belief that mentally retarded persons biologically beget more retarded is being challenged by some researchers.[30]

Child Molestation. Child molestation may occasionally occur, since some retarded adolescent boys seek other children, either boys or girls, to explore what has been forbidden to them in past development. It is difficult to determine the actual number of child molestation events, since they are hidden by fears and shame of parents of the retarded and those of the children who have been approached. Retarded adolescents are guarded and deterred from approaching children and, contrary to popular belief, child molesters of normal intelligence are a much more common problem.[31]

Adulthood and the Middle Years. The mildly retarded adult often disappears into the general population after leaving an institution. There are instances when even the severely and moderately retarded couple after counseling are able to marry or live together as married.[32] However, this is not the usual pattern. The self-image of retarded persons is often confused, since they are not always accepted, treated, or respected as adults. Basic vocational and work programs aim to make them independent, but often retarded persons can not leave home and establish their own relationships and famlilies.[33] Earlier experiences in school also contribute to decreased self-esteem as retarded persons are put in low-status occupational tracks and observe that others do better than they.[34]

Retarded individuals must deal with all the issues of the middle years that confront the general population. Women undergo changes of menopause, usually in a simpler copy of the ordinary pattern, and usually with a sense of relief from the burden. Masturbatory activity may increase. The fight to retain youth that is seen in the general population is less notable in the retarded population, and they do not seem to experience the other conflicts and concerns attendant with aging.

Aging. Similar patterns of aging occur as in the general population, including decreased energy and spheres of activity and responses to all the physiologic changes that accompany old age.[35]

NURSING IMPLICATIONS

The focus of this section will be on sex education and counseling of younger retarded individuals from childhood through adolescence, rather than throughout the life span. Sexual problems have their inception during these formative years, and it is during this time that the nurse's teaching and counseling can help the retarded attain or maintain sexual health.

Assessment
Parents may be and often should be involved in the assessment process, depending on age and level of retardation of the individual, since they are able to contribute information about behavior, learning needs, and problems as they perceive them. They also may be able to help the nurse obtain information from the retarded person and decrease his or her anxiety. Their own self-esteem increases with their active role in helping their child.[36] Parents are seen before the child, and most prefer to be present when the child is seen. Younger children and more severely retarded adolescents are usually willing to

have the parents present.[37] However, the nurse must be sensitive to the retardate's wishes since, as with other individuals, sharing of sexual information may be difficult with parents listening.

During the assessment interview, the nurse observes how the parents and the retarded person perceive the developing sexuality and how the family interacts with and their relationship with the retarded person—whether supportive, punitive, interested, or uninterested. The nurse also explores their goals and problems in relation to independent living, vocation, and sexual expression and what is presently being done to achieve these goals and cope with problems.

Pattullo[38] stresses that sexuality should be put within the framework of other aspects of development to decrease feelings related to expression of sexual concerns. As with normal individuals, other aspects of health and of daily living are explored—a typical day's activity, the opportunities for decision making, and assumption of responsibility (see Chapter 10).

Problems most frequently expressed, especially by the retarded or parents of the retarded living in the community, relate to questions of dating, marriage, parenthood, and birth control (Sterilization or contraception).[39] Masturbation and homosexuality are also sources of concern.[40] The nurse also obtains data necessary to implement the teaching–learning process and identifies in general, if the retarded individual is in the educable group and able to attain or retain information (see Chapter 11).

Planning
After identifying specific problem areas, whether related to behavior or a need for information or counseling, the nurse sets realistic and reachable goals to deal with these unmet needs of the slow learner (and the parents, if they are still involved in care and supervision). The goal of sex education is to develop a positive view and satisfying expression of their sexuality. This in turn will improve self-esteem.

The nurse recognizes, however, that counseling will probably have to be a more directive process than the usual procedure used in counseling and teaching patients/clients.[41] This would include setting of goals even when the retarded person is not able to participate in their identification.

Interventions to Promote Normal Growth and Development of Sexuality

Sensuality. Parents can help in the development of sensuality and growth of care about self and others. This learning begins in infancy when the child is touched, held closely, and cared for in ways that express love and tenderness. A child learns to identify sensory stimuli that produce pleasure and behaves in ways to insure their continuation by control of the environment. Retarded children can develop sensuality by having the same opportunities to receive, give, and learn by playing and "roughhousing" with family and other children, by learning to control elimination, and to tease and be teased by members of the opposite sex. They can be helped to develop friendships with peers, explore their bodies and compare them with those of both sexes, identifying differences and similarities. Perske[42] states that they can learn parts of the body that provide pleasure and gratification; engage in activities, privately and without censure, which help them to know their bodies; and learn to exert control over behavior. They can also learn to take pride in their appearance, i.e., in cleanliness of their hair and clothing.[43]

Feelings. Children are also helped to identify and handle feelings. They need to learn that they are not responsible for feelings that accompany a situation, but the feelings that are expressed are subject to social sanctions.[44] Each time a nurse or parent is aware of situations that would normally elicit an expression of feelings, children should be helped to label whatever they are feeling. Pattullo[45] suggests using diagrams of faces, such as seen in the "Have a Nice Day" buttons. These faces should reflect various feel-ings, from happiness through extreme unhappiness. They are shown to children whenever it appears they are experiencing significant feelings. The children point to the picture that depicts their feeling and the name of the feeling is explored. Children are helped to learn that both their bodies and their words convey ideas to others and that when one names or identifies a feeling, there is little reason to "act out" the communication. Use of mirrors may also be helpful in these situations, so the children can see their expressions.

Decision Making. Retarded children can learn how to develop some degree of control over what happens to them and must be taught responsible decision making—to consider alternatives to any action before acting. Small children begin by being given choice of food, clothes, and play activities. Simple choices can help children learn that they are instrumental in determining what is happening to them. Gradually, choices are made more complex so the children have experiences of relating actions, results, and feelings. This can only be learned slowly through many opportunities.[46]

Behavior modification techniques, such as use of a token economy system as a positive reinforcer, may be used to help the child make decisions. The child decides what he or she will buy with the reinforcers and lives with the results.[47] These early experiences in making choices influence how children express sexual impulses, such as masturbation or sexual activity with others.

Assaultive and inappropriate sexual behavior may be halted by interventions such as differential reinforcement of other behavior (DRO) and social restitution, a procedure whereby the retarded are required to restore the environment to a more favorable condition than before the undesirable behavior.[48]

Interventions to Solve Problems Related to Sexual Behavior

Counseling the Retarded. Kempton[49] describes counseling with slow learners as involving questioning; listening; and getting and giving information, advice, support, and direct help—with love. In the usual counseling process, the client often reflects on past experiences, examines the present, and then discusses the options that affect the future. These procedures are less possible when counseling slow learners. Kempton suggests four steps to the process. First, determine the student's motivation. Why is the student behaving in a certain way? If the retarded person asked to talk to you, why? The counselor evaluates the student behavior and statements in relation to past attitudes and behavior. Second, gather information and discuss the situation with the student. Why is it a problem for the student; is it also presently or potentially one for others? If so, who are they? What are the consequences of the behavior?

Third, discuss the solution and the choices that are available. Which are best for the retarded person; which are best for others? Ask what the retarded individual thinks is the best solution and why. However, the counselor may have to insist on action that is not agreeable or pleasant to the retarded. For example, if a boy wishes to masturbate in public and nothing will dissuade him, he will have to be told that he will be punished if he acts that way. Kempton states that when possible, the retarded person should be told beforehand of the penalty and told why she/he will be punished.

The fourth step in the process is to help the student solve the problem, preferably in a way that is agreeable to both.[50]

Counseling Parents. Parents have all the fears, lack of knowledge, and feelings of inadequacy one finds in any group of parents plus those that characteristically affect parents of the retarded: (1) anxiety about the sexual behavior of young children, such as masturbating in public and approaching and showing affection to adults; (2) fear the children may be sexually molested and, when adults, sexually exploited; (3) anxiety that when the daughter reaches puberty she will become pregnant, adding to the family's burden; and (4) concern that the son who does not have the outlet of intercourse for sexual impulses will be unhealthy, mentally affected, or likely to commit violent crimes.[51]

The counselor reassures parents that children will not suffer if they do not have the opportunity for heterosexual intercourse, that masturbation is a way of relieving sexual tension for some, and that sexual fulfillment is not necessary for health. Parents are also reassured that their loving attention and close family relationship provide much good for sex education. The counselor or teacher builds on their accomplishments and minimizes their deficiencies. It is also emphasized that a different set of sexual values will not be imposed by the counselor on their child and that the child will not be taught a code of sexual behavior different from theirs.[52] For example, those teaching retarded persons that masturbation is an acceptable means of tension reduction will only cause problems if the parents feel it is immoral and if they punish the child for it. Appropriate interventions for various problems—masturbation, homosexual and heterosexual activity—are given in Table 29-1.

Marriage. The question of marriage and parenthood of the retarded plagues parents, teachers, and all associated with their care. Advantages of marriage include companionship, broadening of young people's lives, more opportunity for independent activities, complete expression of sexual needs and a greater sense of accomplishment, security, and self-confidence. Disadvantages include sharing the problems of the retarded with another, stresses on inadequate emotional stability, and inability of the spouse to cope with the retarded individual's physical or mental weaknesses.[53]

Success in marriage may be predicted by identifying: (1) whether a love relationship exists; (2) the ability level of the individuals to cope with their problems and to carry on lasting relationships; (3) the ability of the retardate to take responsibility for home finances and fertility control, and to make de-

TABLE 29–1. COMMON SEXUAL PROBLEMS: ASSESSMENT AND INTERVENTION

Problem	Assessment and Intervention
Masturbation in public (includes touching, rubbing, scratching the genital area)	Determine reason for behavior: possible rash, infection, tight clothing, existence of fear or anxiety due to stress situation. Reassure individual masturbation (in private) is acceptable and normal if he or she enjoys it. Discuss meaning and limitation of privacy—where masturbation is appropriate. Suggest use of alternatives when with others; if used to cope with stress, rubbing Greek worry beads, doodling on a piece of paper. Make sure the person holds to solution or else is punished according to previously set guidelines.
Questioning about morality of masturbation	Assess if individual enjoys it. Reassurance behavior is normal and acceptable if there are other interests and no problems are ensuing. Reassurance that not masturbating is normal—masturbation is a matter of choice.
Persistent masturbation	Assess if individual is happy with life. Is the behavior a crutch and substitute for effort, and accomplishment; a sign of loneliness? Help to develop new interests. Give opportunity to express feelings. Refer for deeper problems.
Compulsive masturbation (stimulates self to orgasm, then resumes activity but without satisfaction or pleasure)	Assess if habit is response to a need that has become a fixed pattern of behavior over which there is no control. Remove from group if necessary. Get specialized attention.
Promiscuous sexual intercourse by girls	Assess if girl is enjoying coitus (ask directly). Take action against those exploiting her. Help girl develop self-esteem and learn to refuse sexual activity if she does not enjoy it. Give help with birth control as appropriate if she is enjoying sexual activity.
Sexual aggressiveness by boys (touching others, sexual intercourse)	Assess if he understands seriousness of acts, if he is imitating others, if he is easily aroused, if girls are being seductive, if he is physically unattractive. Does he masturbate? Tell directly about seriousness of behavior and that people should not be touched. Do not convey idea that person's behavior is sick or evil, only inappropriate. Punish as needed, especially if seriously retarded—make sure he knows he is punished for act, not for being a bad person. Get through that behavior will cause trouble with friends, strangers, police. Get outlet for sexual energy if he is "highly charged" and easily stimulated—physical activity, masturbation, other interests. Help with social skills if boy is acting out desire for attention. Increase self-esteem. Set limits on girls if they are aggressive sexually toward the boy.
Homosexual activity	Assess whether individual has had opportunity to be with the opposite sex and the period of time without contact, the repetitiveness and frequency of the behavior, type of sexual activity (oral, anal, to orgasm, only mutual masturbation), intensity of the relationship, consistent seeking of same sex at social activities, family patterns that encourage homosexual behavior. Teach social skills, give opportunity for heterosexual social interaction. Analyze own feelings and behavior. Are heterosexual relationships discouraged? Should homosexual relationships be permitted? Refer as necessary.

Adapted from: Kempton, Winifred: A Teacher's Guide to Sex Education. *North Scituate, Massachusetts, Duxbury, 1974.*

cisions about usual problems; (4) understanding of and ability to control emotions reasonably well; (5) health problems that may drastically affect or harm the relationship. In addition, if necessary, the couple's parents or others must be willing and able to assume responsibility for both husband and wife.[54] The nurse helps parents and the retarded come to responsible decisions when strong feelings for and against marriage may be expressed.

Parenthood—Conception Control. There is little research on parenting of the retarded. However, the emotional and financial strain of parenting may destroy an otherwise satisfactory relationship. Many retarded persons lack the characteristics necessary for parenting-ability to plan for the future, sound judgment and emotional security, ability to provide for intellectual stimulation and for the child's health needs, and ability to consistently take responsibility for another person. Kempton[55] points out, however, that these qualities may be lacking in normally intelligent persons.

When conception control is prescribed, the nurse makes sure that it is a method that the retarded individual will use, wants to use, and understands how to use.

In the past, the four main methods used to shelter a retarded girl from unwanted pregnancy were sterilization by tubal ligation or by hysterectomy, placement in a protected institutional setting, or, if she lived at home, permitting her no freedom in the community. Now, however, birth control pills and intrauterine devices have been used, with abortion as a backup procedure. Diaphragms, foams, jellies, and condoms may be reliable for some but those with regular sexual activity usually need consistent protection. (See Chapter 19 for discussion of advantages and disadvantages of various conception control methods and Chapter 20 for discussion of abortion.)

The retarded girl must be prepared for any health visit for conception control. She should know the basic facts of sexual intercourse, how one becomes pregnant, what will happen during the visit, and something about the various methods that will be offered her. As much information is given as she is capable of understanding, and if she cannot understand, preparation should be directed toward decreasing her fears.[56]

Teaching the Retarded. One of the basic duties of sex education is helping retarded persons understand their sexual feelings and assuring them that they are natural and good but must be controlled.[57,58] The retarded are also in need of other areas of sex education. Error and confusion about sexual matters appear to be high, especially in those institutionalized. Edmondson and Wish[59] stress that education is essential if understanding of sex is part of normalization of behavior. The teacher works with the parents as well as the retarded individual who is not institutionalized.

Teaching methods discussed in Chapter 11 are appropriate for retarded persons. Understandable vocabulary must be used. Whether teaching or counseling, the nurse must be comfortable with the use of vulgar vocabulary, since the words may be the only ones in the individual's repertoire. It is important to deal with the ideas, not the words. (See Chapter 10 for street words for sexual function and parts.)

Kempton[60] emphasizes that the teacher must be able to relate to the students comfortably. Audiovisual aids are essential. Role play, improvisations, and pantomime may all help clarify and reinforce this information. Behavior modification and value clarification may be useful techniques to present essentially the same information given to normal persons only in a simpler and more repetitive manner.

Teaching content must be concrete since the retarded do not understand abstract concepts. Among mildly retarded individuals, however, marital and prenatal responsibilities are appropriate topics for discussion in sex education programs.

Staff education is also needed. Brantlinger[61] found that negative attitudes of staff of institutions and group homes for the retarded become more liberal and more respectful of the rights of the individual after a 1-day workshop on sex and the handicapped.

Evaluation

Nurses are aware that it will take longer and require more repetition of information and greater patience on their part if goals are to be met. Interventions have been successful not only when the retarded individual is happier, more knowledgeable, or in better control of his or her behavior, but also when parents, family, and the larger society are content and identify the retarded person as a welcome member of society.

MENTAL ILLNESS AND SEXUALITY

Until recently, psychologic theories of mental health and mental illness, especially those derived from psychoanalysis, maintained that mental health is associated with mature sexual functioning and in particular with capacity for orgasm. Mental illness and sexual dysfunction may be associated, if not always in fact, at least at times, in the mind of both physicians and patients/clients.

Mental Illness and Sexual Activity

Physicians and patients appear to believe that sexual activity may be one of several factors contributing to the development or exacerbation of psychiatric disorders. Pinderhughes and associates[62] found that consultant and staff psychiatrists reported that sexual activity could have been a contributing factor in 83 percent of psychiatric conditions listed in a questionnaire sent to them. Thirty-nine percent of 122 psychiatric inpatients also thought sexual activity may have contributed to their illness. Physicians felt that sexual activity might be a contributing factor in anxiety, depression, and schizophrenia.[63]

Patients were less apt to believe that

sexual activity was related to anxiety or depression than physicians, but 47 percent of patients in the schizophrenic group considered sexual activity a contributory cause.

More than two-thirds of the physicians and one-fourth of the patients felt that sexual activity might retard recovery in most categories of psychiatric disorders, while approximately one-fourth of patients with anxiety, depression, or schizophrenia reported retardation of recovery due to sexual activity.[64]

More than four-fifths of the psychiatrists and almost one-half of the patients also believed that psychiatric disorders might interfere with sexual functioning.

Although Masters and Johnson found no psychopathology in their subjects, Derogatis and associates[65] found that individuals with sexual dysfunction had mean psychiatric symptom profiles that ranged one to two standard deviations above normal.

Objective data to support these beliefs are scanty, however, and literature describing the relationships is usually in general terms.

There are few hard data on the physiologic mechanisms involved in various sexual patterns and in each psychiatric disorder. Pinderhughes[66] argues that more attention must be focused on the physiologic bases, correlates, and equivalents of reactions such as comfort, pleasure, anxiety, pain, rage, and love.

Keeping in mind the limitations in available data suggested by Pinderhughes, the rest of this chapter will focus on sexuality and schizophrenia, paranoia, affective (manic–depressive) states, and neurosis. Conception control and the mentally ill woman and the problem of sexual activity in the psychiatric inpatient setting will also be discussed.

Schizophrenia and Paranoia

Folklore and myths about sexuality and schizophrenia abound. Early sexual trauma, sexual abstinence or overindulgence, masturbation, and perverse thoughts or actions have all been suggested as causes of "madness." In fact, schizophrenia is a disorder of the entire personality, not just sexuality.[67] It has been commonly believed that schizophrenics invariably have sex problems, but Kaplan[68] indicates that this is not substantiated by clinical observation or by experiences in treating their sexual disorders. Although schizophrenics may have a high incidence of sexual abnormalities, many function well sexually.

The relationship between sexual difficulties and schizophrenia is complex and variable. Sexual dysfunction is not a symptom of schizophrenia; the conditions are independent. Usually, when the schizophrenic has sexual difficulties, they revolve around the quality of the relationship with the sexual partner or some deviation in sexual aim rather than actual dysfunction.[69] In fact, a sexual disability may defend against a flare-up of the illness.

Characteristically, the schizophrenic's primary symptom is disruption of the thought processes. There may also be increased emotional sensitivity and difficulty in coping with and adapting to anxiety-provoking situations, especially interpersonal relationships. In the preschizophrenic individual, it is fear of intimacy, not inadequate sexual drive per se, that prohibits sexual activity.[70] Some treated patients, however, between bouts of illness are able to establish sound sexual relationships. The severely deranged individual, however, who is left with some degree of constricted or paranoid behavior, may have sexual relationships, but they are often distorted, and the individual whose schizophrenia began in childhood often remains too sick to ever form sexual relationships.[71]

Sexual Behavior. Two different theories make different predictions as to the impact of sexual stimulation on schizophrenics. Psychoanalytic ego psychology predicts greater sexual arousal in the schizophrenics than in normal individuals because of failure of repression and other defenses. In contrast, arousal theories predict decreased responsiveness, because schizophrenics attempt to adapt by inhibiting stimuli through use of avoidance responses. From this standpoint, sexual stimuli should be less arousing for schizophrenics than for normal persons because of schizophrenics' tendency to inhibit and control stimulation.

To test these theories, Garske[72] studied sexual arousal in 14 chronic nonparanoid schizophrenic male outpatients and 16 normal males. The subjects were matched for age, socioeconomic status, and education. Sexual stimuli in the form of pictures were presented and arousal was measured by "looking time." The schizophrenic males looked at the stimuli for significantly longer periods of time than did the normal males, while looking time for neutral stimuli were equal. Garske felt that these results support the viewpoint of ego psychology, since they suggest that schizophrenics are less defensive than normal males in regard to looking at sexual stimuli.

Multiple factors are involved in sexual behavior of the male schizophrenic patient: (1) the type and severity of symptoms; (2) the attitudes of the society in which he lives toward his illness and sexual behavior; (3) state of dopaminergic, serotoninergic, and cholinergic transmission; (4) hormonal factors.[73]

Deviant sexual behavior (with objects rather than persons, sexual acts not associated with coitus, coitus under bizarre conditions such as sadism or fetishism) is the outcome of the schizophrenic's impaired capacity for reality testing.[74] Its sequelae may be depression and suicidal behavior if there is possibility of exposure.

The schizophrenic in psychotic decompensation may also evidence increased masturbatory behavior and sexual obsessions ranging from concerns over impotence or frigidity to Don Juan fantasies. Somatic preoccupations occur. They may reflect change in body imagery and attempts to attribute the psychologic symptoms to physical disorders. Vague genital concerns are common.[75] Schizophrenic women may have genital hallucinations or delusions of change in the size and shape of the genitalia or delusions of changing sex. In other ways, males and females behave similarly, with the exception that women are more likely to retain interest in the opposite sex.[76]

Previously shy individuals may attempt to establish interpersonal relationships or prove sexual prowess by hypersexual behavior. Inappropriate sexual judgment involving a bizarre or idiosyncratic frame of reference may appear. The person may claim some special sexual ability or imagine that "I have love to give everybody" and act out accordingly. Inappropriate sexual behavior may be the person's response to early psychotic changes. Females may be exploited sexually, but the promiscuity is not due to heightened sexual drive but to passive involvement.[77]

Schizophrenics may also have incestuous, murderous, or forbidden sexual and aggressive impulses. These surface as the individual's defensive structure crumbles and reflect this breakthrough.[78] Homosexual tendencies and concerns may be associated with all psychoses, but it is most common in paranoia.[79]

Marital Relationships. Marital relationships of schizophrenics have been described as chaotic and unrewarding. As was mentioned earlier, the very severe schizophrenic is not likely to marry or seek out sexual relationships. However, other schizophrenics marry and establish families.

In a group of nine women, Dupont and Grunebaum[80] found that cessation of sexual intercourse played an important part in the marital breakdown associated with the wife's psychosis. The women seemed to seek husbands with similar personality characteristics—hard-working, soft-spoken, passive men who had difficulty expressing anger or sexual feelings and who were likely to participate in any bizarre sexual behavior exhibited by their wives.

In contrast, some couples report feelings of love and mutual understanding, growing out of a psychotic experience and their attempts to deal with it. The psychiatric therapy helped the couples work together as a team, sharing feelings, responsibilities, and problems, suggesting that the nonpsychotic spouse should be actively engaged in the treatment process.[81]

Treatment. If sexual dysfunctions exist, therapy is not usually advisable during the recovery phase of schizophrenia.[82] Moreover, the therapist must be careful that therapy does not remove defenses of emotional detachment often used by schizophrenics. Touching, caressing, abandonment, and openness between partners emphasized by sex therapy may be extremely threatening to those who need to maintain tight control on their emotions. Sexual symptoms sometimes serve as a defense against schizophrenia, and abrupt remission of impotence and premature ejaculation in the male or orgasmic dysfunction and vaginismus in the female may precipitate an acute schizophrenic episode.[83]

Drug therapy of acute schizophrenic episodes involves use of the major tranquilizers.[84] These provide rapid, effective relief of symptoms, but side effects include alteration of sexual function. Adverse reactions, among others, include abnormal lactation, weight gain, gynecomastia, menstrual irregularities, false results in pregnancy tests, impotency in men, and increased libido in women.[85] Some of these symptoms may occur with administration of other phenothiazines such as prochlorperazine (Compazine) and thioridazine hydrochloride (Mellaril)[86] (see Chapter 30).

Patients may report painful orgasm. Priapism, sustained erection, requires urologic consult and surgery. Other side effects, however, disappear with drug discontinuation.[87] Some patients found that sexual activity was helpful in dealing with extrapyramidal drug side effects.

Although neuroleptic drugs may cause change in sexual function, many patients may actually function better sexually because of reduction of psychotic anxiety, thought disorganization, fear of physical intimacy, and other symptoms that compromise sexuality.[88]

Manic–Depressive Disorders

The relationship between depression and sexual dysfunction has been known since antiquity. While sexual disturbances frequently follow depressive reactions, the affective response to any continued sexual disturbance, with its chronic assault on self-concept, frequently is depression.[89] Thus, sexual disturbances may be the outcome or the etiology of depression.

In the affective disorders such as manic–depressive psychosis, sexual drive frequently increases with mood elevation and decreases with mood depression,[90] so that in the severely depressed person, sexual activity is the furthest thing from the mind, and even moderately depressed persons lose interest in sexual activity and are difficult to arouse sexually.[91] In 249 patients with a diagnosis of manic–depressive disease, 63 percent reported decrease in sexual function. Eighty-three percent of the males and 53 percent of the females reported decreased libido, while 8 percent of the group reported increased sexual function.[92]

In contrast to other reports Watson and Bamber[93] found that sexual and marital functioning may continue in the presence of significant depression.

Stress and Depression. Kaplan[94] states that any severe emotional state adversely affects sexuality. Crises such as divorce, job loss, or legal proceedings may cause depressive reactions. The mechanism for decreased sexual interest is not known, but several are postulated. A purely psychogenic reaction may be involved, since the person in crisis is directing all energies toward mastering difficulties.

The profound physiologic and endocrine changes that accompany depression and fatigue states may also contribute to decreased sexual interest in several ways: by lowering androgen (testosterone) levels,[95] increasing plasma cortisone levels which has an anti-androgen effect, and change in levels of neural transmitters in the brain that effect sexual behavior. Serotonin appears to decrease sexual activity while norepinephrine has the reverse effect. It is postulated that brain catecholamines decline during depression.

Treatment. Mild depressive reactions may occur in response to sexual inadequacy and disappear quickly when the symptoms are relieved by various therapies. However, when the low sexual interest results from depression, the prognosis for sex therapy is poor, since depression impairs libido and responsiveness even if there are no other impediments to good function.[96] Therapy must be directed toward relief of depression, which may in turn increase sexual responsiveness.

Neurosis

At one time, many clincians equated sexual difficulties with neurosis; the impotent male or nonorgasmic female was considered sick. However, at the present time, many recognize that this is not so and that those who cannot function sexually are not necessarily neurotic. The two problems may exist independent of each other and are not necessarily related. While some sexual difficulties may be symptomatic of underlying emotional problems, some highly neurotic individuals have superb sexual functioning.[97]

There is evidence, however, that anxiety and at times clinical anxiety neurosis may be related to sexual dysfunction. Derogatis[98] reports that the diagnosis of anxiety neurosis was the most frequent one identified in a sample of males with potency disorders and speculates that this same disturbance may produce frigid, unresponsive females.

The hypothesis that unconscious conflict is related to the etiology of sexual problems has much value. Kaplan points out that some patients harbor unconscious fears that they will be subjugated or humiliated by the lover or abandoned and thus destroyed after the establishment of a satisfying sexual life. Others may fear failure and disappointing the partner.[99] In either situation, it is less painful to experience sexual failure than to contemplate the possible outcomes of sexual activity.

The obsessive–compulsive personality has a high risk of sexual problems because of fear of losing control, the need to deny spontaneity or pleasure, proneness to spectatoring and perfectionistic trends leading to anxiety or depression. The borderline personality also has a variety of sexual problems, often multifactorial because of relationship problems.[100]

Sexual conflicts may also be associated with the onset of symptoms of obsessional neurosis. Goodwin and associates[101] reviewed 13 studies of patients with this diagnosis and found that symptoms appear as a group and often include violent, sexual, and "disgusting" images. The precipitating events thought to be related to the onset of symptoms included pregnancy, childbirth, and other "sexual factors."

Sexual Activity and the Mentally Ill Inpatient

Overt sexual behavior of psychiatric inpatients take place, but little, if any, information is present in psychiatric textbooks or monographs on sexuality, and guidelines with regard to staff reaction are minimal.[102] This is unfortunate, since both professional and nonprofessional staff may react negatively to the behavior.

Studies by Akhtar[103] and associates and by Modestin[104] indicate that younger, single patients or those more mentally subnormal were more likely to exhibit overt sexual behavior. Incidents range from masturbation, kissing, holding, embracing to actual sexual intercourse between patients of the opposite sex. Homosexual behavior was infrequent. Attitude of staff was negative. Nurses who usually discovered the activity reacted with anger or with disbelief based on denial and embarrassment.

Some provocative questions are raised by the findings: Should sexual activity be allowed on the ward? Or should it be discouraged or treated as a symptom of psychopathology? Which patients are to be "treated" for the behavior and which ones are to be allowed to express their natural biologic drives? While the hospital setting provides a haven from society, it often subtly mirrors the same social values and attitudes. On one hand, proper ideas of conduct are held up as desirable and patients are treated as responsible persons capable of and motivated to normalizing their relationships. However, when patients attempt to meet sexual needs, health professionals are at a loss as to the best response. Akhtar implies that some sexual activity might be tolerated but identifies limitations.

Findings from a study of 13 inpatient couples where both partners had a psychotic disorder and where a sexual partnership was established indicate, however, that these relationships were not positive. There were few affectional bonds or ability to form object relationship. Emotional flatness, jealousy, distrust, and suspiciousness were evident. The duration of the relationship was short and termination seemed to increase severity of the patient's mental condition.[105] There may not be characteristics of true love.

Sexual activity between inpatients should be discouraged if one or both are either (1) legally minor, (2) a nonconsenting adult, (3) mentally deficient, (4) delusional or in other ways grossly disorganized in affect and behavior, (5) receiving significant amounts of psychotropic medications, or (6) acting out in the classic sense of the term.[106] In addition, the risk of pregnancy must be considered, since female patients are frequently without contraceptive protection and have unwanted pregnancies more often than other women.[107,108]

Intervention. Krietner[109] feels that intimacy among patients should be dealt with on a case-by-case basis but clear principles must be kept in mind. All parties, including the staff, should be aware of ward guidelines, discuss them, and apply them directly. Staff should be aware that hospital relationships may have a positive effect on patients and that staff have an important role to play in these relationships. General guidelines can be formulated with the help of patients in the unit. He feels that if the problem is dealt with clearly and directly, it will not be compounded and can be used therapeutically.

"Aggressive" sexual behavior toward staff and appropriate nursing interventions are discussed in Chapter 14. However, extremes of behavior may occur in the psychiatric setting. Undressing or open masturbation of excited and regressed patients should be handled firmly. As in any other extreme in behavior, the patient is isolated, given the opportunity to verbally express needs, and tranquilized if necessary. Autoerotic activities, in the opinion of Akhtar and his associates,[110] should be treated with discretion and benign neglect if they are done privately and appropriately. In different settings, where patients are present more than 2 or 3 weeks, emotional relationships between patients based on mutual awareness and regard may be permissible.

Some health professionals may vehemently disagree with any suggestion that sexual activity be allowed in the inpatient setting. Certainly the possibilities for abuse and potential harm to patients are great. Still, as health professionals are recognizing that conjugal visits are beneficial for inpatient medical or surgical patients, and as loving relationships are seen to develop in long-term inpatient settings, such as nursing homes, perhaps the value of sexual activity may be recognized for the psychiatric inpatient as well.

Mental Illness and Conception Control

As was mentioned earlier, women with psychiatric disorders have more unwanted pregnancies and make less effective use of conception control methods than nonpsychiatric women, and many of the mentally ill women feel that the pregnancy contributed to their emotional breakdown. Their ineffective use of contraception was primarily due to motivational patterns of excessive dependency needs, passive–aggressive expression of ambivalence toward men, and excessive use of denial.[111]

Grunebaum and associates[112] found that 21 psychiatric inpatients tended to have little family planning information at the time of their marriage. The women patients, however, saw the need for family planning information and strongly endorsed seeing a doctor about family planning methods. Some requested that the person be a woman. Interestingly, only 1 of 21 patients in Grunebaum's study stated that a physician talked to her about family planning methods.[113]

Providing conception control information may be difficult because there are few family planning services for psychiatric patients; the women do not seek information or have unpredictable and episodic contacts.[114] Among more disturbed women there may be fears and fantasies, distorted feeling and behavior, or diffuse and irrational desires for pregnancy and motherhood making contraception difficult. Those with low intelligence may have difficulty understanding information given.[115] Suspicions and doubts about methods, the "unnaturalness" of birth control, and guilt about use may deter others. Guilt about abortion is more common among emotionally disturbed women.[116] (See Chapter 20.)

NURSING IMPLICATIONS

Pinderhughes and associates[117] reported that 52 percent of patients who talked with psychiatrists about sex found it helpful, with the highest percentage in the psychoneurotic categories. However, 66 percent of patients in all categories believed that doctors should discuss sexual functioning with other patients who had the same problem.[118] Unfortunately, there is no agreement on the nature, content, or usefulness of these discussions among psychiatrists. At the present time, the nurse's role in teaching and counseling the psychiatric patient about sexuality is also poorly described in the literature. However, the nurse spends the most time with the individual and the family, is faced with dealing with acting out sexual behavior, and has the most opportunity to clarify misinformation and teach about sexuality. Family planning information is shared with the patient and she is helped to choose the method that is acceptable for her. (See Chapter 19.)

Nurses need to inquire about the drug effects since men with psychotic illness may not feel comfortable discussing the topic or are too disorganized to recognize or report dysfunction. Before therapy is initiated, assessment is made of sexual function and previous sexual problems. Patients are reassured that changes are reversible with decreased dose, change to other drugs or to drug discontinuation.

NOTES

1. Nirje B: The normalization principle. In Kugel RB, Shearer A (eds): Changing Patterns of Residential Services for the Mentally Retarded. Washington, D.C., President's Commission on Mental Retardation, U.S. Gov't Printing Office, 1976, pp 232–239
2. Pattullo AW: The socio-sexual development of the handicapped child. Nurs Clin North Am 10:361–372, 1976
3. Nirje B: The normalization principle. In Kugel RB, Shearer A (eds): Changing Patterns of Residential Services for the Mentally Retarded. Washington, D.C., President's Commission on Mental Retardation, U.S. Gov't Printing Office, 1976, p. 232
4. Kempton W: A Teacher's Guide to Sex Education. North Scituate, Massachusetts, Duxbury, 1974
5. Ibid, p 4
6. Johnson WR: Sex education of the mentally retarded. In de la Cruz FF, LaVeck GD (eds): Human Sexuality and the Mentally Retarded. New York, Brunner/Mazel, 1973, pp 58–60
7. Kempton W: A Teacher's Guide to Sex Education. North Scituate, Massachusetts, Duxbury, 1974, p 6
8. Bernstein N: Intellectual defect and personality development. In Bernstein N (ed): Diminished People. Boston, Little, Brown, 1970, pp 165–199
9. Ibid, p 173
10. Ibid, p 174
11. Craft A, Craft M: Sexuality and mental handicap: A review. Brit J Psych 139: 494–505, 1982
12. Kugel R, Shearer A: Toward further change. In Kugel RB, Shearer A (eds): Changing Patterns of Residential Services for the Mentally Retarded. Washington, D.C., President's Commission on Mental Retardation, U.S. Gov't Printing Office, 1976, pp 373–377
13. Nirje B: The normalization principle. In Kugel RB, Shearer A (eds): Changing Patterns of Residential Services for the Mentally Retarded. Washington, D.C., President's Commission on Mental Retardation, U.S. Gov't Printing Office, 1976, p 338
14. Hall JE, Morris HL: Sexual knowledge and attitudes of institutionalized and noninstitutionalized retarded adolescents. Am J Ment Defic 80:382–387, 1976
15. Edmonson B, Wish J: Sex knowledge and attitudes of moderately retarded males. Am J Ment Defic 80:172–179, 1975
16. Small IF, Small JG: Sexual behavior and mental illness. In Freedman AM, Kaplan HI, Sadock BJ (eds): Comprehensive Textbook of Psychiatry II, 2nd ed. Baltimore, Williams and Wilkins, 1975, pp 1500–1509
17. Pattullo AW: The socio-sexual development of the handicapped child. Nurs Clin North Am 10:362, 1976
18. Saunders EJ: The mental health professional, the mentally retarded and sex. Hosp Comm Psychiatry 32:717–721, 1981
19. Morgenstern M: The psychological development of the retarded. In de la Cruz FF, LaVeck GD (eds): Human Sexuality and the Mentally Retarded. New York, Brunner/Mazel, 1973
20. Pattullo AW: The socio-sexual develop-

ment of the handicapped child. Nurs Clin North Am 10:363, 1976

21. Bernstein N: Intellectual defect and personality development. In Bernstein N (ed): Diminished People. Boston, Little, Brown, 1970, p 175

22. Pattullo AW: The socio-sexual development of the handicapped child. Nurs Clin North Am 10:366, 1976

23. Bernstein N: Intellectual defect and personality development. In Bernstein N (ed): Diminished People. Boston, Little, Brown, 1970, p 180

24. Kreutner AK: Sexuality, fertility and problems of menstruation in mentally retarded adolescents. Pediat Clin North Am 28:475–480, 1981

25. Pattullo AW: The socio-sexual development of the handicapped child. Nurs Clin North Am 10:366, 1976

26. Bernstein N: Intellectual defect and personality development. In Bernstein N (ed): Diminished People. Boston, Little, Brown, 1970, p 181

27. Ibid

28. Ibid

29. Ibid, p 182

30. Saunders EJ: The mental health professional, the mentally retarded and sex. Hosp Comm Psychiatry 32:719, 1981

31. Ibid, p 183

32. Nirje B: The normalization principle. In Kugel RB, Shearer A (eds); Changing Patterns of Residential Services for the Mentally Retarded. Washington, D.C., President's Commission on Mental Retardation, U.S. Gov't Printing Office, 1976, p 233

33. Ibid, p 237

34. Bernstein N: Intellectual defect and personality development. In Bernstein N (ed): Diminished People. Boston, Little, Brown, 1970, p 181

35. Ibid, p 194

36. Pattullo AW: The socio-sexual development of the handicapped child. Nurs Clin North Am 10:369, 1976

37. Ibid

38. Ibid

39. Kempton W: A Teacher's Guide to Sex Education. North Scituate, Massachusetts, Duxbury, 1974, p 105

40. Ibid, p 107

41. Ibid, p 105

42. Perske R: About sexual development: An attempt to be human with the mentally retarded. Ment Retard 11:6–8, 1973

43. Nirje B: The normalization principle. In Kugel RB, Shearer A (eds); Changing Patterns of Residential Services for the Mentally Retarded. Washington, D.C., President's Commission on Mental Retardation. U.S. Gov't Printing Office, 1976, p 236

44. Pettullo AW: The socio-sexual development of the handicapped child. Nurs Clin North Am 10:366, 1976

45. Ibid, p 367

46. Ibid

47. Ibid, p 368

48. Polvinale RA, Lutzker JR: Elimination of assaultive and inappropriate sexual behavior by reinforcement and social-restitution. Ment Retard 18:27–30, 1980

49. Kempton W: A Teacher's Guide to Sex Education. North Scituate, Massachusetts, Duxbury, 1974, p 104

50. Ibid, p 105

51. Ibid, p 127

52. Ibid

53. Ibid, p 111

54. Ibid

55. Ibid, p 112

56. Ibid, p 118

57. Ibid, p 135

58. Smigielski PA, Steinmann MJ: Teaching sex education to multiply handicapped adolescents. J School Health 51:238–241, 1981

59. Edmonson B, Wish J: Sex knowledge and attitudes of moderately retarded males. Am J Ment Defic 80:179, 1975

60. Kempton W: A Teacher's Guide to Sex Education. North Scituate, Massachusetts, Duxbury, 1974, pp 80–97

61. Brantlinger E: Measuring variation

and change in attitudes of residential care staff toward the sexuality of mentally retarded persons. Ment Retard 21:17–22, 1983

62. Pinderhughes CA, Grace EB, Reyna LJ: Psychiatric disorders and sexual functioning. Am J Psychiatry 128:1276–1283, 1972

63. Ibid, p 1278

64. Ibid, p 1279

65. Derogatis LR, Meyer JK, King KM: Psychopathology in individuals with sexual dysfunction. Am J Psychiatry 138:57–63, 1981

66. Penderhughes CA, Grace EB, Reyna LJ: Psychiatric disorders and sexual functioning. Am J Psychiatry 128:1278, 1972

67. Donlon PT: Sexual symptoms of incipient schizophrenic psychoses. Med Aspects Hum Sexuality 10:69–70, 1976

68. Kaplan HS: The New Sex Therapy, New York, Brunner/Mazel, 1974, p 490

69. Verhulst J, Schneidman B: Schizophrenia and sexual functioning. Hosp Comm Psychiatry 32:259–262, 1981

70. Donlon PT: Sexual symptoms of incipient schizophrenic psychoses. Med Aspects Hum Sexuality 10:70, 1976

71. Kaplan HS: The New Sex Therapy, New York, Brunner/Mazel, 1974, p 492

72. Garske JP: Effects of sexual arousal on schizophrenics: A comparative test of hypotheses derived from ego psychology and arousal theory. J Clin Psychol 33:105–109, 1977

73. Nestoros JN, Lehman HE, Ban TA: Sexual behavior of the male schizophrenic: The impact of illness and medications. Arch Sex Behav 10:421–442, 1981

74. Sadoff RL: Other sexual deviations. In Freedman AM, Kaplan HI, Sadock BJ (eds): Comprehensive Textbook of Psychiatry II, 2nd ed. Baltimore, Williams and Wilkins, 1975, p 1539

75. Donlon PT: Sexual symptoms of incipient schizophrenic psychoses. Med Aspects Hum Sexuality 10:70, 1976

76. Gittleson NL, Dawson-Butterworth K: Subjective ideas of sexual changes in female schizophrenics. Br J Psychiatry 113:491–494, 1967

77. Donlon PT: Sexual symptoms of incipient schizophrenic psychoses. Med Aspects Hum Sexuality 10:70, November 1976

78. Simons RC, Pardes H (eds): Understanding Human Behavior in Health and Illness. Baltimore, Williams and Wilkins, 1977, pp 593–597

79. Donlon PT: Sexual symptoms of incipient schizophrenic psychoses. Med Aspects Hum Sexuality 10:70, 1976

80. Dupont R, Grunebaum H: Willing victims: Husbands of paranoid women. Am J Psychiatry 125:151–159, 1968

81. Dupont R, Ryder RG, Grunebaum HU: An unexpected result of psychoses in marriage. Am J Psychiatry 128:735–739, 1971

82. Kaplan HS: The New Sex Therapy. New York, Brunner/Mazel, 1974, p 495

83. Ibid, p 497

84. Donlon PT: Sexual symptoms of incipient schizophrenic psychoses. Med Aspects Hum Sexuality 10:70, 1976

85. Physicians Desk Reference. Oradell, New Jersey, Baker, 1978, p 1615

86. Ibid, pp 1455–1456

87. Mitchell JE, Popkin MK: Antipsychotic drug therapy and sexual dysfunction in men. Am J Psychiatry 139:633–637, 1982

88. Nestoros JN, Lehman HE, Ban TA: Sexual behavior in the male schizophrenic: The impact of illness and medications. Arch Sex Behav 10:436, 1981

89. Meier G: Interdigitation of mental health and family planning services. Fam Plann Perspect 5(3):182–186, 1973

90. Donlon PT: Sexual symptoms of incipient schizophrenic psychoses. Med Aspects Hum Sexuality 10:69, 1976

91. Kaplan HS: The New Sex Therapy, New York, Brunner/Mazel, 1974, p 475

92. Cassidy WL, Flanagan NB, Spellman M, Cohen ME: Clinical observations in

manic-depressive disease. JAMA 164:
1535–1546, 1957

93. Watson JP, Bamber RWK: Some relationships between sex, marriage and
mood. J Internat Med 8, (Suppl) 3:14–9,
1980

94. Kaplan HS: The New Sex Therapy,
New York, Brunner/Mazel, 1974, p 475

95. Ibid, p 474

96. Ibid, 475

97. Ibid, p 482

98. Derogatis LR: Psychological assessment of sexual disorders In Meyer JK
(ed): Clinical Management of Sexual
Disorders. Baltimore, Williams and
Wilkins, 1976, pp 35–73

99. Kaplan HS: The New Sex Therapy.
New York, Brunner/Mazel, 1974, p 483

100. Satterfield SB, Stayton WR: Understanding sexual function and dysfunction. Top Clin Nurs 1:24–25, 1980

101. Goodwin DW, Guze SB, Robbins E: Follow-up studies in obsessional neurosis.
Arch Gen Psychiatry 20: 182–187, 1969

102. Akhtar S, Crooker E, Dickey N,
Helfrich J, Rheuban WJ: Overt sexual
behavior among psychiatric inpatients.
Dis Nerv Syst 38:359–361, 1977

103. Ibid, p 360

104. Modestin J: Patterns of overt sexual interaction among acute psychiatric inpatients. Acta Psychiat Scand 64:646–
659, 1981

105. Velek MV, Lane TA: Heterosexual relationships of psychiatric inpatients established during their treatment. Internat J Soc Psychiatry 27:111–118, 1981

106. Akhtar S, Crooker E, Dickey N, et al:
Overt sexual behavior among psychiatric inpatients. Dis Nerv Supt 38:361,
1977

107. Abernathy V: Sexual knowledge, attitudes and practices of young female
psychiatric patients. Arch Gen Psychiatry 30:180–183, 1974

108. Grunebaum HU, Abernathy VD,
Rafman ES, Weiss JL: The family planning attitudes, practices and motivations of mental patients. Am J Psychiatry 128:741–744, 1971

109. Krietner G: Sexual and emotional intimacy between psychiatric inpatients:
Formulating a policy. Hosp Comm Psychiatry 32:188–193, 1981

110. Akhtar S, Crooker E, Dickey N,
Helfrich J, Rheuban WJ: Overt sexual
behavior among psychiatric inpatients.
Dis Nerv Syst 38:361, 1977

111. Grunebaum HU, Abernathy VD,
Rafman ES, Weis JL: The family planning attitudes, practices and motivations of mental patients. Am J Psychiatry 128:741, 1971

112. Ibid

113. Ibid, p 743

114. Meier G: Interdigitation of mental
health and family planning services.
Fam Plann Perspect 5(3):183, 1973

115. Ibid

116. Ibid, p 184

117. Pinderhughes CA, Grace EB, Reyna LJ:
Psychiatric disorders and sexual functioning. Am J Psychiatry 128:1279,
1972

118. Ibid, p 1280

Chapter 30

Drugs That Affect Sexuality

WILLIAM D. BALL

Despite the use of substances with pharmacologic activity throughout human history, remarkably little is known with any certainty regarding the interaction of chemical agents and sexuality. To a large degree, social attitudes have prohibited detailed, controlled investigations into the nature of human sexual experience until very recently. Consequently, much of the information in this area remains mythologic, anecdotal, and poorly documented at best.[1-4]

Scientific research in this area is in its infancy and largely experimental rather than clinical. Generalizations from these data to effects in the context of life experience are generally unjustified. It is becoming increasingly clear that sexual response and its modification depend on a very complex interaction of hormonal, neurologic, psychologic, social, and physical factors. A particular sexual response may not be reproducible if any of these factors is altered. Considering the effects of chemical agents, as we do in this chapter, cannot be done in an isolated manner without realizing that drugs act within this complex context and their effects can be modulated widely by variations in this context.

Perhaps of the greatest interest throughout history have been those chemical agents that could possibly positively affect the sexual experience by enhancing desire, sensation, or performance. The endless search for the true aphrodisiac has been a major instigating factor in the widespread recreational nonmedical use of psychoactive drugs. It is clear that most popular information in this area is almost entirely without substance, as witnessed by the meteoric rise and fall these agents have undergone as the mythology surrounding them has been exposed by experience. In nearly all cases, the actions of these agents have proven to be unreliable, negligible, or in some cases, suprisingly deleterious to the sexual experience, in direct contradiction to popular initial beliefs.

Of major concern to health practitioners are the unintended and usually adverse effects of some medically prescribed drugs on sexual behavior. Such adverse effects have been reported widely with a variety of agents. However, the validity of available data regarding the extent of this problem must be questioned, since most data are derived from voluntary patient reports. In the sensitive area of sexuality, relying on voluntary reports of such problems probably grossly underestimates their true frequency, since patients are usually reluctant and embarrassed to admit sexual difficulties. Frequently, health professionals are reluctant to pursue sexual problems in patients or they may focus their attention on possible psychologic factors instead, ignoring possible drug effects.

A subtler but perhaps more significant

511

concern is the indirect effect some drugs may have on sexual attitudes, mores, and in turn, behavior. The advent of oral contraceptives, with virtually absolute efficacy, served to relieve a great deal of anxiety surrounding nonprocreative sexual activity and coincided with dramatic changes in public attitudes and apparent changes in sexual behavior.

It is evident that drugs can alter all aspects of the sexual experience.[5] The impact of drugs on sexuality, although still largely uninvestigated, must be considered carefully when we observe, evaluate, or counsel patients in sexual health or illness.

EFFECTS OF APPROVED SOCIAL DRUGS ON SEXUALITY

Alcohol

Perhaps the most astute and comprehensive observation concerning the effects of alcohol on human sexuality was made by Shakespeare in 1606:

> MACDUFF: What three things does drink especially provoke?
>
> PORTER: Marry, sir, nose-painting. sleep and urine. Lechery, sir; it provokes and unprovokes. It provokes the desire, but it takes away the performance: therefore, much drink may be said to be an equivocator with lechery: it makes him and it mars him; it sets him on; and it takes him off; it persuades him, and disheartens him; makes him stand to and not stand to; in conclusion, equivocates him in a sleep, and, giving him the lie, leaves him.
>
> *Macbeth*, Act 2, Sc. 3

There is little doubt that alcohol is the most common social lubricant, serving to relieve the tension and anxiety that may surround many social interactions and reducing inhibitions that may restrain individuals from expressing sexual or other desires. The sensation of relaxation and disinhibition that alcohol produces is shared by many substances that generally depress the central nervous system (CNS). Substances like alcohol that affect higher cortical centers of the CNS before producing marked effects in the cerebral and cerebellar areas associated with sensory and motor control are likely to be attributed with aphrodisiac properties. Although it cannot be stated with certainty, it is likely that alcohol and similar substances do not inherently provoke or increase sexual desire (libido). However, the relationship of alcohol and overall sexual responsiveness has been investigated.

In a questionnaire survey, Athanasiou, Shaver, and Tavris[6] found that of the men and women sampled, 45 and 63 percent, respectively, reported that alcohol enhanced sexual pleasure, 13 and 11 percent reported that it had no effect, and 42 and 21 percent reported that it decreased pleasure. Three recent studies investigated alcohol's effects on objectively measured sexual arousal in college students. Farkas and Rosen[7] monitored penile tumescence in response to an erotic film at four different blood alcohol levels, 0 mg%, 25 mg%, 50 mg%, and 75 mg%. Although a slight facilitation in amplitude of penile tumescence was observed at the low blood alcohol concentration (25 mg%), a significant negative linear trend was observed with the rate and extent of tumescence, decreasing with rising alcohol levels. Briddell and Wilson[8] found similar results. Wilson and Lawson[9] used vaginal pressure pulse recordings to measure sexual arousal in female college students at similar blood alcohol concentrations and found a similar negative relationship. At variance with these findings are consistent reports of progressively increased sexual arousal by the study subjects with advancing alcohol concentrations. Although it is clear that many people believe alcohol promotes sexual arousal and pleasure, it cannot be concluded whether this is a result of preconceived expectations of the subjects or a separation of subjective experience from objective signs of arousal.[10]

The effects of alcohol and other drugs on physiologic aspects of sexual function are much more apparent in males, since the necessity of erectile function for successful male sexual function provides an obvious physical index. Data from the previously mentioned studies and observations of sexual function in alcoholics clearly indicate that acute and chronic alcohol intoxication adversely effects male sexual function. This may account for the much lower percentage of males favoring alcohol in the survey by Athanasiou and associates.

As blood alcohol concentrations rise acutely, there is likely to be progressive impairment of sensation, motor abilities, and neural reflexes critically involved in erection and ejaculation, decreasing capacity for effective sexual function. Chronic alcoholism is associated frequently with impotence, which may persist despite sobriety. Unlike acute ingestion, chronic alcohol intake appears to lower plasma testosterone,[11] apparently by accelerating elimination and decreasing production. Alcoholic males who develop cirrhosis are particularly likely to develop hypogonadism and gynecomastia, with lowered testosterone levels and high levels of estrogenic substances.[12] It is well known that chronic alcoholism is associated with severe peripheral neuropathies. Despite prolonged abstinence, only about one-half of alcoholic males who complain of impotence will show improvement in sexual function. The effects of chronic alcoholism on libido, responsiveness, or sexual function in females are essentially unknown.[13]

EFFECT OF NONAPPROVED SOCIAL DRUGS ON SEXUALITY

Opiates (Heroin, Illicit and Licit Narcotics)

As with other popular drugs of abuse, opiates have enjoyed a reputation as enhancers of sexual pleasure. Quite to the contrary, virtually all available information indicates that they seriously impair sexual function. In small doses they may initially act as disinhibiting agents, as seen with alcohol and other CNS depressants. However, it appears that as tolerance and dependence develop, sexual function suffers.

Cushman[14] found a high incidence of complaints of reduced libido, impotency, and retarded ejaculation among heroin abusers. He found these problems to be rapidly reversible with abstinence or, in most cases, with replacement by methadone maintenance. However, methadone maintenance is associated with adverse sexual effects similar to those of heroin, and sexual complaints are the major reason most patients withdraw from methadone maintenance programs. Also, withdrawal from heroin or methadone is associated with a high incidence of premature ejaculation.[15] It is not clear whether this merely reflects preexisting poor sexual adjustment of drug addicts[16] or an aspect of a drug withdrawal or abstinence syndrome.[17]

Chronic heroin and methadone use are associated with reduced function of secondary sex organs. Serum testosterone, ejaculate volume, and sperm motility are all reduced. Interestingly, one study found these effects to be much more pronounced in patients receiving methadone than in heroin addicts.[18] In this study, 75 percent of methadone clients reported that methadone affected their sexual performance to a greater degree than heroin, particularly when they initially entered the methadone maintenance program. The relative effect of heroin and methadone cannot be precisely stated, since it is unclear whether pharmacologically equivalent doses of the two agents were employed in these studies.

Nearly all heroin addicts and patients on methadone maintenance report a substantial reduction of libido but for strikingly different reasons. Among heroin users, the most common reason given for reduced sexual activity was that it took too much time away from drug-seeking behavior. In contrast, failure to maintain an erection during intercourse was the most common reason among methadone receivers.

Some concern has been expressed that methadone may affect fertility due to low ejaculate volumes and sperm motility.[19] This remains to be investigated.

Heroin addicts show a partial decrease in gonadotropin release, which may be partially responsible for some of the reported sexual disturbances. Also, amenorrhea, infertility, reduced libido, and spontaneous abortion are frequent in addicted women and may be evidence of diminished release of pituitary gonadotropins.[20]

Interestingly, the administration of narcotic antagonists (particularly cyclazocine) to addicts has led to markedly increased libido and improvement in sexual function. This is probably due to precipitation of opiate withdrawal with removal of their depressant effects on sexuality and the autonomic nervous system hyperactivity that is common in withdrawal.[21] This phenomenon has not been observed when these agents are given to nonopiate-dependent individuals.

Marijuana

More than any other illicit social drug, marijuana has received consistent, widespread support as a drug of considerable aphrodisiac powers. Nonusers strongly associate marijuana with sexual permissiveness and promiscuity among users, while users generally laud its positive effects on sexual performance and pleasure.[22,23] There is little doubt that in small doses characteristically found in social use, marijuana has considerable disinhibiting effects. However, larger doses, as with other CNS depressants, may depress sexuality generally. The Indian Hemp Commission of 1894 reported that hemp drugs have "no aphrodisiac power whatever; and, as a matter of fact, they are used by ascetics in this country with the ostensible object of destroying sexual appetite."

In association with its disinhibiting effects, marijuana generally induces a number of subjective changes that frequent users report render the sexual experience more pleasurable and exciting:

1. One's sense of touch is more intense and stimulating.

2. One's skin feels warm, tingly, and flushed.

3. The immediate emotional impact of the experience is much greater.

4. Emotional warmth and affection toward one's partner appear to be stronger.

5. The sex act appears to last longer than clock time indicates.

6. One feels more relaxed, freer, more "natural."

7. The sex act becomes a total entity in itself, a totally involving experience.

8. Orgasm is more intense than usual.

These effects are heavily dependent on dosage as well as the set and setting of use.[24] Careful questioning of users refutes the idea that marijuana is per se a sexual stimulant. Rather, as with food, the sensory response to the experience is enhanced and the stimulation results from the anticipation of this augmentation.[25] Also, positive effects on sexuality are reported much more commonly by frequent than infrequent (less than weekly) marijuana users.[26] It may be that these effects are "learned" behavior, part of the cultural milieu of chronic marijuana users, or a pharmacologic effect that requires repeated administration to be maximally apparent.

Chronic, high-dosage use of marijuana by male subjects has recently been associated with sexual dysfunction and failure of secondary sex organs, with oligospermia, gynecomastia,[27] and decreased plasma testosterone[28] in some reports. Effects of this nature are probably not seen unless daily, excessive use continues for several months.[29,30]

The association of marijuana use with sexual permissiveness has received considerable support from studies and surveys that reveal that sexual activity is much greater among frequent marijuana users. Marijuana users are much more likely to have engaged in premarital sex, to have had a greater number of sexual partners, and to have had earlier initial sexual experiences than nonusers. This strong relationship has led a number of observers to conclude that marijuana causes permissive sexuality. However, there are no data to support this contention. It appears more likely that liberal sexual behavior is merely one of the nontraditional values and activities tolerated or embraced by a subculture of which drug use is only another component.[31]

Sedative–Hypnotics

A variety of sedative–hypnotic agents that have established medical uses are abused and misused widely to produce intoxication, general relaxation, and relief of tension. At times, some of these agents have received public attention as potential aphrodisiacs, subsequently undergoing a period of rapid increase in use.

A dramatic recent example of this phenomenon centered around the nonbarbiturate sedative hypnotic methaqualone (Quaalude, Sopor). In the early 1970s methaqualone abuse swept the United States. It rapidly became the hottest drug on the streets, following popular rumors of its mystical sexual properties.[32] It was widely touted as the "love drug" or "orgy drug" and associated with wild sexual behavior. It is clear that in common with other central nervous system depressants, methaqualone and other sedative–hypnotics are effective disinhibitors. Disinhibition is commonly followed by lethargy, loss of coordination, and other effects that may interfere with sexual interest and function. Also, in terms of special aphrodisiac properties, methaqualone ranks with other depressants. Among those who have actually experienced the conjunction of methaqualone and sex, the drug receives very low ratings. At present, use of this drug seems to be decreasing, and claims for its special sexual properties are seldom heard. Also, aphrodisiac effects have never been identified secondary to medical use of the drug.

Thus, methaqualone serves as a classic example of the mythology that can contribute to the abuse of CNS depressants that have enjoyed the reputation as sexual enhancers almost exclusively among the inexperienced.[33]

Cocaine and Amphetamines

Cocaine, a local anesthetic, is a potent CNS stimulant renowned for its aphrodisiac qualities; it is often referred to as the "champagne" of sexual drugs.[34] Taken in small doses, usually intransally, it produces euphoria, a sense of well-being, loss of fatigue, and heightened sensory awareness, all of which may contribute to greater appreciation of a sexual experience. Larger doses, particularly by the intravenous route, result in intense CNS stimulation similar to the rush seen with intravenous heroin and somewhat "orgasmic" in quality. In some persons, this experience may serve as a substitute for rather than an enhancer of sexual pleasure and disturb the interpersonal communication that is important to a satisfying sexual experience.

Amphetamines, although having a less elegant reputation, produce effects quite similar to those of cocaine due to CNS stimulation. The effects observed are dose related as well, with smaller doses likely to vitalize some aspects of sexual experience, while larger doses may produce distracting agitation.[35]

Both cocaine and amphetamines have potent systemic sympathomimetic (adrenergic agonist) effects, which may account for the frequent observation of a delay in achieving orgasm and ejaculation.[36]

As with other drug abusers, chronic, high-dose amphetamine abusers have a relatively high incidence of sexual disturbances and complaints.[37] However, recent studies[38] have failed to support the contention that chronic amphetamine use is either a sexual substitute or contributes directly to sexual disturbances. Rather, both durg use and sexual pathology seemed to result from common, yet unidentified, personality variables. In one survey of abusers of oral amphetamines, females frequently reported disturbances in sexual function and libido, while males were unaffected.[39]

Amyl Nitrite

Amyl nitrite is a potent peripheral vasodilator used medically in the treatment of angina pectoris (ischemic heart pain). The drug is commercially available in fragile, cloth-covered glass vials, which are crushed to release the volatile drug. Inhalation of the vapors produces a rapid vasodilation with reflex tachycardia and headache (due to extracranial vasodilation). In recent years, this product has seen little use, since sublingual nitroglycerin tablets are nearly as rapid and effective and less likely to produce severe hypotension from excessive vasodilation. However, more recently, amyl nitrite (known as "poppers" or "snappers") has become an extraordinarily popular "sex drug," especially among male homosexuals.[40]

The usual pattern of use is for one or both partners to inhale the drug as orgasm approaches. This is reputed to produce a more powerful, sensual orgasm. It can only be speculated as to how a vasodilator might result in such effects. The abrupt drop in blood pressure may produce behavioral and perceptual changes secondary to changes in brain perfusion. Its hemodynamic effects may produce pleasurable changes in genital blood flow. However, loss of erection may occur. Systemic hypotension may cause faintness and syncope.

Women apparently do not find amyl nitrite very satisfactory, in general. Also, the reported effects are not appreciated by all male users.[41] The changes in cerebral circulation may alter consciousness in such a way that the person may lose awareness of his environment. More experience with amyl nitrite may quickly erode its current image as a potentiator of the orgasmic experience.

LSD and Other Hallucinogens

Many of the hallucinogens resembling LSD (lysergic acid diethylamide), such as psilocybin, dimethyltryptamine (DMT), and mescaline (synthetic peyote), are purported to have aphrodisiac properties as confirmed by users' opinions.[42,43] Undoubtedly, sexual experiences under the influence of these drugs must be different than usual, consider-

ing the somatic, perceptual, and psychic phenomena that these agents produce.[44] The effects again appear to be dose related, with more generous quantities of hallucinogens bringing about loss of bodily control and redirecting one's attention from sexual desire into mysticism, internal absorption, and universal communion.[45] Thus, some users report aphrodisiac effects while others report opposite effects.[46] Hollister[47] reports that "many of my experimental subjects have told me that while they had thoughts of sex while under the drug, the idea of being able to accomplish the act seemed preposterous." Thus, it is undoubtedly true that hallucinogens influence perception of a variety of experiences, sexual and otherwise, and that the nature of this influence is highly variable. There is no evidence that hallucinogens directly stimulate sexual desire, although in one animal study LSD was reported to enhance sexual activity. Also, LSD acts in a fashion similar to serotonin, a neurotransmitter that appears to play some role in sexual function.[48]

Cantharides (Cantharis, Cantharidin)

Cantharides ("Spanish fly") is a powdered drug derived from the crushed, dried Spanish fly or beetle *Cantharis vesicatoria*. This drug has an intensely irritant action on mucous membranes and is a potent systemic poison. Despite its status as a legendary sexual stimulant, taking internally, it can produce severe illness and death.[49] Also, the drug produces bladder irritation and inflammation with increased genital circulation. Priapism also has been reported. These sensations may be interpreted as signs of sexual arousal, although changes in libido are not evident.

Yohimbine

Yohimbine, an alkaloid derived from the West African tree *Corynanthe yohimbe,* has complex pharmacologic actions including alpha-adrenergic blocking effects. This produces a mild peripheral vasodilation and parasympathetic dominance of the autonomic nervous system. There is conflicting evidence regarding its reputed action as an aphrodisiac ingredient in the commercial preparation Afrodex.* The two available controlled studies[50,51] lack any statistical analysis of significance, and a recent review of these studies[52] failed to resolve the controversy surrounding this product.

EFFECT OF THERAPEUTIC AGENTS ON SEXUALITY

It is clear from available data that drugs prescribed for the treatment of medical illness may have significant adverse effects on sexuality.[53] As a corollary, it has been observed that these adverse effects may have a significant impact on patient acceptance of and compliance with the prescribed regimen. One clinician responsible for a large outpatient clinic in the Veterans Administration noted that among male patients, impotence was the most important cause of failure to take medications.[54] Thus, to assure successful therapy of medical conditions as well as preventing or alleviating sexual complications of drug therapy, we must be very aware of the nature of the interaction of drugs with sexuality.

Drugs may alter sexuality in a number of ways. As we have seen with the abuse of psychoactive agents, depressants, and stimulants, effects on the CNS may alter libido, function, and perception of sexual experience. A variety of medicinal agents also influence the autonomic nervous system (ANS), which is instrumental in sexual function. The reliance of sexual function upon the ANS activity has been described adequately only in males.[55]

Parasympathetic (cholinergic) stimulation is responsible for producing erection by causing dilation of penile arteries and ve-

*Afrodex (product of Bentex Pharmaceutical Company) contains nux vomica extract, 5 mg; methyltestosterone, 5 mg; and yohimbine, 5 mg.

nous constriction. Drugs that interfere with parasympathetic impulses (anticholinergics, ganglionic blockers) may induce erectile failure. Sympathetic (adrenergic) impulses produce emission of sperm from the testes and prostatic fluid from the seminal vesicles. Ejaculation, the projection of this mixture from the penis, is a result of parasympathetic stimulation. Thus, adrenergic and ganglionic blockers may impair ejaculation and even produce retrograde ejaculation (ejaculate expelled into the bladder) or produce painful ejaculation.

Some agents may alter sexual behavior by hormonal actions, influencing the production or activity of estrogenic and androgenic substances that modulate sexual behavior. In patients with erectile failure (impotence), it may be difficult to separate drug-related from psychogenic factors. However, organic causes, such as drugs, tend to produce more consistent failure under all circumstances—all partners, with masturbation, and during sleep. Also, organic impotence tends not to be associated with significant life events, is preceded by uninterrupted normal erectile function, and is characterized by intact libido.[56] Among organic causes, drug-related erectile failure may be identified by rapid alleviation, in most cases, upon discontinuation of the offending agent. In contrast, disease states, such as diabetes mellitus or multiple sclerosis, produce generally progressive and permanent impairment of erectile function.

Antihypertensives
Virtually every agent used in the chronic management of hypertension has been associated with sexual dysfunction. Many of these agents produce vasodilation and/or decreased cardiac output (reducing blood pressure) by acting upon the sympathetic nervous system peripherally or in the CNS. Also, some of these drugs have other depressive affects on the CNS that may influence sexual behavior. It should be recognized that hypertensive patients may have sexual dysfunction as a manifestation of the disease process.[57]

Guanethidine (Ismelin). This drug is a potent adrenergic blocker that, among antihypertensives, is most frequently associated with sexual dysfunction. It is clear that adrenergic blockade could be responsible for reduction or absence of ejaculate with normal libido and normal erection, as is most commonly observed.[58] However, instances of erectile failure and loss of libido are more difficult to explain, as the drug is generally devoid of anticholinergic, ganglionic blocking, or CNS activity.

Reserpine (Serpasil). This drug is a relatively weak antihypertensive that depletes norepinephrine and dopamine from adrenergic neurons in the CNS and peripherally and thus can interfere with emission in males. Its use as an antihypertensive, at least alone in therapy, has declined markedly as a result of frequent and severe mental depression that results when adequate antihypertensive doses are prescribed. Thus, reserpine often not only interferes with emission in many patients, but produces impotence and loss of libido probably as a result of its CNS effects. Also, through alterations of CNS transmitters, particularly dopamine, reserpine can produce anovulation, galactorrhea, and amenorrhea.[59]

Methyldopa (Aldomet). Methyldopa affects adrenergic neural transmitters in the CNS and ANS, producing moderate vasodilation and some CNS depression (usually drowsiness). Recent reports indicate that sexual dysfunction may be frequently associated with this drug. Newman and Salerno[60] reported that 7 of 27 hypertensive patients receiving methyldopa developed sexual dysfunction manifested as either loss of libido, erectile failure, or ejaculatory difficulties, which reversed within 2 weeks of discontinuation. Alexander and Evans[61] noted that when they carefully questioned their patients, the incidence of such effects was even higher, pointing out that voluntary questionnaires may dramatically underestimate the true incidence of such problems.

Colindine (Catapres). Clonidine inhibits CNS sympathetic activity, producing moderate vasodilation, and has antihypertensive efficacy and toxicity similar to that of methyldopa.[62] Claims by the manufacturer that clonidine lowers blood pressure "with little risk of impairing sexual function" are not supported by available data. Impotence and retrograde ejaculation in men and inability to achieve orgasm in women can occur in patients treated with clonidine. Also, the incidence of sexual dysfunction caused by clonidine and methyldopa appear to be similar.[63]

Propranolol (Inderal). This drug is an effective CNS and peripheral blocker of beta-sympathetic receptors that produces mild vasodilation and decreased cardiac output. Although adverse sexual effects were long believed to be very rare with propranolol, recent reports of impotence and, less commonly, loss of libido, have contradicted this notion.[64] The CNS actions of propranolol can produce a variety of behavioral problems including insomnia, nightmares, and depression that may be associated with sexual dysfunction. There are many new beta-sympathetic receptor blocking agents on the market, such as metoprolol (Lopressor), atenolol (Tenormin), and timolol (Blockadren) that do not have as prominent CNS effects as propranolol and may be less likely to have adverse effects on sexuality.

Spironolactone (Aldactone). This is an aldosterone-antagonizing diuretic agent with mild antihypertensive activity. This agent has a variety of endocrine effects, probably due to its steroid chemical configuration, which confers antiandrogenic activity upon the substance.[65] In males, spironolactone is associated frequently with estrogenlike feminizing effects such as gynecomastia with painful nodularity. Although this can occur at all dosages,[66] it is particularly common with higher dosages. Loss of libido and impotence are reported, although less commonly than gynecomastia.[67] In women, spironolactone can induce breast soreness and menstrual irregularities, including amenorrhea. Although these effects are documented in only a handful of cases, their incidence may be quite high. These effects appear to be slowly reversible over several months.

Phenoxybenzamine (Dibenzyline). This alpha-adrenergic receptor blocking agent can lower blood pressure by producing vasodilation in skin and mucosal and visceral vasculature. Inhibition of ejaculation has been reported in several patients.[68]

There are isolated case reports that implicate a variety of other antihypertensive agents, such as hydralazine (Apresoline), prazosin (Minipres), and hydrochlorthiazide, although the etiologic connections in these cases are generally tenuous.[69,70]

Antipsychotic Tranquilizers

Of the major antipsychotic tranquilizer groups, the phenothiazines are probably the most widely used. Chlorpromazine (Thorazine) is perhaps the best known example of this group. Phenothiazines possess a variety of actions that can affect sexual behavior. Many of these agents have potent anticholinergic effects that may produce impotence or ejaculatory difficulties. Also, they are potent peripheral alpha-adrenergic blockers, which may affect emission. Potent actions on neurotransmitters in the CNS alters many forms of behavior, as well as sexual. Also, these drugs interfere with gonadotropin release from the hypothalamus, producing a variety of frequent endocrinologic side effects, including galactorrhea, amenorrhea, and anovulation.

Thioridazine. Thioridazine (Mellaril), the most potent anticholinergic and alpha-adrenergic blocker of this group, is probably the antipsychotic most frequently associated with sexual dysfunction. One recent study[71] reported a 60 percent incidence of difficulties in 57 male patients. Although impotence was frequent in this group, the most consistent

effect was a marked reduction or absence of ejaculate at orgasm and painful ejaculation. A third of these patients had retrograde ejaculation. Similar ejaculation difficulties are reported very infrequently with a variety of other phenothiazines—mesoridazine (Serentil), chlorprothixene (Taractan); chlorpromazine (Thorazine)[72]; and piperacetazine (Quide).[73]

Among women, amenorrhea and other endocrine side effects may be as common with thioridazine use as ejaculation difficulties among men.[74] This appears to be secondary to increased levels of prolactin and a loss in the normal cycling of luteinizing hormone and estrogens.[75] Males may exhibit reduced serum testosterone levels while receiving phenothiazines.[76]

The majority of sexual difficulties associated with phenothiazines other than thioridazine consist of loss of libido and impotence or endocrine side effects (galactorrhea, amenorrhea).[77]

Antidepressants

Depression is usually accompanied by decrease in libido and sexual activity and, in some cases, impairment of function. Treatment with antidepressants usually restores normal sexual behavior as depression resolves. However, sexual dysfunction can be a manifestation of antidepressant therapy as well.

Tricyclic Antidepressants. The tricyclic antidepressants, represented by amitriptyline (Elavil), imipramine (Tofranil), desipramine (Norpramin), and others, are the most commonly used antidepressant agents. Among other actions, these agents tend to have potent anticholinergic effects. Thus, a fair incidence of impotence and ejaculatory difficulties might be expected. Recent surveys indicate that delay in orgasm and ejaculation is very common in men and that many women experience delay in achieving orgasm.[78] Although impotence is indicated to be common in some reviews, as would be predicted, there are little data in support of this observation.

Several newer antidepressants, such as trazodone (Deseryl) and mianserin, have greatly reduced anticholinergic and sedative actions and may be expected to interfere less with sexual function.

Monoamine Oxidase Inhibitors. Monoamine oxidase inhibitors (MAOI), represented by phenelzine (Nardil), tranylcypromine (Parnate), and pargyline (Eutonyl), are potent antidepressants generally reserved for recalcitrant cases due to frequent adverse effects and many drug interactions. The primary action of these drugs is to block the action of monoamine oxidase, which metabolizes sympathomimetic amines (norepinephrine, dopamine, epinephrine, 5-hydroxytryptamine), resulting in an accumulation of these compounds. A variety of sexual disturbances have been attributed to the use of MAOIs, including impotence and delayed ejaculation in men and difficulty in achieving orgasm in women.[79]

Cancer Chemotherapeutic Agents

The majority of cancer chemotherapeutic agents are cytotoxic to normal host cells as well as malignant cells. Most agents have greater activity in cells that are proliferating rapidly. Among host cells that proliferate rapidly are the germinal cells involved in spermatogenesis (as well as the cells of the bone marrow and gastrointestinal tract). Consequently, temporary sterility is commonly associated with the use of these agents. Azoospermia, lasting at least several years, with intact libido and sexual potency has been observed after combination regimens for lymphoma. Gynecomastia has been described as a complication of chemotherapy. In female patients cytotoxic-induced gonadal damage includes amenorrhea and menopausal symptoms.[80]

Some chemotherapeutic agents, such as vincristine, cause a great deal of neurotox-

icity, represented as disorders in consciousness (e.g., agitation, seizure, depression) and peripheral neuropathies (e.g., paresthesias, decreased deep tendon reflexes). Alterations in sexual function secondary to these effects have not been noted in most reviews; however, one investigator reported frequent impotence in a large study of the therapeutic use of vincristine.[81]

Drugs That Affect Brain Amines (Neurotransmitters)

The exact role of brain amines in controlling or modifying sexual behavior and function is not clear, although it is apparent that they perform some important functions. Studies in experimental animals have found that increased brain serotonin (5-hydroxytryptamine) has an inhibitory effect on sexual activity.[82] However, studies with L-tryptophan, a serotonin precursor, in psychiatric patients[83] and case reports in supposed normal individuals[84] have shown opposite results.[85]

L-Dopa. L-Dopa (Dopar, others) is a dopamine precursor used in the treatment of Parkinson's disease. Many reports of increased sexual behavior among patients treated with L-dopa[86] have led investigators to posit that L-dopa may have aphrodisiac properties and have value in the treatment of psychogenic impotence. However, it is not clear whether the effects observed in Parkinsonism are due to aphrodisiac action or are secondary to general functional improvement from the treatment of Parkinsonism.[87] A pilot study in sexually impotent patients revealed a mild transient effect on sexual function and libido in a portion of the patients.[88] Among psychiatric patients with prior sexual maladjustment, L-dopa appeared to increase the aberrancy of their sexuality.[89] Most studies of these effects are very poorly controlled and poorly evaluated.[90] Also, it is important to recognize that L-dopa therapy can produce a variety of psychiatric side effects of which changes in sexuality may be only one facet.[91]

Hormones and Hormonal Antagonists

Hormones play extremely vital roles in sexual function and behavior, and compounds that alter hormone levels or effects can have dramatic effects on sexuality. The use of estrogens for women and androgens for males with impaired sexual responsiveness or desire is very popular. The evidence that they are of any benefit except in clear cases of deficiency is scanty.

Testosterone. Testosterone and its derivatives, singly or combined with other agents, have been prescribed widely to restore flagging sexual potency and interest in aging males and to treat impotence. The usefulness of these agents in the presence of hypogonadism is clear. Substantial evidence is not available for their use in more nonspecific conditions. Most studies are not well designed and lack firm criteria for evaluating changes in sexual function and behavior.[92]

Testosterone inhibits the release of luteinizing hormone (LH) and follicle-stimulating hormone (FSH) and can produce azoospermia secondary to this effect. This action is being exploited in ongoing investigations of testosterone and its derivatives as male contraceptives agents.[93] Paradoxically, some anabolic testosterone derivatives, widely used by athletes to enhance muscle growth and endurance, have produced impotence and loss of libido as well as azoospermia.[94] This effect is secondary to gonadotropin inhibition and conversion of androgens to estrogen if given in large doses chronically.

Clomiphene Citrate. Clomiphene citrate (Clomid), a nonsteroid triethylene derivative, has a combination of interesting effects. Its antiestrogenic action causes FSH and LH levels to rise, resulting in stimulation of ovulation in women. In males, clomiphene produces a significant rise in testosterone levels. In a small study of patients with psychogenic (nonorganic) impotence, the drug was essentially without beneficial effect.[95]

Uremic patients, who frequently have hypogonadism with oligospermia secondary to decreased serum testosterone levels, respond to clomiphene with increases in gonadotropins and testosterone levels. Libido and sexual potency are improved, while the effects on spermatogenesis are variable.[96]

Other Estrogenic or Antiandrogenic Drugs. Drugs that have estrogenic or antiandrogenic effects have been shown to suppress sexual function and behavior in males. These drugs have been used somewhat successfully to control hypersexual or deviant sexual behavior in males. Progestogens, such as medroxyprogesterone, have libido-reducing qualities in both males and females, producing a marked reduction in circulating androgens. Estrogens reduce libido in males but produce feminization (e.g., gynecomastia) and a variety of disturbing (e.g., nausea) and dangerous (e.g., cardiovascular disease) side effects. Cyproterone acetate, a drug that competitively inhibits androgen action, has demonstrated beneficial effects in male and female sexual deviants.[97, 98] It is not clear if this drug will cause feminization of males.

Diethylstilbestrol (DES), a synthetic compound with estrogenic activity, has been used as a postcoital contraceptive, an antitumor agent against prostatic and breast cancer, and to maintain pregnancies which are threatened by spontaneous abortion. For the latter use, not only is there no evidence of efficacy, but studies have revealed significant risk to the offspring of mothers who receive DES during pregnancy. Many of the female offspring have vaginal adenosis and some have developed vaginal carcinoma. Male offspring have developed hypoplastic testicles, epididymal cysts, and other urologic abnormalities.[99]

Oral Contraceptives. Our understanding of gonadotropin–hormone interactions in the ovulatory cycle of females has produced perhaps the most significant pharmacologic agents affecting sexuality—the oral contraceptive. The most effective of these agents combine estrogens and progestogens. This combination, taken continuously, inhibits FSH and LH release from the pituitary, which is responsible for ovarian follicle development and release. Some products use sequential rather than combined estrogen and progestogen to more closely mimic natural hormone levels. These agents block FSH secretion and alter LH secretion patterns and are somewhat less effective. More recently, the "mini" pill, which contains small amounts of progestogen only, has been released in an attempt to reduce adverse effects thought to be associated with estrogens and larger doses of progestogens. These agents do not alter FSH or LH levels markedly and may act by inhibiting sperm penetration into the cervical mucus or interfering with uterine implantation. Several clinical trials of a "morning after" pill consisting of large doses of DES have shown it to be effective, although there is some concern over the association of this drug with uterine cancer in offspring.[100]

The impact of oral contraceptive agents on sexual attitudes and behavior have not been adequately assessed. Such assessment is obviously methodologically problematic or perhaps impossible, considering how closely the inception and proliferation of these agents were linked to other major social and nonsexual changes in society. Although a cause and effect relationship between widespread oral contraceptive use and major shifts in sexual practices and attitudes is highly suspected, it may never be proven.

Some of the more direct effects of oral contraceptives on sexual behavior and function have been the subject of much investigation.[101] In particular, the effects of oral contraceptives on female libido have been a major subject of interest, since it is known that progestogens can impair libido, while estrogens have a minor role in maintaining libido. In a comprehensive review of the literature on this subject, Dennerstein and Burrows[102] concluded that in the vast majority of oral contraceptive users there is no measurable effect. A small proportion (5 percent)

experience a decrease in sexual desire and psychologic depression. However, another small segment of the population seems to experience greater pleasure in spontaneity of sexual behavior. It has not been determined whether this is a pharmacologic effect of the pill or the result of preexisting attitudes and emotional makeup of the patient. In a recent study it appeared that oral contraceptives inhibited a natural rise in the rate of female-initiated sexual activity that occurs around the time of ovulation.[103] No adequately controlled studies have evaluated the relative contribution of progestational and estrogenic substances, although it is the clinical impression of several investigators that depression and reduced libido are more common with the more strongly progestational products.[104]

Women with irregular or difficult menses often receive oral contraceptives in order to stabilize and reduce the distress of their menstruation. In some of these patients and patients with normal menses, the discontinuation of oral contraceptives after usually 1 or more years of use is followed rarely (1 to 2 percent) by a prolonged period of amenorrhea and, in some cases, galactorrhea. This appears to be due to the slow resolution of the prolonged suppression of pituitary function (FSH and LH secretion) in these patients.[105,106] The occasional case of associated galactorrhea may be secondary to suppression of release of prolactin-inhibiting factors, although this has not been investigated. Although sequential products probably interfere less with LH secretion, there is no firm evidence that the risk of this problem is any less with these products.[107] It is important to distinguish postpill amenorrhea from other causes of amenorrhea (e.g., pituitary adenoma, hypoadrenalism, and hypothyroidism). The vast majority of patients return to normal menstrual cycles spontaneously within 6 months, although some may resolve only after several years.[108] Treatment may be undertaken to stimulate ovulation with agents such as clomiphene citrate (Clomid) should spontaneous resolution not occur.

Bromocriptine (Parlodel). This drug is an ergot alkaloid derivative whose primary action is that of a dopamine receptor agonist in the CNS, producing effects of a prolactin-release inhibiting factor. In patients with galactorrhea and amenorrhea associated with elevated prolactin levels, the drug has proven remarkably effective. It is being investigated for use in a variety of other disorders involving dopamine (e.g., Parkinsonism) and tropic hormone release (e.g., acromegaly and Cushing's syndrome). Since this agent has restored gonadal function in males with galactorrhea and hyperprolactinemia, it has recently undergone preliminary trials in male infertility associated with high normal or slightly elevated serum prolactin levels. The reduction in prolactin levels with the use of this agent was associated with a rapid rise in the depressed testosterone levels seen in these patients. In several oligospermic patients, adequate spermatogenesis returned.[109]

Cimetidine (Tagamet). Cimetidine is an antagonist of the histamine H_2 receptor. The H_2 receptor for histamine is partially responsible for stimulating gastric acid secretion and is not antagonized by usual antihistamines. Cimetidine, by inhibiting this effect of histamine, has found great use in the treatment of duodenal ulcer and related conditions. There are many reports of loss of libido and erectile dysfunction that progressed to complete impotence in several male patients receiving cimetidine. In some cases, this persisted after discontinuation. Also, breast soreness and gynecomastia have been reported. The mechanism for these reactions is not clear, although an antiandrogenic effect has been found in animals, while gonadotropin levels have been elevated in some studies involving humans. In one study[110] of usual therapeutic doses of cimetidine in men, a mean reduction in sperm count of 43 percent occurred in association with a variety of gonadotropin abnormalities. The implications of this finding in terms of the possible long-term effects of cimetidine on male fertility have not been evaluated.

Ranitidine (Zantac). Ranitidine, a new histamine H_2 receptor antagonist, appears to have much less antiandrogenic effect than cimetidine, and several patients have experienced relief of impotence and breast changes when switched from cimetidine to ranitidine.[111]

Miscellaneous Agents

There are several agents for which only one or two isolated case reports of effects on sexuality exists:

Clofibrate (Atromid), a hypolipidemic agent, was reported to have been associated with erectile impotence in three male patients. This resolved within 3 to 4 weeks of stopping the drug and returned promptly when therapy was reinstituted in one patient.[112]

Disopyramide (Norpace), an antiarrhythmic that resembles quinidine, was associated with erectile impotence in one male patient while receiving 300 to 400 mg of the drug per day. This problem resolved with a reduction in dosage.[113]

Nitrates (nitroglycerin and pentaerythritol tetranitrate) provided dramatic relief of apparent atherosclerotic impotence in one patient.[114]

Fenfluramine (Pondamin), a nonamphetamine anorexiant with sedative properties, was associated with two cases of impotence in a study of 36 patients,[115] although a much higher frequency was reported in another study.[116]

Zinc, a cofactor in spermatozoal enzymes, was found to increase sperm motility and count in males with infertility associated with reduced seminal zinc levels.[117]

Chlordiazepoxide (Librium), a benzodiazepine sedative, has been associated with a delay or failure to ejaculate without erectile impotence in a single case report.[118] Interestingly, chlordiazepoxide and other members of this drug group have been used to treat sexual disorders in which anxiety is a strong component.[119]

Epsilon aminocaproic acid (Amicar), an inhibitor of fibrinolysis used to promote clotting in conditions such as hemophilia, has been associated with inhibition of ejaculation without impotence in 4 of 25 patients in 1 series.[120]

NURSING IMPLICATIONS

Although physicians select the drugs they feel will have the greatest therapeutic effect, nurses may have the responsibility of administering the medication and/or responding to patient's/clients' questions about the effects or the side effects of the drugs.

Assessment

Patients/clients may suspect that a medication is causing sexual dysfunction but may not directly seek information. Statements such as, "This pill makes me feel different" or "I'm not as good as I used to be before taking this medication" may be subtle clues that the person is experiencing sexual difficulties and suspects the drug as the etiologic factor. Some persons may directly question if the medication has sexual dysfunction as one of its side effects. The nurse who is knowledgeable about drugs and sexuality will be alert for possible problems when individuals indicate that they are taking drugs with high potential for compromising sexual health and will question them about side effects at each visit. The nurse ascertains if there is association between the initiation of drug therapy or an increase in dosage and dysfunction, remembering that stresses in the sexual relationship or other health deviations may be the underlying cause, rather than the medication.

Planning

Some physicians believe strongly that sexual dysfunctions as a consequence of certain drug therapies are not indications for discontinuance of the medication and that the overall benefit to the patient must be the ultimate criterion in any decision to change dosage or discontinue a medication. The nurse identifies the physicians' viewpoints in this regard as it applies to each patient when planning interventions. A few physicians may be adamant in their refusal to change medication, even after the nurse has communicated the patient's concerns about sexuality. Others may alter either dosage or drug, thereby solving the problem. If no change will be made, the nurse plans to help the patient/client accept the therapeutic regimen and cope with the sexual dysfunction.

Intervention

Controversy exists about telling clients of drug side-effects, some health professionals arguing that sexual dysfunction occurs because the client expects it to occur (self-fulfilling prophecy).[121] To avoid this "psychologic set" the nurse assures the client that although side-effects may occur, they do not do so in every case and the physician can make adjustments in medication dose or substitute another drug if necessary. Noncompliance with the medical regimen may be a tragic consequence of altered sexual response. Depending on the value nurses put on sexual function, they may either be sympathetic to individuals' desire to regain optimal sexual response or they may have difficulty helping the persons who decide to discontinue a drug because of its adverse effects on sexuality.

Nurses help patients/clients identify and clarify their feelings about the drug's side effects, provide information, and at times act as an intermediary between physician and patient to help both come to a mutually agreed-upon therapeutic decision.

When persons decide to continue the medication, nurses are the empathic presence who help them verbalize and work through their feelings and accept the loss of a part of their lives that may have been highly valued. Alternate forms of sexual expression are suggested when appropriate. Sexual partners must also be included in the discussion, since their response to altered sexuality often is the difference between patient acceptance of therapy or its rejection.

Individuals who use drugs socially are taught about their potential for causing sexual dysfunction as well as about other physiologic, psychologic, and legal ramifications of their use. A threatening, punitive approach to teaching is self-defeating so information is given in a straightforward, nonemotional manner. Referral is made to community mental health and drug abuse services and Alcoholics Anonymous when severe drug dependence or addiction exists. Nurses' associations have developed peer-assistance programs to help the drug-dependent nurse.

Evaluation

The patient's expression of satisfaction with the sexual life style and with the effects of therapy and compliance with the drug therapy are indications that adjustment has been made.

NOTES

1. Hollister LE: Drugs and sexual behavior in man. Life Sci 17:661–668, 1975
2. Freedman AM: Drugs and sexual behavior. In Sadock BJ, Kaplan HI, Freedman AM (eds): The Sexual Experience. Baltimore, Williams and Wilkins, 1976, pp 328–334
3. Jarvik ME: Drugs and sexual functioning. In Jarvik ME (ed): Psychopharmacology in the Practice of Medicine. New York, Appleton, 1977, pp 115–123
4. Sandler M, Gessa GL (eds): Sexual Behavior: Pharmacology and Biochemistry, New York, Raven, 1975
5. Bancroft JHJ: Evaluation of the effects of drugs on sexual behavior. Br J Clin Pract 30 (Suppl):83–90, 1976
6. Athanasiou R, Shaver, P, Tavris C: Sex. Psychol Today 4(2):37–52, 1970
7. Farkas GM, Rosen RC: The effects of ethanol on male sexual arousal. J Studies Alcohol 37:265–272, 1976
8. Briddell DW, Wilson GT: The effects of alcohol and expectancy set on male sexual arousal. J Abnorm Psychol 85:225–234, 1976
9. Wilson GT, Lawson DM: Effects of alcohol on sexual arousal in women. J Abnorm Psychol 85:489–497, 1976
10. Munjack DJ: Sex and drugs. Clin Toxicol 15:75–89, 1979
11. Gordon GG, Altman K, Southren AL, Rubin E, Lieber CS: Effect of alcohol (ethanol) administration on sex-hormone metabolism in normal men. N Engl J Med 295:793–798, 1976
12. Lloyd CW, Williams RH: Endocrine changes associated with Laennec's cirrhosis of the liver. Am J Med 4:315–330, 1948
13. Lemere F, Smith JW: Alcohol-induced sexual impotence. Am J Psychiatry 130:212–213, 1973
14. Cushman P: Sexual behavior in heroin addiction and methadone maintenance. NY State Med J 72:1261–1265, 1972
15. Mintz J, O'Hare K, O'Brien CP, Goldschmidt J: Sexual problems of heroin addicts. Arch Gen Psychiatry 31:700–703, 1974
16. Mathis JL: Sexual aspects of heroin addiction. Med Aspects Hum Sexuality 4:98, 1970
17. Cushman P, Dole VP: Detoxification of rehabilitated methadone maintenance patients. JAMA 226:747–752, 1973
18. Cicero TJ, Bell RD, Wiest WG, et al: Function of male sex organs in heroin and methadone users. N Engl J Med 292:882–887, 1975
19. Ibid, p 886
20. Mirin SM, Meyer RE, Mendelson JH, et al: Opiate use and sexual function. Am J Psychiatry 137:909–915, 1980.

21. Freedman AM, Fink M, Sharoff R, Zake A: Cyclazocine and methadone in narcotic addiction. JAMA 202:191–194, 1967

22. Gay GR, Sheppard C: Sex-crazed dope fiends—myth or reality. Drug Forum 2:125–140, 1973

23. Goode E: In Gross LM (ed): Sexual Behavior, Current Issues. Flushing, New York, Spectrum, 1974, pp 166–167

24. Ibid, p 167

25. Zinberg NE: Marijuana and sex. N Engl J Med 291:309–310, 1974

26. Goode E: In Gross LM (ed): Sexual Behavior, Current Issues. Flushing, New York, Spectrum, 1974, pp 166–167

27. Harman J, Aliapoulios MA: Gynecomastia in marijuana users. N Engl J Med 287:936, 1972

28. Kolodny RC, Masters WH, Kolodner RM, Toro G: Depression of plasma testosterone levels after chronic intensive marijuana use, N Engl J Med 290:872–874, 1974

29. Kolodny RC, Toro G, Masters WH: Normal plasma testosterone concentrations after marijuana smoking. N Engl J Med 292:868, 1975

30. Mendelson JH, Kuehnle J, Ellingboe J, Babor TT: Plasma testosterone levels before, during and after chronic marijuana smoking. N Engl J Med 291:1051–1055, 1974

31. Goode E: In Gross LM (ed): Sexual Behavior, Current Issues. Flushing, New York, Spectrum, 1974, pp 166–167

32. Inaba DS, Gay GR, Newmeyer JA, Whitehead C: Methaqualone abuse, "luding out." JAMA 224:1505–1509, 1973

33. Gay GR, Newmeyer JA, Elion RA, Wieder S: Drug-sex practice in the Haight-Ashbury or the "sensuous hippie." In Sandler M, Gessa GL (eds): Sexual Behavior: Pharmacology and Biochemistry. New York, Raven, 1975, pp 63–79

34. Gay GR, Smith DE: A free clinic ap-proach to drug abuse. Prev Med 2:543–553, 1973

35. Kramer JC, Fishman VS, Littlefield DC: Amphetamine abuse. JAMA 201:305–309, 1967

36. Gay GR, Newmeyer JA, Elion RA, Wieder S: Drug-sex practice in the Haight-Ashbury or the "sensuous hippie." In Sandler M, Gessa GL (eds): Sexual Behavior: Pharmacology and Biochemistry. New York, Raven, 1975

37. Bell DS, Trethowan WH: Amphetamine addiction and disturbed sexuality. Arch Gen Psychiatry 4:74–78, 1961

38. Greaves G: Sexual disturbances among chronic amphetamine users. J Nerv Ment Dis 155:363, 1972

39. Bossop MR, Stern R, Connell PH: Drug dependence and sexual dysfunction: A comparison of intravenous users of narcotics and oral user of amphetamines. Br J Psychiatry 124:431–434, 1974

40. Everett GM: Amyl nitrite ("poppers") as an aphrodisiac. In Sandler M, Gessa GL (eds): Sexual Behavior: Pharmacology and Biochemistry. New York, Raven, 1975, pp 97–98

41. Gay GR, Smith DE: A free clinic approach to drug abuse. Prev Med 2:543–553, 1973

42. Gay GR, Sheppard C: Sex-crazed dope fiends—myth or reality. Drug Forum 2:125–140, 1973

43. Gay GR, Newmeyer JA, Elion RA, Wieder S: Drug-sex practice in the Haight-Ashbury or the "sensuous hippie." In Sandler M, Gessa GL (eds): Sexual Behavior: Pharmacology and Biochemistry. New York, Raven, 1975, pp 63–79

44. Hollister LE: Chemical Psychosis, LSD and Related Drugs. Springfield, Illinois, Thomas, 1968

45. Gay GR, Newmeyer JA, Elion RA, Wieder S: Drug-sex practice in the Haight-Ashbury or the "sensuous hippie." In Sandler M, Gessa GL (eds): Sexual Behavior: Pharmacology and Bio-

chemistry. New York, Raven, 1975, pp 63–79

46. Gay GR, Sheppard C: Sex-crazed dope fiends—myth or reality. Drug Forum 2:125–140, 1973

47. Hollister LE: Chemical Psychosis, LSD and Related Drugs. Springfield, Illinois, Thomas, 1968

48. Jarvik ME: Drugs and sexual functioning In Jarvik ME (ed): Psychopharmacology in the Practice of Medicine. New York, Appleton, 1977, pp 115–123

49. Craven JD, Polak A: Cantharidin poisoning. Br Med J 2:1386–1388, 1954

50. Miller WW Jr: Afrodex in the treatment of male impotency: A double-blind-cross-over study. Curr Ther Res 10:354– 359, 1968

51. Sobotka JJ: An evaluation of Afrodex in the management of male impotency: A double-blind-cross-over study. Curr Ther Res 11:87–94, 1969

52. Roberts CD, Sloboda W: Afrodex vs. placebo in the treatment of male impotence: Statistical analysis of two double-blind-cross-over studies. Curr Ther Res 16:96–99, 1974

53. Slag MF, Morley JE, Elson MK, et al: Impotence in medical clinic outpatients. JAMA 249:1736–1740, 1983

54. Marshall EF: Why patients do not take their medications. Am J Psychiatry 128:656, 1971

55. deGroat WC, Booth AM: Physiology of male sexual function. Ann Intern Med 92 (part 2):329–331, 1980

56. Levine SB: Marital sexual dysfunction: Erectile dysfunction. Ann Intern Med 85:342–350, 1976

57. Bulpitt CJ, Dollery CT, Carne S: Change in symptoms of hypertensive patients after referral to hospital clinic. Brit Heart J 38:121–128, 1976

58. Bauer GE, Hull RD, Stokes GS, et al: The reversibility of side effects of guanethidine therapy. Med J Aust 1:930–933, 1973

59. Weiner N: Drugs that inhibit adrenergic nerves and block andrenergic re-ceptors. In Gilman AG, Goodman LS, Gilman A (eds). The Pharmacological Basis of Therapeutics, 6th ed. New York, Macmillan, 1980, pp 176–210

60. Newman RJ, Salerno HR: Sexual dysfunction due to methyldopa. Br Med J 4:106, 1974

61. Alexander WD, Evans JI: Side effects of methyldopa. Br Med J 2:501, 1975

62. Mroczek WS, Leibel B, Finnerty FA Jr: Comparison of clonidine and methylodopa in hypertensive patients receiving a diuretic. Am J Cardiol 29:712–717, 1972

63. Anonymous: Clonidine (Catapres) and other drugs causing sexual dysfunction. Med Lett 19(20):81–82, 1977

64. Burnett WC, Chahine RA: Sexual dysfunction as a complication of propranolol therapy in men. Cardiovasc Med 4:811–815, 1979

65. Loriaux DL, Menard R, Taylor A, Pita JC, Santen R: Spironolactone and endocrine dysfunction. Ann Intern Med 85:630–636, 1976

66. Zarren HS, Black PM: Unilateral gynecomastia and impotence during low-dose spironolactone administration in men. Milit Med 140:417–419, 1975

67. Greenblatt DJ, Koch-Weser J: Gynecomastia and impotence, complication of spironolactone therapy. JAMA 223:82, 1973

68. Ricordan JF, Walters G: Effects of phenoxybenzamine in shock due to myocardial infarction. Br Med J 1:155–158, 1969

69. Slag MF, Morley JE, Elson MK, et al: Impotence in medical clinic outpatients. JAMA 249:1736–1740, 1983

70. Anonymous: Drugs that cause sexual dysfunction. Med Lett 25(641):73–76, 1983

71. Kotin J, Wilbert DE, Verburg D, Soldinger SM: Thioridazine and sexual dysfunction. Am J Psychiatry 133:82–85, 1976

72. Ibid, p 84

73. Jeffries   JJ: Piperacetazine-induced

failure to ejaculate. Can Psychiatr Assoc J 19:322–323, 1974

74. Kotin J, Wilbert DE, Verburg D, Soldinger SM: Thioridazine and sexual dysfunction. Am J Psychiatry 133:82–85, 1976

75. Beumont PJV, Gelder MG, Freiser HG, Harris GW, MacKinnon PCB, Mandebrote BM, Wiles DH: The effects of phenothiazines on endocrine function—I. Br J Psychiatry 124:413–419, 1974

76. Beumont PJV, Corker CS, Freiser HG, Kalakowska T, Mandebrote BM, Marshall J, Murray MAF, Wiles DH: The effects of phenothiazines on endocrine function—II. Br J Psychiatry 124:420–430, 1974

77. Kotin J, Wilbert DE, Verburg D, Soldinger SM: Thioridazine and sexual dysfunction. Am J Psychiatry 133:82–85, 1976

78. Couper-Smartt JD, Rodham R: A technique for surveying side effects of tricyclic drugs with reference to reported side effects. J Int Med Res 1:473, 1973

79. Barton JL: Orgasmic inhibition by phenelzine. Am J Psychiatry 136:1616–1617, 1979

80. Shalet SM: Effects of cancer chemotherapy on gonadal function of patients. Cancer Treat Rev 7:141–152, 1980

81. Holland JF, Scharhau C, Gailani S: Vincristine treatment for advanced cancer: Cooperative study of 392 cases. Cancer Res 33:1258–1264, 1973

82. Hyyppa MT: L-Tryptophan and sexual behavior. Br Med J 2:1073, 1976

83. Doust JWD, Huszka L: Amines and aphrodisiacs and chronic schizophrenia. J Nerv Ment Dis 155:261–264, 1972

84. Oswald I: Sexual disinhibition with L-tryptophan. Br Med J 2:1559, 1976

85. Hyyppa MT, Falck S, Aukia H, Rinne U: Neuroendocrine regulation of gonadotropin secretion and sexual motivation after L-tryptophan administration in man. In Sandler M, Gessa GL (eds): Sexual Behavior: Pharmacology

and Biochemistry. New York, Raven, 1975, 307–314

86. Bowers MB Jr, Van Woert M, Davis L: Sexual behavior during L-dopa treatment for Parkinsonism. Am J Psychiatry 127:1691–1693, 1971

87. Ibid

88. Benkert O, Crombach G, Kockoff G: Effect of L-dopa on sexually impotent patients. Psychopharmacol Bull 23:91–95, 1972

89. Angrist B, Gershon S: Clinical effects of amphetamines and L-dopa on sexuality and aggression. Compr Psychiatry 17:715–722, 1976

90. Hyyppa MT, Falck SC, Rinne U: Is L-dopa an aphrodisiac in patients with Parkinson's disease? In Sandler M. Gessa GL (eds): Sexual Behavior: Pharmacology and Biochemistry. New York, Raven. 1975, pp 315–327

91. Shapiro SK: Hypersexual behavior complicating levodopa (L-dopa) therapy. Minn Med 56:58–59, 1973

92. Jakobovits T: The treatment of impotence with methyltestosterone thyroid (100 patients—double blind study). Fertil Steril 21:32–35, 1970

93. Mauss J: Investigations on the use of testosterone oeranthate as a male contraceptive agent. Contraception 10:218–289, 1974

94. Fraiser SD: Androgens and athletes. Am J Dis Child 125:479–480, 1973

95. Cooper AJ, Ismail AAA, Harding T, Love DN: The effects of clomiphene in impotence, a clinical and endocrine study. Br J Psychiatry 120:327–330, 1972

96. Lim VS, Fang VF: Restoration of plasma testosterone levels in uremic men with clomiphene citrate. J Clin Endocrinol Metab 43:1370–1377, 1976

97. Cooper AJ, Ismail AAA, Harding T, Love DN: The effects of clomiphene in impotence, a clinical and endocrine study. Br J Psychiatry 120:327–330, 1972

98. Saba P, Salvadorini F, Galeone F, Pel-

licano C, Rainer E: Antiandrogen treatment in sexually active abnormal subjects with neuropsychiatric disorders. In Sandler M, Gessa GL (eds): Sexual Behavior: Pharmacology and Biochemistry. New York, Raven, 1975, pp 197–204

99. Stillman RJ: In utero exposure to diethylstilbestrol: Adverse effects on the reproductive tract and reproductive performance of male and female offspring. Am J Obstet Gynecol 142:905–921, 1982

100. Swerdloff RS, Odell WD, Bray, GA, et al: Complication of oral contraceptive agents—A symposium. West J Med 122:20–49, 1975

101. Gambell RD Jr, Bernard DM, Sanders BI, Vanderberg N, Buxton SJ: Changes in sexual drives of patients on oral contraceptives. J Reprod Med 17:165–171, 1976

102. Dennerstein L, Burrows G: Oral contraception and sexuality. Med J Aust 1:796–798, 1976

103. Adam DB, Gold AR, Burt AD: Rise in female-initiated sexual activity after ovulation and its suppression by oral contraceptives. N Engl J Med 299:1145–1150, 1978

104. Dennerstein L, Burrows G: Oral contraception and sexuality. Med J Aust 1:796–798, 1976

105. Golditch IM: Postcontraceptive amenorrhea. Obstet Gynecol 39:903–907, 1972

106. Hanson FW: "Post-pill" amenorrhea diagnosis and management. Postgrad Med 55:156–162, 1973

107. Golditch IM: Postcontraceptive amenorrhea. Obstet Gynecol 39:903–907, 1972

108. Ibid, p 907

109. Saidi K, Wenn RV, Sharif F: Bromocriptine for male infertility. Lancet 1:250–251, 1977

110. Van Theil DH, Galaver JS, Smith WI Jr, Paul G: Hypothalamic–pituitary–gonadal dysfunction in men using cimetidine. N Eng J Med 300:1012–1015, 1979

111. Jensen RT, Collen MJ, Pandol SJ, et al: Cimetidine-induced impotence and breast changes in patients with gastric hypersecretory states. N Eng J Med 308:883–887, 1983

112. Schneider J, Kaffarnik H: Impotence in patients treated with clofibrate. Atherosclerosis 21:455–457, 1975

113. McHaffie DJ, Gius A, Johnson A: Impotence in patients on disopyramide. Lancet 1:859, 1977

114. Mudd JW: Impotence responsive to glyceryl trinitrate. Am J Psychiatry 134:922–924, 1977

115. Hollingsworth DR, Amatruda TA: Toxic and therapeutic effects of EMTP in obesity. Clin Pharmacol Ther 10:540, 1969

116. Sproule BC: Treatment of the grossly obese with a high dosage of fenfluramine. S Afr Med J 45(suppl):46, 1971

117. Caldamore AA, Freytag MK, Cockett ATK: Seminal zinc and male infertility. Urology 13:280–281, 1979

118. Hughes JM: Failure to ejaculate with chlordiazepoxide. Am J Psychiatry 121:610–611, 1964

119. Mareksha S, Harry TVA: Lorazepam in sexual disorders. Br J Clin Pract 29(7):175–176, 1975

120. Evans BE, Aledor LM: Inhibition of ejaculation due to epsilon aminocaproic acid. N Eng J Med 298:166–167, 1978

121. Fuentes RJ, Rosenberg JM: Sexual side-effects. RN 46(2):35–41, 1983

ANNOTATED BIBLIOGRAPHY

This section is organized by chapters rather than alphabetically for ease in identifying sources.

Chapter 1. Boston Women's Book Collective: Our Bodies, Ourselves, 2nd ed. New York, Simon and Schuster, 1976

>Covers all aspects of sexuality from a woman's perspective. Many useful references.

Chapter 2. Kalisch BJ, Kalisch PA: Improving the Image of Nursing. American Journal of Nursing 83:48–52, 1983

>Summary of the authors' comprehensive study of the image of nursing as portrayed by the media with suggestions for improving the profession's image.

Chapter 3. Masters WH, Johnson VE: Human Sexual Response. Boston, Little, Brown, 1966

>The report giving the first objective data obtained about human sexual responses in a laboratory setting. Discussion of normal response and changes that occur during pregnancy and with aging. A historical first in studying sexuality.

Chapter 4. Money J: The development of sexuality and eroticism in humankind. The Quarterly Review of Biology 56:379–403, 1981

>As the title suggests, a comprehensive review of biopsychosocial factors that impact on sexuality and sexual behavior.

Chapter 5. Saghir M: Homosexuality. In Green R, Weiner J (eds.) Methodology in Sex Research, Rockville, Drug Abuse and Mental Health Administration, U.S. Department of Health and Human Services, Public Health Services, National Institute of Mental Health, 1980

>Describes research needed on homosexuality and methodologic problems that exist. Entire book contains excellent information about sex research.

Chapter 6. Damrosch SP: How nursing students' reaction to rape victims are affected by a perceived act of carelessness. Nursing Research 30:168–170, 1981

>Study investigating attitudes that blame the victim for the rape.

Chapter 7. Selekman J: The development of body image in the child: A learned response. Topics in Clinical Nursing 5:12–21, 1983

>Clear delineation of factors that impact on body image development.

Chapter 8. Moving into the second stage: An interview with Betty Friedan. Nursing Outlook 29:666–669, 1981

>A leader of the feminist movement gives her views of future actions needed to ensure women's rights.

Chapter 9. Oppenheimer C, Catalon J:

Counseling for sexual problems: Ethical issues and decision making. The Practitioner 225:1623–1633, 1981

Discussion of pertinent ethical issues that should be considered by the sex counselor, teacher when working with the client.

Chapter 10. Mitchell JR: Male adolescents' concern about physical examination. Nursing Research 29:165– 169, 1980

Raises questions about problems occurring when female practitioners do physical examination on male adolescents.

Chapter 11. Journal of School Health 51, 1981

Entire issue devoted to problems of sex education in the home and school.

Chapter 12. Kaplan HS: The New Sex Therapy. New York, Brunne/Mazel, 1974

Not a new book but comprehensive discussion of sexual dysfunction and the treatment.

Chapter 13. Izard CE: Human Emotions. New York, Plenum, 1977, pp 385–450

In-depth discussion of the concepts of shame, guilt, and morality.

Chapter 14. Assey JL, Herbert JM: Who is the seductive patient. American Journal of Nursing 83:530–532, 1983

Profile of the seductive patient and nursing interventions.

Chapter 15. Pediatrics Clinics of North America 28, 1981

Issue devoted to sexual problems of infants and children.

Chapter 16. Strahle WM: A model of premarital coitus and contraceptive behavior among female adolescents. Archives of Sexual Behavior 12:67–89, 1983

Theoretical model to account for all variables that affect adolescent use and nonuse of contraception.

Chapter 17. MacPherson K: Menopause as disease. The social construction of a metaphor. Advances in Nursing Science 31:84–88, 1981

A different approach to viewing menopause.

Chapter 18. Masters WH, Johnson VE: Sex and the aging process. Journal of The American Geriatrics Society XXIX:385–390, 1981

Masters and Johnson discuss not only physiologic changes, but also their views of psychosocial impact on sexuality of older age.

Chapter 19. Williams D, Swicegood G, Clark MP, Bean FD: Masculinity–femininity and the desire for sexual intercourse after vasectomy: A longitudinal study. Social Psychology Quarterly 43:347– 352, 1980

Interesting study; its findings may help identify men who are at high risk for sexual problems after vasectomy.

Chapter 20. Smith ED: Abortion: Health Care Perspectives. Norwalk, Appleton-Century-Crofts, 1982

Discussion of all aspects of abortion as an accepted intervention for problem pregnancies.

Chapter 21. Reamy K, White SE, Daniell WC, LeVine ES: Sexuality and pregnancy. Journal of Reproductive Medicine 27:321–327, 1982

Prospective study of 52 married couples in relation to sex enjoyment, coital frequency, and orgasm as pregnancy progressed.

Chapter 22. Clinical Obstetrics and Gynecology 26, 1983

Entire issue devoted to sexually transmitted diseases and their treatment regimens.

Chapter 23. Frontiers in Radiation Therapy and Oncology 14, 1980

Entire issue devoted to sexuality and the cancer patient.

Chapter 24. Zussman L, Zussman S, Surley R, Bjornson E: Sexual response after hysterectomy—oophorectomy: Recent studies and reconsideration of psychogenesis. American Journal of Obstetrics and Gynecology 140:725–729, 1981

Review of 9 research studies related to sexual response after hysterectomy. Findings indicate physiologic changes may be implicated in sexual dysfunction.

Chapter 25. Miller S, Szarz G, Anderson L: Sexual health care clinician in an acute spinal cord injury unit. Archives Physical Medicine

and Rehabilitation 62:315–320, 1981

Describes activities of sexual health care clinician in dealing with spinal cord injured persons.

Chapter 26. Krosneck A, Podolsky S: Diabetes and sexual dysfunction: Restoring normal ability. Geriatrics 36:92–100, 1981

Discussion of causes of sexual dysfunction in diabetes including possible physiologic changes resulting in females' dysfunction.

Chapter 27. Papadopoulos C, Larrimone P, Cordin S, Shelley SI: Sexual concerns and needs of the post-coronary patient's wife. Archives of Internal Medicine 140:38–41, 1980.

Study involving 100 wives of coronary patients: Implications for teaching and counseling of patients and spouses.

Chapter 28. Waltzer WC: Sexual and reproductive function in men treated with hemo-dialysis and renal transplantation. The Journal of Urology 126:713–716, 1981

Comprehensive review of the literature and research related to dialysis and transplantation and sexuality.

Chapter 29. Craft A, Craft M: Sexuality and mental handicap: A review. British Journal of Psychiatry 139:494–505, 1982

Comprehensive review of all aspects of sexuality as they relate to the mentally handi-

capped, with an extensive
bibliography.

Chapter 30. Anonymous: Drugs that cause
sexual dysfunction. Medical
Letter 25(641):73–76, 1983

A concise, up-to-date, well-
referenced list of drugs and
the specific sexual dysfunctions with which they have
been associated.

APPENDIX—SEXUAL HISTORY: CONTENT OUTLINE

An outline prepared by the Group for Advancement of Psychiatry based on the sexual performance evaluation questionnaire of the Marriage Council of Philadelphia (which is affiliated with the Division of Family Study, Department of Psychiatry, University of Pennsylvania School of Medicine) indicates the lines of inquiry to be considered in obtaining a sexual history. It is not intended as a questionnaire to which patients should be subjected. Depending on the individual clinical situation, one or more lines of inquiry in this comprehensive review of possible topics could be sufficient and appropriate.

I. Identifying data
   A. Patient
      1. Age
      2. Sex
      3. Marital status (single, number of times previously married, currently married, separated, divorced, remarried)
   B. Parents
      1. Ages
      2. Dates of death and ages at death
      3. Birthplace
      4. Marital status (married, separated, divorced, remarried)
      5. Religion
      6. Education
      7. Occupation
      8. Congeniality
      9. Demonstration of affection
      10. Feelings toward parents
   C. Siblings (as indicated)
   D. Marital partner
      1. Age
      2. Marital status (number of times previously married if divorced), widowed
      3. Place of birth
      4. Religion
      5. Education
      6. Occupation
      7. Cultural background
   E. Children
      1. Ages
      2. Sex
      3. Assets
      4. Problems

II. Childhood sexuality
   A. Family attitudes about sex
      1. Degree of parents' openness or reserve about sex
      2. Parents' attitude about nudity and modesty
      3. Behavior about nudity and modesty: (a) parents, (b) patient
   B. Learning about sex
      1. Asking parents about sex: (a) which parent, (b) answers given, (c) at what age, (d) nature of questions, (e) feelings about it
      2. Information volunteered by parents: (a) which parent, (b) what information, (c) at what age, (d) feelings about it
      3. Explanations by either parent (indicate which parent or parent substitute): (a) sex play, (b) pregnancy, (c) birth, (d) intercourse, (e) masturbation, (f) nocturnal emissions, (g) menstruation, (h) homosexuality, (i) venereal disease, (j) age at the time of each explanation, (d) feelings about such learning
   C. Childhood sex activity
      1. First sight of nude body of same sex: (a) age ("how young"), (b) feelings, (c) circumstances
      2. First sight of nude body of opposite sex: (a) age ("how young"), (b) feelings, (c) circumstances
      3. Genital self-stimulation: (a) age ("how young") *before adoles-*

534

cence at first occurrence, (b) manner, (c) orgasm? (how often?), (d) feelings (pleasure, guilt), (e) consequences if apprehended

4. Other solitary sexual activities (bathroom sensual activity regarding urine, feces, odors)

5. First sexual exploration or play (playing doctor) with another child (possible reply may be *never*): (a) age; (b) sex and age of other child; (c) nature of activity (looking, manual touching, genital touching, vaginal penetration, oral–genital contact, anal contact, other); (d) feelings (pleasure, guilt); (e) consequences if apprehended (what and by whom)

6. Other episodes of sexual exploration or play with other children *before adolescence* (subcategories as in 5 above)

7. Sex activity with older persons: (a) at what ages, (b) ages of other persons, (c) nature of activity, (d) willing or unwilling, (e) force or actual attack involved? (f) feelings

D. Primal scene

1. Parents' intercourse: (a) hearing, (b) seeing, (c) feelings

2. Other than parents: (a) hearing, (b) seeing, (c) feelings

E. Childhood sexual theories or myths

1. Thoughts about conception and birth

2. Functions of male and female genitals in sexuality

3. Roles of other body orifices or parts (such as umbilicus) in sexuality and reproduction (such as oral impregnation, anal intercourse, and birth, pregnancy by kissing)

F. Other childhood sexuality

III. Onset of adolescence

A. In girls

1. Preparation for menstruation: (a) informant, (b) nature of information, (c) age given, (d) feelings about way in which the information was given, (e) about the information itself

2. Age: (a) at first period, (b) when breasts began developing, (c) of appearance of pubic and axillary hair

3. Menstruation: (a) regularity (initial, subsequent, present), (b) frequency, (c) discomfort? (d) medication? (e) duration, (f) hygienic method (Kotex, tampons), (g) feelings about first period (surprise, distaste, interest, anticipation, guilt, shyness), (h) about subsequent periods

B. In boys

1. Preparation for adolescence: (a) informant, (b) nature of information, (c) age given

2. Age: (a) of appearance of pubic and axillary hair, (b) change of voice, (c) of first orgasm, (d) with or without ejaculation, (e) frequency of orgasm, (f) for how many years?

3. Emotional reaction: (a) to early or delayed onset of adolescence, (b) to first orgasm

IV. Orgastic experiences

A. Nocturnal emissions (male) or orgasm during sleep (female)

1. Frequency: (a) premarital, (b) postmarital

2. Accompanying dreams

B. Masturbation

1. Age when begun

2. Ever punished?

3. Frequency per week: (a) during teens, (b) during 20s, (c) during 30s, etc.

4. Method: (a) usual, (b) others tried, (c) others used

5. Marital partner's knowledge of past or present masturbation

6. Practiced with others: (a) before marriage, (b) with spouse
7. Emotional reactions
8. Accompanying fantasies

C. Necking and petting ("making out")
   1. Age when begun
   2. Frequency
   3. Number of partners
   4. Types of activity

D. Intercourse (see also section IX below)
   1. Frequency of occurrence
   2. Number of partners
   3. Kinds of partners (fiancee, lover, friend, prostitute, unselective)
   4. Contraceptives used
   5. Feelings about premarital intercourse: (a) for girls, (b) for boys, (c) for different ages

E. Orgastic frequency (overall)
   1. During teens
   2. During 20s
   3. During 30s
   4. During 40s, etc.

V. Feelings about self as masculine/feminine
   A. The male patient
      1. Does he feel masculine?
      2. Popular?
      3. Sexually adequate?
      4. Any feelings about being a "sissy"?
      5. Does he feel accepted by his peers (belongs to a group)?
      6. Feelings about: (a) body size (height, weight, etc.), (b) appearance (handsomeness, virility), (c) voice, (d) hair distribution, (e) genitalia (size, circumcision, undescended testicle, virility, potency, ability to respond sexually), (f) cross-dressing (any experience in doing so)
   B. The female patient
      1. Does she feel feminine?
      2. Popular?
      3. Sexually adequate?

4. Was she ever a "tomboy"?
5. Does she feel accepted by her peers (belongs to a group)?
6. Feelings about: (a) body size (height, weight, etc.), (b) appearance (beauty); (c) breast size, hips; (d) distribution of hair; (e) cross-dressing (any experience in doing so)

VI. Sexual fantasies and dreams
   A. Nature of sex dreams
   B. Nature of fantasies
      1. During masturbation
      2. During intercourse

VII. Dating
   A. Age ("how young")
      1. First date
      2. First kissing: (a) lips, (b) deep
      3. First petting or "making out"; feelings
      4. First going steady; feelings
   B. Frequency: feelings about frequency of dating

VIII. Engagement
   A. Age (formal or informal?)
   B. Sex activity during engagement period
      1. With fiancee: (a) kissing, (b) petting, (c) intercourse
      2. With others: (a) number of persons, (b) frequency, (c) nature of activity

IX. Marriage
   A. Vital statistics
      1. Date of marriage
      2. Age: (a) interviewee, (b) spouse
      3. Spouse's occupation
      4. Is spouse present at interview?
      5. Previous marriage(s): (a) interviewee, (b) spouse
      6. Reason for termination of previous marriage (death, divorce): (a) interviewee, (b) spouse
      7. Number, sex, and ages of children from previous marriage: (a) interviewee, (b) spouse
   B. Premarital sex with spouse (if not previously covered)

1. Petting: (a) frequency, (b) feelings about it
2. Intercourse: (a) frequency, (b) feelings about it
3. Contraceptives (identify kind used, if any)

C. Wedding trip (honeymoon)
   1. Social and geographic particulars: (a) where, (b) duration, (c) generally pleasant or unpleasant?
   2. Sexual considerations: (a) frequency of intercourse, (b) was sex pleasant or unpleasant? (c) was the wife aroused? (d) was orgasm achieved (occasionally, always, never)? (e) was spouse considerate? (f) any complications (impotence, frigidity, pain, difficulty in penetration, honeymoon cystitis)?

D. Sex in marriage
   1. General satisfaction or dissatisfaction
   2. Thoughts about general satisfaction or dissatisfaction of spouse

E. Pregnancies
   1. Number
   2. At what ages
   3. Results (normal births, cesarean delivery, miscarriages, abortions)
   4. Effects on sexual adjustment (fear of pregnancy)
   5. Number wanted and number unwanted
   6. Sex of child wanted or unwanted

X. Extramarital sex
   A. Emotional attachments
      1. Number of different attachments
      2. Frequency of contacts
      3. Feelings about extramarital emotional attachment
   B. Sexual intercourse
      1. Number of different partners
      2. Frequency of incidents

   3. Feelings about extramarital intercourse
   C. Postmarital masturbation
      1. Frequency
      2. How recent?
   D. Postmarital homosexuality
      1. Frequency
      2. How recent?
   E. Multiple sex ("swinging")

XI. Sex after widowhood, separation, or divorce
   A. Outlet
      1. Orgasms in sleep
      2. Masturbation
      3. Petting
      4. Intercourse
      5. Homosexuality
      6. Other
   B. Frequency of past or current resort to outlet
   C. Feelings about such experiences

XII. Sexual variants and sexual disorders
   A. Homosexuality
      1. First experience: (a) age ("How young"), (b) age and number of persons involved, (c) how often repeated, (d) nature of activity (looking, manual, oral, anal), (e) active or passive (in seeking the activity, in performance)? (f) circumstances (childhood sex play, seduction by elders)
      2. During and since adolescence: (a) patient's age, (b) age and number of persons involved, (c) frequency, (d) recency, (e) nature of activity (looking, manual, oral, anal), (f) usual circumstances (at movies or gay bars, in public toilets or turkish baths, with minors), (g) penalties (blackmail, being "rolled," being arrested), (h) interest or desire and whether fulfilled or unfulfilled
   B. Sexual contact with animals
      1. When: (a) childhood, (b) adolescence, (c) since adolescence
      2. Nature of contact: (a) vaginal

penetration, (b) anal penetration, (c) licking by animal, (d) masturbation on or off an animal
3. Frequency
4. Recency
5. Feelings about sexual contact with animals

C. Voyeurism
1. Interest or pleasure in looking at objects connoting sex (genitals, nudes, etc.): (a) in childhood, (b) in adolescence, (c) since adolescence, (d) frequency, (e) recency, (f) circumstances, (g) consequences, (h) arousal or masturbation while looking
2. Sexual interest or pleasure from looking into mirror: (a) in childhood, (b) in adolescence, (c) since adolescence, (d) frequency, (e) recency
3. Interest in pornographic pictures: (a) in childhood, (b) during adolescence, (c) since adolescence, (d) frequency, (e) recency, (f) feelings about them (pleasure, disgust), (g) response (arousal, masturbation)
4. Peeping: (a) in childhood, (b) in adolescence, (c) since adolescence, (d) frequency, (e) recency, (f) circumstances (in bathhouses, public toilets, lighted windows at night, by use of field glasses, etc.), (g) consequences if apprehended, (h) feelings about peeping

D. Exhibitionism (deriving pleasure from displaying genitals)
1. To whom: (a) children, (b) adults
2. When: (a) in childhood, (b) in adolescence, (c) since adolescence, (d) frequency, (e) recency, (f) circumstances (in bathhouses, public toilets, lighted windows at night, etc.), (g) consequences if apprehended; (h) feelings about exhibitionism

E. Fetishes, transvestism
1. Nature of fetish (underwear, other clothing, objects of sexual attraction): (a) when adopted, (b) sexual behavior associated with it (such as masturbation), (c) frequency, (d) recency, (e) consequences
2. Nature of transvestite activity: (a) when adopted, (b) sexual behavior associated with it, (c) frequency, (d) recency, (e) consequences

F. Sadomasochism
1. Nature of activity: (a) pain inflicted, (b) pain undergone, (c) means employed
2. Sexual response: (a) to activity itself, (b) to fantasies of such activity
3. Frequency
4. Recency
5. Consequences

G. Seduction and rape
1. Has the patient seduced or raped another person? (a) frequency, (b) recency, (c) circumstances, (d) consequences
2. Has the patient been seduced or raped? (a) frequency, (b) recency, (c) circumstances, (d) consequences

H. Incest
1. Nature of sex play or sexual activity with: (a) brother, (b) sister, (c) mother, (d) father, (e) son, (f) daughter, (g) other
2. Period of activity: (a) in childhood, (b) in adolescence, (c) since adolescence
3. Frequency
4. Recency
5. Consequences

I. Prostitution
1. Has patient accepted or paid money for sex: (a) when in life? (b) frequency, (c) recency

2. Has patient "rolled" someone or ever been "rolled"?
3. Feelings about prostitution
4. Types of sexual practices: (a) actual, (b) tolerated, (c) preferred
5. Types of clients accepted or partners paid for

XIII. Certain effects of sex activities
  A. Venereal disease
    1. Age ("How young") of learning about venereal disease
    2. Venereal disease contracted: (a) gonorrhea (when, treatment, effects), (b) syphilis (when, treatment, effects); (c) other (when, treatment, effects)
  B. Illegitimate pregnancy
    1. Having an illegitimate pregnancy (female patient): (a) how often, (b) at what age, (c) disposition of pregnancy (miscarriage, abortion, adoption, marriage, kept baby, kept baby without marriage), (d) feelings about it
    2. Causing an illegitimate pregnancy (male patient): (a) how

often, (b) at what age, (c) disposition of pregnancy, (d) feelings about it
  C. Abortion
    1. Why performed?
    2. At what age(s)?
    3. How often?
    4. Before or after marriage?
    5. Circumstances: (a) who, (b) where, (c) how
    6. Feelings about abortion: (a) at the time, (b) in retrospect, (c) anniversary reaction

XIV. Use of erotic material
  A. Response to erotic or pornographic literature, pictures, movies
    1. Sexual pleasure arousal
    2. Mild pleasure
    3. Disinterest
    4. Disgust
  B. Use in connection with sexual activity
    1. Type of material
    2. Frequency of use
    3. Use accompanying or preceding: (a) intercourse, (b) masturbation, (c) other sexual activity

Index